HANDBOOK OF PSYCHIATRY · 4
THE NEUROSES AND PERSONALITY
DISORDERS

HANDBOOK OF PSYCHIATRY

General Editor: Professor M. Shepherd

Edited by: Professor N. Garmezy, Dr. L. A. Hersov,
Professor M. H. Lader, Professor P. R. McHugh,
Professor G. F. M. Russell, Professor J. K. Wing,
Professor O. L. Zangwill

Assisted by the Editorial Board and International
Advisory Board of *Psychological Medicine*

Volume 1: General psychopathology
Edited by M. Shepherd and O. L. Zangwill

Volume 2: Mental disorders and somatic illness
Edited by M. H. Lader

Volume 3: Psychoses of uncertain aetiology
Edited by J. K. Wing and L. Wing

Volume 4: The neuroses and personality disorders
Edited by G. F. M. Russell and L. A. Hersov

Volume 5: The scientific foundations of psychiatry
Edited by M. Shepherd

Handbook of
PSYCHIATRY
Volume 4

THE NEUROSES
AND PERSONALITY
DISORDERS

Edited by
Gerald F. M. Russell
and
Lionel Hersov

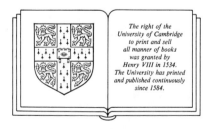

The right of the
University of Cambridge
to print and sell
all manner of books
was granted by
Henry VIII in 1534.
The University has printed
and published continuously
since 1584.

CAMBRIDGE UNIVERSITY PRESS
Cambridge
London New York New Rochelle
Melbourne Sydney

Published by the Press Syndicate of the University of Cambridge
The Pitt Building, Trumpington Street, Cambridge CB2 1RP
32 East 57th Street, New York, NY 10022, USA
296 Beaconsfield Parade, Middle Park, Melbourne 3206, Australia

© Cambridge University Press 1983

First published 1983

Printed in the United States by
Vail-Ballou Press, Inc., Binghamton, NY

Library of Congress catalogue card number: 82-25498

British Library cataloguing in publication data

Handbook of psychiatry.
Vol. 4: The neuroses and personality disorders

1. Psychiatry
I. Russell, Gerald F. M.   II. Hersov, Lionel
616.89   RC454

ISBN 0 521 24221 5 hard covers
ISBN 0 521 28537 2 paperback

1) Psychiatry

v

Contents

Contents

Contents

Contributors

John Bancroft, MD, MRCP, FRCPsych,
Clinical Consultant, MRC Reproductive Biology Unit,
and
Hon. Senior Lecturer, Department of Psychiatry, University of Edinburgh,
Centre for Reproductive Biology,
37 Chalmers Street, Edinburgh EH3 9EW

Ian Berg, MD, FRCP (Edin.), FRCPsych,
Consultant in Child and Adolescent Psychiatry, Leeds AHA(T) and Yorkshire RHA,
and
Senior Clinical Lecturer, University of Leeds,
Department of Psychiatry, University of Leeds,
15 Hyde Terrace, Leeds LS2 9LT

Klaus Bergmann, MD, ChB, FRCPsych,
Consultant Psychiatrist, Bethlem Royal Hospital and the Maudsley Hospital,
The Maudsley Hospital,
Denmark Hill, London SE5 8AZ

George W. Brown, PhD,
Professor of Sociology, Bedford College, University of London,
and
External Staff, MRC
Department of Sociology, Bedford College,
Regent's Park, London NW1 4NS

P. G. Campbell, MA, BM, BCh, MPhil, MRCP, MRCPsych,
Consultant Psychiatrist, Friern Hospital and University College Hospital,
31 Cholmeley Park, Highgate, London N6 5EL

R. H. Cawley, BSc, MB, PhD, FRCP, FRCPsych,
Joint Professor of Psychological Medicine, King's College
Hospital Medical School and the Institute of Psychiatry,
Institute of Psychiatry,
De Crespigny Park, Denmark Hill, London SE5 8AF

J. R. W. Christie Brown, MA, BM, BCh, MRCP, FRCPsych,
DPM,
Consultant Psychiatrist, the Maudsley Hospital,
The Maudsley Hospital,
Denmark Hill, London SE5 8AZ

Anthony Clare, MD, MPhil, MRCPI, MRCPsych,
Professor of Psychological Medicine,
St Bartholomew's Hospital Medical College,
West Smithfield, London EC1

Brian Cooper, MD, FRCPsych, DPM,
Head, Department of Epidemiological Psychiatry,
Zentralinstitut für Seelische Gesundheit,
D-6800 Mannheim 1, J5, Federal Republic of Germany

J. E. Cooper, BM, FRCP, FRCPsych, DPM (Lond.),
Professor of Psychiatry, University of Nottingham,
University Department of Psychiatry, Mapperley Hospital,
Porchester Road, Nottingham

John Corbett, MRCP, FRCPsych, DCH,
Physician, the Bethlem Royal Hospital and the Maudsley
Hospital,
The Maudsley Hospital,
Denmark Hill, London SE5 8AZ

Antony D. Cox, MB, MPhil, MRCP, FRCPsych,
Consultant Child Psychiatrist, the Bethlem Royal Hospital
and the Maudsley Hospital,
The Child and Adolescent Department,
The Maudsley Hospital,
Denmark Hill, London, SE5 8AZ

Michael J. Crowe, DM, MRCPsych,
Consultant Psychiatrist, the Bethlem Royal Hospital and the
Maudsley Hospital,
The Maudsley Hospital,
Denmark Hill, London SE5 8AZ

Padmal de Silva, MA, MPhil,
Lecturer in Psychology, Institute of Psychiatry,
and
Senior Clinical Psychologist, the Bethlem Royal Hospital
and the Maudsley Hospital,
Department of Psychology,
Institute of Psychiatry,
De Crespigny Park, Denmark Hill, London SE5 8AF

P. T. d'Orbán, MB, ChB, FRCPsych, DPM,
Consultant Forensic Psychiatrist, Royal Free Hospital and
the Home Office,
Academic Department of Psychiatry,
Royal Free Hospital,
Pond Street, London NW3 2QG

Griffith Edwards, DM, FRCP, FRCPsych,
Professor of Addiction Behaviour, Institute of Psychiatry,
Addiction Research Unit,
Institute of Psychiatry,
101 Denmark Hill, London, SE5 8AF

Ann Gath, DM, MRCPsych, DPM, DCH,
Consultant Child Psychiatrist, West Suffolk Hospital,
Department of Child Psychiatry,
West Suffolk Hospital,
Bury St Edmunds, Suffolk IP33 2QZ

M. G. Gelder, DM, FRCP, FRCPsych,
Professor of Psychiatry, University of Oxford,
Warneford Hospital,
Headington, Oxford OX3 7JX

Chirsty Gillies, RGN, RMN,
Clinical Specialist Sister,
Department of Psychiatry,
Institute of Psychiatry,
De Crespigny Park, London SE5 8AF

David Goldberg, DM, FRCP,
Professor of Psychiatry, University of Manchester,
Withington Hospital,
Manchester M20 8LR

Philip Graham, FRCP, FRCPsych,
Walker Professor of Child Psychiatry,
Department of Child Psychiatry,
Institute of Child Health,
The Hospital for Sick Children,
Great Ormond Street, London WC1N 3JH

John Gunn, MD, FRCPsych,
Professor of Forensic Psychiatry, University of London,
Institute of Psychiatry,
De Crespigny Park, London SE5 8AF

Lionel Hersov, MD, FRCP, FRCPsych, DPM,
Consultant Psychiatrist, the Bethlem Royal Hospital and the
Maudsley Hospital,
and
Senior Lecturer and Honorary Consultant, The Royal
Postgraduate Medical School and Hammersmith Hospital,
London,
Children and Adolescents' Department,
The Maudsley Hospital,
Denmark Hill, London SE5 8AZ

Christopher Howard, BM, BCh, MPhil, FRCPsych,
Senior Lecturer in Psychiatry, Royal Free Hospital School of
Medicine,
and
Honorary Consultant Psychiatrist, Royal Free Hospital,
Academic Department of Psychiatry,
Royal Free Hospital,
Pond Street, London NW3 2QG

R. E. Kendell, MD, FRCP, FRCPsych,
Professor of Psychiatry,
Edinburgh University Department of Psychiatry,
Royal Edinburgh Hospital,
Edinburgh EH10 5HF

Israel Kolvin, MD, FRCPsych, DipPsych,
Professor and Consultant in Child and Adolescent
Psychiatry,
Nuffield Psychiatry Unit, Fleming Hospital and University
of Newcastle,
Fleming Memorial Hospital,
Great North Road, Newcastle-upon-Tyne NE2 3AX

Malcolm Lader, DSc, PhD, MD, FRCPsych,
Professor of Clinical Psychopharmacology, University of
London,
Institute of Psychiatry,
De Crespigny Park, London SE5 8AF

William Alwyn Lishman, MD, FRCP, FRCPsych,
Professor of Neuropsychiatry, University of London,
Institute of Psychiatry,
De Crespigny Park, London SE5 8AF

Mavis Macguire, Dip. Social Studies, Cert. Mental Health,
Senior Social Worker,
Academic Department of Psychiatry,
Royal Free Hospital,
Pond Street, London NW3 2QG

E. Moran, MA, MB, FRCP, FRCPsych, DPM,
Senior Consultant Psychiatrist,
Department of Psychiatry,
Enfield District Hospital,
Chase Farm Hospital,
The Ridgeway, Enfield, Middlesex EN2 8JL

Charlotte Munday, MBAOT, SROT,
Examiner for College of Occupational Therapists,
previously District Head
Occupational Therapist, North Camden, London,
6 Ryland Road, London NW5 3EA

Issy Pilowsky, MD, ChB, FRANZCP, FRCPsych, FRACP,
DPM,
Professor of Psychiatry,
The University of Adelaide,
Department of Psychiatry,
Adelaide, South Australia 5000

David C. R. Pitcher, MB, BS, MPhil, FRCPsych, DPM,
Senior Lecturer, The Royal Free Hospital School of
Medicine,
and
Consultant Psychiatrist, the Royal Free Hospital and Friern
Hospital, London,
The Royal Free Hospital School of Medicine,
at Friern Hospital,
Friern Barnet Road, London N11 3BP

Naomi Richman, MSc, FRCPsych,
Senior Lecturer and Honorary Consultant Psychiatrist,
Department of Psychological Medicine,
The Hospital for Sick Children,
Great Ormond Street, London WC1N 3JH

Derek Ricks, MD, MRCPsych, DPM,
Physician, Handicapped Children's Service, Harper House,
Radlett, Herts,
and
Consultant in Mental Handicap, Department of Paediatrics,
University College Hospital,
Harperbury Hospital,
Harper Lane, Shenley, Radlett, Herts WD7 9HQ

Gerald F. M. Russell, MD, FRCP, FRCP Ed, FRCPsych,
Professor of Psychiatry, University of London,
Institute of Psychiatry,
De Crespigny Park, London SE5 8AF

David Shaffer, MRCP, FRCPsych,
Professor of Clinical Psychiatry and Pediatrics, College of
Physicians and Surgeons, Columbia University, New York
City,
722 West 168th Street, New York, NY 10032

Nancy Swift, MD, BSc, FRCPsych, DPM
Late Consultant Physician, the Maudsley Hospital, London,
and
Honorary Consultant Psychiatrist, Royal Free Hospital,
London,
366 Finchley Road, London NW3 7AJ

Eric A. Taylor, MB, MRCP, MRCPsych,
Senior Lecturer in Child and Adolescent Psychiatry,
Institute of Psychiatry,
De Crespigny Park, London SE5 8AF

A. Wakeling, PhD, MB, ChB, FRCPsych,
Professor of Psychiatry, Royal Free Hospital School of
Medicine,
Royal Free Hospital
Pond Street, London NW3 2QG

Henry Walton, MD, PhD, FRCP, FRCPsych,
Professor of Psychiatry,
Department of Psychiatry, University of Edinburgh,
Royal Edinburgh Hospital,
Edinburgh EH10 5HF

D. J. West, MB, ChB, MD, PhD,
Professor of Clinical Criminology,
and
Director, Institute of Criminology, University of
Cambridge,
7 West Road, Cambridge CB3 9DT

Sula Wolff, BM, BCh, FRCP, FRCPsych, DCH,
Consultant Child Psychiatrist and Part-time Senior
Lecturer, Royal Hospital for Sick Children and Department
of Psychiatry, University of Edinburgh,
Department of Psychological Medicine,
Royal Hospital for Sick Children,
3 Rillbank Terrace, Edinburgh EH9 1LL

Foreword

The idea of this handbook originated from a survey of the available British books on psychiatry in the late 1960s (1). It became apparent then that the post-war development of the subject as a major, independent branch of medicine had been accompanied by a spate of textbooks and specialized monographs from the rapidly increasing number of academic and clinical departments. The time seemed ripe 'to compile the comprehensive authoritative multi-authored handbook which has yet to appear in this country' (2).

In the event almost another decade was to pass before the enterprise was to be realized. During this time the climate of opinion has come to favour the appearance of a representative statement of what has been termed the 'Maudsley' approach to psychological medicine. Modern British psychiatry, as Lord Taylor has pointed out, is 'largely the product of the Maudsley Hospital' (3). It embodies not so much a national school of opinion as a continuation of the broad, central tradition of psychiatric theory and practice which originated on the European mainland, was transported through the psychobiology of Adolf Meyer to North America and returned to Europe via the United Kingdom, where its pre-eminent representative has been Sir Aubrey Lewis (4). At its core is an adherence to the principles of scientific enquiry in clinical and basic research, with due acknowledgement of the role played by social and psychological investigation as well as by the natural sciences.

The prospects for the production of a handbook were further improved by the creation in 1969 of *Psychological Medicine,* a journal devoted to research in the field of psychiatry and the allied sciences, which brought together an editorial board which has played an important part in this undertaking. The participation of the journal's international advisory board also helped to ensure a wide base for the work which, from its inception, has received sympathetic encouragement from Cambridge University Press.

Why call a handbook what is clearly so much more than a manual or guide which can be held in the hand? If the term is a misnomer it is one which has been blessed by tradition and usage. In the German-speaking countries, where so many of the roots of modern psychiatry are embedded, a *Handbuch* is much weightier than a *Lehrbuch* and the massive volumes associated with the names of Aschaffenburg and Bumke exemplify the fruits of German scholarship at its most diligent. The format has, of course, been applied to other medical disciplines in other languages, largely to meet a need which has been clearly expressed in the preface to the *Handbook of Clinical Neurology,* now comprising some forty volumes: 'only a Handbook designed on the principle of exhaustive, critical, balanced and comprehensive reviews written by acknowledged experts, is in the position of reflecting the state of neurology in the second half of the twentieth century' (5).

While the *Handbook of Psychiatry* has a similar objective, it is less expansive in content and more ambitious in form. An encyclopaedic compilation of all the theories and speculations which impinge on contemporary psychiatry would call for more than forty volumes, but would become outdated very soon. Here we have preferred to concentrate on the fabric of psychological medicine and the loom of observations and concepts on which it has been woven. Accordingly, volumes 2–4 contain the clinical substratum of the subject, flanked by one volume devoted to general psychopathology and another to the various scientific modes of enquiry on which the discipline is founded.

A full list of contents, with titles of chapters and names of authors, is provided in each volume. An outline of the material contained in all five volumes is as follows:

All the volumes are self-contained and edited separately, but they are intended to reinforce one another.
Every effort has been made to avoid overlap and
duplication of material and the inclusion of cross-ref-
erences, some in the text and others at the back of
each volume, should facilitate the process of integration. The whole is designed to be more than the sum
of its parts.

Michael Shepherd
Institute of Psychiatry
October 1980

References
(1) Shepherd, M. (1969) British books on psychiatry, I & II. *Brit-
     ish Book News*, Feb/Mar., pp. 85–8 and 167–70
(2) (1980) Psychiatry: personal book list. *Lancet*, i, 937
(3) Taylor, Lord (1962) The public, parliament and mental health.
     In *Aspects of Psychiatric Research*, ed. Richter, D., Tanner,
     J. M., Taylor, Lord & Zangwill, O. L., p. 13. London: Oxford
     University Press
(4) Shepherd, M. (1977) *The Career and Contributions of Sir Aubrey
     Lewis*. Bethlem Royal & Maudsley Hospitals
(5) Vinken, P. J. & Bruyn, G. W. (1969) Preface to *Handbook of
     Clinical Neurology*, vol. I, p. v. Amsterdam: North Holland

Preface

Our aim in planning this volume of the *Handbook of Psychiatry* has been to produce a text which would be of help to clinicians. Neurotic and personality disorders are so ubiquitous that every practising doctor will be called upon to treat and advise patients presenting with symptoms which will elicit one or both of these diagnostic labels. Such an exercise in labelling is deceptively simple and is, moreover, of limited value. The more comprehensive assessment of the patient, and the design and execution of an effective course of treatment will tax even the experienced and skilled clinician. Accordingly, this volume is aimed at those clinicians who are most likely to have responsibility for the continued care of this group of patients. They will mainly be psychiatrists and general practitioners, but included also are those physicians willing to accept a therapeutic role for some of their patients complaining of bodily symptoms without an adequate physical basis to account for them. It is hoped that clinicians other than doctors – nurses, psychologists, social workers, and occupational therapists – often called upon to treat these patients, may also benefit from reading this book.

We sought to attach equal importance to the assessment and the treatment of patients with neurotic and behavioural disorders. Accordingly an attempt has been made to provide as much guidance on effective methods of treatment as current knowledge permits. Simple and specific remedies may not

always be available. For this reason it is often necessary to rely on a carefully planned programme of
management. Thus, much attention has been devoted
to general aspects of treatment, including the role of
the multidisciplinary therapeutic team and the value
of an eclectic approach.

The structure adopted for this book is principally one of separate sections describing salient
symptoms, syndromes, and types of disordered personality. This approach runs the risk of suggesting a
wider separation between these sections than is warranted by the clinical facts. Care is therefore taken to
emphasize the overlap of symptoms and syndromes,
and the intermeshing that almost always occurs
between personality structure and neurotic symptom
patterns. We hope that this need to emphasize the
individual nature of the patients' afflictions has been
facilitated by the liberal use of clinical histories,
another feature of this volume. It is also the intention
that the case histories should enliven the text, and
illustrate the clinical complexities which often occur
in practice. Whereas the main body of the book consists of a series of chapters describing syndromes and
disorders, the first three chapters have been devoted
to the general issues which deserve prior discussion
under the main headings of causal factors, the clinical assessment of the patient, and principles of treatment.

An attempt has been made to integrate within
this volume of the *Handbook* the relevant areas of child
and adolescent psychiatry and adult psychiatry. This
aim may have been over-ambitious and it proved
necessary to devote one chapter to disorders specific
to childhood. But elsewhere in this volume the
authors have taken care to describe the manifestations of the syndromes in children as well as in adults

and have sought to identify the childhood antecedents of the disorders of later onset. They have, moreover, indicated whether the symptoms or disorders
of childhood have a favourable outcome or reappear
in adulthood. Finally, there has been a thorough
treatment in several chapters of the repercussions on
the children of parents afflicted with various neurotic
symptoms or disturbances of personality.

This volume is one of a series comprising the
Handbook of Psychiatry. Its subject matter – the neuroses and personality disorders – has been carved out
from the corpus of psychiatric knowledge in a manner which is inevitably imperfect. There are, as a
result, uneasy lines of separation between this volume and the others. For example, the reader concerned with obtaining an overall view of the affective
disorders will, of necessity, have to combine material
from this volume and from volume 3, *Psychoses of
Uncertain Aetiology*, on the functional psychoses.
Similarly, for a full understanding of alcohol and drug
dependence, the relevant chapters on the organic
psychoses in volume 2, *Mental Disorders and Somatic
Illness*, will have to be studied in conjunction with
those in this volume. Nevertheless it is our hope that
this volume *The Neuroses and Personality Disorders*,
achieves a great measure of coherence and independence.

It remains for us to thank the authors for their
painstaking work and especially for their forbearance
and diligence in adhering to the broad editorial
guidelines. We are grateful to Mrs Deanna Voos and
Miss Pamela Richards for their help in coordinating
the work of the editors and authors.

Gerald Russell
Lionel Hersov

PART I
Concepts, assessments, and treatments

1
Concepts
and classifications
Aetiology

1.1.1
Concepts
and classification
R. H. CAWLEY

1.1
Classification

In its simplest usage the term *neurosis* denotes a class of mental disorders which have no known or suspected basis in organic pathology and where the victim recognizes his unwanted feelings, thoughts, and other experiences as personal and subjective: in this sense he retains 'insight' and his appraisal of the external world is unimpaired. Among the principal manifestations some – such as morbid anxiety – are exaggerations of universal experience, while others – such as phobias and compulsions – though less common are readily comprehensible to healthy people, and yet others – such as hysterical conversion symptoms – are alien to normal experience. Accompanying these symptoms, and perhaps eclipsing them in importance, distortions in behaviour and social adaptation may occur, sometimes leading to prolonged or recurrent difficulties, most notably in the interpersonal sphere. In addition there may be a sense of discontent, inner conflict, pain, or distress. The illnesses are classified according to their main clinical features.

Personality disorders are separately classified but not sharply differentiated. The main emphasis is on the habitual style of behaviour and adaptation, which is seen as abnormal in such a way as to cause suffering, continuous or recurrent, on the part of the person affected or on the part of others or both. The pattern generally becomes established and recognizable by the time of adolescence, and continues throughout life with variations according to circumstance and ageing. Occasionally it is acquired as a result of brain damage following trauma or disease. The abnormality may take the form of a gross deficiency or exaggeration of certain modes of psychological functioning, or the balance between different aspects may be disturbed. Personality disorders are classified according to the predominant behavioural pattern.

The Ninth Revision of the International Classification of Diseases (World Health Organization, 1978) makes separate provision for Neurotic Disorders (300), Personality Disorders (301) and a number of other categories of non-psychotic mental disorders in adults, viz., Sexual Deviations and Disorders (302), Alcohol dependence syndrome (303), Drug dependence (304), Non-dependent abuse of drugs (305), Physiological malfunction arising from mental factors (306), Special symptoms or syndromes not elsewhere classified, including anorexia nervosa, specific disorders of sleep and of eating, and psychogenic pain (307), Acute reaction to stress (308), Adjustment reaction (309), Specific non-psychotic mental disorder following organic brain damage (310), Depressive disorder not elsewhere classified (311), Psychic factors associated with systemic diseases (316).

The standard descriptive classifications and descriptions of non-psychotic mental disorders raise a great many questions. By contrast the psychotic disorders appear to form a series of natural groupings: when these are removed from the arena of mental disorder (and when mental retardation is also excluded) what remains is a heterogeneous assemblage of symptoms, syndromes, illnesses, dispositions, and reactions in which it may be thought that order can be imposed only in the most arbitrary fashion. Yet order must be sought: it is necessary to describe, characterize and classify, for only by so doing can we claim systematic knowledge of the vast majority of those people whose predicaments constitute the subject matter of psychiatry. They experience non-psychotic mental disorders by virtue of impairment of some part of their mental function which leads either to specific syndromes or to severe emotional distress, persistent or recurrent low-grade morbidity due to a range of bodily symptoms and anxieties, chronic unhappiness, significant problems of living, and some varieties of antisocial behaviour. Some of these people see psychiatrists: a very much larger number are frequent attenders at their general practitioners' surgeries; some are on the books of social workers and other members of the helping professions; a proportion of them remain – at least

for long periods – out of sight of the organized medical and social agencies, though they may enter into the ambit of fringe medicine or receive unwelcome attention from authority. The group of disorders with which we are here concerned – for which the term neurosis is sometimes used in a generic and imprecise sense – is large and very heterogeneous: its boundaries with psychotic disorder are blurred and subject to the vicissitudes of clinical definition. At the other extreme the borderline between the pathological and the normal is arbitrary, depending not only on clinical factors but also on a spectrum of social, cultural, and subcultural phenomena – including, for example, the availability and style of medical care and the prevailing attitudes towards help-seeking from this and other sources.

In some of those affected with non-psychotic mental disorders the manifestations are protean: a range of psychological and somatic symptoms may coexist, relationships may be disturbed and the life style seriously disrupted: consequently it may be difficult to unravel causes and effects, or primary and secondary phenomena. Moreover, in these disorders, social and cultural factors appear to interact with biologically-determined predispositions in a most elaborate and curious way. Such factors appear to influence not only the overall prevalence but also the predominant types of disorder characteristic of a community: they have both pathogenic and pathoplastic effects. Thus anxiety states, dependence on alcohol, and self-poisoning – to cite but a few instances – are significantly commoner in some contemporary societies than in others; and in many European countries the prevalence of conversion hysteria has fallen over the last century whilst that of identified minor affective disorders has mounted.

Four themes, themselves inter-related, link the multiplicity of clinical and other features of the non-psychotic mental disorders: (1) the morbid phenomena can be seen for the most part as *quantitative deviations* from the phenomena of normal living; (2) the diversity of individual and unique patterns of psychological functioning can be comprehended only by a systematic approach to the appraisal of *personality* in terms of traits, dimensions, categories or dynamics; (3) ecological variables are of central importance, so that the degree of harmony or disorder in *adaptation to environment* (including most prominently the human environment) assumes a crucial role; and (4) variables in the course of *psychological development* are important in that patterns of behaviour, adaptation, and subjective and objective response are influenced by the biological processes of growth, maturation, and ageing, and by the processes of emotional and cognitive learning which become established as experience accumulates. Modern studies of neurosis and personality disorder could be set out as a series of variations on these four cardinal themes, which are closely interwoven with some of the main threads running through the history of psychiatry and psychology.

The term neurosis, introduced by Cullen in 1772, referred to a large group of diseases attributed to malfunction of the nervous system: its original meaning is not relevant to contemporary usage. But among the disorders we now call neurotic some – for example depression, hysteria and addictions to various substances – have been recognised since the earliest times, some – like hypochondriasis in men and 'the vapours' in women – became fashionable in the eighteenth century, others – such as neurasthenia – were described in the mid-nineteenth century, and yet others – anxiety neurosis, sexual deviations and disorders – did not emerge until the late nineteenth century or later. In this aspect of medicine even more than any other, social history has shaped the style of medical belief and practice. With the growth of humane interest in the mentally ill which took place after the Inquisition and became established at the end of the eighteenth century, medicine came to concentrate on the floridly insane: the larger numbers of the less disturbed continued in their own communities without special provision or concern. The era of demonology was ending but it was superseded by an efflorescence of cults and quackery. The misery was largely spurned by the medical establishment, for medical science could offer no solutions. Later it came about that the severely ill, housed in asylums, became the concern of the alienists of the day: the small proportion of neurotic people who came to medical attention received it from physicians in private consulting rooms. Then there developed a tendency to differentiate these types of practice respectively as 'psychiatry' and 'psychological medicine': this distinction, never complete, is now obsolescent but that between psychotics and neurotics has persisted, for social as well as medical reasons.

Our present understanding of psychosis stems from systematic observation of hospitalized patients which led through the classificatory systems of the nineteenth century to the Kraepelinian era, when the development of a natural classification of the func-

tional psychoses opened the way for further developments. This story, similar to those for other fields of medical progress, is in sharp contrast to the history of our understanding of neuroses, where prejudice, opportunism and therapeutic fervour provided stronger passions to shape the course of events. The sequence and interplay of forces is well described in the authoritative histories of Zilboorg and Henry (1941) and Ellenberger (1970). They relate how Anton Mesmer established himself in Paris in 1776 and how the reputation of mesmerism as a treatment for a wide range of afflictions then became widespread until the effective components of 'animal magnetism' were eventually recognized and defined as hypnotism by Braid in 1843. Thus the scene was set for the gradual introduction of hypnosis into the thinking and practice of other innovators who gave impetus to the process which ended the neglect of the great mass of neurotic patients. Some thirty years later Charcot's work at the *Salpêtrière* sought detailed appraisal of the neurophysiological concomitants of hypnosis. Meanwhile the different and more fruitful approach of the Nancy school, in which Liébeault had established unpretentious routines for achieving substantial therapeutic effectiveness, led Bernheim in 1886 to postulate that psychological rather than neurological mechanisms were responsible for the induction of hypnosis. He emphasized the crucial role of suggestibility not only in treatment by hypnosis but also in the genesis of a wide range of normal and abnormal behaviours. Freud, who visited Bernheim in 1889, was much influenced by the climate of opinion which was gradually coming to recognize the value of the new 'psychotherapeutics' as a method of investigation. From another angle Janet undertook detailed clinical studies in hysteria and related disorders and urged the importance of the 'automatic' psychology – exclusion of certain functions from the field of consciousness – in the neurotic person. The psychoanalytic movement took shape in the last decade of the nineteenth century with Freud's paper with Breuer on unconscious hysterical mechanisms in 1893 and with the publication of *The Interpretation of Dreams* in 1899. Since that time the history of our concept of neurosis has been deeply interwoven with the development of dynamic psychiatry, which lays so much emphasis on the strength of the individual's past experience as a force governing his present behaviour and feelings.

The four cardinal themes of personality characterization, psychological development, adaptation to environment, and the continuity between the normal and the abnormal have been illuminated by the development of psycho-analytic theory and its derivatives, which has carried forward the notion of an explanatory psychopathology as a necessary supplement to descriptive psychopathology for understanding the phenomena of neurosis. Freud developed a great explanatory system, which signified a tremendous advance in thinking – even though its very wide claims are perhaps its main weakness: whatever purports to explain all explains nothing. We have reached a stage in the growth of our understanding about neurosis at which no discussion is complete if it fails to recognize the salience of dynamic psychiatry and the contribution made by psychoanalytic theory: yet no discussion is adequate if restricted to this view of the subject, or if dominated by abstraction beyond the reach of what can be observed.

But the history of our four themes has another side which commands scrutiny. Before the latter half of the nineteenth century the subject matter of psychology had belonged to the province of philosophers and logicians. Though there had been penetrating analyses of human experience and perception, and though many of those contributing to the literature were medical graduates, these studies were not concerned with developing a body of knowledge fitted for practical use. Modern scientific psychology is generally regarded as having emerged with the application of principles of physics and sensory physiology to psychological concepts most particularly by the contributions of Fechner, Helmholtz, and Wundt in the 1860s, these developments eventually leading to Wundt's establishing the first psychological laboratory, at Leipzig in 1879. Meantime the *Origin of Species* had been published in 1859 and not long afterwards Darwin had published his book on *Expression of the Emotions in Man and Animals* (1872) This was of very great significance in opening the subject of emotion and motivation to scientific inquiry and in inaugurating the discipline of comparative psychology. Before the theory of evolution animals were thought to be automata whereas men had souls, but now the laws governing mental functioning in man and animals became a legitimate topic for scientific inquiry. A further thread appeared in the fabric as Galton applied newly acquired statistical concepts to explore the basis for a scientific psychology which was much concerned with recognizing and characterizing certain human faculties or individual differences: his *Inquiries into Human Faculty and its Development,* published in 1883, displayed his deep concern with the problems of natural selection and the consequences of Darwin's theories. The nature–nurture issue made its appearance on the scene, later to become intensified in the debate on the relative contributions of constitutional and exogenous factors to personality formation. But Galton's work had little immediate effect on scientific psychology which, following the recognition of the potential for animal studies, was moving away from introspection and individual psychology to a greater emphasis on objectifiable behaviour and the search for general laws. James and Lange in 1884/5 independently developed their general theory relating emotional feeling to physiological events. The growth of those aspects of experimental psychology which have a bearing on human psychological disorder became thereafter increasingly concerned with physiological psychology and with behaviourism – the latter approach being crystallized in a paper written by Watson in 1913. Subsequently the emerging concepts of the psychophysiology of behaviour converged with those of the Russian school of objective psychology which had taken shape in the 1860s with the work on the foundations of reflexology by the physiologist Sechenov and gained momentum with Pavlov's work on classical conditioning and experimental neuroses in the first two decades of the present century. The development of tests for measuring human behaviour gave impetus to improved methods of investigating human abilities, and this was subsequently extended by the application of multivariate statistics to data on personality traits in order to define independent 'dimensions' of personality.

Thus it becomes clear that the growth of modern psychology, unrelated to psycho-analytic theory, has led to developments which provide a framework for exploring the four cardinal themes, viz. theories of personality, psychological development, adaptation to environment, and continuities between the normal and the abnormal.

The theoretical basis of the non-psychotic mental disorders can therefore claim two broadly distinct ancestries, in dynamic psychiatry, and in experimental psychology. In a general way these correspond respectively to the 'subjective' psychologies, which include a major concern with the data of conscious experience and of meaning, and to the objective psychologies in which the data of behaviour and mechanisms are subsumed into an observational science and in which psychophysiological correlations are sought. The distinction persists in present-day theory, research, and therapeutic emphases in the non-psychotic mental disorders, though there is much overlap. Current empirical knowledge goes some way towards providing a synthesis and, where disparities persist, blurs the boundary between the dynamic approach and that which is based upon more stringent theories of emotional and cognitive processing: attempts are made to bridge the gap both in investigative work and in therapy. Many questions remain unresolved from either vantage point – for example the relative roles of personality make-up and recent stress in the presence and form of symptoms, crucial to the question of differentiation between personality disorder and neurotic illness.

Meanwhile the term 'neurosis' remains unsatisfactory because its usage may be extensive or intensive: it may include or exclude personality disorders and the other syndromes listed on pp. vi and vii. Its reference may be to a series of symptoms, syndromes, and personality variants, and in addition it may be held to subsume the supposed aetiology, pathogenesis, or mechanisms of such states, in terms of faulty learning, social maladjustment, or intra-psychic processes. It has come to carry so many contradictions that its specificity can be no more than a pretence; and with this in mind some authorities hold that modern psychiatry would have much to gain if this term were to be abandoned in favour of less pretentious epithets such as 'nonpsychotic mental disorders' or 'abnormal emotional reactions'. In its defence it may be argued that the word 'neurosis' is to be avoided only through great striving: its usage is justified by long tradition and broad consensus and, all in all, it is as good a term as any for a very large class of phenomena. This utilitarian view has been adopted by contributors to the present volume.

The neuroses and personality disorders can be described in a strictly medical framework, in which distinct illnesses or handicaps are operationally defined, admittedly sometimes in an arbitrary fashion, in terms of symptoms and signs, functional disability, and perhaps also by recourse to suspected aetiology or pathogenesis. Alternatively emphasis may be placed on psychological variables: for example the disorders are conceptualized sometimes as due to aberrant personality function consequent upon defects incurred during the course of psychological development and maturation, and sometimes as the result of faulty learning and consequent failure in

cognitive and emotional processes. Respective theoretical standpoints then define the psycho-dynamic and the behavioural (learning theory) formulations of the disorders. A further possibility is that the aberrations may be viewed from a social perspective, with emphasis on ecological rather than on individual variables: the problem then becomes focused on the social stresses which have provoked particular reaction patterns, and the concept of social deviance may be invoked together with the related concepts such as illness behaviour (chap. 6.2, 6.3, 8.2, 8.8, 8.9), and the social response to labelling whereby under certain conditions the very recognition of a pattern of behaviour as deviant promotes a sequence of events which themselves encourage or limit styles of behaviour, setting up vicious circles which may explain much of the observed abnormality. Among these contrasting theoretical formulations no single one is adequate to do justice to the phenomena and their personal, social, and situational contexts, and the diversity is such that at present it seems unlikely that any unified approach will ever encompass the whole range of abnormal behaviour and feelings subsumed under the heading of the non-psychotic mental disorders. To comprehend them it is necessary to enter simultaneously into medical, psychological, and social concepts, theories, and evidence: these are complementary perspectives rather than competing solutions. Meanwhile classifications are necessarily arbitrary: definitions are incomplete, nomenclature tends to be confused and distinctions remain blurred. The best nosology is likely to be the one which achieves the greatest reliability while attaining the greatest validity in terms of clinical usefulness and predictions concerning course, treatment, and outcome. It also follows that treatment – which at its best will be justified by empirical validation – should not slavishly follow diagnostic categorization. In the non-psychotic mental disorders even more than any other field of medicine, the clinician does well to remember that he is treating individuals rather than abstract entities.

It is likely that in due course a dimensional or multi-axial approach to the characterization of neurotic and personality disorders and related handicaps will lead to an improved nosology. Meanwhile classification according to predominant symptom or behavioural feature, however unsatisfactory, comes nearer than any other to acceptable levels of reliability and validity. It is employed in the *Ninth Revision of the International Classification of Diseases*, and detailed definitions of categories are set out in the *Glossary* (World Health Organization, 1978). Its principles are followed in this book although a number of categories of non-psychotic mental disorder are combined when they appear to form natural groupings of symptoms or syndromes.

The remainder of the present chapter is devoted to the classification of emotional and conduct disorders in children, an examination of associations between disorders in childhood and adult life, and consideration of aetiological factors in neuroses and personality disorders. Chapter 2 is concerned with a detailed examination of methods of clinical assessment of patients, and in chapter 3 the principles of treatment are reviewed under the several headings appropriate for the main methods. The remainder of this book is devoted to a series of accounts of the symptoms and syndromes, grouped in the way which has appeared to the authors to be the most realistic, convenient and natural arrangement. Disorders specific to childhood are set out in chapter 4; and chapters 5, 6 and 7 are concerned with the common neurotic disorders. Chapter 8 focuses on the complex and heterogeneous group of conditions in which mental disorders present, through the operation of a variety of mechanisms, with bodily complaints. Sexual disorders and deviations are described in chapter 9, and chapter 10 is devoted to those habit disorders in adult life which result in dependence on alcohol, drugs and gambling. The last two chapters are devoted to the two main groups of personality disorder: sociopathic (antisocial) personalities and the so-called inadequate personality disorders in which the patients present, for the most part, not with specific symptoms or antisocial behaviour but with a range of problems of everyday living and social and interpersonal adjustment.

1.1.2
Classification of psychiatric disorders in children*

DAVID SHAFFER

1. Introduction

The classification of child psychiatric disorders has changed considerably in the past decade. The 8th Version of the International Classification of Diseases provided only one code for the psychiatric disorders of childhood. The 9th Version provides 20 and there are 34 conditions listed as originating in childhood in the 3rd Version of the American Pyschiatric Association Diagnostic and Statistical Manual (DSM–III) (American Psychiatric Association, 1980).

The classification systems in most common use in child psychiatry (ICD–9 and DSM–III) are based on descriptions of behavioural or emotional phenomena rather than on causes or psychopathological processes. Although conditions with similar clinical features may have both different causes and natural histories, this basis for classification has proved surprisingly robust and, in the light of the paucity of our knowledge about cause, is also realistic. The phenomenological approach, which avoids speculation about aetiology or inference about dynamic mechanisms, allows communication between professionals who may hold very different views on these issues. It also gives momentum to the process of trial and error by which the usefulness and validity of diagnostic entities is explored by research.

The usefulness of a diagnosis is limited by the

* This work was supported in part by NIMH Psychiatry Education Grant MH07715–19 and by a grant from the William T. Grant Foundation.

reliability with which it can be communicated from one professional to another. Agreement between professionals is in part a function of the skill and diligence with which clinical information is elicited and interpreted and in part the way in which entities are decribed and classified. Features of a classification system which enhance reliability include:

(a) clear non-inferential descriptions of clinical entities

(b) the avoidance of overlap between a sufficient criterion for one condition and any criterion required for another

(c) the provision of detailed glossary descriptions for each condition

Reliability is also increased if the classification system is not unduly long or complex and if it is conveniently displayed. Ideally, the diagnostic process involves a scanning of all diagnostic possibilities ending with the application of the diagnosis that 'best fits' the case. If the diagnostic possibilities are too numerous or difficult to discern, then different users are likely to choose different 'best fits' for similar clinical problems.

The value of a diagnosis can be measured by how much it tells us about cause, course, or treatment. Classification systems evolve as knowledge is acquired. Symptomatically different conditions which are found to share a common aetiology, prognosis or response to treatment may ultimately be grouped together just as diagnostic groupings with similar clinical features but with varied antecedents, prognosis or treatability may come to be differentiated into more meaningful sub-groups.

This dynamic process of 'lumping' and 'splitting' is at work in both the ICD and DSM classification systems and will be described in more detail below.

2. Major diagnostic groups

Most children who are referred to a child psychiatric clinic fall into one of the following categories:

(1) Children with a *conduct disorder* whose behaviour is seen as troublesome to others and not conforming to expected social norms. The children may fight with their peers or siblings, disobey their parents, teachers or other caretakers, or steal. Their disobedience my take the form of disruptive behaviour in the classroom, running away from home, precocious indulgence in alcohol or addictive substances, and sexual promiscuity. Approximately three

out of four of the children will be boys, (Rutter, Tizard & Whitmore, 1970) and they are likely to come from homes in which there is marital disharmony (Rutter, 1971) and many closely spaced male siblings (Jones, Offord & Abrams, 1980). Their parents are likely to use inconsistent but harsh disciplinary methods including physical punishment (Martin, 1975), and many will have provided the children with inadequate supervision (McCord, McCord & Howard, 1961). About one in three of the children will be doing poorly in their schoolwork (Berger, Yule & Rutter, 1975). The prognosis for about half of these children appears to be poor. When they grow up they will be more likely to have an antisocial personality pattern and to suffer from schizophrenia than children without a conduct disorder (Robins, 1978). However, though all adults with antisocial personality disorder will have shown signs of a conduct disorder in childhood, most (50–60 per cent) conduct-disordered children will grow up without appreciable psychiatric problem.

(2) Children who suffer subjective distress from a variety of *emotional problems.* They may be afraid of strangers or of separating from their parents. They may be depressed or withdrawn or show obsessional rituals or thoughts. Unlike adults with an affective illness their mood states are likely to fluctuate, and vegetative symptoms such as insomnia or anorexia will be uncommon. (Hersov, 1977). These disorders are evenly distributed between the sexes, and their families do not show any characteristic form of disturbance (Rutter, Tizard & Whitmore, 1970). On the basis of admittedly very few follow-up studies, their prognosis appears to be good. No more of these children will experience psychiatric problems in adulthood than children without psychiatric problems (Rutter, 1972).

(3) Children with a *mixture of conduct and emotional problems.* They will get into trouble *and* experience emotional symptoms such as depression or anxiety. Many adolescents who attempt suicide will have a history of antisocial behavior (Shaffer, 1974; Chiles *et al.,* 1980). This group resembles the conduct-disorder group in several respects. Most are boys, they show a high proportion of learning difficulties and many come from stressed homes and families (Rutter, Tizard & Whitmore, 1970).

(4) Children referred to a psychiatric clinic because of a significant *developmental delay* in some complex neurological function. These will include children with a speech or language disorder and chil-

dren who have shown a delay in acquiring normal sphincter control, that is, children with enuresis and encopresis. Most of these disorders run in families and occur predominantly in boys. Many of the children will eventually acquire largely normal function in the delayed area. Associated psychiatric disorders are common in all of these conditions.

(5) There are also children and adolescents with relatively *uncommon, discrete* symptomatic patterns which nearly always originate in early life. These include: *infantile autism,* or pervasive developmental disorder, which is characterized by onset before 30 months of age, a profound language disturbance, social avoidance, bizarre and repetive mannerisms, and a need for sameness; *Gilles de la Tourette syndrome,* characterized by chronic multiple motor and vocal tics with a waxing and waning course and a frequent association with non-specific neurological abnormalities (Shapiro *et al.,* 1973). *Anorexia nervosa,* which usually has its onset in adolescence, occurs

more often in girls, and is characterized by an elective refusal to eat based on a belief by the patient that he or she is overweight.

(6) Finally, there will be children who develop disorders which occur most characteristically in *adults,* for example, children with *depression,* children with isolated *phobias* and *obsessional* disorders and children with *schizophrenia.* The clinical features of these children will resemble those found in adults with the same condition.

3. Diagnostic systems

Two closely related systems are widely used to code and classify the conditions listed above. These are the 9th Version of the International Classification of Diseases, (ICD–9) and the Third Diagnostic and Statistical Manual of the American Psychiatric Association (*DSM–III*).

These two systems show a number of similarities, but also some important differences.

Table 1.1.2.1. *Comparison of child psychiatric disorders in ICD-9 and DSM-III: conduct disorders*

ICD-9		DSM-III	
Code	Diagnosis	Code	Diagnosis
312	*Disturbance of conduct not elsewhere classified*		
312.0	Unsocialized disturbance of conduct	312.00	Undersocialized aggressive conduct disorder
		312.10	Undersocialized non-aggressive conduct disorder
312.1	Socialized disturbances of conduct	312.23	Socialized aggressive conduct disorder
312.2	Compulsive conduct disorder		
312.3	Mixed disturbances of conduct and emotions		
312.8	Other		
312.9	Unspecified		
314.0	*Hyperkinetic syndrome of childhood*		
314.0	Simple disturbance of activity and attention	314.01	Attention deficit disorder with hyperactivity
314.1	Hyperkinesis with developmental delay	314.00	Attention deficit disorder
314.2	Hyperkinetic conduct disorder	314.80	Attention deficit disorder residual type
314.8	Other		
314.9	Unspecified		

3.1. *Similarities*

(a) Both provide a classification of conditions and not of individuals.

(b) Both disregard the *age* of a patient. Diagnostic entities which are similar in children and adults are given similar codes.

(c) Both offer various diagnostic subcategories (see tables 1.1.2.1 and 1.1.2.2) for the large undifferentiated conduct disorder and emotional disorder groups.

(d) Both use a behavioural descriptive approach with definitions for each diagnosis appearing in especially prepared glossaries (American Psychiatric Association, 1980; World Health Organization, 1978).

(e) Both allow conditions to be described at a greater and lesser degree of specificity. The most specific diagnoses are designated with a four- or five-digit code. Each of these specific diagnoses is subsumed under a more general grouping which in ICD–9 is indicated by a three-digit code. DSM–III has adopted certain different subclassifying assumptions but retains broad numerical compatibility with ICD–9.

(f) Both systems provide essentially similar codes for the diagnosis of well-established and well-defined conditions such as infantile autism, Tourette's syndrome, anorexia nervosa, and isolated disorders with physical manifestations, such as enuresis, encopresis, and stuttering.

3.2. *Differences*

There are differences in the way that broad diagnostic categories are subdivided, in the format and style of the accompanying glossaries, and in the provision that is made for the organization of codes.

Diagnostic subgroupings

(i) *Conduct disorders.* Both systems distinguish between socialized and unsocialized conduct disorder (Hewitt & Jenkins, 1946). Socialization is inferred if a child or adolescent seems able to form good and lasting peer relationships, even if with bad companions, and is capable of showing guilt or remorse. In DSM III, conduct disorders are further categorized into aggressive and non-aggressive types as indicated by a history of physical violence against persons or property. ICD–9 provides a further subcategory for compulsive stealing or kleptomania.

It is not clear that these subdivisions are clinically useful. It is difficult for a clinician to be certain about guilt or remorse and the evidence that the socialized and unsocialized subtypes of disorder differ in outcome is contradictory (Robins, 1966, Field, 1967; Henn *et al.*, 1980). Differences between aggres-

Table 1.1.2.2. *Comparison of child psychiatric disorders in ICD-9 and DSM-III: emotional disorders*

ICD-9		DSM-III	
Code	Diagnosis	Code	Diagnosis
313	*Disturbance of emotions specific to childhood and adolescence*		
313.0	With anxiety and fearfulness	309.11	Separation anxiety disorder
		313.00	Over-anxious disorder
		313.23	Elective mutism
313.1	With depression and misery	313.89	Reactive attachment disorder of infancy
		313.82	Identity disorder
313.2	With sensitivity, shyness, and social withdrawal	313.22	Schizoid disorder of childhood or adolescence
		313.21	Avoidant disorder of childhood or adolescence
313.3	Relationship problems		
313.8	Other or mixed		
313.9	Unspecified		

sive and non-aggressive conduct disorders may represent differences of degree rather than any more fundamental division (Farrington, 1978).

(ii) *Hyperkinesis or attention deficit disorder.* DSM–III differentiates between hyperactivity and inattention, and suggests that inattention is the primary abnormal psychological process. The condition is, accordingly, designated 'attention deficit disorder'. Although activity and attention may be distinguished under laboratory conditions their differentiation at a clinical level is not easy. Parents and teachers who use the term 'hyperactivity' will often be describing a range of behaviours including *inappropriate* attention and activity as well as, or instead of, an *excess* of activity or *inadequate* attention.

(iii) *Emotional disorders.* Neither system differentiates phobic, obsessive compulsive, conversion, or clear depressive disorders occurring in childhood from the same disorders in adults. However, each system makes a somewhat different provision for the *emotional disorders* that are *characteristic* of childhood. Children with these disorders usually show a mixed clinical picture, with elements of anxiety, dysphoria, and social withdrawal (Hersov, 1977). ICD–9 classifies these children according to the predominance of any one of these features, and also provides a further subcategory for children with relationship difficulties that are not associated with more general conduct problems (see table 1.1.2.2).

DSM–III provides a series of specific diagnoses for the emotional disorders. These include *separation anxiety disorder*, characterized by children who experience anxiety when separated from their parents or other major attachment figure; *over-anxious disorder* for children who show both situational, object fears and anxiety about their social or academic competence; *reactive attachment disorder of infancy* in which the clinical features of apathy and withdrawal are associated with a history of social deprivation; *identity disorder* describes adolescents who experience distress and uncertainty about their social relationships, sexual orientation, religious and ethical values, career goals, and so on.

Shy children with impaired social relationships are categorized as *'emotional disorder with predominant withdrawal'* in ICD–9 and in DSM–III as either *'Anxiety disorder of childhood and adolescence'*, which describes shy, socially anxious children, initially hesitant but nevertheless capable of forming adequate social relationships, or *'schizoid disorder'*, which is applied to withdrawn, aloof children who show no

apparent interest in making friends and appear to obtain no pleasure from usual peer contacts.

Both systems provide categories for children who show person-specific relationship difficulties, such as defiance of parents, temper tantrums, or sibling rivalry, but who show no other evidence of antisocial disorder. In ICD–9, these are grouped as *'emotional disorder with relationship problems'* and in DSM–III as *'oppositional disorder'*.

There is as yet little evidence to support the differentiation of many of these conditions. For example it is not known whether children who show brief fluctuating dysphoric states differ in their family history, responsiveness to treatment, or biological correlates from children who show more persistent or severe depression. The diagnosis of 'reactive attachment disorder' is likely to be difficult to make in infants, and it is not clear whether it could – or should – be reliably differentiated from the cognitive effects of social deprivation. 'Identity disorder', described in DSM–III, has not been the subject of any systematic study, and many of its features are normal in adolescence.

(iv) *Psychotic conditions* are coded in broadly compatible ways in both system (see table 1.1.2.3). However, the nomenclature differs for autistic conditions in which the onset is thought to have occurred *after* the age of 30 months. In ICD–9 such conditions are grouped as *'disintegrative psychosis'* in DSM–III as *'pervasive developmental disorder'*.

3.3. *Reliability*

The reliability of these two systems has been studied empirically (Sturge *et al.*, 1977; Cantwell *et al.*, 1979). Agreement between users is excellent for certain well-defined conditions such as infantile autism but is satisfactory for the more common conduct and emotional disorder problems *only* when the diagnosis is considered at a more general, three-digit level. Agreement between users is much less adequate for specific subtypes of disorders that have been considered above.

3.4. *Glossary differences*

The style of the accompanying glossaries differs markedly. The ICD–9 glossary is generally brief, providing an outline of predominant symptoms. The DSM III glossary is laid out with highly specific, sufficient, and necessary criteria for each disorder. It can be argued that the provision of very precise criteria will maximize the compatibility of diagnostic practice in different centres and will, therefore, increase reliability. However, several problems can also be expected to follow from the highly specific approach. First, the empirical basis for the specific diagnostic criteria is generally lacking, yet the didactic tone and high degree of specificity of the glossary may mistakenly lead the clinician into accepting their validity. Secondly, if the diagnostic guidelines are followed too literally, many patients will be found not to fulfil criteria, with the result that there will be a high proportion of patients who are undiagnosable in terms of the specific criteria.

One of the consequences of the refinement and the expansion in number of many diagnostic categories (that is, the 'splitting' process) is that any one child may meet criteria for several different diagnoses. ICD–9 provides no guidance about which diagnosis is to be treated as the primary one. DSM–III directs that the condition which led to the clinical referral should be regarded as primary.

Despite certain drawbacks, both ICD–9 and DSM–III represent a very considerable advance, and both systems offer the promise of stimulating valuable research into the classification of childhood disorders.

Empirical approaches to classification. The diagnostic entities that are coded in ICD–9 and DSM–III have their origins in clinical observation and description. One of the problems of this approach is that clinical stereotypes become fixed, and clinicians continue to recognize only those conditions and patterns of pathological phenomena that they have been trained to recognize. This may in turn inhibit the process of discovering new diagnostic entities and criticizing those that have already been established.

An alternative approach that has been used by some research psychologists has been to examine empirically how signs and symptoms coexist in disturbed children. A variety of statistical approaches has been used in this process (see a review by Achenbach, 1980). Although the statistical approaches have differed, the essential procedure has been to examine inventories of signs or symptoms derived from children being treated or assessed in a mental health service and then to examine how the behaviours and symptoms aggregate together.

A large number of studies of this sort have been carried out, and these consistently reveal two broad groupings of symptoms which coincide closely with the 'conduct disorder' and 'emotional disorder' categories described above. Depending largely on the statistical procedure that is adopted or the data upon which the analysis has been undertaken, these broad categories can be seen to be made up of further subcategories. Normative data, taking into account age and sex, can be obtained and it is then possible to determine the extent to which a child deviates from the norm on all or any of these subgroupings or factors. Using this information, a profile can be con-

Table 1.1.2.3. *Comparison of child psychiatric disorders in ICD-9 and DSM-III: psychotic disorders*

ICD-9		DSM-III	
Code	Diagnosis	Code	Diagnosis
299	*Psychosis with origin specific to childhood*		
299.0	Infantile autism	299.0	Infantile autism
		299.01	Infantile autism residual state
299.1	Disintegrative psychosis	299.91	Childhood onset pervasive developmental disorder residual state
		299.8	Atypical psychosis
299.8	Other	299.81	Atypical psychosis-residual state
299.0	Unspecified		

structed for an individual child to delineate a pattern of deviance. Such profiles can be considered as equivalent to diagnoses.

The value of these diagnostic profiles has yet to be established. Problems in their use include the fact that uncommon conditions may not be well represented in the data base from which the profiles are derived and information on the validity of the profiles, that is, whether they reflect basic differences in aetiology or early experiences, natural history, and responsiveness to treatment, or only differences in current symptomatology has only started to be acquired (see Gould *et al.*, 1980).

Conclusions. The critics of diagnosis and classification commonly focus on the problems of labelling, and on the use of a 'medical model' for conditions which may seem to have little in common with those biological abnormalities that we associate with physical illness.

However, *labelling,* that is, describing a patient with a diagnosis which carries with it pejorative implications and negative predictions which come to pass only through the effect of a self-fulfilling prophecy, is largely a product of inefficient diagnosis rather than an inevitable consequence of the diagnostic process. For example, if the diagnosis of hyperactivity subsumes a broad range of conditions with different outcomes and responses to treatment then it

will have limited value as a guide to treatment and should be used with this limitation in mind. One of the causes of diagnostic inefficiency will be unreliability. A disorder that is defined ambiguously is more likely to embrace a mixed class of conditions and, therefore, be less useful in making predictions of treatment and outcome. To the extent that both DSM–III and ICD–9 aim at more restrictive diagnoses and greater reliability, it must be hoped that this danger will be reduced.

A second objection to classification is that it embraces the 'medical model', although there seems to be little agreement on precisely what is meant by this term (see Rutter & Shaffer, 1980). If the medical model implies that a condition that is diagnosed is ultimately defined by a biological abnormality, then it is clear that most psychiatric disorders of childhood do not in our present state of knowledge fulfil such criteria even though it is highly likely that they may come to do so in due course. However, a disease can be viewed more broadly as a collection of morbid clinical phenomena which are likely to occur together and, in the knowledge of which, certain predictions can be made.

Knowledge about the diagnostic entities of childhood has certainly advanced to a point where diagnostic concepts which fulfil these criteria can be made with considerable value to both clinician and patient.

1.2
Aetiological factors more relevant for adult disorders

1.2.1.
Psychogenesis

P. G. CAMPBELL

Psychogenesis is one of those many words in psychiatry which one can easily learn to use but be hard pressed to define. The word has no clearly agreed range of application and many textbook writers avoid any attempt at a definition. 'The origins and development of mental processes' is how Rycroft (1972) puts it, but this meaning as genesis-*of*-psyche is probably obsolete. Genesis-*by*-psyche is more widespread now, usually with implications of 'causation by psychological factors', a meaning Kraepelin acknowledged to be current (Lewis, 1972). 'Psychogenic', the adjective, is defined by Rycroft as 'qualifier of illness and symptoms assumed to be of mental origin', but some authors have used it less selectively so that it becomes synonymous with 'mental' or 'psychological', or something vaguer still. Mayer-Gross, Slater, and Roth (1969), for example, consider the question of whether '. . . psychotic states . . . may arise under severe psychogenic stresses'.

Historical background
A detailed historical survey of the concept of psychogenesis has been written by Sir Aubrey Lewis (1972). He attributes its introduction into psychiatry to Sommer in 1894, who sought to distinguish a group of 'psychogenic' cases from what he saw as the larger category of hysteria: 'We are dealing with morbid states (*Krankheitzustände*) which are evoked by ideas (*Vorstellungen*) and can be influenced by ideas'. Sommer regarded the operative ideas as arising within

the body of the affected person or his environment; he stressed the physical factor and regarded exaggerated suggestibility as an indispensable feature of every psychogenic condition. The concept underwent various mutations through successive editions of Kraepelin's textbook and was further modified under the influence of other German authors, notably Birnbaum (who dealt with it as part of his construct of psychosis and stressed special predisposing factors such as constitution and the role of pathoplastic factors), Bonhoeffer and, later, Gruhle, Braun, Jaspers, and Pinder. The term was used in England in the 1930s but it was undefined. In America, under the influence of Hoch and Meyer, its meaning became less restricted. Lewis distinguishes three main views during the last thirty years, which he names the Orthodox, deriving from early German conceptions and particularly developed in Scandinavia following a review by Wimmer and Faergeman's concept of 'psychogenic psychosis'; the Nihilist, represented by Ey in France, who repudiated psychogenesis for mental disorders; and the Catholic, represented by the psycho-analytic and Meyerian schools, whose followers related the concept to all mental disorders. Ending with a list of contemporary definitions which range from the laconic (for example, Kind's of 1966 that 'We shall consider "psychogenic causation" as implying causation by exogenous mental influences') to the convoluted, Lewis complains that they show 'the same shimmering ill-focused quality'. He concludes:

> Robert Sommer rendered psychiatry a disservice when he coined the word 'psychogenic' and so gave currency to a confused but speciously attractive and convenient concept. The subtle arguments of French and German disputants have shown it to be at the mercy of inconsistent theoretical positions touching on the fundamental problems of causality, dualism, and normality. It would be as well at this stage to give it decent burial, along with some of the fruitless controversies whose fire it has stoked.

The obviousness of mental causation

The newcomer to psychiatry may find it odd that there should have been so much dispute about the role of psychogenesis in the causation of mental disorders. Can one even conceive of mental illness which is not in some way coloured or created by mental factors or the mind? Practical experience with patients may well seem to provide a compelling case for mental causation, especially so in neurosis. The patients' preoccupations centre on the personal details of their lives, their present circumstances, past experiences, and expectations of the future. The precipitation and progress of their illnesses seem closely bound up with events and with upheavals in personal relationships, to the extent that the latter may often seem to be 'the real problem'. Often there are histories of emotional deprivation or other adversities so that the observer may feel that he, too, might have had a breakdown if he had had to endure the same disadvantages. In other cases, where the patient appears to have been overwhelmed by adversity of no more than normal proportions, the observer may be struck by the patient's feebleness of resistance, and his apparent ease of transition to (and reluctance to give up) a sick and defeated role. In such cases one thinks naturally of psychological personality factors like motivation, self-sufficiency, and self-esteem. A deeper look at the patient's difficulties will quickly reveal mental and perhaps social mechanisms whose operation or decompensation seem at first sight to go far towards explaining the origins of the breakdown.

There are other considerations, too, which weigh in favour of an obvious role for psychogenesis. We all know that mental disorder may be linked to changes in society, such as the association of suicide with the economic depression of the 30s, or 'shell-shock' with the first world war. Recent research has substantiated the role of life-events in preceding and probably precipitating mental disorder. Mass hysteria is a term of everyday language, and other kinds of communicated mental aberration such as *folie à deux* or cultural fashions in hysterical symptomatology, suicide methods or drug abuse are well known. We know, too, that in most types of mental disorder, and especially in the neuroses and personality disorders, physical causes have not been identified. Often these abnormal developments or deviations seem no more than exaggerations of normal mental life and behaviour. Lately we have been reminded how easily labels of 'illness' can be used for political ends, and popular writers such as Goffman, Laing, Szasz and Scheff have given currency to the view that the phenomena of 'mental illness' are largely or even entirely the consequences of social processes of labelling, alienation, and invalidation.

To some people it is obvious that the important

questions about understanding and alleviating mental disorder lie mainly in the psychological and psychosocial realm. For them, the avenues to clinical understanding will lie primarily in an exploration of the sufferer's subjective world, as it is experienced and remembered, and of the social milieu of people, events and culture which have shaped that world. Much emphasis will probably be given to the events and circumstances which have preceded and precipitated the development, aggravation, or relapse of the patient's disorder, and quite often the patient's behaviour and anamnesis will be the only source of information. To the question, 'why did Mr Jones have a breakdown?' a simple answer in terms of distressing personal experiences such as a recent bereavement, marital upheaval, or some other conflict will often provide an answer that suffices for casual conversation. Such precipitating events will very often be easy to recognize, and a more detailed unravelling of the patient's memories will readily yield patterns of experience in his history which give meaning to the current content of his preoccupations, and the strengths and weaknesses of his personality. Thus far, psychogenic explanations may well appear good enough to make the breakdown intelligible. But suppose we ask further simple questions, like:

(1) Why couldn't Mr Jones cope with these distressing events when other people can?

(2) Why did his mental disturbance take the particular form, severity and time-course that it did (and why did he respond to treatment in that particular way)?

(3) To what extent could his behaviour, perhaps altered as a result of incipient illness, have had any part to play in bringing about the events which seemed to trigger his manifest disorder?

(4) Why did it happen now rather than, say, six months ago, or five years ago when something very similar happened to him?

(5) How likely is it that he will have another breakdown, and how can one prevent it happening?

A comprehensively 'psychogenic' description of mental causation would be one that satisfactorily answered all such questions in terms of psychological processes, and if it were to claim special merit, these processes would not be susceptible to other languages of explanation. Furthermore, the description of causes should be able to specify to what extent each causal process was sufficient, necessary, or con-tributory, and in medical terms whether they were aetiological, pathogenic, or pathoplastic (a distinction often overlooked, but emphasized by Cooper and Shepherd (1970), following Griesinger).

The problem of susceptibility

Some of the questions illustrated above may be more easily answered in purely psychological terms than may others, depending on the case and the theoretical beliefs of the observer. A major stumbling-block, of course, is the role played by individual susceptibility, which has itself to be explained in psychological terms if a notion of pure psychogenesis is to be retained. As Lewis (1972) illustrates, constitutional vulnerability of the patient has had to be included as a qualifying limitation of most formulations of psychogenesis, from Sommer onwards. An example of the problem in psycho-analysis is the question of what determines the patient's particular pattern of ego mechanisms. One way to cut through the difficulty at a stroke is to deny any demarcation between mental disorder and normal life. Berke (1972), for instance, is quoted as observing that 'Insanity is synonymous with behaviour or experience that is "unacceptable" within a given cultural framework'. On such a basis, mental disorder is to be explained, not as a development in the individual patient, but solely in terms of other people's reaction to, and interaction with, the person who is stigmatized by his family or by society at large as 'mentally ill'.

Recognition of the aetiological importance of contributory social factors in some mental disorders is now so general that belief in 'psychosociogenesis' is likely to be commoner than acceptance of purely intrapsychic theories of causation. A detailed discussion of the issues involved in examining the role of psychosocial causation is included in Brown and Harris' (1978) report of their research into the social origins of depression in women in Camberwell and the Outer Hebrides. They provide a schematic outline of the contributing roles of *provoking agents, vulnerability factors,* and *symptom formation factors,* and are forthright in identifying the limitations and areas of uncertainty in their model.

Delineating psychogenic disorders

One of the major concerns of writers on psychogenesis has been to single out types of disorder where a psychogenic basis is particularly prominent.

Much of the debate has centred on psychosis. Neuroses and personality disorders tend to be assigned to the more psychogenic end of the spectrum, but there are many disorders, including depression, anxiety states, alcohol and drug dependence, anorexia nervosa, or the more severe obsessional disorders where some cerebral rather than purely mental level of organization is postulated to be a necessary component.

In the course of these disputes, the notion of psychogenesis has become diffused so that one can understand it, in so far as it has any claim to be a formal or scientific term, only in a very general way. The concept implies the existence of a relationship between an emergent phenomenon y, and an antecedent or accompanying phenomenon x. The exact nature of x and y, and the nature of the relationship between them, have not been agreed on.

The emergent phenomenon Y

Y may be an illness, a disease, or individual symptoms or signs. In Ey's view (Lewis 1972), Y encompasses normal mental activity but not illness. Fish (1974) is quite definite that the emergent phenomena are psychological and states that 'a psychogenic disorder is one in which a psychological trauma has given rise to a psychological abnormality'. He then goes on to distinguish hysterical disorders as a subgroup of psychogenic disorders (thereby reversing Sommer's initial hierarchy). Others, however, are equally insistent that the emergent phenomena are physiological changes or even structural physical disease. Cobb (1963), for instance, claims that the triumph of psychogenesis has been the demonstration of the 'psychological and physical mechanisms by which emotional stimuli can be turned into disorders of function and thereby inevitably into structural changes'. Terms like 'psychogenic headache' (commonly attributed to spasm of the scalp muscles) or Sim's (1968) 'psychogenic fever' illustrate the ambiguity. Both are recognized to be associated with objectively recognizable manifestations, yet are designated as phenomena created by the sufferer's mind.

Antecedent and accompanying phenomenon X

The range of processes and phenomena which have been at one time or another implicated in producing the observed disorder is very wide. It encompasses *external* (or interactive) events, relationships, upbringing, social class and culture, and *internal* agents such as attitudes and personality,

unconscious conflicts, mechanisms of defence, personal construct systems, and behavioural conditioning. Vague terms like stress or trauma are also used, whose spatial location inside or outside the patient is uncertain.

The relationship between X and Y

Though commonly regarded as in some way causal, the relationship may be defined instead as not causal but meaningful, a distinction stressed by Jaspers (1963). It may be claimed that the connection is to be comprehended rationally, or empathically, or perhaps by special techniques such as the psychoanalytic study of free association. Often the exact nature of the relationship is left undefined, or is referred to in terms of the question-begging concept of 'reaction'.

The continuing usefulness of the term

The very vagueness of the terms 'psychogenesis' and 'psychogenic' may partly account for their continuing use. They offer a kind of buffer, to stop a train of thought rolling beyond the rails of commonsense wisdom into areas of uncharted terrain; the user can stay within the familiar confines of his experience that, of course, there are connections between what people feel and say and do, and the events and experiences that shape their lives. In this way, some kinds of illness or symptoms, perhaps even physical changes, become more accessible to everyday ratiocination and 'understanding'. If we agree to call something 'psychogenic' there may be, too, a tacit assumption about what we are *not* going to talk about, such as physical entities like the brain and its neuronal circuits and neuro-transmitters or putative cerebral lesions or pathophysiology. In this way we can declare a determination to stick to the world of everyday experience and the psychological insights embodied in ordinary language.

As well as designating boundaries for thought, the words may also serve a purpose for indicating territorial domains for action. A physician or surgeon who describes his patient's symptoms as 'psychogenic' not only distinguishes them from symptoms of what he recognizes as physical disease but may also be indicating a feeling that they ought to be the concern of somebody else, like a psychiatrist or a social worker.

Bodily symptoms

The reasons for making such an attribution to psychogenesis when symptoms are referred to the body can vary, as is illustrated by Slater's (1965) examination of the diagnosis of hysteria in a neurological hospital. Absence of demonstrable physical pathology, or inadequate pathology (as in psychogenic or 'functional' overlay), visible signs of mental disorder, multitudinous symptoms, emotional underreaction or over-reaction or other histrionic behavioural traits, atypicality or anatomical impossibility of symptoms, conformity with stereotype notions of hysteria or psychosomatic disorders, or relationship in time or place to distressing events or particular circumstances are among possible reasons. Sometimes there are implications that the symptoms are unduly magnified or feigned or that they arise by suggestion, imitation, or motivation for gain. Psychiatrists, too, have called such symptoms psychogenic, for reasons which, besides ones already listed, may include claims to recognize mechanisms of secondary gain, conversion, or dissociation, or the use of the language of bodily illness to coerce a helping response from other people. The fallibility of such diagnoses is inevitable, given that the presence or absence of physical pathology can no more accurately be appraised by examination of the mental state, than can the operation of the mind of a conscious patient be explored by physical investigations. Since all symptoms are mental phenomena, whatever else they may be, the notion of a psychogenic symptom is arguably tautologous. Symptoms which are not referred to the body, bodily symptoms not explained by demonstrable physical events or pathology, bodily symptoms attributed to mental upheaval, or demonstrable physical changes believed to be the manifestation of mental processes are just some of the phenomena commonly called psychogenic: they are not synonymous.

Defining territories

The territorial imperative, that the patient's problems have to be categorized in a way that allows some doctor or other person to be designated as the proper person to deal with them, is a practical necessity. For the psychiatrist, the question of whether or not a disorder is psychogenic, may arise in territorial negotiations not only with physicians and surgeons but also with other mental health professionals.

Many people seem to believe that if a disorder is psychogenic it demands psychological intervention, such as some form of psychotherapy and hence, perhaps, a psychotherapist or psychologist and not a medically-orientated psychiatrist (or general practitioner) within too easy reach of a prescription pad. To some the logic of such a view is inescapable, but to others it is indefensibly specious: it overlooks the possibility that mental processes put in motion by psychological events in a susceptible individual may acquire an autonomy, a degree of irreversibility by events or further experiences, and even perhaps a pathophysiological momentum which take the process of illness, for a time at least, beyond the reach of purely psychotherapeutic or social intervention. Such possibilities are catered for if, for instance, one uses (as did Brown and Harris, 1978) a concept like 'clinical depression', but are not adequately acknowledged if terms like 'unhappiness,' 'distress' or 'illness behaviour' are preferred because of their freedom from medical overtones. The obverse view can be just as inhumane, namely that when a patient's illness is *not* psychogenic psychotherapeutic help can be dispensed with. The treatment received by patients with unequivocally physical disease or psychosis may appear to be organized along lines which give only secondary consideration, if any, to the non-diseased parts of their subjective mental world. One sad result is that services designated to provide psychotherapy tend, with some notable exceptions, to be reserved for the patients with the least disabling illness.

The conceptual problems of psychogenesis are not new at all, but they may have acquired a new urgency. With the increasing participation of non-medical disciplines in the field of mental health and the increasing self-determination of paramedical disciplines has come an eagerness to reject what are believed to be 'medical' models of illness practised by doctors (often characterized in rather simplistic terms as 'organic' models), in favour of psychological, sociological, family-orientated, and 'antipsychiatric' models (Siegler & Osmond 1966). At one level the argument is still metaphysical, but at another there are major practical and professional issues at stake. The territorial limits of psychiatry and of treatment with drugs are two such concerns. Linked with these issues is the question of who should have responsibility and appropriate professional status and reward for the care of those troubled people now designated as psychiatric patients.

1.2.2
Factors in the social environment

GEORGE W. BROWN AND
BRIAN COOPER

Scope and definitions

Discussion of the causal significance of environmental factors for the neuroses is hampered by vagueness and ambiguity – to some extent unavoidable – in the relevant concepts. In this brief contribution we are concerned, not with the direct influence of changes in the physical environment or in physical activity, but rather with how individuals perceive and react emotionally to such changes: in other words, with man's capability to give meaning to his environment and to himself. This use of the term 'social' is artificially restrictive since in modern society many physical, chemical, and biological characteristics are socially determined. We do not wish to assert that these are never of relevance for the aetiology of neurosis. However, clinical experience and research findings alike indicate that the environmental factors most important in neurotic illness are those which impinge on the individual through his awareness of the world and particularly through personal contacts and interaction with other individuals or groups. Such aspects are often referred to collectively as the 'psychosocial environment'. We prefer not to use this term, since it may lead to confusion between objectively verifiable features of the environment and their subjective interpretation.

The task of aetiology may be defined as that of identifying noxious agents by establishing their connections with the occurrence of disease. Study of the intervening physiological and psychological processes leading to manifestations of disease (pathogenesis) is not strictly part of aetiology, though it can of course greatly reinforce causal inference when applied within an aetiological framework. Aetiological agents include both those which operate over the longer term, or at some point in the individual's past, to increase proneness to a given disease or to disease in general (vulnerability or predisposing factors) and those which operate at or shortly before the onset of illness (provoking or precipitating factors). The same predisposing factors may be involved in emotional disorders of childhood or in adult neuroses, whereas the provoking factors must by definition be operative in that part of the life span in which the disorder occurs.

'Neurosis' we shall take to be a broad descriptive term as outlined in the section on concepts and classification (chap. 1.1) at the beginning of this chapter. Clinical descriptions in most classifications, such as in the Glossary accompanying the International Classification of Diseases (World Health Organization, 1978) do not permit any clear differentiation between conditions said to be reactive to stressful events and those said to occur in the absence of such events. We shall not make any assumptions as to which forms of neurotic illness are 'reactions' and which are not, but instead shall try to assess the scientific evidence bearing on this question.

Much of the evidence is derived from community studies, in which depressive states have been found to constitute the most frequent form of mental disturbance. While a case has been made for regarding some of these conditions as milder analogues of affective psychosis, the majority conform more closely to clinical descriptions of 'depressive neurosis' (ICD category 300.4). Research into the aetiology of this group may be taken as illustrative for the neuroses generally, bearing in mind that the formation of symptoms in each diagnostic group must be determined by relatively specific factors, causal or pathoplastic.

Social and familial correlates of neurosis

Neurotic illness – unlike, for example, schizophrenia or chronic alcoholism – is not as a rule accompanied by gross disturbances in social adaptation. Nevertheless, a number of controlled studies have shown neurotic illness to be associated in the general population with a relative excess of family and social problems. Cooper (1972) compared a sample of general practitioners' patients suffering from chronic depressive or anxiety neuroses with a comparison series of individually matched patients and found among the former an increase in difficulties related to finances, living conditions, occupation, social contacts, and care of children. These findings have since been replicated by other workers. Weissman and Paykel (1974) reported the performance of acutely depressed women to be less adequate in respect of all social roles than that of a group without depression. There is evidence that the risk of neurotic illness is increased among the spouses of neurotic patients, as well as more generally within their nuclear family groups. In a recently-reported Australian study (Henderson *et al.*, 1980) an inverse relationship was found between the presence of neurotic symptoms and the strength of established social bonds; in particular, of close affectional ties.

These findings serve to demonstrate associations between clinical and social variables, but not the nature of the underlying causal relationships. Causal significance can only be attributed to a social concomitant of disease, if it is known to have been present before the illness-onset. A first step, therefore, in testing any environmental hypothesis is to establish the temporal relationship between exposure to the factor in question and the inception of illness. For this reason, research into the environmental causes of mental illness has in recent years become concentrated increasingly on the investigation of life changes and life events, whose occurrence can be reliably identified and accurately dated.

Investigation of life changes and life-events

A number of different research strategies may be adopted in studying the aetiological and prognostic significance of life-events. Certain types of stress-situation may be singled out, such as bereavement, premature birth, or enforced rehousing. The illness-experience of groups exposed to such risk factors can then be examined either retrospectively or prospectively. Alternatively, exposure to a wide range of life-events may be summarized and quantified, using some form of standard schedule, and this exposure then related to the occurrence, either of all illness-episodes or of some relatively specific type of illness, such as myocardial infarction or depressive illness. In this rapidly developing field of research, workers are still largely preoccupied by methodological issues;

in particular, by problems of measurement. The general requirements for investigations of this kind cannot be fulfilled by clinical studies alone, but call for epidemiological techniques. Moreover, the association between events and illness-onset must be elaborated by introducing additional variables into the analysis; in other words, a causal model must be constructed.

Towards an aetiological model of depression

A systematic attempt has been made to construct such a model for depressive illness, making use of data from clinical and social research (Brown & Harris, 1978). The occurrence of life-events such as change of job, birth of a child, or learning of a husband's infidelity was established for the period preceding onset of the depressive disorder. The *severity* of each event was assessed in terms of the extent to which it was judged to have threatened the individual's social adjustment and equilibrium, and the duration of this threat.

The basic findings for occurrence of life events among the group of depressed female patients treated by psychiatrists and a group of 'normal' women (i.e., excluding all psychiatrically-ill women found in a random sample) living in the same area of London are summarized in Fig. 1.2.2.1.

When all events are considered there is a steep rise among the patients in the rate of events in the three-week period before illness-onset, but no difference other than this (Fig. 1.2.2.1A). However, when only severely threatening events, having long-term implications for the affected persons, are distinguished from other events this picture changes dramatically (Fig. 1.2.2.1B). There is still a sharp rise in the three-week period before illness-onset, but a higher rate of severe events throughout the whole of the previous 10 months can be observed. Severe events form only one-sixth of the total of events and *no* other type of event shows an association with onset of illness (Fig. 1.2.2.1C). Only a certain type of event – that which is seriously threatening to the individual – appears capable of bringing about depression.

In all, 61 per cent of the patients, compared with only 20 percent of the 'normal' women, reported at least one severe event in the period covered at interview. Statistical analysis of the data indicated that such severe events had been of causal significance in 49 per cent of the patient-group, and that the 'brought-forward time' – the notional period of time by which life events advance the onset of illness, on average – was just over two years.* This latter finding suggests that severe events do not simply trigger off depressive illness in persons who are already at the point of breaking down, but have a strongly formative influence on the development of the illness.

Description of the individual events leaves little room for doubt that loss and disappointment are the central features. Typical events included: being given notice to quit from a post held for many years, because

*The 'brought-forward time' is an estimate of the mean time-interval between the point of onset of an illness provoked by life-events and the hypothetical point in time at which the illness would have occurred 'spontaneously' – that is, in the absence of such events. While this value obviously cannot be measured directly, it can be estimated from the distribution of life-events among members of a population who manifest the illness in question and those who do not. For technical reasons the value so obtained will as a rule be an under-estimate of the 'true' brought-forward time (Brown & Harris, 1978, pp. 116–29).

Fig. 1.2.2.1. Rate of events in 16 three-week periods before onset (patients) or interview (normal women) by severity of threat.

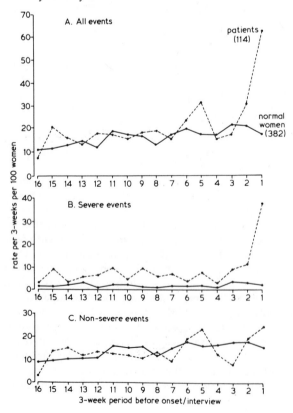

the firm was moving its premises, having a husband lose his job in a context of financial difficulties, making a change of house that could not be afforded in order to get away from difficult neighbours, having a husband go to prison, a marital separation, and the death of a parent.

In addition to such well-defined events, which could be fairly accurately pin-pointed in time, 47 per cent of the patient-group as compared with only 17 per cent of the healthy women were found to have been labouring for at least two years under one, or more than one, major social difficulty – mostly involving problems centred on marriage, care and upbringing of children, finances, housing conditions, or conditions in the neighbourhood. Problems of physical health appeared to lead only seldom to depression, unless some kind of acute crisis had intervened, or financial or other difficulties had been caused by chronic illness and disability. When life-events and ongoing difficulties were grouped together as 'provoking agents', the difference between patient-group and healthy women was increased: three-quarters of the former, as against only one-third of the latter, reported either a severe life-event or a major social difficulty, or both, within the relevant period.

To bring these findings into perspective, it must be emphasized that in most instances neither life-events nor social difficulties of the kind reported lead to depressive illness; from the research data it could be estimated that such provoking agents had been followed by a clinically significant depression in only about one-fifth of the persons exposed to them. The obvious explanation is that this proportion represents a minority of the population which for some reason is susceptible, or predisposed, to depressive illness. It should not, however, be concluded that the predisposition is necessarily genetical or otherwise constitutionally determined; on the contrary, the evidence suggests that, here also, social factors are involved. The probability of developing a depressive state in the face of one or more provoking agents was found to be increased if one or more of the following 'vulnerability' factors was also present: (i) lack of an intimate, confiding relationship with husband or man-friend; (ii) presence at home of three or more children under 14 years; (iii) a history of loss of the mother, by death or separation, before the age of 11. In addition, lack of paid employment appeared to be important for those women who had no intimate, confiding relationship.

This heterogeneous group of indices, which

probably reflects some common underlying factor, is convenient but in no sense definitive. The crucial point is that certain background factors in the life of women appear to increase their risk of developing a depressive illness in the face of severe life-events or major social difficulties – or, stated more positively, certain background features may help to protect women from the worst effects of such provoking agents.

The vulnerability factors so far identified are to some extent linked with social class. Thus, working-class women have been shown to have an increased frequency of depressive illness and to be more likely than other social class groups to display one or more 'vulnerability' factors (Brown & Harris, 1978). However, some of the social class differences in morbidity could also be attributed to a higher incidence of provoking agents among working-class women. In the rural community studied, social class differences appeared to be less important than the degree of integration into the traditional way of life based on small-scale farming and churchgoing. Those who had

moved furthest from traditional patterns were most likely to have experienced severe life-events or major social difficulties, and displayed more evidence of vulnerability.

On the basis of their research findings, a causal model of depression has been constructed, incorporating both provoking agents and vulnerability factors, together with a group of putative 'symptom-formative' or pathoplastic factors (see Fig. 1.2.2.2).

Social causation: specific or general?

The question must now be posed: how specific is this causal model? Is it valid only for depressive neurosis, or for all types of depressive illness; or is it common to all forms of neurotic disorder?

The conceptual and methodological problems involved do not permit these questions to be answered firmly. The classification of depressive illness remains unsettled after half a century of controversy (Kendell, 1968). In this context, the importance must be stressed of maintaining, for research purposes, as sharp as possible a distinction between the

Fig. 1.2.2.2. Schematic outline of causal model (shown in capitals) and theoretical interpretations (shown in small type).

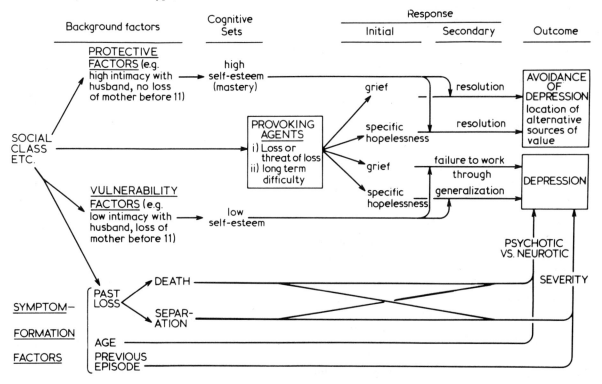

clinical symptomatology on the one hand, and the aetiological and background features of illness on the other. In the previously mentioned study of depressed women, in which this condition was carefully observed, patients receiving diagnoses of 'psychotic' and 'neurotic' depression respectively did not show any significant difference in their pre-morbid experience of life-events and social difficulties (Brown *et al.*, 1979). Comparison of depressed patients with severe life-events or major social difficulties ('reactive') and those with neither ('endogenous') revealed only a slight tendency for the latter to manifest more psychotic symptoms. Apart from age, the only important characteristic differentiating between patients with psychotic and those with neurotic depression was a more frequent history of past death of a close member of the family in the former group. Incidence of provoking agents did not differentiate between the two groups. The evidence thus suggests that such provoking agents play a similar role in the aetiology of depressive neurosis and depressive psychosis, but that the predisposing factors differ between these two diagnostic categories.

This finding is not the only one to challenge the widespread assumption that psychotic depression is fundamentally endogenous, whereas neurotic depression is largely reactive. Similar conclusions were reached by Leff and colleagues (1970), Paykel and colleagues (1971), and Thomson & Hendrie (1972). In general, the types of life-event associated with the onset of depressive disorders, attempted suicide, and neuroses in general practice appear to be broadly of the same kind, namely loss or threat of loss, in contrast with events producing schizophrenia, which appear to be best defined as incidents producing strong emotion of any kind.

Much less is known about the aetiology of other forms of neurosis, characterized by acute anxiety, phobias, obsessional-compulsive symptoms, and so on, than about that of depression. Some recent research findings suggest that life-events are often important in the genesis of anxiety and phobic conditions but that these events less often involve clear-cut loss or disappointment than those preceding depression and more often present the individual with a problem whose resolution is still in the balance (Finlay-Jones & Brown, 1981).

It thus appears probable that the form of the psychiatric disorder is to some extent influenced by the nature of the provoking agent and partly by underlying pathoplastic factors. That family influ-

ences are important in all these conditions is now widely accepted. Epidemiological research has shown, for example, that phobic anxiety, in its distribution in the general population, tends to cluster within families. The nature of these influences, however, has still to be established. Lader & Marks (1972), at the end of a comprehensive review, could only conclude that:

> Why internal triggers start the clinical anxiety in the first place is usually a mystery . . . It is sometimes suggested that the triggers to clinical anxiety are in fact not internal but external, in the form of ubiquitous stimuli like light to which anxiety has been conditioned. The search for consistent stimuli of this kind does not usually result in evidence which fits clinical facts convincingly.

It might have been more prudent to conclude that the necessary research has not yet been undertaken. There is a dearth of controlled or comparative studies, analogous to those described above for depression, which could tell us what exposure to social stress-situations characterizes persons suffering from anxiety or phobic neuroses, when compared with matched groups in the general population.

1.2.3

Genetic and chromosome disorders

DAVID C. R. PITCHER

Genetics

Genetic disorders include those produced by gross chromosome abnormalities and by single genes of large effect resulting in Mendelian dominant, recessive, or X-linked conditions. For the most part these conditions exert effects on personality of a secondary nature, as in the deviation of personality seen in a gradually developing Huntington's chorea. Their primary effects are usually associated with specifiable pathological processes and are qualitatively distinct from the normal. In the population at large, however, personality traits vary from individual to individual in a quantitative manner, as does stature and intelligence, their distribution conforming mathematically to a 'normal' or Gaussian curve. Deviant individuals whose disorder is not due to specific causes such as disease or injury are those at the extremes of this distribution, the genetic contribution to which will be due to a number of genes, each of small effect but operating cumulatively and subject to the influence of the environment, which provides a further source of variation. Using this model, the neuroses can be understood as maladaptive reactions to which some personalities are more vulnerable than others.

The evidence for genetic factors in personality disorders and the neuroses derives mainly from twin, family, and adoption studies. Comprehensive reviews of the subject include those by Slater and Cowie (1971) and Shields (1973). In some cases studies in animal behaviour genetics provide at least theoretical support to the findings in human beings (Slater & Shields, 1969).*

Monozygotic (MZ) twins are genetically identical, whilst dizygotic (DZ) twins share, on average, only half their genes. Resemblances between MZ twins in excess of those between DZ twins will support a genetic hypothesis. Differences between members of a MZ twin pair must be due to factors in the environment – including an interaction between the twins themselves. Comparisons between MZ twins reared together and those reared apart may reveal both genetic and environmental influences on their development. Environmental influences contributing to differences between twins begin at conception. *In utero,* one twin may enjoy a greater share of the placenta than the other, and this and other more complex differences may be reflected in differences in antenatal development – differences in birthweight, for example – that may be crucial for subsequent development. Apart from these latter factors, there appears to be no evidence of any special hazard in twinship itself, since twins as such are not found to suffer from mental or other disorders more frequently than single conceptions.

Twin studies (Shields, 1962, 1973) confirm that MZ pairs are consistently more alike than DZ pairs in physique, intelligence, and temperament. Separated pairs of MZ twins are only to a limited extent less alike than those reared together. Their similarity is reflected in their rate of development in infancy and childhood; in specific talents and learning disabilities; and in measurable physiological variables, such as specific drug effects and the rate of metabolism of certain drugs, the rate of habituation of the galvanic skin response, and both the resting electrical activity of the brain and evoked EEG potentials. At the end of their life span MZ twins remain more alike than DZ twins in their longevity and their manner of ageing.

Personality disorders

Evidence of the genetic contribution to personality disorder comes mainly from studies of criminality, male homosexuality, and alcoholism. Slater (1962) found a tendency for male homosexuals to be born to older mothers, and Heston and Shields (1968) found higher concordance rates among MZ than

---

* Genetic factors in mental handicap are described elsewhere (See vol. 3, chap. 36 and vol. 5, chap. 3).

among DZ twins; but the evidence from a number of studies overall is inconclusive.

Regarding adult crime, Slater and Cowie (1971) reviewed a number of studies, beginning with those of Lange (1931), in which concordance rates are higher for MZ than for DZ twins. MZ:DZ differences are not always statistically significant, which emphasizes the importance of environmental factors, but genetic factors are reflected in greater MZ:DZ differences when persistent psychopathic offenders are considered as a separate group. Among the latter, MZ pairs are more likely to be concordant with respect to the nature of their criminality: for example, sexual offences or violence, and the pattern of their criminal careers. Christiansen (1974), in a study based on the Danish national twin register and criminal records, found a concordance rate of 52 per cent among MZ twins and of 22 per cent among DZ twins. Shields (1976), reviewing the work of others, reports the findings among Danish adoptees of an incidence of criminality of 21 per cent among those subjects of whom only the biological father had a criminal record. When neither or both of the biological and adoptive fathers had a criminal record the incidence among the adoptees was 10 per cent and 36 per cent respectively.

Further support for the influence of heredity in what he calls psychopathic spectrum disorders (including criminality, alcoholism, and hysterical character disorder) comes from a study by Schulsinger (1972). He studied the incidence of mental disorder in the biological relatives of 57 psychopathic adoptees and an equal number of matched controls. Mental disorders of all kinds were more common among 305 biological relatives of the index cases than among other groups; but when psychopathy was taken alone it was found to occur in 9.3 per cent of biological fathers of the index cases as compared with a maximum of 1.9 per cent among other fathers.

Clearly, however, environmental influences play a part in criminal or psychopathic behaviour, and they appear to be much more important in juvenile than in adult delinquents. Among the juvenile delinquents, concordance rates for MZ and DZ twins are barely different. These findings, and the much lower incidence of criminality among women – which contrasts with the greater MZ:DZ differences in their concordance rates for criminality, suggest that adult criminals, especially women, constitute a very deviant group, among whom genetic factors may play a role distinct from that operating in delinquency in younger groups.

The likelihood that a proneness to alcoholism (or complete abstinence) might have a partly genetic basis is supported by animal studies (see Shields, 1973). Goodwin and colleagues (1973, 1974), in a study of the biological sons of alcoholic fathers, found a raised incidence of alcoholism in these sons whether or not they had been adopted away. Kaij (1960) in a study of 214 twin pairs, in which at least one twin of each pair was a registered alcoholic, found a higher concordance among MZ (53.5 per cent) than DZ pairs (28.3 per cent), and the concordance rates increased with the severity of alcohol abuse. The findings of Partanen and colleagues (1966) suggest that genetic factors may operate most strongly in alcoholism of early onset, whereas in older age groups age itself, marital status, and urban residence play an increasingly important part.

Neurosis

Shields (1962) found a higher incidence of neurosis in those members of separated twin pairs reared in lower socio-economic circumstances but also that neurosis correlated with measures of introversion. A number of family studies have shown fair agreement in finding a higher than average incidence (15 per cent) of anxiety neurosis among first-degree relatives of anxiety neurotics, but with an especially high concordance between mothers and sons. Slater and Shields (1969) studied 146 same-sexed MZ and DZ twins treated at the Maudsley Hospital for personality disorders and neuroses. The diagnoses were made 'blind', without a knowledge of the diagnosis in the co-twin or the zygosity of the pair. These findings indicate a degree of genetic specificity for anxiety (Table 1.2.3.1). Similar results were found for at least some personality disorders: for example, those in which antisocial, obsessional, or schizoid traits predominate. Neuroses such as neurotic depression were less often concordant, and there were no MZ:DZ differences.

Hysteria is a diagnosis often made on unsatisfactory criteria. Ljunberg (1957) in a family study of hysteria found a low rate in first-degree relatives and that a proportion of his index cases had suffered a cerebral injury. Slater (1961), in a twin study of patients with a hospital diagnosis of hysteria, failed to find a similar disorder in either 12MZ or 12DZ co-twins. It is probable that specific genetic factors play little or no part in hysteria but that hysterical symptoms occur as a reaction to stress, including that produced by organic and functional disorders.

Regarding obsessive-compulsive states, Slater and Cowie (1971) reviewed a number of family and twin studies and concluded that obsessionality is distributed quantitatively and normally in the population, on a polygenic basis, with a high correlation between traits and symptoms in reaction to stress.

Considering the neuroses together, while the genetic contribution appears to be high in obsessional neurosis or anxiety (including phobic) neurosis, the same does not apply to all neurotic disorders. However, while the presence or severity of neurotic symptoms seems to be very much related to environmental stress, the nature of a neurotic reaction when it does occur is more likely to be determined by hereditary factors. These hereditary or constitutional factors cause some individuals to be more neurotically predisposed than others, so that less stress is required to cause breakdown in these more vulnerable subjects.

The evidence is quite clear that genetic influences are important over a wide range of abnormalities of personality and behaviour, but this has to be weighed against the evidence of dissimilarity between related individuals. Perhaps paradoxically, 'genetic studies often help to elucidate the importance of environmental factors' (Shields, 1973). Most behaviour, normal or otherwise, results from an interaction between the environment and an orga-

Table 1.2.3.1. *Psychiatric diagnosis and concordance in same-sexed twins*

	MZ	DZ
Anxiety state in proband	$N = 17$	$N = 28$
Any diagnosis in twin	*47%*	*18%*
Same diagnosis in twin	*41%*	*4%*
Other neurosis in proband	$N = 12$	$N = 21$
Any diagnosis in twin	*25%*	*24%*
Same diagnosis in twin	*0%*	*0%*
Personality disorder in proband	$N = 33$	$N = 35$
Any diagnosis in twin	*55%*	*29%*
Same diagnosis in twin	*33%*	*6%*
All probands	$N = 62$	$N = 84$
Any diagnosis in twin	*47%*	*24%*
Same diagnosis in twin	*29%*	*4%*

Data from Slater & Shields (1969).
Reprinted here by permission of Royal College of Psychiatrists, London.

nism whose constitution is laid down on a genetic basis: 'Nowadays there are no hereditarians, only environmentalists and interactionists' (Slater & Shields, 1969).

Chromosome abnormalities

Autosomal defects are usually severe, or lethal *in utero*. Sex chromosome anomalies, on the other hand, are compatible with life and usually produce only minor physical defects, but may give rise to mental disability in the form of disorders of character and personality. Comprehensive reviews of the subject include those by Slater and Cowie (1971) and by Pitcher (1981).

These anomalies occur in about 0.5 per cent of the newborn, of which about 25 per cent are mosaic individuals, with two or more cell lines that differ in their chromosome complement. Karyotypes 47XXX in females and 47XXY (associated with Klinefelter's syndrome) and 47XYY in males occur with an about equal frequency (0.1 per cent). Karyotype 45X (associated with Turner's syndrome) is much less common in the newborn (about 0.03 per cent) but is probably the commonest anomaly at conception: an association with physical defects contributes to the very high pre- and post-natal mortality (Polani, 1977). Polysomies involving more than three sex chromosomes, for example 48XXYY, 49XXXXY, and so on, are very rare, and in general produce more severe effects. The phenotypic effects of mosaic genotypes are generally less severe but depend upon the proportion of abnormal cells and the tissues affected. Morphological aberrations of the X or Y chromosomes also produce phenotypic effects. Variants of Turner's syndrome may be associated with structural abnormalities of the X chromosome, and there is evidence that Y chromosome abnormalities may affect personality and behaviour.

The 47XXX and 47XYY genotypes are not associated with somatically distinct phenotypes. Among other genotypes, somatic effects include some or all of the stigmata of Turner's syndrome in 45X girls and of Klinefelter's syndrome in males with extra X chromosomes (commonly 47XXY). Both X and Y chromosomes have a quantitative effect on height: 45X girls are short and both 47XXY and 47XYY males are taller than average. None of these effects is invariable, however, and, when the somatic and mental effects are taken together, sex chromosome anomalies do not produce a simple stereotype comparable, for example, to that found in Down's syndrome.

Evidence associating sex chromosome anomalies with mental disorder derives mainly from a comparison of their incidence among the newborn with their prevalence in special groups of children or adults. The increased risk of mental illness in 47XXX females (Barr *et al.*, 1969) and 47XXY males (Nielsen, 1969) implies effects that make emotional adjustment precarious. No specific form of neurotic or psychotic disorder applies but some authors believe that in many of these cases psychoses are reactive or psychogenic in origin and have a relatively good prognosis.

Extra sex chromosomes appear to affect intelligence adversely in a quantitative manner. Mean intelligence is usually low in the normal range, except for individuals with three or more supernumary sex chromosomes, who may be more severely affected. Triple-X females and 47XXY males suffer an increased risk of mild subnormality but their presence in an institution is likely to be influenced by illness or disorders of behaviour independently of their subnormality. In Turner's syndrome non-verbal skills are impaired (Money, 1975), whereas males with Klinefelter's syndrome tend to display poor speech development in childhood and to have a deficit in verbal intellectual skills as adults (Nielsen, 1972; Theilgaard, 1972).

In respect of other personality characteristics, little has been described of 47XXX females. Girls with Turner's syndrome and Klinefelter males may react adversely to their anatomical abnormalities and hormonal deficits but these effects are amenable to modification by judicious timing of hormonal therapies and appropriate counselling. 45X females have a normally feminine orientation but with a low libido. Phlegmatic and stoical qualities of temperament are held to promote their social adjustment and to reduce the incidence of overt psychological disorder, which is acknowledged to be low (Money & Mittenthal, 1970). Males with Klinefelter's syndrome, on the other hand, are frequently maladjusted. They tend to be infantile in character and temperamentally unstable, especially with respect to their precarious masculinity which may be due to hypogonadism (Nielsen, 1969, 1972; Myhre *et al.*, 1970; Theilgaard, 1972; Beumont *et al.*, 1972). Among 47XYY males, disorders of sexual development, including hypogonadism, have been identified in a minority of cases: the majority have no physical abnormality. The association of this genotype with abnormalities of behaviour is now well recognized.

Interest in heritable factors in crime has a long history and was revived in the 1960s by the finding of a significantly higher than expected frequency of 47XYY and 48XXYY males in the British special hospitals for dangerous or criminal patients (see Pitcher, 1981). These findings have been confirmed in later studies and apply also, but to a lesser extent, to 47XXY males. Criminality in these men is significantly more common independently of factors such as poor intelligence and low socio-economic status (Witkin *et al.*, 1976). The possibility of an association of sex chromosome disorders with female criminality is an area for further research.

The mechanisms by which chromosomal anomalies operate to exert their effects are as yet obscure. Direct evidence of brain dysfunction derives mainly from the finding of clinical neurological abnormalities (including frank epilepsies, but mostly equivocal findings of hypotonia, intention tremors, asymmetric reflexes and the like) and anomalous electrical activity in the brains of 47XXY and 47XYY males. Abnormal EEG findings are not invariable, however, and tend to be non-specific: frankly epileptic records are uncommon. Heterochromatin effects are discussed by Polani (1977). The heterochromatin portions of chromosomes are those which remain condensed and highly stainable in interphase nuclei. There is evidence that heterochromatin effects – which may apply especially to sex chromosomes, and more especially to extra sex chromosomes – include effects on the transcription ('copying' of genetic information) of constituent and neighbouring genes, and on cell growth and metabolism. Space does not permit a detailed account of heterochromatin and its effects but it is such as to provide a theoretical as well as an evidential basis upon which to conclude that many of the disorders observed in association with chromosome abnormalities might be expected and are not merely chance findings.

1.2.4
Biological landmarks: adolescence, climacteric, old age

A. WAKELING

Introduction

Adolescence, the climacteric, and old age are important periods in an individual's life cycle. Each is characterized by biological change which imposes specific maturational tasks on the individual. In addition, these periods are associated with marked life change requiring adaptation to altered circumstances and adjustments in self-concept and identity. They are periods of stress which have particular relevance to the consideration of personality adjustment and the development of neurotic disorder in adult life.

The profound biological events of puberty occur throughout adolescence. There is rapid physical change and a need to integrate sexual development with the emerging personality and acquire a sense of personal identity. It is a critical period for personality growth and is associated with marked emotional turmoil.

The climacteric is the period of involution and the alterations at this time assume psychiatric importance chiefly for women. The biological events associated with the menopause and the effects of middle age on the woman's social role may combine to increase her vulnerability to psychoneurotic disorder.

Old age is a time of general decline affecting both physical and psychological functioning and the capacity to adapt to life change. During this period of life personality quirks may become accentuated and there is a high incidence of psychiatric disorder.

Adolescence

Adolescence is a period of varied duration that starts with the onset of puberty and ends with the completion of sexual development and epiphyseal fusion. It is a period of rapid biological, psychological, and sexual maturation. Biologically there is a marked increase in height, weight, and musculature and the development of adult sexual characteristics. Excretion of androgens increases in both sexes, more in boys than in girls, and there is a large rise in oestrogens in girls. These hormonal changes have a marked psychological effect on sexual drive and libido with an increase in heterosexual interest and activity during the course of adolescence (Schofield, 1965).

In addition to rapid psychosexual development adolescence is also characterized by an accelerating cognitive growth. An important aspect of this is the increased ability for abstract conceptualization. This is related to the adolescent's characteristic preoccupations with broad religious and philosophic issues and with notions concerning the meaning of life and his own identity. This emerging cognitive development is also associated with questioning and criticizing established authority and power. An important related theme is concern with establishing a sense of personal identity or sense of self (Erikson, 1965). The adolescent becomes intensely bound up with thoughts of who he is and what he is to become. In this context attempts are made at separation from parents and there is a greater identification with peer groups. The adolescent gradually begins to explore different social roles and modes of behaviour.

At the end of adolescence the individual should have developed a sense of personal identity and achieved some emotionally secure autonomy with a loosening of ties with parents. He should have achieved peer-group integration and friendships, and some mastery over genital sexuality. Adolescence is thus a period of rapid change and development associated with marked psychological upheaval and turmoil.

In terms of personality development, Offer (1969) has shown that the great majority of adolescents pass through this period smoothly without undue disruption and with good adjustment. Nevertheless, for some adolescents, factors operating throughout adolescence may confirm or accelerate processes of personality maladjustment that first appeared before puberty. Poor parent–child relationships, inadequate, deviant, or abnormal peer groups can all affect in varied ways the complex maturational processes of adolescence and may lead to distortions of personality at this time, or predispose to the later occurrence of psychoneurotic disorder. For instance, failure to master genital sexuality may lead to sexual anxieties which can suppress sexual functions and which may contribute to other neurotic disorders, such as anxiety states or obsessional neuroses. Deviations from norms in terms of physical development may lead to sensitivity about body shape or size or other aspects of physical appearance. Such handicaps may be overcome with adequate personal, family, and peer-group interactions, but they may persist or remain dormant and become a focus for the occurrence of neurotic disorder in adult life.

The marked psychological upheaval and turmoil during adolescence is associated with the common experience of mild psychiatric symptoms such as rapid mood oscillations, anxiety, tension, and sensitivity. Rutter and co-workers (1976) suggest that up to one-half of all adolescents experience symptoms of this sort at some time. These symptoms, which may in some cases resemble neurotic states seen in adults, are generally transient in nature, are non-handicapping, and remain unreported or undetected. Nevertheless adolescence is associated with an increased prevalence of defined psychiatric disorder and a change in pattern of disorder in comparison with earlier age periods. Prior to puberty psychiatric disorders are commoner in boys than girls, while in early adolescence the ratio is nearly equal; in adult life they are much commoner in women, with affective disorders predominating. Depressive illness and affective disorders are uncommon prior to puberty but much commoner during adolescence, again showing the beginning of a shift towards the adult pattern.

Neurotic disorders appearing during adolescence are generally similar to disorders occurring in adult life. The commonest are some kind of affective disorder such as depressive illness or anxiety neurosis. Hysterical neurosis and specific phobias do occur during adolescence but are relatively uncommon.

Whether there is any specific relationship between the developmental turbulence of adolescence and the increased prevalence of psychiatric disorder at this time remains uncertain. The fact that psychiatric disorders, when they occur, are similar in pattern and course to those occurring in adult life suggests that the causes are not to be found solely in terms of developmental crisis. Factors related to con-

stitution, childhood and parent–child interactions are all implicated (Graham & Rutter, 1977).

Climacteric

The menopause has long been regarded as a period when women are particularly vulnerable to stress and to the development of psychological disturbance. The term menopause refers to cessation of menses which occurs for the majority of women between the ages of 45 and 50. This is a clearly defined point which may occur suddenly or follow cycles of gradually increasing intervals. The menopause has often been confused in the literature with the climacteric (Greene & Cooke, 1980). The term climacteric is a more general one and refers to the involution of the ovaries and the various hormonal changes associated with this event. They occur over a period of some years prior to the menopause and continue for some years after (Studd *et al.*, 1977). The climacteric thus refers to the life period from the late thirties to the early fifties, although these age limits are somewhat arbitrary.

It was previously thought that a specific type of depressive illness, so-called involutional melancholia, was directly associated with the menopause. This diagnostic category is now subsumed under the rubric depressive psychosis and Winokur (1973) has demonstrated that although the latter rises in frequency with increasing age there is no specific menopausal association. This lack of association between the menopause and depressive psychosis probably also holds true for other psychotic illnesses such as schizophrenia (Christie Brown & Christie Brown, 1976).

A number of studies, however, have clearly documented a rise in minor psychiatric and somatic symptomatology among women in the general population at the climacteric (Neugarten & Kraines, 1965; Jaszman *et al.*, 1969; Thompson *et al.*, 1973; McKinlay & Jeffreys, 1974; Ballinger, 1975). The symptoms most commonly reported are: anxiety, irritability, depression, fatigue, tiredness, headaches, insomnia, palpitations, and hot flushes. The vasomotor changes resulting in hot flushes show an unequivocal association with the menopause and are experienced by the majority of women particularly during the first two years after the last period. There is a general tendency for the increase in the other symptoms to occur prior to the menopause in the early period of the climacteric. There is no evidence to suggest a specific menopausal pattern nor that the symptoms themselves are distinguishable from similar symptoms occurring at other times. In some women the symptom pattern is similar to that of depressive or anxiety neurosis.

Traditionally this increase in psychiatric symptoms during the climacteric has been attributed to the endocrine changes occurring at the menopause, although there is little direct evidence to support this. Treatment with oestrogen replacement regimes suggests that whilst flushing can be clearly related to oestrogen lack, no such certainty appends to the psychiatric symptoms. Response of these symptoms to hormone therapy is variable and often no better than that of the placebo (Christie Brown & Christie Brown, 1976).

In addition to the endocrine changes, there are marked life changes occurring during the climacteric which can have a profound effect on adjustment and self-esteem. Changes in maternal role, the growing up and moving away of children, illness or death of parents, waning sexual interests of husbands all require some readjustment and may contribute to the increased psychiatric morbidity during this period of life. The menopause itself signals the end of reproductive capacity and may for some women have important symbolic or psychological meaning. A recent study by Greene and Cooke (1980), using a life-event model and multivariate analysis, suggested that life stress had a significantly more powerful influence on the increase in psychiatric symptoms at the climacteric than did the menopause.

Furthermore there is evidence to suggest that women who develop psychiatric symptoms during the climacteric constitute a psychologically vulnerable group in that they are more likely to have had prior psychiatric disturbance (Ballinger, 1976). It would seem therefore that the increase in psychiatric morbidity at the climacteric results from the interaction of a number of factors including endocrine and physical events, coincidental life changes, and specific personality and constitutional factors.

Old Age
(1) *Physical and psychological aspects of ageing*
With ageing there is a decline in both physical and mental health. There are characteristic physical changes of ageing related to physical appearance and physiological functioning. There is a decrease in physiological adaptability leading to diminished physical resilience. The psychological consequences of ageing lead to a decrease in psychological resilience. With ageing there is a diminution in cognitive functioning, some restriction in the emotional and motivational aspects of personality, and impairment in social competence (Post, 1965). Memory declines with age and there is a general tendency to retain longer material acquired in early life. There is a reduction in short term retention and recall which underlines the poor memory for recent events characteristic of ageing. Learning ability and the capacity for assimilating new experiences correspondingly decline sharply with increasing age. There is also a diminution of sensori-motor performance.

Emotionally there is a general tendency as people grow older to turn inwards; a move towards a greater introversion. With the diminished capacity for new learning there develops a greater mental rigidity, a greater fixity of belief and opinion, a narrowing of outlook. There is a general tendency towards a more worried, anxious demeanour, an increasing concern over bodily function, and an emotional overreaction to stress. There is also a diminution of outwardly directed drives such as the sexual drive.

Socially there is a process of disengagement and withdrawal and in general a diminished interest in other people. In addition, there is a loss of status associated with ageing. Retirement may reinforce the reduction in status as well as contribute to economic decline and to the loss of contact with other people.

These psychological and social processes of disengagement and withdrawal can be regarded as adaptive to old age and many individuals adjust well to the effects of senescence. For others however, particularly those with pre-existing personality vulnerability, these age-related changes increasingly impair the capacity to deal with life stress, leading either to exacerbation or the appearance of psychiatric disorder.

(2) *Ageing and disorder of personality*
Ageing has an adverse effect on individuals with severe disorders of personality of the passive, dependent, or inadequate kind. Such people often become unable to sustain independent lives in the community and permanent care is necessitated. However, with the waning of outwardly directed drives the severity of psychopathic disorder as a rule diminishes with increasing age. Aggressive and impulsive behaviour tends to stabilize and a diagnosis of psychopathic disorder is seldom made in an elderly patient.

An important aspect of ageing is that psychological and personality change can lead to an exaggeration and caricaturing of lifelong personality traits with the development of senile character disorders. Individuals who develop such disorders in general have personality defects which in adult life were slight or modified but become amplified with increasing age. Thus, isolated suspicious individuals may become habitually suspicious and overtly paranoid, seeing the world as a totally hostile place. A lifelong concern about bodily health may turn into hypochondriacal preoccupations. Introverted individuals may gradually become totally isolated and lead hermit-like existences. Irascible, self-centred and argumentative individuals may with ageing become cantankerous, hostile people totally unable to achieve any adequate relationships. Old age may also release sexually deviant tendencies previously held in check.

(3) *Old age and neurosis*

Associated with the psychological changes of ageing there is a trend among the elderly towards developing mild states of depression and anxiety. These minor mood disorders are often short-lived and fluctuating, and precipitated by specific events. They seldom come to the attention of the psychiatrist although they may produce intense distress to the individual for brief periods. The proportion of patients with diagnosed neurotic illness however decreases dramatically in old age (Meyer, 1974). This decrease is not strictly a phenomenon of old age, as it starts in middle age. Many of the patients with neurosis seen in late life are those with a previous history of recurrent neurotic episodes or those with chronic neurotic conditions. Nevertheless there are individuals with apparently good previous adjustment who develop neurotic illness for the first time in late life. Situational crises, social and economic difficulties, physical ill health, and personality vulnerability exacerbated by ageing have all been implicated as aetiological factors in these patients.

The decline in neurotic illness presenting in late life suggests that age may have a mitigating effect on these syndromes. This certainly seems to be the case with obsessional and hysterical neuroses. When hysterical conversion symptoms occur in the elderly they tend to do so in the setting of other psychiatric or physical illness. Typical obsessive compulsive symptoms are encountered infrequently in the elderly and when they occur are usually part of an affective disorder in an obsessional personality. The commonest symptom pattern of neurotic illness in the elderly is that of an affective disorder with an admixture of depressive, anxiety, and hypochondriacal symptoms.

1.2.5
Organic factors
WILLIAM ALWYN LISHMAN

Organic influences entering into the aetiology of the neuroses and personality disorders can run a considerable risk of being overlooked. The association is rare in relative terms, other factors being more commonly and obviously related to the genesis of such conditions. Moreover, organic psychiatric disorders usually carry distinctive hallmarks by way of clouding of consciousness or cognitive impairments; when these are lacking one turns less readily to search for brain malfunction. Thus clinical traditions, coupled with the comparative dearth of knowledge concerning cerebral substrates for emotional disorder and personality dysfunction, have conspired to lower vigilance for possible organic contributions in this group of disorders.

Yet both neurotic states and personality disorders can owe much to organic factors – either intrinsic brain disease, or somatic pathologies which serve to compromise brain function. The relationship may be of so direct a nature that the organic influences on the mental state transcend in large measure differences in constitution and background, leading to similar forms of disturbance in widely dissimilar persons. The characteristic changes in personality which follow frontal brain lesions are an obvious example. States of heightened tension seen with thyrotoxicosis are another. Where the link is very close, treatment directed other than at the fundamental cause may be destined to be fruitless.

In other examples we see an interaction, the organic contribution serving to accentuate or liberate preformed tendencies in the individual. The patient who becomes seclusive in the early stages of dementia, or presents with depression while harbouring a cerebral tumour, is likely to be illustrating multifactorial causation. He may be reacting to subjective awareness of cognitive decline, or in Goldstein's (1942) terms reflecting 'the struggle of the changed organism to cope with the defect and to meet the demands of the milieu with which it is no longer equipped to deal'. Such reactions may not always be accompanied by detectable cognitive changes, and may antedate other clear clinical evidence of the organic nexus of the problem.

Brief consideration of some of the known organic provoking factors will serve to illustrate the range and scope of such situations. The possible role of covert brain pathology in relation to certain forms of neurosis and personality disorder will also be discussed.

The primary senile and pre-senile dementias usually declare themselves with failure of memory and intellect. But in the elderly, in particular, there may be a phase in which other symptoms hold the foreground of the picture. Ill-founded anxiety, restlessness, or persistent hypochondriasis may be the presenting features, the cognitive impairments not being obvious until carefully sought out. Thus it is axiomatic to beware of neurotic developments first manifesting themselves in middle or late life, or when decisive provoking life-events cannot easily be discerned.

Personality changes may likewise figure prominently. An accentuation of premorbid traits – suspicion, egocentricity, withdrawal – is common in senile dementia. Where the frontal lobes bear the brunt of the early pathology, as in Pick's disease, lack of social control may be the opening manifestation. In Huntington's chorea premonitory changes in personality – moroseness, apathy and irritability – are well recognized for their import by those who have practical dealings with communities where the disease is rife (Lyon, 1962).

Cerebral tumours may sometimes present with neurotic symptoms or change of disposition. Depression and anxiety are not uncommon. More elaborate developments with obsessional and hysterical features may emerge before focal signs are apparent. Slow-growing tumours in the frontal or temporal lobes may declare themselves by an insidious alteration in the personality. Thus, when the tumour is in neurologically silent parts of the brain the true diagnosis may be considerably delayed.

A special source of error is the readiness with which such symptoms may be ascribed to current stresses in the life situation. Minski (1933) found that 19 of 58 patients with cerebral tumour admitted to a psychiatric hospital had a clear history of problems antedating their admission – accidents, bereavements, or occupational difficulties. Sometimes the patient's attempts to cope with such stresses may have served to unmask his reduced adaptability.

Post-traumatic neuroses are the most frequent of the psychiatric sequelae of head injury. The degree to which brain damage must be held responsible is, however, much debated. In the early post-traumatic phase a host of quasi-neurotic manifestations are often much in evidence – anxiety, depression, and irritability, often coupled with headache and dizziness. Their frequency and their stereotyped nature would alone suggest that at such a stage they owe much to disturbed brain function. However, long-lasting and floridly elaborated post-traumatic neuroses appear to rest principally on other sets of factors such as the premorbid constitution, current stresses, or problems inherent in litigation. The evidence on such issues is discussed in detail by Lishman (1973). We must recognize, of course, that some head-injured patients will fall in the borderland, with both organic and non-organic aetiological factors operating together and reinforcing one another. Clinical appraisal must attempt to apportion such causative influences in the individual case if treatment and prognosis are to be correctly formulated.

The importance of head injury as a cause of personality disorder is well appreciated, even in cases where intellectual competence is unaffected. Frontal lobe damage is again the classical example. Diminished control over aggression may sometimes be traceable to factors such as alcohol abuse, but in other examples disturbed cerebral function may emerge as the only reasonable explanation.

Intracranial infections must be taken into account, especially encephalitic illnesses in childhood. Encephalitis lethargica was influential in its day in focusing attention on the relationship between brain pathology and 'functional' psychiatric disorders. Obsessional symptomatology could be a striking aftermath, with compulsions, rituals, and complex ruminations. Tics and habit spasms could be severe. A seemingly sensitive period could be discerned – when children or young adults were affected,

the personality could be profoundly altered thereafter. Impulsive over-activity and antisocial conduct could amount in severe examples to a callous, amoral psychopathic development. Other forms of encephalitis appear to be more benign in these respects, but nevertheless residual behaviour disorder can still occur in children (Greenbaum & Lurie, 1948). The possible association of herpes simplex infections with depression and personality disorder, and the curious tendency for depressive reactions to ensue on infections such as glandular fever are discussed by Crow (1978). The mechanisms behind such associations remain unclear, though in the case of herpes simplex infections it has been hypothesized that the link may lie in disturbance of brain monoamine synthesis (Lycke *et al.*, 1974).

Epilepsy has been closely studied in relation to personality disorder. Though still disputed, the balance of evidence supports the view that epilepsy arising within the temporal lobes is unusually prone to be associated with personality difficulties, especially aggressive tendencies of an explosive, immature kind (reviewed by Lishman, 1978). Temporal lobectomy, when it relieves the seizures, may greatly ameliorate the problem.

Of considerable interest is the finding that hyposexuality is commoner in temporal lobe epilepsy than epilepsy arising elsewhere (Shukla *et al.*, 1979). Some 15 per cent of Taylor's (1969) series showed various forms of sexual deviation. Rare examples of fetishism have proved reversible when the discharging focus was excised (Mitchell *et al.*, 1954). Thus, the study of epilepsy continues to reveal much about associations with cerebral malfunction where none might otherwise have been suspected.

Metabolic and endocrine disorders show how readily disturbances of the *milieu intérieur* can lead to emotional symptoms. Uraemia, electrolyte disturbances, and liver disorder are quite regularly associated with states of depression and anergia. Attacks of acute intermittent porphyria are commonly accompanied by florid emotional disorder. But the endocrinopathies perhaps illustrate most impressively the relationship between metabolic disturbances and neurotic symptomatology. Anxiety states may accompany thyrotoxicosis, and lethargic depression may accompany myxoedema. Depression can be severe in Cushing's syndrome and date from early in the illness. In both hypo- and hyperparathyroidism affective disorder can be the presenting feature, the serum calcium level clearly having a decisive influence on mood. With such relatively rare conditions the true diagnosis may be much delayed. Petersen (1968) indeed suggests that hyperparathyroidism should always be considered 'when lack of initiative, depression and thirst appear during a prolonged, insidiously developing and diagnostically unclear change of personality'.

Of toxic disorders alcoholism is the best known in relation to change of personality. It is possible that this may depend on minor degrees of brain damage more often than is commonly supposed (Ron, 1977). A relationship between chronic cannabis intoxication and personality alteration (Kolansky & Moore, 1971, 1972) is a great deal more controversial. Other agents must sometimes be considered when occupational exposure is a risk – lead, mercury, manganese, and carbon disulphide, for example, can lead to distinctive forms of neurotic and behavioural disorder.

Malnutrition may be encountered as a cause of neurotic symptoms, especially among the elderly. Lack of the B vitamins is clearly incriminated as the principal cause. Thus experimental studies have shown that thiamine deficiency can lead over several weeks to depression, weakness, and insomnia, later to forgetfulness and impaired concentration. Less severe but more prolonged deprivation produces emotional instability, moodiness, and depression (Brozek & Caster, 1957). Pellagra, consequent on nicotinic acid deficiency, often shows a long prodromal period of neurotic manifestations which can promptly respond to replacement therapy (Spies *et al.*, 1938). Folic acid deficiency may be related to depression, and at least in epileptics to lethargy, irritability, and personality difficulties (Reynolds, 1967; Reynolds *et al.*, 1970; Snaith *et al.*, 1970). The general undernutrition of anorexia nervosa may contribute to symptoms of depression, irritability, and insomnia which often improve after treatment, resulting in weight gain (see chap. 8.3, pp. 287, 293).

The role of covert brain damage

In addition to the foregoing, where disease processes or deficiencies are ultimately identifiable, it seems likely that a proportion of neurotic and personality-disordered patients may harbour some degree of covert brain pathology. This may have dated from early in life, perhaps from birth injury, but in many cases the cause will be unknown.

Thus, cerebral atrophy has occasionally been revealed by air encephalography in patients with chronically disabling affective and neurotic illnesses (Haug, 1962; Eitinger, 1959). This must raise the possibility that sometimes covert brain pathology has altered the patient's reaction to life stresses and facilitated the development of the neurosis. Hysterical conversion symptoms may also be facilitated by brain damage. Whitlock (1967) found evidence of preceding or coexisting brain disorder much more commonly in such patients than in controls with other forms of neurotic illness.

With regard to personality disorder the principal evidence comes from electroencephalography. A high proportion of patients with disturbed personality are known to have abnormal EEGs, especially those with aggressive antisocial behaviour (Hill & Watterson, 1942). The EEG changes involve the temporal lobes particularly, and are usually of a type reflecting cerebral immaturity or previous cerebral insults. A striking incidence of changes has emerged in persons convicted of murder, increasing in proportion to the senselessness of the crime (Stafford-Clark & Taylor, 1949). Williams's (1969) more recent study has reinforced such findings. Two-thirds of a group of habitually aggressive offenders were found to show abnormal EEGs, compared with only a quarter of persons who had been convicted for an isolated act of aggression. When persons with clinically obvious brain damage were excluded the figures were 57 per cent and 12 per cent respectively. The concept of 'episodic discontrol' described by Mark and Ervin (1970) likewise suggests that some seriously aggressive persons are victims of their disturbed cerebral physiology. A complex interaction can then readily be envisaged between such brain dysfunction and the social disorganisation which it engenders. An important task for the future will be to refine understanding of such dysfunction further, to see how widely it applies, and what may be its origins.

Non-organic aetiological factors in the ill and physically disabled

Finally it may be apposite to stress again that a large amount of neurotic disability among the physically ill may be determined by factors which have little or nothing to do directly with pathophysiological disturbance. Psychological factors will very often need to be taken into account. Physical illness of long duration or with frequent relapses may undermine the patient's confidence; pain readily impairs morale; and physical handicaps, limitations, and disfigurements may have seriously adverse consequences at a purely psychological level. It will not infrequently emerge that such matters as threats to independence, earning capacity, or family life are the important or even the sole determinants of the neurotic responses encountered in the course of physical illness (see chap. 8.1, pp. 276–80.)

(The reader is also referred to volume 2, chapters 1–15.)

1.3
Aetiological factors of special relevance to childhood disorders

1.3.1
Determinants of emotional and conduct disorders in childhood

SULA WOLFF

Introduction: general considerations

Emotional and conduct disorders are the most frequently encountered psychiatric disturbances of childhood and, despite important constitutional, social and medical disadvantages which often contribute to their genesis, the disorders themselves are most helpfully explained on the basis of psychological mechanisms.

Levels of explanation

Causal explanations derive from the scientific study of groups of subjects or phenomena and are the basis for predictions within statistical limits. They provide certainty when groups of children or conditions are under consideration, as in the planning of services, but not when an individual child is the subject of concern. For example, we now know that between four and eight per cent of children in middle childhood have clinically significant conduct disorders, but that among children with serious educational retardation fully one-third are affected.

Advances in knowledge of the causes of emotional and conduct disorders in childhood, derived from epidemiological and clinical studies in the last forty years, help the clinician both in his enquiry and management of the individual case. When faced with a conduct-disordered boy he will always ask about the child's school performance and adjustment. When consulted by a social services department about alternative care arrangements he will give priority to considerations of substitute family care rather than to a children's home because he knows about the potential disadvantages of group care for young children. Clinical interventions are however always taken within a unique set of circumstances and the subjective worlds of child and family are also salient.

For helpful therapeutic interactions with children and families we need a different level of aetiological explanation: the *subjective*. Here, as Toulmin (1970) has made clear, we are in the realm of reason rather than causes, of retrospective explanations for current experiences, and of justification for conduct and intent. If psychiatrists want to be personally helpful to patients they must be as knowledgeable about the subjective explanatory connections patients make between their life experiences, as they are about the scientific causes of psychiatric disorders. The validation of a patient's view of his life and of his retrospective subjective explanations for his predicament, and the knowledge that his behaviour and emotional reactions are understandable consequences of his experiences, improve his self-esteem whatever his age, lower anxiety and contribute to symptom resolution.

Knowledge about cognitive development in childhood (Piaget, 1926, 1929, 1932; Donaldson, 1978; Bower, 1979; Boden, 1979), although based on the study of normal children, has helped us understand that children under the age of seven, when animistic, pre-causal logic is common, tend to interpret adverse life-events differently from older children. This enables the clinician to understand how an individual child is likely to reason things out and on what subjective explanations he bases his fears, his hopes, and his intentions. Adverse events often engender a sense of personal responsibility and hence of more anxiety than in later life.

Other general aspects of subjective experience relate to the child's emotional attachments to other people, to sources of anxiety and how children tend to cope psychologically with excessive anxiety. For example, we now know that when young children lose the people to whom they have formed their primary attachments, depression and anger follow (Bowlby, 1975). Moreover, in childhood, psychological defence mechanisms are much more open to inspection than in adult life. Children often know when they put anxiety-inducing thoughts out of their minds and when other thoughts or activities (such as stealing) take their place, and some children actually tell the clinician about these inner manoeuvres.

Guesses about such defences, in the form of interpretations, are often rewarded by a reduction in anxiety and symptomatic improvement (see chapter 5).

What constitutes a disorder in childhood?
(1) *Normal differences of behaviour*
Items and traits of behaviour characterizing emotional and conduct disorders: fears, anxiety, depression of mood, shyness, with perhaps associated sleeping and appetite disturbances on the one hand and temper tantrums, fighting, disobedience, destructiveness, stealing, lying, truanting, and wandering on the other, may merely reflect particular styles of childhood behaviour that, considering the child's age, sex, and social context are acceptable, congruent with adult expectations, and not at all associated with personal disadvantage for the child. At once it is clear that the frequency and magnitude of each symptom are important and that some symptoms, for example, fears, anxieties, and shyness, are much more likely to be part of an expected behavioural repertoire than, for example, stealing and wandering from home. Age, sex, temperament and culture contribute to individual differences in the behaviour of normal children, but they also predispose disadvantaged children or children under stress towards one or other type of behaviour disorders.

(2) *Childhood behaviour disorders in the community and in clinic populations*
The epidemiological surveys on the Isle of Wight in the 1960s by Rutter, Tizard and Whitmore (1970) have been a landmark.

Children in the community with emotional and conduct disorders were identified using a clinical definition in terms of the presence of 'abnormality of behaviour, emotions or relationships which was continuing up to the time of assessment and was sufficiently marked and sufficiently prolonged to cause handicap to the child himself and/or distress or disturbance in the family or community'. The term handicap was used in the sense of 'any disability which impedes the child in some way in his daily life' (p. 148).

Many causal relationships were identified in this study between social, educational, family and health factors on the one hand and child psychiatric disorders on the other. Of the psychiatrically disturbed children identified in this survey (6.8 per cent of the general child population aged 10 and 11 years) only one in ten had come forward for psychiatric care.

Disturbed children attending a psychiatric clinic differ in a number of ways from similarly disturbed children in the community. In particular, disturbed children attending a clinic have more anxious and more disturbed mothers (Shepherd, *et al.,* 1966).

It has been said that whether a child appears at a child psychiatric clinic or not may depend more on the sensitivity and level of tolerance of his parents, his teachers, and the wider community than on the child's behaviour. Nevertheless, a comparative study of children referred to a child psychiatry department and a matched control group of children attending the same primary school classes, showed highly significant differences between the two groups, both in behaviour and in a number of background factors relating to health and family life (Wolff, 1967; Wolff & Acton, 1968).

It is possible that the causes of emotional and conduct disorders in the community differ from those to be identified in referred children. The differences are, however, likely to be numerical rather than qualitative, and indeed the results of aetiological studies of clinic attenders (Rutter, 1966; Wolff & Acton, 1968) are not at variance with the results of epidemiological surveys.

(3) *Emotional and conduct disorders as part of an interactional process*

While for the purposes of this review the results of epidemiological and of clinical studies will be pooled, it is important to be clear that in children, even more than in adults, pathological behaviour is the outcome of an interactional process.

When a seven-year old, granny-reared from the age of four, joins her father and a new stepmother, is on her best behaviour, eager for affection from her 'new mummy', but starts to steal small amounts of money from her purse, the stepmother, if unsure of her own abilities as a parent and of her new husband's approval, may interpret the conduct disorder as a deliberate attack upon herself and as indicating that her new daughter really resembles her husband's feckless first wife who deserted the family some three years earlier. The stepmother may become hostile and punitive, increasing the child's fears of a further rejection, reinforcing her need to repress even normal displays of oppositional behaviour and increasing even more the child's cravings for affection. In such circumstances the stealing is likely to persist as an avenue for the expression both of cravings and hostile impulses through behaviour she

herself dislikes and which is beyond her control. A mutually reinforcing pattern of interaction between child and stepmother continues.

Children become legitimate patients not primarily because their behaviour lies outside the range of statistical normality for their sex and age, but when for whatever reason it arouses concern or distress in their care-givers or in themselves.

Diagnostic grouping of emotional and conduct disorders in relation to aetiology

The British epidemiological studies (Rutter *et al.,* 1970; Rutter *et al.,* 1975) have shown that, although many disturbed children have a mixed symptomatology of emotional *and* conduct disorders, children with significant conduct disorders differ in many ways from those without. The differences relate to causal and associated factors as well as to outcome. For example, children with conduct and with mixed disorders differ from emotionally disordered children in being more often boys, having very high rates of educational retardation, coming very often from manual working-class families, and coming much more often from families where there is open marital discord.

In clinical practice when one is concerned not only with causes and prognosis, but with aetiology in the wider sense of including individual psychopathology and subjective experience, the above diagnostic dichotomy is less helpful. It now matters a great deal whether manifest symptoms of anxiety or depression accompany aggressive and delinquent behaviour. From the point of view of clinical management the approach to a depressed and solitary twelve-year-old truant whose mother died three months before, will be different from that to a cheery boy who habitually truants in company, is failing educationally and greatly dislikes school.

While some more specific syndromes within the two broad categories of behaviour disorders have been elucidated, for example, school refusal (Hersov, 1976) and types of stealing (Rich, 1956), the field is still wide open both for further exploration of the causes of individual syndromes and of their psychopathology.

The determinants of behaviour are multiple

When children are referred to a child psychiatric clinic the chances are that multiple adverse factors are at play.

(1) *Developmental and intrapsychic considerations: how adverse life circumstances and constitutional handicaps are translated into symptoms*

It is useful to consider two basic processes: privation and excessive anxiety as mediating between adversity or handicap on the one hand and the genesis of emotional and conduct disorders on the other.

(i) *Privation.* Inadequate opportunities for selective human attachments between the ages of six months and three years predispose children to psychiatric disorder, poor language development, and educational failure. Privation of social and especially language stimulation, as happens in children from large and/or economically deprived families and in many children reared in institutions, has its major effect during the pre-school years, contributing to educational failure and secondary behaviour difficulties. Absence of adequate parental role models begins to be harmful from about 3 years of age.

Theoretically these privations can be remedied. But in practice this requires quite exceptional efforts because deprived children become difficult and do not evoke spontaneous positive care.

(ii) *Excessive anxiety.* Because up to the age of 7 or 8 years their reasoning is pre-logical, children are exceptionally prone to anxiety.

In the first two years of total dependency on parents, *parent loss* engenders depression, anxiety, and anger. From 2 years onward, threats of loss, abandonment, or withdrawal of affection, become meaningful and lead to *separation anxiety, shame,* and anger. From about 3 years children can experience *fear of injury*, often with frightening fantasies of being attacked or damaging others. Domestic and street violence, illness and accidents now arouse overwhelming anxieties, expressed as emotional symptoms or risk-taking behaviour, dangerous and aggressive, as if repeatedly to test out the limits of safety. *Guilt* arises at this stage, and is often irrationally harsh because the egocentric child sees himself as the cause of disasters.

At around 5 or 6 years children enter the wider social group. *Stigma* can now be perceived, and *loss of self-esteem* may become an added source of anxiety. Children become aware of handicaps, physical, intellectual, or social, and both guilt and *the anxiety that springs from loss of self-esteem* mediate between the causes of child psychiatric disorder (such as edu-

cational failure, abnormal family composition, living in a children's home, having an alcoholic father) and their symptomatic expression.

A knowledge of psychological defence mechanisms (A. Freud, 1946) is essential to understand how the individual child transforms excessive anxiety into symptoms.

The effect on later development of stressful life events interacting with predisposing or protective factors, and especially the sensitizing effects of adverse events in early childhood have recently been discussed in detail (Rutter, 1981).

(2) *Age, sex, temperament and culture*

(i) *Age.* Developmental disorders, for example of elimination, of language, and of motor skills, are by definition age-related (see p. 41). But other aspects of behaviour also have developmental components. Poor impulse control, characteristic of the first three years, is evident once children are on their feet, and boundless motor energy develops in early childhood. Fears, phobias, nightmares, and night terrors are at their height during the third, fourth and fifth years of life (McFarlane *et al.*, 1954) when there is a growth spurt in children's symbolic functions, as expressed in play, language, and artistic skills. Lability of mood characterizes adolescence, when symptoms of depression, misery, and unhappiness are common (Rutter *et al.*, 1976).

(ii) *Sex.* Among disturbed and non-disturbed children, boys are always found to be more active and overtly aggressive while girls are more often withdrawn and fearful. Hutt (1972) found nursery-school boys not only to be more aggressive but to elicit more aggression from other children than were girls. While some of the sex differences even at this early age are likely to reflect sex-role modelling and cultural differences in social expectations of boys and girls, there is evidence that muscularity and activity-level distinguish between the sexes from early infancy and that activity level itself fosters aggressive behaviour in groups of young children. Boys are constitutionally more predisposed to the development of aggressive behaviours than girls.

(iii) *Temperament.* The New York longitudinal study of children's behavioural styles (Thomas *et al.*, 1968) showed not only that there are individual differences of reactivity present in infancy and relatively stable during early childhood, but that these contribute to parents' reactions and in turn to the child's life adjustment. Some children are temperamentally predisposed to psychiatric disorders. (See also Porter & Collins, 1982.)

(iv) *Culture.* It has generally been assumed that cultural differences of personality reflect the effectiveness whereby parents bring up children in their own image. Freedman (1975) however has speculated that acculturation may not act on 'a universal infant' but that the gene pool of a nation contributes.

Social class differences in child rearing (John & Elizabeth Newson, 1976) help to explain the more aggressive and dependent behaviour of unskilled working-class children, especially boys, who then elicit more criticism at school. Such subcultural factors are not in themselves pathological, but lower the threshold for the effect of other adversities in socio-economically deprived children, especially boys.

Children of immigrant families, especially West Indians and especially girls, are found to have more conduct disorders than white English children. Rutter (1976a) has stressed the lack of early stimulation at home in West Indian children, their educational retardation, their frequent attendance at schools with high pupil turnover, their large family size, frequent family disruption, and reception into care.

(3) *Constitutional impairments of aetiological importance*

The matrix of causes for child psychiatric disorders includes those constitutional impairments which limit a child's development or constrict his adaptive capacities so that he is more likely to develop significant emotional or conduct disorders.

The early EEG studies of aggressive sociopaths (Hill & Watterson, 1942) are congruent with the view that obstetric or very early cerebral trauma is related to psychopathic behaviour in adult life, and the possibility exists that the constitutional factors of aetiological importance for child psychiatric disorders also contribute to pathological aspects of adult personality (see also Quitkin & Klein, 1969).

(i) *Low intelligence.* The aetiological contribution of intellectual retardation to psychiatric morbidity in children was greatly clarified by the Isle of Wight study (Rutter *et al.*, 1970) where full attention was paid to the complex nexus of other disadvantages: educational retardation, socio-cultural deprivation, and physical handicap (especially cerebral palsy) with which low intelligence is often also associated.

Intellectually retarded children were over three times as likely to be psychiatrically disturbed as children in the control group (23.6 per cent, compared with 6.8 per cent), with an excess both of emotional and conduct disorders.

(ii) *Developmental disorders and cerebral dysfunction.* Many children have behaviour disorders and learning difficulties best accounted for on the basis of specific maturational delays. These disorders, which include specific developmental delays of language and language-related educational skills, of mathematical skills, of motor co-ordination, and sphincter control, are discussed elsewhere (see vol. 3). Here we shall summarize the characteristics they share, to clarify how they contribute to the aetiology of emotional and conduct disorders.

They occur in children of all levels of intelligence but are more obvious clinically when the child is clearly of average or superior general abilities but has failed to begin to speak at the normal time, is still speaking indistinctly and clumsily by the time he starts school, or has not mastered early reading and writing skills although a sophisticated thinker and socially competent for his age. Although language is usually fluent by the time he enters school and the child eventually reads well, spelling difficulties sometimes persist into adult life.

Enuresis and encopresis too are often familial and frequently associated with other developmental disorders. Evidence of neurological dysfunction is associated more often with enuresis and encopresis than with other behaviour disorders. But in by no means all enuretic or encopretic children is there clinical evidence for a maturational cause for the symptom. All developmental disorders occur more often in boys than girls, and Rutter and colleagues (1970) argue for a sex-linked predisposition.

There is much overlap between developmental disorders and manifestations of cerebral dysfunction. In the individual case one can often not be sure whether one is dealing with a child with an intact nervous system who is predisposed to maturational delays or whether the child sustained some cerebral trauma *in utero*, at birth, or in early infancy.

Rutter (1977) and Sandberg, Rutter, and Taylor (1978) have rightly argued that, while conduct disorder is often associated with restlessness, over-activity, and poor concentration, there is no evidence that most over-active and distractable children have any organic brain impairment. But (Sandberg *et al.*, 1978; Schachar, Rutter & Smith, 1981) there is a small group of pervasively hyperactive children who as a group have a lower IQ, and are more often educationally retarded. Children diagnosed as hyperkinetic by clinicians also have greater deviance on neurological examination, a higher incidence of perinatal complications, and more impulsivity, over-activity, and inattention than other disturbed children. At times they too develop conduct disorder presumably, as in children with developmental delays, in response to their educational and social failures.

(4) *School failure*

Educational failure is a major cause of conduct disorder in boys. Rutter and colleagues (1970) showed that of severely retarded readers (of whom over three-quarters were boys) one-third had conduct disorders, and that of conduct-disordered children (of whom 80 per cent were boys) one-third were severely retarded readers. The findings were amply confirmed in a deprived inner London Borough (Rutter *et al.*, 1975). Retarded readers tended to come from large families with a family history of educational difficulties. Some schools have consistently high rates of educational failure and conduct disorder, whereas others serving similar neighbourhoods have low rates. In an important study of secondary schools, Rutter, Maughan, Mortimer, and Ousten (1979) showed that the quality of school life itself can foster or, on the contrary, safeguard children from these disorders.

(5) *Physical illness and handicap*

Children with recurrent or chronic physical illness or handicap not affecting the brain (of which asthma is the commonest) have nearly twice as much psychiatric, emotional, and conduct disorder as healthy children (Rutter *et al.*, 1970). Primary school children with reactive disorders attending a psychiatric clinic had many more accidents, hospital admissions, and minor physical disabilities than a matched control group of their school fellows (Wolff, 1981, p. 73).

The privations and stresses imposed by physical illness vary with the child's stage of cognitive and emotional development, with the severity and emotional and social significance of the illness or handicap, with the treatment procedures including

hospitalization needed, and with the parents' reactions (see also Wolff, 1981, pp. 63–85).

(6) *Family disorganization*

(i) *Parental illness, psychiatric disorder, and marital strife*. Although the association between family disorganization and child psychiatric disorders has been known for a long time, the precise features of family life involved, the size of their aetiological contribution, and the mechanisms by which they exert their effect have been greatly clarified during the past fifteen years. Rutter (1966) demonstrated that disturbed children attending a psychiatric clinic were twice as likely to have a parent with chronic or recurrent physical illness or handicap as non-disturbed children attending a hospital or dental surgery. Wolff and Acton (1968) showed that it was sickness of the mother rather than the father that distinguished disturbed primary-school children from controls. Rutter (1966) also found that psychiatric treatment of a parent was three times as common in disturbed as in non-disturbed children (occurring in one-fifth of the disturbed children), and that children are particularly at risk when both parents are psychiatrically ill, when the symptoms of the psychiatric illness involve the child, and, much the most common occurrence, when there is parental personality disorder.

It has been a striking finding (Rutter *et al.*, 1977) that marital discord is predominantly associated with conduct disorders in sons. It is likely that this is because during marital strife the father is generally the more conspicuous aggressor (see pp. 411).

(ii) *Bereavement, illegitimacy and family disruption.* Bereaved children have an excess of conduct and emotional disorders often related to the antecedents and consequences of the death. Only at adolescence is their disturbance related in time to the traumatic event itself (Rutter, 1966).

The parents of a nine-year old adopted boy, *David*, complained of his temper tantrums, aggressive behaviour to other children and 'insensitivity' towards his mother, treated for breast cancer since before the adoption. She was still assailed by doubt whether she should have adopted David at all and, perhaps because her guilt towards him was overwhelming, she found herself hostile and critical instead, firmly believing that his behaviour had caused her recurrent relapses and downhill course. Her own father died of tetanus after a minor accident when she was 10 and she remembered thinking 'thank goodness it's not my mother' (an idea likely to have concealed a contrary feeling, since her mother was a vigorous, competent woman whom she felt she could never emulate).

The father, fully conscious of his own childhood domination by his mother, could understand David's difficulties in terms of insecurity (the boy often stayed with relatives when his mother was in hospital), was extremely supportive of his wife, whose religious faith he had adopted, and stoical about his many household commitments and his own lonely future. At that stage neither parent wanted David seen by a psychiatrist.

After the mother's death when David was 10 the relationship between him and his father deteriorated, in part because the father, now depressed, temporarily lost his authority with his son. David was made anxious by his father's helplessness and began to taunt him, once locking him out of the house. The focus of their troubles was David's aggression at school, his academic failure, and the father's demands for greater effort and achievement. Now that David himself was seen, it became clear that his struggle to cope with only average intelligence in an academic private school contributed to his poor self-esteem, his loneliness, and his high level of anxiety. A brief psychiatric admission for David with psychotherapy for father and son focused on the mother's death, followed by support to the father in finding a small boarding school for the boy led to symptom resolution and improved social relationships.

Other causes of parent loss: illegitimacy, divorce, and separation, are related to one or both parents' poor capacities for rewarding heterosexual attachments and often to more widespread difficulties in intimate relationships. Children from such unions are at risk of developing conduct and emotional disorders because of a variety of interrelated adversities, and again boys are more vulnerable than girls.

Mothers are more often the remaining parent and, if they have parted from an aggressive husband, they often have negative expectations of their sons. All children are biologically programmed to be attached to their parents. When small children have to think badly of an absent parent, who manifestly failed to provide affectionate care for the family, they often become very anxious. Access arrangements between divorced parents in continuing strife can increase a young child's conflicting loyalties and result in overwhelming anxiety.

Moreover, all types of family disruption carry the risk of multiple disrupted primary relationships for the child, since single parents, especially fathers, are dependent on other people (grandparents, other relatives, foster parents, and children's homes) to augment the care they themselves provide.

It is sometimes argued (Rutter, 1976b) that disrupted attachments and their emotional accompaniments are of little aetiological importance and that childhood disturbance can be accounted for entirely by family disharmony and other disadvantages surrounding children from broken homes. In clinical practice, however, of overriding subjective importance for the children themselves is the loss of people to whom they are attached and a lack of trust in their subsequent relationships. Children cared for by grandmothers (or by foster mothers) during their first three or four years often have great difficulty when returning to their natural parents or perhaps a new stepparent. This is especially so when the parents and grandmother are in conflict. Child psychiatrists see many emotionally disordered and conduct-disordered children whose relationship with their current parent figures are interfered with by such disrupted bonds.

(iii) *Substitute care and adoption*. Children in institutional care have very high rates of psychiatric disorder and, like foster children, are over-represented among psychiatric clinic attenders. Children's family experiences prior to their reception into care are thought to contribute to this (Wolkind & Rutter, 1973) but it is likely that there are other important adverse influences, including the child's ongoing disturbed relationships with his family, the many changes of care givers in children's homes, the frequent breakdown of foster placements and the stigma and lack of security which all children in children's homes or foster care suffer.

Adoption is generally accepted as the best alternative for illegitimate children and children who for other reasons require long-term substitute care (Tizard, 1977). The National Child Development Study (Seglow *et al.*, 1972) has shown that the outcome in terms of educational progress and adjustment of illegitimate children who remained with their mothers was worse than that of legitimate children and of children who were adopted. Long-term studies show that adopted children do well in middle childhood with only a slight excess of behaviour disorders, mainly at school and probably due to the fact that adoptive parents tend to be middle class and with superior intelligence, while their children, of average ability, do not match up to their parents' and hence their own educational aspirations. The good adjustment of adoptive children often breaks down at adolescence (Lambert & Streather, 1980). The results of prospective longitudinal studies usually relate to circumstances that no longer pertain and the outcome of adoption in later childhood, now so popular, is as yet unknown.

1.3.2
Problems of predicting disturbances in adulthood from behaviour disorders in childhood

PHILIP GRAHAM

Although early Freudian theory dating from the nineteenth century laid emphasis on events occurring in childhood in the aetiology of adult disorders, the scientific study of continuities and discontinuities between events and disorders in childhood and adulthood has only flourished in the last twenty-five years. Interest in long-term prospective and retrospective studies has grown because of the light it casts both on the aetiology of adult disorders (thus making rational prevention at least a theoretical possibility) and on the natural history of disorders in childhood, thus establishing a long-term prognosis for these disorders and providing a standard against which the effectiveness of intervention can be measured.

Research into the life history of individuals presents special problems both in the collection of data and in their interpretation. It might seem that, to collect information on the origins of adult disorder, the most satisfactory method would be to question affected adults and their relatives about their childhood experiences. The value of such retrospective studies is, however, limited by the distortion to which recollections are subject. A body of work suggests that such distortion affects some memories more than others and that it produces systematic rather than random bias. Thus, anecdotal information suggests that neurotic individuals tend to remember the home atmosphere in which they grew up as more subject to tension than their non-neurotic sibs who, in fact, were subjected to the same domestic influences (Ryle,

1967). Studies comparing later parental accounts with information collected at the time when events actually occurred show that parents are often inaccurate in remembering the dates at which their children acquire the skills of walking and talking (Robbins, 1963). Again, distortion is systematically biased – if a child walked or talked rather early or rather late the parent will recollect more average performance than the child actually showed. However, gross deviations in skill acquisition are likely to be more accurately recalled. More generally, major events are recalled with greater accuracy so that the death of a parent in childhood will be recalled more certainly than parental marital breakdown, and both of these will be remembered more successfully than the details of brief parental separations. Just as pleasant experiences are recalled more easily than unpleasant (Lishman, 1974), so shameful experiences involving, for example, earlier criminal activity are likely to be repressed or the respondent may recollect them very well but choose not to report them. It should also not be forgotten that interviewer bias may affect the way an informant recollects information.

The degree of distortion can be reduced by skilful interviewing. For example, by encouraging an informant to link remembered events with dates that can be established by checking with contemporaneous documentation, it is possible to obtain greater accuracy in the timing of the events. By insisting on obtaining actual examples of events, one can reduce the risk that the informant has a set attitude towards a period of his life which is systematically affecting his recall. However, even with the best available techniques, retrospectively gathered information is of dubious value, and studies that place reliance on information gained entirely in this way must be interpreted with caution.

One technique which employs the retrospective method but reduces the risk of distortion, involves the study of information recorded contemporaneously on individuals identified retrospectively. Thus, Watt (1978) has studied school records of adult schizophrenic patients and has compared remarks made about the personalities of such patients by their teachers with remarks made about control children matched for sex and certain social characteristics. Such studies are limited by the fact that the early data are often recorded rather unsystematically and it is therefore difficult to know whether satisfactory control of social and other factors has indeed been achieved. Nevertheless they have provided valuable information on which more reliance can be placed than on studies relying entirely on long-term recall. They do, however, have an important limitation which lies in the weakness of their predictive power. For example, hypothetically, a retrospective study might reveal that criminal men in their childhood have been separated from their mothers four times more commonly than a control group but if only one out of ten children experiencing this type of separation actually turns out to be criminal in adult life, the fourfold figure is misleading. For information leading to effective prediction it is therefore necessary to turn to prospective studies.

In these studies data can be systematically recorded at the outset on groups of children who can then be followed up later in life. Such studies are highly relevant for predictive purposes. They can be broadly divided into

(1) Studies of children in the general population in which personality and social factors in childhood have been correlated with personality in adolescence and adulthood (Kagan & Moss, 1962). Sometimes measures of outcome include the presence or absence of psychiatric disorders (for example, Thomas & Chess, 1977).

(2) Studies in which disturbed children in the general population have been examined a few years later to determine patterns of deviance (Graham & Rutter, 1973; Gersten *et al.*, 1976).

(3) Follow-up studies of children attending psychiatric facilities. Follow-up may be virtually complete (Robins, 1966) or may be restricted to those people attending a psychiatric facility as adults (for example, Mellsop, 1972; Pritchard & Graham, 1966).

(4) Studies in which children suffering from a particular condition are followed up into adolescence and adulthood.

Before considering such studies in somewhat more detail, some attention should be given to methodological problems involved in carrying them out and to difficulties in interpretation which often arise.

Data are often not recorded on initial attendance as systematically as one would wish. The aims of the follow-up investigators are likely to be unknown to the person making decisions on which data are recorded initially, so that many areas that seem important to the follow-up investigator may not have been recorded at all. For firm conclusions to be drawn success of follow-up must be virtually complete. This is often difficult to achieve because the mobility of the population is high and that of disturbed people in the population even higher. Tracing procedures are increasingly hampered by concerns regarding confidentiality. Such concerns are highly appropriate, but sometimes appear to be overstressed if professional investigators are able to demonstrate the anonymity of their records and the thoroughness of precautions they take to maintain confidentiality.

The interpretation of findings of studies examining child–adult continuity also presents special problems (Graham, 1977). Thus, the same underlying condition may present with different manifestations at different stages. For example, children with epilepsy or autism who are hyperkinetic in early childhood may be hypokinetic in adolescence. This pattern of continuity has come to be known as 'heterotypic' and a pattern showing the same manifestation of behaviour in different life phases as 'homotypic'. Secondly, there are problems in disentangling the continuity of a particular disorder from the continuity of social stresses producing that disorder. A child with a conduct disorder may turn out to be an adult with a particular type of personality. This may reflect either the continuity of the disorder or the different effects of the same social stress acting first upon a child and later upon an adult. Thirdly, the finding of a degree of continuity of a particular disorder in one social setting should not be readily generalized to a different social setting. A child with a learning problem may have a much better prognosis in a society where the demand for unskilled labour is high than in another setting where literacy is a requirement for most forms of employment. Finally, a level of continuity from childhood may be misleading in terms of the contribution of earlier problems to the spectrum of disorders later on. Most disturbed pre-school children may develop problems in mid-childhood, for example, yet most children with disorders of mid-childhood may not have shown any serious behaviour problems before they went to school.

Continuity of temperament and personality

Results of longitudinal studies mainly embarked upon in the 1930s with subsequent follow-up twenty or thirty years later have been summarized by Kohlberg and co-workers (1972). In general, they show weak continuity of personality traits from childhood into adulthood. Those involved in the studies did not have the development of adult psychopathology as a primary interest so that it is not possible to draw conclusions from them about personality traits in childhood predisposing to adult psychiatric illness.

A more recent study with perhaps greater relevance to psychiatry is that recently summarized by Thomas and Chess (1977). In this study, the mothers of 141 children from mainly middle-class homes in New York were interviewed regarding their child's everyday behaviour from two to three months onwards. The descriptions provided by the parents were rated on nine different categories (activity level, rhythmicity, approach withdrawal, adaptability, threshold of responsiveness, intensity of reaction, quality of mood, distractability, and attention span and persistence). Subsequently, it was shown that children who developed behaviour problems later on had demonstrated characteristic temperamental patterns earlier in their lives. Children with 'active' symptoms had been 'difficult' babies – highly active and irregular in their habits, whereas children with 'passive' symptoms had in their fourth and fifth years shown low activity, withdrawal responses, and poor persistence. Subsequently, Thomas and Chess have followed their children up into adolescence and have found continuity of temperament especially for activity levels and adaptability. So far no clear-cut patterns have emerged predicting adolescent disturbance from earlier temperamental attributes. However, a review of studies of temperamental characteristics in infancy, hyperkinesis, and conduct disorders in school-age children and sociopathy in adolescence and adulthood suggests that a significant level of continuity between these various conditions exists (Graham, 1970). Difficult babies and young children are prone to develop conduct disorders especially if they meet with negative parental attitudes (Graham *et al.*, 1973). Other studies now to be discussed suggest that conduct disorder is a frequent precursor of adult aggressive personality disorder.

In her thirty-year follow-up study of children referred to a child guidance clinic in St Louis in the 1930s, Robins (1966) found that children who at that time showed conduct disorders were disadvantaged in later life in a variety of ways. They were especially likely to develop 'sociopathic personality' defined as 'gross repetitive failure to conform to societal norms in many areas of life, in the absence of thought disturbance suggesting psychosis' and this was reflected in higher rates of criminal activity, marital breakdown, and occupational failure when comparisons were made with a control group of people who had, as children, attended the same schools. Children with

conduct disorders are also more likely to develop a range of psychiatric problems later in life including schizophrenia, hysterical disorders, and alcoholism. Summarizing her work on this and other cohorts more recently, Robins (1978) proposes that a number of reasonably firm conclusions can be drawn regarding the best predictors from conduct disorder in childhood. It appears that all types of antisocial disorder predict anti-social disorder, but that the greater the variety of antisocial behaviour shown by a child the more likely he is to develop antisocial problems in adulthood. However, most anti-social children do not become antisocial adults.

Nevertheless, virtually all anti-social adults are found to have a history of anti-social behaviour in childhood. In predicting which anti-social children do become antisocial, characteristics of the child's behaviour – the range and seriousness of his misdemeanours – are the best predictors, whereas family background, socio-economic status and type of child rearing are of little predictive value.

These conclusions are substantially supported by studies by other workers. Thus, Mellsop (1972), studying people who had, as children, attended a department of child psychiatry, found that those with symptoms of conduct or personality disorders, fared worse in later life than those attending with other conditions. Overall, about 12 per cent of people who had attended the child psychiatric service were in touch with adult mental health services later in life, compared with an expected rate of 3 per cent – 4 per cent. Social factors, such as socio-economic status, and the child coming from a broken home, did not distinguish cases from controls. However, the presence in childhood of a disease or disorder of the central nervous system worsened prognosis as did the existence of a learning problem in the child. Similarly, in shorter-term studies (Gersten *et al.*, 1976; Graham & Rutter, 1973), conduct disorders have been found to have a poorer prognosis than neurotic problems. Roff (1974) compared 150 people who had attended a child guidance clinic with three different outcomes in adulthood – 'normal', 'bad conduct', and 'neurotic'. People whose adult outcome involved antisocial activity had more neglectful and rejecting parents and had been more exposed to physical violence. However, these are factors likely to be associated with the development of antisocial behaviour, and it is unclear whether the presence of these factors improved prediction once the type of disorder shown by the child had been taken into account. In previous work, Roff (1972) had demonstrated that low popularity with other children was negatively correlated with delinquency outcome, particularly in children from socially advantaged backgrounds. Low peer acceptance appears less important in children from less privileged backgrounds in whom a range of other factors may be significant.

Recent work (Sandberg *et al.*, 1978) has suggested that the delineation of a hyperkinetic syndrome distinct from conduct disorder presents many difficulties and it is therefore not surprising that the follow-up findings on children with this syndrome are similar to those in conduct-disordered children. Indeed, as suggested earlier, a number of children diagnosed as showing the hyperkinetic syndrome in early childhood are identified with conduct disorders in school and later develop evidence of sociopathic personality (Mendelson *et al.*, 1971; Minde *et al.*, 1972). Nevertheless, it is of interest that children with severe over-activity in mid-childhood do appear to have such a poor outlook, and this suggests, though firm evidence is not available, that over-active children with a conduct disorder fare at least as badly as children with conduct disorder and a normal activity level.

Evidence regarding the outcome of children with neurotic or emotional disorders and the antecedent difficulties of adults with neurotic disorder is less clear-cut. In the Robins (1966) study cited earlier, it was found that children with neurotic disorders fared just as well in adulthood as did normal control children drawn from the same school population. This finding is supported by other medium and long-term studies suggesting that neurotic children at least have a better outlook than those with antisocial disorders. However, Waldron (1976) claimed to have found sizeable differences between neurotic children and controls when they were followed up into their twenties. There were various deficiencies in this study including a rather low follow-up rate, but evidence from general population medium-term studies (Graham & Rutter, 1973) also suggests that even if the long-term outlook of such disorders is good, a high proportion (about 50 per cent) of ten- and eleven-year-old children with neurotic disorders are still showing significant problems three and four years later. Further, certain types of childhood and early adolescent phobic states, for example, those associated with school refusal, may persist to late adolescence and adult life in the form of agoraphobia (Berg *et al.*, 1974) or work phobia (Pittman *et al.*, 1968), though, because these studies are retrospective, the degree to which this occurs is unclear.

The antecedents of adult neurotic disorder appear to vary with the condition in question (Mellsop, 1973). Probably most adults with affective disorders have no history of psychiatric attendance in childhood, although insect and animal phobias are likely to have commenced in early childhood and agoraphobia may begin in mid or late adolescence (Marks, 1969). The prediction of neurotic disorder has not been adequately investigated, but the work of Roff (1974) suggests that if both parents have nervous peronalities, and if the mother is neurotically over-involved with her child's development, neurotic symptoms in the child are more likely to persist.

Most physical conditions, such as asthma and eczema, to which psychological factors are frequently strongly linked as precipitants have a good prognosis and are rarely seen in adulthood. However, non-specific abdominal pain is an example of a common condition in childhood in which persistence into adulthood is relatively frequent. Christensen and Mortensen (1975), for example, found 53 per cent of children with abdominal pain still to have significant gastro-intestinal symptoms when followed up as long as thirty years later. The adults had usually been diagnosed as suffering from 'irritable colon' and complained of continuing abdominal discomfort and variation in bowel habit. Apley and Hale (1973) found a similar level of persistence of abdominal pain into adult life. Investigations of links between psychosomatic relationships in childhood and adult life are, however, few in number, and, in particular, there is a lack of information on childhood antecedents of peptic ulcer, coronary artery disease, and the physical disorders of adult life in which stress is thought to play a particularly important part. One group of investigators (Butensky *et al.*, 1976) has however confirmed that personality characteristics of coronary-prone individuals do occur in childhood, though whether their presence predicts the later development of coronary artery disorder is quite unclear.

Lack of information about precursors of psychosomatic disorders mainly occurring in adult life is paralleled by paucity of data concerning the outcome of developmental disorders largely limited to childhood. The most comprehensive follow-up study of encopresis (Bellman, 1966) suggests that, after two years, faecal soiling was no longer present in over half a sample of children referred with encopresis, and was practically absent by 16 years.

Longer-term follow-up of encopretic children would be of interest but does not seem to have been reported. There is a similar lack of information on the outcome of enuretic children, although Bindelglas and Dee (1978) reported outcome in 29 adult men aged sixteen to twenty-five years who had been treated for this condition in childhood with imipramine. One young man still wet the bed occasionally, but none had any serious form of psychiatric disorder. This finding calls in question the value of enquiring about the presence of enuresis in childhood in adults being interviewed for the presence of psychiatric disorder.

Conclusions

Despite the general belief that the roots of adult psychiatric disorder are laid down in childhood, there is remarkably little evidence that this is the case. The one clear exception lies in the area of childhood anti-social disorder and adult sociopathic personality where close and important links have been clearly established. From the point of view of prevention, it seems likely that measures reducing serious conduct disorder in childhood would have a real impact on the prevalence of adult personality disorders manifesting seriously aggressive behaviour. However, it seems unlikely from existing knowledge that preventive measures taken in childhood could reduce the rate of adult neurosis to a significant degree.

1.4
Aetiological factors (non-organic) relevant to mental handicap (mild degrees)

1.4.1
Maladaptive responses of parents to mentally handicapped children: the paradoxical effects of parental concern

DEREK RICKS

The tragic impact on any family of a mentally handicapped child is profound. It generates feelings which permeate all current and future relationships between family members, their child and indeed all individuals, professional and lay, who are involved in the child's care. The aim of this section is to outline those feelings and relationships as they affect the efforts of the family to cope with their child's handicap and to help him progress. An additional objective is to alert the reader to the many ways in which the distress, anger and bewilderment of the family may present.

This presentation takes the form of a series of paradoxes. The family's response may at once make them dependent upon, yet resistive to, professional counselling. Their anxious concern may compel them to seek solutions and reassurances so widely that their efforts undermine an already failing self-confidence. Above all they want to rear their handicapped child as normally as possible, but, finding this often makes life more difficult for him, they learn, with bewildered misgivings, that to help him they may have to behave in an obviously abnormal way. In short their burden is not only the array of distressing emotions each family member feels but the contradictory effects of their struggle to overcome this distress, and to care for and bring up their child. To provide any supportive service for such a family the doctor must be sensitive to these paradoxes. Usually the family are not aware of them, certainly not initially, although they interfere quite seriously with the progress of their child.

1. Medical advice and parental self-confidence

Few people appreciate the array of conflicting feelings generated in parents by the realization that their baby may be mentally handicapped. Even when it confirms previous warnings following complications of birth or pregnancy, it is a shock. All accompanying feelings will be intense and the parents will be at once vulnerable and so acutely sensitive, yet numbed and so may respond more to attitudes, registering *how* reassurance or explanations are given rather than *what* is said. Atmosphere rather than information may colour their recollection of the crisis. A variety of reactions may overwhelm them, first one then another dominating. The fact that their child is mentally handicapped may affront them arousing a sense of shame. Being disabled and vulnerable, he will appeal as pitiable and dependent. They have happily anticipated a normal child and will feel a profound sense of loss, alternating with, or combining with, anger that their prospective child is being denied to them. All these feelings will be initiated and experienced in a medical setting. Inescapably, the doctor will be an integral part of that experience whether he shocks them with the diagnosis, hitherto unsuspected, or confirms suspicions dreaded for some time earlier. From then on, doctors inevitably assume an ambiguous role. As a major part of the setting in which the tragedy was enacted they are to some extent regarded as to blame, yet on them the parents depend for an explanation of the tragedy, for advice on how or indeed if to accept its consequences, and for instruction on how to cope with them. The doctor in this crisis can be immensely supportive or damaging.

His impact is unavoidable. Advice on fulfilling this role is outlined elsewhere in the *Handbook* (see vol. 2, chap. 16 and vol. 3, chap. 39). Here the main point is that the distinctive role doctors assume at this crucial stage influences the degree to which parents see their child as a 'medical' problem and hence that their efforts should be medically guided thereafter. Effective medical support depends on helping parents to keep this in proportion – always remembering that 'medical', i.e. physical disabilities are emotionally more acceptable. Initial difficulties in keeping this in perspective may afterwards seriously distort the efforts of the family to help their child.

They may seek, through diets or drugs, medical solutions as cures for his handicap, knowing these to be effective remedies in some cases about which they read. They may be convinced that distorted behaviour or delay in development is associated with medical features, such as trace elements, and place great faith in mineral supplements and food preparation, or in sleep needs, and organize the family life around their affected child's enforced rest periods, or in sensory deprivation, and exhaust themselves in protracted intensive programmes of stimulation. They may seek medical guidance in even the most everyday aspects of child rearing such as what, or how often, he should eat or drink, what he should wear, whether he should watch TV or how far he should sit from the set. Examples are endless. All illustrate the not uncommon, and by no means abnormal, response of parents who see their child's handicap too rigidly and far too extensively as a medical phenomenon.

A combination of factors may account for this. Early intense experiences in a medical setting may lead the parents, subconsciously or indeed openly, to regard doctors as accountable for the tragedy, and, holding them responsible, expect them to understand and remedy virtually all manifestations of the handicapping condition. With his failure to meet these needs, confidence in their doctor dwindles or collapses and they may ignore or neglect his advice on legitimate medical precautions, such as anticonvulsant therapy. Failure of their doctor may be all the more painful for those parents whose defence against the acceptance of a handicapped child as their own has been to share him with a protective paternal figure external to the family. To find that his doctor has feet of clay may well destroy their trust in all doctors, leading them to embrace any one of a whole range of agencies offering remedies and support, some of which may be excellent, some highly suspect. The point to emphasize is the obligation of the doctor to keep his role in perspective, to know his own limits but to retain the trust and confidence of the family in his care. This can be best achieved by frank, careful explanation of how their child's disability genuinely affects his everyday activities and in what aspects it appears to be irrelevant. Parents inevitably are overwhelmed by the handicapping condition; they need help to see their child as a person, disabled in some ways but not to a degree which need dominate their care of him nor their feelings for him. As the clinical nature of his disabilities are understood and kept in perspective the family should be encouraged to seek their own solutions as they bring up their child. If advice is given on what to promote and what to avoid, it is imperative to explain why and what seems reasonable to expect or to risk.

Crucial early emotive experiences often develop an overdependence on medical judgement in parents who later may equally unwisely reject it. The doctor can all too easily reinforce this by clinging to the prescribing role which may well be expected and indeed pressed on him. This is the paradox to be avoided by adopting an explanatory advisory role. The family needs fortifying in confidently accepting the handicapped member as *their* child and *their* responsibility. Some families cannot; this must be respected.

2. Team support and parent consistency

To accept responsibility for rearing their handicapped child, his parents need support – not only the support afforded by their growing self-confidence and realistic appreciation of his handicap – but practical advice and aids in day-to-day management. Advice of this nature touches on a variety of needs in the same child, for example, encouraging speech, correcting posture, stabilizing gait and so on. Each need may be catered for by a different specialist, such as a physiotherapist or speech therapist or advisory teacher; advice on aids or grants may be sought from occupational therapists or social workers. So several people may visit the family and though each has a recognized role, the parents understandably will discuss other broader topics with them all and press for advice. With a commendable expansion of community handicap teams, a diversity of advice, both professionally intended and gratuitous, is becoming commonplace.

Parents react accordingly and very often become confused, much to the detriment of their handicapped child. Since this array of support usually intensifies while the child is two to five years old, it is likely to occur at the very stage when the need for his consistent management is greatest. As with the normal child, the pre-school period is often the time the mentally handicapped child is most prepared to try, is least socially aware of his own handicap, and is more physiologically flexible (with some notable exceptions). He is then at his most vulnerable to changes in handling, indecisive control, or fluctuating stimulation. At this age, his parents, comparing him with normal toddlers beginning to walk, talk, or play, feel at their most helpless. With increasing

urgency they seek ways of promoting those simple skills that appear so effortlessly in his contemporaries. They seize on each practical or unpractical tip, whoever supplies it and however casually. They compare one person's advice with that of another and cross-question all those helping them. In so doing they often acquire a reputation for playing one professional against the other.

In the same way as sensible caring parents of a handicapped child often establish an ambivalent dependence on their doctors, so they can equally easily develop, with the team helping them, working relationships that complicate and confuse their own efforts. At an earlier stage, coping with the realization of handicap promoted dependence on medical advisers which could easily prevent their gaining what they most needed at that time – confidence in their own ability to care for their child. If confident, the parents want to act, yet don't know what to do. Their need at this stage is for practical advice to reach realistically accessible aims. To achieve this, they must work together in a consistent manner not only with each other but with their team of professional advisers. A second paradox arises. The parents' sense of urgency and purpose may well compel them to use the multidisciplinary but fragmented support which they receive in such a way that it disrupts the coherent consistent programme they and their child need. Again, the paradox can arise with stable, caring, and conscientious parents who interact with competent and equally caring professional staff. The remedy, discussed at length elsewhere in the *Handbook* (vols. 2.16 and 3.39), is to ensure at least periodic frank and forthright meetings between members, reviews, clear agreement on aims, and above all involvement and consultation with the parents themselves.

3. Conscientious concern and parent anxiety

As their child grows up, the family, now it is to be hoped effectively supported by a team of professionals, try to help him to acquire skills he lacks and to keep his behavior and demands within reasonable limits. Yet often the limits such a family sets itself inexorably become what others would regard as unreasonable. Parents of the mentally handicapped accept quite extraordinary burdens of care and distort the whole life-style of themselves and their normal children to accommodate the needs of their affected child. In so doing, they may hinder his progress not merely through their own increasing weariness, but in ways which can specifically aggravate their child's disability. A few examples are given to emphasise the major point which is to alert the doctor to this common, tragic consequence of compassionate over-conscientious management.

The dilemma of making disabilities worse by trying too hard to correct them occurs over the whole range of handicapping conditions. The mother with the retarded hyperactive child is exasperated by his behaviour, which disrupts her domestic routine and wreaks chaos in her home. When, as he trips, grabs, or bumps his way around the house, he perpetrates some particularly annoying disaster, her spontaneous fury erupts but many times she will suppress it or any reprimand which will relieve it because, knowing that he is retarded, she feels he could not help it and, particularly if he is diagnosed as brain-damaged, her conscience will deter her. Inevitably her child will repeatedly irritate her in this way and on each successive occasion she will suppress her reaction until her patience snaps, she reprimands him severely, and is promptly overwhelmed by a sense of guilt at his distress, or more significantly by her own shame in not tolerating his disability. So she compensates by indulging the same activity thereafter until the process repeats itself. For such a child, who above all needs clear and consistent limits to help him remember what behaviour is acceptable, her reactions are disastrous since for him acts previously permissible suddenly evoke a brief, hostile response which is then dropped. A similar dilemma arises in the child with serious language disorders who is frequently socially impaired, not simply because he cannot communicate but because, for a number of reasons, he resists eye-to-eye or face-to-face contact. If such contact is forced on him he becomes acutely disturbed. Many parents of such children find his apparent personal indifference to them almost intolerable and if their conscientious concern compels them to attempt to 'get through to him', they will persist vigorously in trying to establish facial contact. The resulting increased evasiveness of their child may well spur them on to progressively disastrous efforts. A further example is afforded in the spastic retarded child. His spasticity handicaps him whenever he attempts to move, by promoting a rapid rise in tone and distorting the directions of his movement by reflex patterning. The earlier he is given opportunity and practice to offset these disabilities the better, but his efforts not only need such opportunities, afforded by his mother's frequent handling, but also practice in a relaxed state. If he is excited or

frightened his raised level of arousal aggravates his spasticity. He needs every chance to adjust his posture through handling and cuddling that he can see coming and quietly enjoy. Any mother, worried about such a child's motor defects, yet struggling to suppress her anxiety and handle him as advised, often runs into trouble. When she picks up her baby his behaviour is likely to contrast sharply with the snuggling, smiling response which she anticipates or sees in other babies. Her child may stiffen with spasm, throw out his arms, screw up his face, flush, or stare blankly. This is an alarming experience often suggesting to the conscientious mother that she is 'doing it wrong'. So she picks him up less often. This worries her further, not least because with less practice he is more prone to spasm. Far from developing as a mutually enjoyable interaction, picking him up is left to the last minute so that mother, either in a hurry or tense with obligation, may well lift him suddenly with little warning or reassurance further promoting the spasm which alarms her. Nor are these difficulties restricted to parents with a young handicapped child. As he grows older into adolescence and adult life the pressures of his care increase. The dependent child becomes the heavier adult, lifted by ageing, more feeble parents; the boisterous child is so able physically to assert himself as an adult that he can dominate the family routine. It is remarkable how often and to what extent parents tolerate the burden he imposes by excusing his behaviour as childlike – which in many ways it is. It may be that only by regarding him as still a child can his parents draw on resources enabling them to continue his care. Unfortunately, regarding him as a child, they treat him as one with the limited expectations, patience, and comforting indulgence that would be appropriate were he much younger. Inevitably he expects this and becomes steadily more dependent and demanding.

The same paradox emerges: the strenuous effort of fond and conscientious parents intensifying the problems they are struggling to contain. Such a deteriorating situation is most likely when the family is isolated; encouraging contact and discussion with other similarly struggling parents will usually be a most effective remedy since shared perspectives of what is tolerable are likely to be more realistic. To establish and maintain in parents a balance between enough enthusiasm to persevere and a relaxed realism which avoids the pitfalls of over-conscientious effort is the essence of supportive counselling. (See also chapter 3.3.3 of this volume.)

4. Natural responses and parent perplexity

Trying so hard to care for their child and to cope with his tantrums or reduce his disability may result in the contradictory results outlined above. These results are, however, consequences of conscious, indeed over-conscientious effort and can be recognized as such. By comparing their plight or expectations with that of other parents, or through counselling, or through simply taking stock together enforced through exhaustion the family can be made aware of their own dilemma and, it is to be hoped, take steps to remedy it. Such steps may be painful, since for many parents trying less strenuously means caring less devotedly. A far more disabling paradox, and one more difficult to remedy, results from parents' responses to their handicapped child of which they are unaware because they are the same spontaneous and in no way self-conscious or over-conscientious reactions with which they relate to their normal children in identical circumstances. A remarkable fact, illustrated below by a few examples, is how often such prompt intuitive reactions appropriate to the normal child are not only inappropriate to the handicapped child in the same situation but aggravate his disability and reduce his competence to cope with that situation.

Retarded children with motor defects afford some examples. The child with ataxia needs a great deal of confidence to attempt weight-bearing and the experience which will enable him to compensate for his low tone and lack of balance. Simple tips on his handling and arranging his surroundings can help this but above all his apprehension needs to be overcome and this can be most effectively achieved by confident handling. The immediate and quite natural response of parents to their weaving, stumbling, ataxic child is to hover anxiously near and to reach impulsively to support him as his balance fails. This undermines his confidence and deflects his vision so he falls more readily; in doing so his parents' anxiety is reinforced and so is their inappropriate behaviour. Athetoid children are similarly vulnerable. Their defective striatal control prevents their organizing in a smooth sequence those gradations of tone and movement which enable the normal child to execute fluently everyday motor skills such as washing, dressing, or feeding oneself. To be effectively co-ordinated these movement sequences need to be automatic, as becomes painfully apparent to all of us as we later learn to write, swim, or drive a car. Hence the athetoid child's efforts need to be just as auto-matic, which means as unselfconscious as possible. Yet he is a child who by his involuntary movement draws the attention of the whole family to his efforts. They wait tense and expectant for him to knock over or spill whatever he reaches for – tension readily communicated to him and frequently reinforced by his parents' spoken approval and relief at success or cautionary warning as he begins to jerk. Either response focuses his attention on his movement and disrupts it, often promoting further exasperated comment. Similar disabling interactions occur with parents whose child has a severe communication handicap. However sensibly such parents understand their child's poor comprehension and appreciate the need to keep to the same short statements in standard situations, they behave quite differently at times of stress when the desire to communicate with their child is at its most urgent. At such times the parents act normally, that is, they will expand the simple intended message to give it emphasis. Listening to any mother with an active 'helpful' toddler in a supermarket is a very revealing experience in this context. As he starts to put unwanted articles into the trolley she may smile, telling him 'no' but if he persists and her anger mounts she will tell him a great deal more, changing not only her tone but the information she conveys. Unless it is pointed out to them, parents are unaware how much they rely on verbal control of their children, control which is intensified by the use of more rather than fewer words.

Just as the apprehensive ataxic child needed confidence and his parents' spontaneous response undermined it, so the athetoid child's efforts provoke their attention, which unsettles him, while to the non-communicating child at crucial times they expand and complicate rather than reduce and simplify what they say. Yet these are all natural spontaneous responses, presumably effective in normal child-rearing. Parents of handicapped children eventually realize that in so many circumstances treating him like other children does not work. Appreciating that they are resorting to 'unnatural' reactions may worry them considerably quite apart from their discomfort at treating their handicapped child so differently from his siblings. One of the most supportive contributions of the doctor to such a family is to explore these reactions and help parents not only to accept them as effective but to see them as a testimony to their own normality rather than to their inadequacy as parents.

The contradictory effects of parents' responses

towards, and efforts on behalf of, their mentally handicapped child are regrettably rarely recognized as the paradoxical consequences of normal people's attitude to an externally imposed tragedy. Although a great deal of depressed, defensive, and unrealistic behaviour may develop – behaviour which could be labelled as a psychiatric disorder – it is the author's belief that in the vast majority of cases this is the consequence, and indeed the measure, of the severity of this tragedy. It is not simply that such a tragedy becomes recognized as open-ended, indeed never-ending, but also that it undermines and distorts fundamental parent/child relationships. To have an abnormal child is not only a profound personal disaster for any parent, it condemns parents to rearing experiences which are themselves disastrous and which their struggle to correct may aggravate, all for reasons of which they are unaware. The stress and sadness of this experience testifies to the highly abnormal demands made on any family in bringing up and caring for their mentally handicapped child. Parents report that in some ways the experience is an enriching one. It is one obligation upon all professionals to safeguard this, but a greater one to respect how fundamental and frightening are the dilemmas such a child imposes and their paradoxical consequences which, once recognized, can be effectively resolved.

2
Methods of interview and assessment

2.1
The assessment of neurotic and personality disorders in adults

P. G. CAMPBELL AND
GERALD F. M. RUSSELL

The assessment of neurotic and personality disorders will be considered here mainly from the clinical viewpoint as part of the general psychiatric or medical assessment. The focus will primarily be on individual interviews as the means of assessment. Other methods used for more specialized purposes in clinical practice or research, such as joint interviews, questionnaires, and structured rating schedules, will be referred to in other chapters, where appropriate.

The assessment is relevant to all patients, not just those whose primary disorder is neurotic or personality-related. In many patients other priorities will seem at first to be more pressing, such as the assessment of psychotic symptoms or of signs of physical disease. The detailed characterization of neurotic symptoms or of personality traits may then have to be temporarily demoted in priority. It is important, however, that such demotion should not be permanently maintained. Neurotic symptoms, not recognized at presentation, may appear later. Personality factors, too, will have a crucial influence on later progress. Beyond the boundaries of specialist psychiatry, the need for assessment of neurotic and personality disorder extends across the whole range of clinical medicine. Such problems will greatly affect the quality and degree of the patient's distress and disability, as well as his relationships with doctors and other helpers, his needs for treatment and his capacity to benefit from it.

The aims of assessment

A major purpose for the clinician is to formulate and test hypotheses about what is troubling the patient (in terms of both the form and content of his disorder) and what treatment, if any, is required. By evaluating probabilities about the patient and his world the doctor seeks guidance towards appropriate choices from the limited range of management options open to him. A summary of these hypotheses is recorded as a descriptive *diagnosis* of the form of the patient's mental disorder and as a wider-ranging and more detailed *formulation*. In addition, the assessment serves at least three other purposes in varying measure, which may be named as (a) therapeutic, (b) research, and (c) educational; only the therapeutic will be further considered here but the other two should not be overlooked as part of the potential yield of every assessment.

(1) Diagnosis

The formal diagnosis should serve as a means of bringing to bear on the patient's individual disorder professional knowledge accumulated from psychiatric experience and research. The aim is to categorize patterns or *syndromes* of mental disorder so that the doctor's appraisal can be set within a wider framework of psychiatric knowledge and can be reliably communicated. In this task, the assessor avoids value judgements and claims of special insight or intuitive understanding in favour of descriptive technical terms which embody broad, but testable, hypotheses open to criticism or revision.

In the poorly demarcated field of neurosis and personality disorder many clinicians will readily acknowledge the limited value of diagnosis alone. In contrast to psychotic illness, where abnormal processes of mental function seem easily inferred from unusual behaviour and utterances, these disorders may seem insubstantial and hard to pin down. The assumption implicit within formal diagnosis, that a patient's disorder can be validly categorized by doctors in terms of the form of mental aberration displayed, without regard to social and economic background, education, intelligence, or volition, may seem extremely questionable. Except in those cases of severe or 'pure' syndromes of neurosis, the diagnosis is likely to give a very puny characterization of what is wrong. The patient may suffer various kinds of symptoms and other adversities which either do not lend themselves easily to brief summary of their form or could equally well be summarized in different ways. Diagnostic terms used clinically tend to be imprecisely defined and several are used casually in everyday language, sometimes (as in the case of 'neurotic' or 'hysterical') in ways different from the psychiatric. Often the patient's symptoms seem so closely bound up with events in his social history and with his current relationships, conflicts, and attitudes that it may be hard to see them as evidence of pathology in any distinctly medical sense. In such cases they may invite interpretation (particularly by people who are not psychiatrists) as personal signals of emotional turmoil, social disharmony or demand for help, more closely akin to the phenomena of ordinary human unhappiness than to signs of malfunction in mind or brain. Deviations from individual or population norms will commonly appear quantitative rather than qualitative in form. Unless the assessor knows how the patient functioned in the past and is familiar with the expectations of his social culture it may be impossible to estimate how large or abnormal these deviations are. The patient's degree of concern about his symptoms or about himself may appear more remarkable than the actual symptoms or any manifest abnormality of personality as a whole. Factors other than simply the degree of deviation will determine whether the patient seeks medical help. Still others will determine whether he ever gets to see a psychiatrist, and different psychiatrists may respond to patients with similarly-named disorders in very different ways.

Familiar as such limitations are in this area, psychiatrists continue to regard diagnosis as important and useful, seeing it as an exercise which meaningfully indicates the broad orientation of medical experience and expectation about different forms of disorder. It may not yield precise compass-bearings towards knowledge of causes, optimal remedy or outcome but this is also likely to be true of very many common physical disorders which doctors treat.

(2) Formulation

The weakness of diagnosis alone in the assessment of neurosis and personality disorder makes it all the more important to prepare a carefully detailed formulation. This summarizes, besides the descriptive diagnosis, salient features of the patient's history and mental state, a provisional 'explanation' identifying possible causal factors, plans for future action, and a prediction of outcome. Due attention can be given to individual factors and to the importance of social and physical dimensions as well as the psychological. The formulation can be set out under the following headings:

(i) *History:* a brief summary of salient points

(ii) *Findings* on examination: mental state and physical examination

(iii) *Diagnosis* or *differential diagnosis*, in descriptive terms*

(iv) *Aetiological, pathogenic and pathoplastic factors,* psychological, social, physical

(v) *Further investigations,* psychological (most commonly further interviews), social, physical

(vi) *Management and treatment,* psychological, social, physical

(vii) *Prognosis:* predictions about future progress and response to treatment (not just 'good' or 'bad')

An alternative method of formulation is now provided by the problem-oriented approach to medical records (POMR). The patient's difficulties are recorded as active or inactive *problems* on an initial *problem list* which can be repeatedly revised and kept up to date. History and initial examination are recorded as a *data base* and proposals about further investigations, treatment, and explanations given to the patient are recorded separately for each problem as an *initial plan,* each followed by systematic *progress notes.*

(3) *Therapeutic aims and the fostering of communication*

A further aim is to give help directly to the patient by means of the assessment process itself, either by using the interview(s) to foster a good relationship as a basis for future treatment or to give the patient a new awareness of his difficulties. Sullivan (1954) has particularly emphasized this purpose of the psychiatric interview; a single assessment interview can be followed by major changes in the patient even when no further treatment is given. In psychiatric interviewing assessment and therapy are closely interwoven.

Participant observation. During the interview the assessor seeks to obtain objective information by methods which are reliable and without bias. But the interviewer is not just a neutral, non-participant observer. Beside this *objective focus,* therefore, at least two other foci of observation may be important in the assessment of neurotic and personality disorder. The *empathic focus* provides the interviewer with a means of fostering the communication process and may give a deeper insight into the patient's predica-

* For purposes of communication, diagnosis should be stated in the standardized nomenclature of the International Classification of Diseases (1978)

ment. By trying to put himself in the patient's shoes, so to speak, the interviewer hopes to understand more of what the patient is experiencing and attempting to communicate (or to conceal or deny). The *interactional focus* is different again. From this viewpoint the events of the interview and the patient's behaviour may be seen as the outcome of the interaction between him and the interviewer in the particular context and environment of the assessment. The interviewer may hope to understand more about the patient's capacities and difficulties in social relationships by evaluating the interview in these terms. His own emotional reaction to the patient may be informative from both the empathic and interactional viewpoints, though the validity of such intuitions may at times be questionable. Different assessors may want to give different weight to these three kinds of viewpoint. Fruitless arguments about their relative value are common. Each may have its own particular values and deficiencies.

The three types of focus can be illustrated by a case example (patient 1): the interview was recorded on videotape:

The patient was a 46-year-old divorcee who was attending a psychiatric day hospital for treatment of depression. She was interviewed by the female registrar responsible for her care, who was trying to explore why the patient was not making progress. The interview began quietly and amicably, the patient describing her continuing feelings of tension and despondency. The registrar proceeded to more searching questions about the patient's lack of progress. The patient became increasingly agitated, insisting she was not getting any help from the staff. The interview dragged on, the patient becoming first noisily tearful and then screaming at the interviewer, so that it was difficult to terminate the session.

Objectively, an observer of the recording could recognize that the patient showed evidence of a depressive mood state. *Empathically,* one could feel with her the distress of believing the staff (including her interviewer) were not making adequate or appropriate efforts on her behalf. Equally, one could empathize with the doctor's feelings of helplessness (which she admitted later) when confronted by the patient's negative attitudes. *Interactionally,* the interview appeared to be aggravating the patient's distress. As the patient became more animated, the interviewer became less so, with a bodily posture and facial expression that could be read as boredom or resignation, her head several inches lower in her chair than at the start of the interview. Later the patient poured paint over the registrar's car.

The psychiatric interview
(1) *Variations of method: frameworks*
In the absence of an established corpus of scientific knowledge about the most valid method of conducting an assessment, prevailing fashions, local

traditions, imitation, and personal choice usually seem to be important factors in determining the variety of methods used. One might expect that different methods will vary in usefulness according to the individual characteristics of assessors, patients, the settings in which they meet, and the treatment decisions to be made. A demonstration of the wide range of individual variations in technique even within a narrowly definable type of practice is given by Glover (1955) who distributed a questionnaire about working habits to British psycho-analysts. The interview may be more or less structured or unstructured, directive or non-directive. One or more interviews of variable duration may be employed as standard practice. The patient may be interviewed alone, conjointly with other family members or even in a group, by interviewers working alone or with other observers or participants present.

In Britain the format used by most psychiatrists is based on the scheme of examination developed and taught at the Maudsley Hospital. Mayer-Gross, Slater and Roth (1969) set it out in detail (and attribute its origins to a publication by Kirby in the USA in 1921). A more recent revision has been published in a booklet by the Institute of Psychiatry (1973). The scheme is objective, comprehensive, and flexible. It owes much to the *psychobiological* approach of Adolf Meyer but is not tied to any particular theoretical model. It is a framework for recording information about the patient in terms of the history and the mental state examination.

Another exposition is given in a textbook by Leff and Isaacs (1978), which incorporates the standardized terminology of Wing's Present State Examination (Wing *et al.*, 1974). This approach raises the question of what kind of evidence is to be regarded as relevant and useful. Should the assessment be concerned primarily with what are claimed to be 'the observable phenomena of mental illness' (Leff & Isaacs, 1978)? Or is there an important role also for other kind of data which are more personal, subjective, and intuitive?

The more structured schemes of assessment carry a number of advantages. They ensure a wider and systematic screening of the patient's history and mental state and they tend to achieve greater reliability. Thus, fully structured schemes are particularly valuable in research. A major advantage of the Maudsley scheme is that it encourages the interviewer to record in detail the evidence presented by the patient and other informants. A less formal approach can easily be misleading if reported information, observations, and inferences are mixed haphazardly together.

The structured clinical schemes can also be criticized, though more perhaps for abuses of them than for intrinsic faults. They are intended as frameworks for structuring information rather than programmes for interrogation, but the beginner may be tempted to follow their sequence over-rigidly when interviewing. More fundamental a problem is that they cannot easily be married to the general medical history used by other doctors. Medical students and non-psychiatrists may regard these frameworks as providing an exercise only for psychiatrists, which find no ready application outside the specialty. They have also been criticized for providing a too narrowly 'medical' perspective, with undue emphasis given to detecting abnormality *in* the patient, whilst neglecting disturbances of social interaction which may be especially important in the field of neurosis and personality disorder.

Confident familiarity with a framework such as the Maudsley scheme is an essential requirement for the psychiatrist. He should learn to use it intelligently, adapting it as required for special purposes or problems, but retaining its overall form as an indispensable basis for communication with colleagues.

(2) *The components of the psychiatric interview*

Under this heading will be considered the interviewer's actions in performing the interview. They will, of course, be clearly evident to the patient and can therefore affect him beneficially or adversely. The components to be considered are

  (i) the three stages of the interview
  (ii) the time taken by the interview(s)
  (iii) the recording of the interview.

(i) *The three stages of the interview*. It is useful to regard every interview as having a beginning, a middle, and an end, each with its own purpose and requirements.

The first part or beginning of the interview is concerned with establishing some personal contact or *rapport* with the patient. The interviewer will identify himself and his role and, if other staff have to be present, he will introduce them by name and explain their presence. It is appropriate to anticipate the anxiety frequently felt by patients at the prospect of a psychiatric consultation and offer sympathy and reassurance. Background information already known to the interviewer can be briefly outlined and the purpose and duration of the interview mentioned. Sometimes the patient has not realized that he was to see a psychiatrist or he has anxieties about confidentiality or other issues. Time may need to be spent talking about these problems before the interview progresses further. The interviewer needs to help the patient to verbalize obvious doubts.

The middle part is concerned with eliciting detailed information. The aim will be to help the patient talk freely on important matters. A balance will be needed between non-directive encouragement and directive guidance, as will be discussed in later sections of this account.

The ending requires some statement by the interviewer to summarize what has been learned or to point the way to an agreement with the patient about what is to be done. The *exposition* to the patient (Fletcher, 1979) is often neglected. There is no need to say more than is readily acceptable to the patient but it is important that he should be left with some positive sense of what has been achieved and what is planned.

Neglect of the beginning and ending of interviews is a common fault. Often the novice interviewer plunges into a disjointed and inconsequential interrogation which is liable to alienate the patient. Alternatively, he may feel unable to halt the patient's flow of talk once he has found something to talk about. The exposition may be confined to vague platitudes which extricate the interviewer but do little or nothing to relieve the patient or answer his uncertainties.

(ii) *The time taken by the interview(s).* Closely linked with questions about how wide should be the scope of an interview is how much time should be devoted to it. In clinical practice no strict limit need exist. The conventional duration of about an hour is commonly justified as being about as much as a disturbed or distressed patient can comfortably endure. But it is important that the more-or-less ritualized clinical practice of performing 'an assessment' by one or more interviews within a particular time-period is not equated with assessment in the broader sense. To meet clinical diagnostic or therapeutic aims the assessment of neurotic and personality disorder has no obvious limits to its scope or duration other than those imposed by practical constraints. The problem is that no detail of the patient's past or present functioning, as seen from the psychological, social or physical viewpoints can be presumed to be of such little relevance that it can be totally ignored. Thus the assessment may be viewed as a continuous process, and as information about the patient increases, hypotheses about him and his difficulties can be further tested, refined, and brought up to date.

(iii) *Recording of information.* The keeping of proper records is an essential element of good medical practice, but the method adopted may affect the assessment process. Most assessors make notes during the interview but this can inhibit the patient from revealing intimate details. Some interviewers prefer to write notes only after the end of the interview, but detailed factual information may be lost in this way. Inspection of hospital psychiatric records may reveal extensive recording of the patient's account with little or no detail about the interviewer's assessment, or his treatment decisions or communications to the patient. The more positive virtues of verbatim note-taking are stressed by Finesinger (1948) who showed how the discipline of writing down every word spoken by both the patient and the interviewer can serve as the basic framework for a method of psychotherapy. It is also a valuable means of recording finer shades of meaning of the patient's utterances, thus indicating the subtler, albeit less reliable, features of his mental state (see patient 2, below).

(3) *Contents of the interview*

The contents of the interview will be summarized according to the framework of the Maudsley scheme published by the Institute of Psychiatry (1973), and summarized in modified form in an appendix at the end of this chapter.

History-taking. The exact order in which the history is elicited need not matter provided it can be related to a structure suitable for record-making. Many clinicians like to offer the patient time to expand on his present problems before proceeding further to biography. Alternatively, and particularly if time is limited, one may ask the patient to name his major complaints and their duration before stopping him in order to proceed through the family history and the rest of his personal history, assuring him that it will be helpful to get a background picture first before hearing more about the present situation. The exercise of relating his biography may be fairly easy for the patient and can help to establish rapport with the interviewer. The patient then feels more able to talk freely about his present preoccupations when attention once more is focused on them at a later stage.

Present illness. This is an exploration of the problems experienced by the patient, allowing him as much spontaneous description as possible, and recording his story largely in his own words. He is encouraged to describe the severity and effects of his symptoms, their mode of onset and subsequent course, situational and temporal relationships, other accompanying symptoms, and treatment already received.

The patient's *biography* is obtained in order to establish his background as provided by the following: his *family history* from both the hereditary and environmental points of view; the *personal history* in chronological order with emphasis on the important landmarks of his life, and the patient's adjustment in the educational, occupational, sexual, and marital spheres. The patient's *medical and psychiatric history* before the onset of his current illness is obtained, including any antisocial behaviour or use of alcohol and drugs. The patient's *personality* prior to the onset of his current illness should be assessed mainly from information given by close and reliable informants (which should be recorded separately), but his own account may be usefully informative.

An account of the patient's *current life situation* and a *review of recent events* and of *the past year* complete the initial history. The inclusion of these details emphasises the importance of relating the patient's presenting problems to significant *life-events,* and to his social and economic circumstances.

The mental state. The examination of the patient's mental state consists of the interviewer's observations and evaluation of his appearance, behaviour, and mental functioning. A common mistake arises from muddling the history and mental state with each other: for example, the interviewer's observations may be included in the record of the patient's history, whereas they should await the presentation of the mental state. It is commonly said that the history provides a longitudinal perspective of the patient's life, and the mental state, a cross-sectional view of his current mental functioning. Useful though this three-dimensional metaphor is, it has its limitations.

The assessment of the patient's mental state starts from the moment of the first meeting with the patient. Much evidence will emerge in the relating of the history. Specific screening questions may be needed to reveal evidence of major symptoms not reported spontaneously by the patient, such as depression, suicidal preoccupations, anxiety, phobias, obsessions, or depersonalization. Sometimes there will be obvious signs, such as the physical manifestations of depression or anxiety, the reddened, abraded hands of the compulsive handwasher, tell-tale features of alcoholism or drug abuse, weight disorder, old scars at the wrist of previous self-injury. Inconsistencies between the patient's verbal report and observed behaviour may be especially noteworthy.

Often, however, gross evidence of disorder is lacking and the beginner may tend to under-report findings on examination. The evidence is commonly 'softer' than the florid disturbances of psychosis, but this should not deter the interviewer from attempting to evaluate in detail the patient's state of mind; a comment that it is 'normal' betrays a lack of attention to the individual information elicited. His dress, demeanour, and general behaviour may be informative about his life-style or recent upheavals. Besides exploring the details of the major symptoms elicited in the course of history-taking or a screening enquiry, the interviewer will need to explore the content of the patient's preoccupations, to elicit what particular ideas, visual images, and other fantasies of past, present or future adversity trouble him. The precise personal meaning of the words he uses will need to be known in order to understand what is on his mind, for it is not enough to assume that the patient's attribution of labels to his thoughts and feelings corresponds with the interviewer's use of such terms. In addition to depression or anxiety, other components of his affective state such as resentment, inner conflict, and shame may be especially important. The evaluation will include some attempt at assessing the patient's credibility as a historian, and evidence of denial, resistance, or other possible mechanisms of defence.

Exploration of intellectual capacities may be important. Educational and occupational history and the patient's apparent verbal fluency and capacity for conceptualization may provide valuable evidence of problems related to intelligence. Special intellectual strengths and weakness may emerge. Formal testing of memory, orientation, intelligence, and general knowledge is commonly omitted if the patient's disorder is clearly a neurosis or personality disorder. Yet it can be important to include such testing in the examination for the useful information it occasionally provides. Impairment of concentration by anxiety or depression may provide further evidence of their severity. In cases of drug or alcohol abuse or possible physical disease, such testing assumes greater priority.

In exploring the patient's preoccupations and attitudes, the interviewer will give special attention to the patient's own appraisal of his problems and to all the aspects of his wishes, intentions, and capacity for change which are often generally subsumed under the title of motivation. Does he hope for things to be done to him or does he want assistance in changing himself? Has he come mainly to please somebody else? Was his decision to see a psychiatrist a sign that he had already made positive efforts to alter his predicament? His manner of relating to the interviewer may point to the ease or difficulty of achieving a therapeutic alliance in attempts at treatment.

Physical examination. A physical examination may be best done at the first assessment, since it can present more of an embarrassment if left until later. Unless recently performed by other doctors, physical examination may be especially important where there are prominent physical symptoms, suspicions of drug or alcohol abuse, or where treatment with anti-depressants, β-blockers, or anti-alcohol drugs is contemplated. If there is a suspicion of physical illness it is best to proceed quickly to the necessary physical investigations rather than to allow them to drag on indefinitely. It may yet be desirable to carry out a physical examination at a later assessment if the patient develops new or distressing bodily symptoms. The psychiatrist's concern for all aspects of the patient's health is likely to have a beneficial effect upon him, quite apart from the intrinsic and immediate value of the examination itself.

(4) Interviewing techniques

There is no one method of interviewing which is appropriate to all psychiatric patients: the method must be tailored to suit the needs of the individual. Nevertheless there are a few general principles which are especially relevant to the assessment of patients with neurosis or personality disorder.

The conversational approach. Much of the art of good interviewing is to conduct a personal conversation with the patient, without subjecting him to the discomfort of an interrogation or of being put on trial. The clinician should employ language which is most conducive to the patient's comfort and understanding, namely layman's language adapted to his educational and social background. The conversation taking place should be friendly and informal, the interviewer listening attentively to the patient's account of his symptoms, problems, and his explanation of their origin. For example, a middle-aged lady working as a secretary may complain that her employer has unreasonably burdened her with excessive work and has become impatient and difficult to work with. She explains that, as a consequence, she has become miserable, feels constantly exhausted, and is worried that her post and security are threatened. The interviewer will nod encouragement as she unfolds her story and will not cast doubt on her account of the circumstances. At the same time, and while keeping an open mind about the actual role played by the employer, he will consider the possibility that the patient has developed a depressive state which is primarily responsible for any difficulties she may have encountered at work. The totality of these observations may point towards a minor depressive syndrome with origins other than those identified by the patient. The conversation continues, allowing the patient to express her subjective view of her problems, while simultaneously the clinician makes his assessment of the symptoms and circumstances. The one conversation therefore embodies two different aspects: the patient's subjective view and the clinician's objective appraisal. As discussed by Watzlawick and co-workers (1968), what the patient communicates is much more than just the content of his talk. The interviewer needs a 'third ear' to be able to detect not only the relative emphasis, order, and omissions in the patient's account but also more subtle nuances of feeling displayed in the telling.

The patient will often present with symptoms referred to the body. It is necessary that no major demarcation should be made between 'organic' and 'functional' symptoms: the distinction presupposes an assessment of the significance of the patient's complaints. All symptoms, whether or not due to demonstrable physical disease should be recognized as psychological phenomena. Thus if the patient determinedly presents symptoms as evidence of physical disorder, for example, questioning should start with a thorough exploration of the bodily experience; further enquiry about psychosocial implications and consequences can proceed in a symptom-oriented way without the patient feeling he is being accused of being 'mental' or of having imaginary symptoms. The clinician's wider explorations may be assisted with questions such as the following. 'These pains which have gone on for so long must have caused you much distress . . . Have they interfered with your sleep? . . . Have they made you feel miserable at times? . . . or caused you to weep? . . .'

In other cases, too, questions may usefully be presented in an appropriate social context, on the patient's own territory as it were. For example, the clinician wishing to find out whether a student suffers from depression, loss of interest, or impaired concentration, may choose not to ask direct questions about these symptoms, but will instead enquire more tangentially about his progress with his studies and examinations. Another useful method of prompting the patient to describe spontaneously the severity of his symptoms is to ask how he spends his spare time. The patient may then reveal how his symptoms and personal problems have interfered with his normal way of life.

Although the danger of putting 'leading' questions to the patient is well known, it still bears repetition. Balint's (1957) description of GPs 'organizing' their patients' diverse symptoms by responding selectively to those suggesting a possible organic basis may be highly relevant to psychiatry too, when the assessor may give undue attention to symptoms which conform to expectations of psychiatric phenomenology and nosology. In treating neurosis, particularly, it is common to find that the patient's difficulties can initially be regarded as 'illness' but that the distinction from personality disorder becomes blurred as more is known. His difficulties may well take on a different appearance as at least partly predictable and habitual patterns of response to the conflicts and disappointments of everyday life. The initial appearance of discreteness in the form and development of his symptomatology may then seem in retrospect to have been a result of insufficient and biased information. On the other hand, the interviewer is supposed to know more about describing the varieties of human feeling and distress than the patient. Though he will not want to put words into the patient's mouth he can often help communication by demonstrating simple understanding of how the patient is likely to feel. For example when broaching a sensitive or potentially embarrassing area such as a young woman's sexual difficulties the interviewer may assist her to volunteer information with a question such as 'I would guess that your problems have caused difficulties with the physical . . . the sexual . . . side of your marriage . . . ?' It may even be advisable to make a preceding apology such as 'Forgive me for asking you a personal question, but it may be important . . . '. Another difficult area is that of suicidal intent, especially when the genuineness of threats has to be assessed. It is useful to ask the vague question 'Have you ever felt desperate?' The word 'desperate' is ambiguous and the patient may indeed interpret it as meaning 'suicidal' or merely 'frustrated'. The way he chooses to interpret the question will itself be informative. At other times it is helpful to conduct the interview with the minimum of questions. Other verbal statements may be less controlling and intrusive, such as general requests ('Tell me about your marriage'), promptings ('I haven't a picture yet of how life has been for you recently'), or summaries ('So there's always been some friction with your husband about the children?').

All these methods of interviewing which encourage spontaneity on the part of the patient carry a number of advantages. They serve to promote the patient's comfort and reduce any resentment from having to undergo a psychiatric examination. Greatest credence will also be given to problems the patient mentions or elaborates on spontaneously. The method also serves to facilitate the detection of the 'soft signs' of the mental state, for example the use of mechanisms of denial or the presence of ambivalence.

A *case example* (patient 2) will illustrate how an oblique approach might usefully reveal information held back by the patient:

The patient was the 19-year-old daughter of a medical practitioner. She had had anorexia nervosa for an indeterminate time and neither she nor her father seemed able to date the onset of weight loss. 'We did not notice when it happened', they said. The subject was changed to that of her amenorrhoea which she could date to two years previously. The interview went as follows:
Clinician: You must have consulted a doctor when your periods stopped?
Patient: Yes . . . I saw a gynaecologist . . . He weighed me . . . What a shock . . . 6½ stone . . . I did not tell them . . .
Clinician: Who do you mean?
Patient: My parents.
Clinician: What else did this doctor say?
Patient: He said I was underweight . . . I should eat more . . . but he did not stress it . . . at least not much.
Clinician: How do you feel about not having periods?
Patient: I'd like them to come back. to be normal again . . . I think . . . but yet they can be a nuisance.

This conversation was most valuable in eliciting spontaneously that the weight loss had been of over two years' duration and that the patient had purposely endeavoured to conceal it from her parents (who seemed to collude in denying that a problem existed). Similarly she made excuses for not heeding the gynaecologist's advice. She also betrayed ambivalence about returning to her former health and resuming menstruation.

A symptomatic approach. A general view of the psychosocial nature of symptoms may be obtained by using the symptoms themselves as a starting point. This approach may be seen in part as an alternative method to the encouragement of spontaneity described above, or the two may be combined, one or two of the main presenting symptoms being fully explored. The enquiries proposed should not, however, be used as a scheme for interrogation. The basic information about symptoms called for in medical texts often comprises no more than:

(1) quality of the experience,
(2) location, if referred to the body,
(3) severity,
(4) onset and time-course (including presence or absence now),
(5) aggravating and relieving factors,
(6) accompanying symptoms.
    Further exploration might include:
(7) the degree of disability caused by the symptom,
(8) previous occurrence of anything similar,
(9) what the patient thinks it is due to and what should be done about it,
(10) recent attempts at treatment (including self-treatment).

Further enquiries may be directed at elucidating contributory physical, social, or psychological factors and mechanisms. Appropriate enquiries for eliciting direct links are:

(11) relationship of onset and progress to outside events,
(12) reasons for the patient presenting *now* with the symptoms.

Finally, there may be indications for exploring the more elusive and theoretical mechanisms underlying the expression of symptoms in their particular form:

(13) Does the patient's account appear to ring true?
(14) Does the symptom serve a communicational purpose by mobilizing help and allowing the patient to claim the privileges of invalidism?

(15) Are there other rewards or reinforcements for it?
(16) Could it be induced by suggestion or other iatrogenic mechanisms?
(17) Does it have symbolic or cultural significance?

(5) *Evaluating and directing the interview*
Abstraction and inference. Evaluation of the evidence is an intrinsic part of the assessment. In clinical interviewing, most of this processing of the data will be performed during the time spent with the patient. In this way, the experienced clinician identifies the areas of enquiry he needs to explore and, at the appropriate moment, steers the interview towards them. Thus, the process of evaluation influences the kind of data obtained. The diagnostic task of weighing the evidence about the patient and his functioning commonly involves several stages of abstraction and inference. The first may be to infer from what the patient says and does that he is experiencing or displaying certain nameable symptoms and signs. The second is to study the pattern of symptoms and their reported evolution over time and so make hypotheses about the descriptive diagnosis in terms of normality or of a syndrome of neurosis or personality or other disorder. A third stage may be to identify possible aetiological, pathogenic, or pathoplastic factors in the recent or more remote past. This stage or earlier ones may include further abstractions according to theoretical allegiances of the interviewer.

Each stage of inference and abstraction is liable to error and disagreement unless they are performed according to standard rules, such as those embodied in the International Classification of Diseases. Even though these rules do not demand particular theoretical loyalties of the user, many psychiatrists seem to prefer their own personal categories. Disagreements arise not only because words are differently used, but because the phenomena described are often quantitative and not readily susceptible of the categorical designation of everyday language. Crippling as these uncertainties and disagreements about the meaning of words have been in the pursuit of research into neurosis and personality disorder, they do not have to matter to the clinician who bases his practice on his own perception and experience, and places little value on the reports of others. The personal meaning of the concepts he uses to organize his thinking about his patients may be precisely what allows them to be of greatest use as intermediaries in his decisions about treatment. Since communicated knowledge about neurosis and personality disorder is so lacking in many of the areas of uncertainty he faces daily alone, he may feel he has little other choice.

As a general rule, the higher the order of abstraction used, the less easy it will be for others to translate the description back into the phenomena observed. Many of the terms in current use are so abstract that they lack any generally accepted descriptive or explanatory power, other than perhaps in conveying something about the user's attitude. Neurotic, disturbed, psychopathic, regressed, manipulative, hysterical, acting out, attention-seeking, immature, dependent, are just a few examples of popular words with mainly pejorative overtones. All are probably best avoided in favour of more descriptive alternatives.

The doubtful validity of abstractions is further illustrated by the common problem of inferring more or less intentionality or motivation to the patient's behaviour. Many assessors seem incautious about such attributions and appear over-ready to equate effects with causes (for example, the patient's disorder distresses his mother. Inference: he behaves in an ill way in order to hurt her). In this area psychiatry may at times seem extraordinarily cruel.

Perhaps the commonest method of simplifying the task of assessment is to rely on 'clinical impression'. In the absence of any other widely accepted or proven method of recognizing neurosis or personality disorder, the role of individual judgement and clinical experience cannot be lightly dismissed, and such an approach may be the highest expression of the clinician's art. There must be a danger, however, that impressionistic appraisal is performed superficially or incautiously, with an over-readiness to act on far-reaching conclusions from limited data.

Deciding on priorities. It is helpful to think of the task of assessment as having certain priorities which can be investigated hierarchically and sequentially. At first meeting, for instance, exclusion of psychosis and of physical illness, and assessment of possible suicidal risk or any other immediate physical, social, or psychological hazard take obvious precedence. The next priority is the delineation of major syndromes of neurosis, the recognition of which is described in the other chapters of the present volume. The diagnosis of personality disorder is multidimensional and requires the clinician more than ever to take a global view of his patient: a decision may need to be

deferred until more can be known, probably with the help of other informants.

The assessment of personality disorder. The assessment of personality disorder presents special problems because of the uncertain validity of the concept, its commonly negative connotations, and the need for a greater degree of retrospective evaluation than in the recognition of neurosis. The theoretical problems of the concept, its demarcation from neurosis and its subclassifications are examined in chapter 1.1.1. The term will be used here in a descriptive sense, broadly following Schneider's (1950) characterization.

Evidence suggesting a descriptive diagnosis of personality disorder may emerge from many areas of the history. Likely indicators of disorder include one or more of the following: recurrent failures and conflicts in interpersonal relationships, marked overdependence on others, frequent changes of employment, repeated brushes with the law or other authorities, recurrent episodes of aggressive or impulsive behaviour, multiple drug abuse, repeated self-injury or overdoses, repeated medical or surgical investigations of unexplained physical symptoms, longstanding instability of mood, marked tendencies to perfectionism or other obsessional traits, excessive introspectiveness and aloofness, recurrent behavioural disorder or neurotic symptoms arising in response to the usual stresses of life (Campbell & Russell, 1982).

Such evidence may at times be open to interpretation as the manifestation of recurrent social difficulties or episodes of neurosis rather than of any enduring and definable psychological propensity. Two diagnoses may be appropriate (as now sanctioned by ICD–9), a syndrome of neurosis to designate current symptoms, and a type of personality disorder for persistent morbid behavioural traits. If we understand personality to mean the constellation of attitudinal, behavioural, and physical characteristics which constitute a person's individuality as seen by others and himself, the patient must be limited in his capacity to know or describe this. His view of himself may be distorted by mental disturbance; other aspects of his current predicament may colour his account of himself. A depressed patient, for example, will commonly describe himself as habitually unhappy and a failure. Information from others, therefore, is likely to be essential in order to gain a reliable picture of how the patient usually behaves.

There will be a strong temptation to make

inferences about the patient's previous personality from observations of his current behaviour, particularly if the patient is seen daily over several days, as, for example, during a hospital admission. Words like manipulative, attention-seeking, or immature often spring readily to mind. In psychiatry, however, it is essential to remember that a person may, for all sorts of reasons, behave in a way that is atypical of him. Attempts to validate an attribution of personality disorder should always be pursued with care, and in the absence of strong evidence it is best to reserve judgement.

Therapeutic implications of diagnosing personality disorder. Neurosis is often taken to represent a discontinuity in the patient's mental functioning, whereas personality disorder implies continuity. The apparent difference between them may possibly stem more from the different view-points from which we can choose to view mental turmoil than from a real difference in the nature of disorder. The distinction commonly carries other implications. For instance, attributions of personality disorder tend to carry with them negative connotations of chronicity or unresponsiveness to treatment. There is a temptation to see the patient in terms of unfavourable stereotypes which may well mean that too little attention is paid to his individual strengths and weaknesses. Furthermore, if the patient's difficulties are considered intrinsic to his personality, the particular factors which led to his current distress and search for help may be given too little importance. Treatment, if pursued, may be directed towards grandiose notions of reconstructing the personality rather than towards the alleviation of factors associated with current disequilibration or the provision of future potential support. For many patients diagnosed as having personality disorders, there appear to be periods of time or particular environments in which their suffering or the suffering they cause to others is greatly diminished or absent. The clinician may do well to try to identify from the history and from the progress of an open-ended assessment the necessary conditions for such relative well-being, and thus strive to attain the more limited goals which may suffice to re-establish a tolerable normality. To this end it may be helpful to construct a life chart as a means of identifying meaningful patterns of development and change, or a significant temporal relationship between events and symptoms. Three vertical columns are used to record the sequence over time of (1) symptoms, (2) life-events, and (3) medical and other interventions. By this means, significant correlations can often be seen which might not otherwise be evident.

Summary and conclusions

The evaluation of neurotic and personality disorders is an essential part of the general psychiatric and medical assessment. It is more elusive and difficult than the evaluation of psychotic disorders because of the limited value of expressing neurotic and personality deviations in terms of descriptive diagnoses. These deviations are more often quantitative than qualitative, and their appearance and fluctuations are often closely interwoven with significant life-events and situations. The discussion has been confined to the use of the psychiatric interview. The interview is a means of obtaining detailed information about the patient and assessing diagnosis, causation, pathogenesis, and pathoplastic factors. But the value of the psychiatric interview extends beyond this, to include an essential therapeutic component, not only in evaluating therapeutic possibilities in the light of the information obtained, but also as a direct result of the interaction between psychiatrist and patient.

Among the components of the psychiatric interview, the introduction and the conclusion have been stressed because in practice they are often neglected and are crucial in establishing good rapport with the patient. There is no ideal method of conducting the interview, but it is recommended to rely as much as possible on the 'conversational' method which allows the patient maximum spontaneity. A systematic exploration of symptoms might be confined to those of greatest relevance, though a judicious combination of both methods is usually necessary.

The appraisal of the interviewer's observations should in the first instance be expressed according to standard rules such as recognized classifications of disorders, but it will also be necessary to go beyond this in order to do justice to the individual nature of the patient and his disorder, while exercising caution in matching the conclusions to the available evidence. In particular a careful assessment of the patient's premorbid personality is essential, as well as an appraisal of the role of previous events and the current life situation.

Thus the psychiatric assessment must be flexible and modified according to circumstances. It is always helpful, however, for the interviewer to have in mind a suitable frame of reference. He may depart from it from time to time in the course of the interview, but it will prove most useful in reminding him of areas of enquiry that may initially have been omitted. It will also lend structure to the recording of his observations and inferences. Such a framework is summarized in the appendix that follows.

Appendix

History
Reason for referral
Complaints
Present illness
Problems experienced, severity and effects, mode of onset and subsequent course, situational and temporal relationships, accompaniments, treatment already received. (The present illness may alternatively be recorded at the end of the history so that it can be seen against the background of other historical information.)

Personal biography
Family history. Father, mother, and siblings: biographical details. Where brought up and by whom. Family history of mental disorder and psychiatric treatment, other illnesses. Family relationships and atmosphere. Separations and bereavements – dates and reaction. Current contact with family.

Personal history. Early development: Mother's pregnancy; birth, infancy, milestones. *Childhood health:* including behaviour disorders, neurotic symptoms. *Education:* Schools and college attended, scholastic attainments. Interests. Relationships, behaviour. *Adolescence:* Changes in attitudes, relationships, behaviour. *Occupations:* Detailed history, including military service. Reasons for changes. Satisfaction. Income. Relationships to colleagues and superiors.

Ambitions. Dates and nature of most recent employment. Time off through illness.

Sexual history. Puberty, menarche, menstrual history. Sexual education. Masturbation. Hetero- and homosexual experience, fantasies, inclinations. Sexual relationships, satisfaction, or difficulties. Contraception. Pregnancies. *Marital history:* Biographical details, occupation and health of spouse or cohabitee. Children. Quality of relationship.

Medical history. Serious illnesses, operations, head injuries, hospital admissions, past and current treatment. Relationship with general practitioner.

Previous mental health. Details of previous treated or untreated psychiatric disorders; duration, precipitating factors. Treatment; efficacy and by whom.

Antisocial behaviour: Delinquent or criminal behaviour, convictions.

Drug use and abuse: Alcohol, tobacco or other drugs of dependence. Hypnotics, tranquillizers, analgesics. Past and recent use.

Personality before illness
(1) Capacity for interpersonal relationships: ease, intimacy. (2) Attitudes to self. Strengths, weaknesses. Future ambitions. (3) Moral attitudes and standards. (4) Mood and temperament. (5) Hobbies and other leisure interests. (6) Fantasy life, dreams. (7) Reactions to stress, disappointment, or frustrations.

Current life situation and review of past year
Housing, domestic relationships, financial situation, job opportunities, social life, emotional support, contact with helping agencies. Recent conflicts, disappointments, bereavements, or other changes and upheavals. Recent physical health.

Mental state assessment in neurosis and personality disorders
General appearance and behaviour
These include dress, posture, demeanour, motor activity, manner towards interviewer (and accompanying relatives or others), credibility as historian, consistency of verbal and non-verbal behaviour.

Form of talk
Spontaneity, flow, speed, quantity, coherence, relevance.

Mood
Quality, severity, constancy, reactivity. Associated evidence of affective disturbance.

Preoccupations and other content of thought
These include suicidal ideas or intent, obsessions, phobias, hypochondriacal or other morbid ideas and attitudes.

Abnormal perceptions and sensations
These include depersonalization, illusions, vivid imagery.

Cognitive functions
These include attention and concentration, language functions, intelligence.

Insight and appraisal of illness
These include beliefs about nature and origins of problems, wishes about treatment, motivation for change, denial, and other mechanisms of defence.

2.2
Clinical assessment of the emotionally disturbed child and his family
ANTONY D. COX

The aims of a clinical assessment

Clinical assessment should produce information which enables the clinician to make decisions about treatment. It follows that clinical assessment must continue throughout therapy. Knowledge about the status of problems and the progress of treatment ideally produce continuously re-evaluated hypotheses which are tested by further investigation and by modification of the therapeutic approach.

This section concentrates on those initial contacts with a child and his family which lead to the first substantive formulation about the referred problem and the first treatment decisions. Contacts will be necessary on several occasions and relevant persons outside the immediate family must also be approached.

At the point of referral the Child Psychiatric team is relatively ignorant of the problem; the child and his family are relatively ignorant of the range of treatments. If treatment is warranted, the team and the family need to collaborate. Therefore assessment must also prepare for intervention. It should facilitate therapy: not prejudice it.

Diagnostic considerations

(a) Most symptoms and behaviours indicative of psychiatric disorder in children are quantitatively rather than qualitatively different from behaviours displayed in the normal course of life and development. (Rutter, Tizard & Whitmore, 1970). Whether

intervention is merited must be decided from knowledge of the age and sex of the child, the cultural appropriateness of the behaviour, (Cox & Rutter, 1976) and from criteria of severity. The best criteria are persistence and impact: whether the behaviour or emotional state persistently produces personal suffering, restriction of social life, interference with normal development, or adverse affects on others. (Rutter *et al.*, 1970). Handicapping symptoms rarely exist in isolation: six or more are commonly present in a child with a psychiatric disorder. (Rutter, Cox, Tupling, *et al.*, 1975a). Certain symptoms, such as disturbance of peer relationships, are better indices of the presence of a disorder than others, for example, nail biting (Rutter *et al.*, 1970).

(b) Most symptoms and behaviour indicative of psychiatric disorder in children are manifest during interactions with others and are influenced by those interactions (Cox & Rutter, 1976). Two corollaries are that (1) what happens may differ with different situations, and (2) referral means that there is a dysfunction in the web of relationships surrounding the child and not necessarily in the child himself. Thus in making an appraisal it is necessary to obtain information from a variety of sources and by a variety of means. Anything that is observed may be relevant, not just what occurs in the consulting room. There must be understanding of why there has been a referral and why it has occurred at this point in time.

(c) Most psychiatric disorders in children are multifactorial in origin. If the assessment is to suggest the best mode and point of intervention there must be distinctions (1) between factors which have precipitated the problem and those which are maintaining it, and (2) between factors acting directly on the index child and those mediated through parents or others. It is also helpful to formulate the problem from a variety of different theoretical standpoints.

(d) Such a formulation should start with descriptive statements and progress to more inferential ones. At the beginning is a brief summary of the data which contribute to the subsequent hypotheses about aetiology, views of prognosis, and plans for treatment. The first axis diagnosis using the multi-axial system is intended to be descriptive (Rutter, Shaffer, & Sturge, 1975b) and is therefore conveniently appended to an initial outline of child characteristics, behaviour, and symptoms. Major factors which research confirms as often causal can then be listed: such as those in the child, the family, and the social circumstances as well as any life events. Thereafter, hypotheses about why matters are in their present state can be placed under different conceptual headings: genetic, developmental, psychodynamic, behavioural, and family or systems theory. The formulation logically concludes with prognosis and plans for intervention.

Modes of assessment

Reports. Reports can usefully be taken from the referred child, parents, other family members, teachers, and other professionals concerned with the child. The methods can vary in their degree of structure and standardization. The main techniques are interviews, questionnaires, diaries, and free written reports.

Interviews with parents or adults can cover a wide range of items relatively efficiently, including uncommonly occurring events or behaviour (Cox, 1975). The information must be viewed with caution, because retrospective recall is frequently biased and inaccurate: more so for distant happenings (Hart, Bax & Jenkins, 1978). Behavioural sequences and contingencies are not reliably reported even when they are recent (Douglas, Lawson, Cooper & Cooper, 1968) and some qualitative aspects of interactions cannot be obtained. Individual children may give more reliable data on their feelings, attitudes, and peer relationships (Rutter & Graham, 1968): they may reveal significant items kept secret by parents. The more people present in the interview the more limited the range and detail of the reports, but the more that can be observed of interactions.

Although quick and efficient, questionnaires only cover a limited range of items and with little detail. They are also subject to bias that cannot be so readily checked as in an interview. If standardized they are useful for registering change (Cox, 1975).

The great value of a diary is that it can be prospective. However, since diaries are usually completed by untrained observers (the parents) the recordings may be delayed and inaccurate and can cover only a limited range of events (Cox, 1975).

Observation. Any person in the child's circle may usefully be observed in interaction with the child or another. Various interviews, for example, family and marital interviews, provide settings in which observations can occur. Because of situational variation, observation in different settings and at different times is important.

Like interviews and other reports observation schemes can be more or less structured or standardized. Vital but infrequent events may not happen while the observer is present but direct observation is the best way to obtain details of behavioural sequences and contingencies, non-verbal behaviour, and patterns of communication (Cox, 1975). It is crucial to the assessment of the mental state of both children and parents. Standardized observations such as those which occur during psychological assessment are valuable for comparative purposes, but because they are necessarily structured, behaviour may be very different from that occurring naturally. Less structured observations such as might occur in a family interview at home tend to provide opportunities for a more limited but more natural range of responses. If the observer is more active, as in an interview, he will be less accurate in observation and recording. More immediate records are more accurate (May & Miller, 1977).

Techniques in commonly used modes of assessment

Interviews with parents. Parents will report most problems spontaneously, so they should be encouraged to talk (Rutter & Cox, 1981; Cox, Hopkinson & Rutter, 1981; Rutter, Cox, Egert, Holbrook & Everitt, 1981; Cox, Rutter & Holbrook, 1981), since this also facilitates the expression of feelings and attitudes. It is necessary to probe for details of problems: contingencies, frequency, impact, course, and so forth, (Cox, Rutter & Holbrook, 1981), and later in the interview checks should be made for problems not spontaneously mentioned. If detailed descriptions of behaviour and events are requested, their reporting often gives good information on feelings, as well as events and behaviours. A responsive and sympathetic manner combined with an attentiveness to areas of concern to the parents probably facilitates both expression of emotion and co-operation in therapy (Duehn & Proctor, 1977). If necessary, information about feelings and more intimate or threatening matters can be obtained by direct request (Rutter & Cox, 1981; Hopkinson, Cox & Rutter, 1981; Rutter, Cox, Egert, Holbrook & Everitt, 1981; Cox, Holbrook & Rutter, 1981). Reflection of feelings may also promote emotional expression; however, too much disclosure of feelings or intimate matters at the first interview may produce anxiety so that the parent does not return a second time. Family life and relationships can be probed by asking about who does what, and with whom, and by asking about areas of disagreement and dissatisfaction, for example, child rearing (Brown & Rutter, 1966; Rutter & Brown, 1966). An active interview technique promotes subsequent co-operation in therapy (Heilbrun, 1974).

Interviews with children. Children have usually been brought to the clinic, they have not chosen to come. It is important to understand how they see the referral and explain what is intended (Cox & Rutter, 1976). The interviewer needs to lead the child into, and support him in, communication. The mode of communication must be adjusted to suit the age, development, and personality of the child: the appropriate admixture of play, drawing, and talk. Indirect and implicit approaches to feelings through play or discussion of others are usually more effective than a head-on technique. Confidentiality should be clarified. The most important function at the initial interview with the child is often engagement with a view to therapy, rather than the discovery of data contributing to the formal diagnosis: this latter usually comes mostly from the parental interview (Rutter, Tizard & Whitmore, 1970). However, the interview with the child is crucial in the diagnosis of certain mental states: psychoses of childhood or adult type, depression, and hyperkinetic syndromes. For the latter, tasks which assess attention and distractibility are useful.

Family interviews. A wide variety of techniques is currently used (Haley, 1976; Satir, 1964) but in most the interviewer takes an active role from the outset: engaging all family members, demonstrating that he values everyone's communications, and promoting interaction. Talk about the referred problem often starts a session. Discussion between pairs of family members may be used. There is variation in the extent to which it is recommended that historical data are brought in. Techniques include construction of a family tree actively employing all family members, and exploring the development of the parents' relationship. Sculpting can produce useful hypotheses about family divisions and alliances. Standard family tasks are also available.

Questionnaires. The most commonly used questionnaires are the teachers' scales devised by Rutter (1967), Stott (1963), and Conners (1969). There are also parent questionnaires. In clinical as opposed to research use these can point to areas of difficulty and be used

to assess change. They do not substitute for interviews with the appropriate teachers.

Diary. It can be helpful to ask parents to record the occurrence and duration of certain events (for example, temper tantrums), their context, and the parents' own response. Usually a report of only one or two types of events can be requested.

Neurological screening of the child. With younger children a neurological screening examination can be performed in the context of play: only baring arms and legs and removal of shoes and socks is necessary. The main items are movements of the eye, tongue, and face; testing of hearing and vision; distal limb power, tone, and coordination; posture, gait, and balance; deep tendon reflexes; plantar responses and fundal examination. Neuro-developmental features also requiring assessment are speech and language, clumsiness, visuo-motor disabilities, mirror movements, and involuntary movements. (Cox & Rutter, 1976).

Observation. Observation is a vital component of all interviewing; however, it is difficult to observe all that is happening, especially if more than one person is interviewed. It is useful to have a colleague observing through a one-way screen or by means of closed circuit TV. In certain circumstances more systematic observation, with or without an interviewer, can aid the assessment, for instance, in the classroom or of parent(s) and child at play in clinic or home.

Choice and ordering of modes of assessment

Every type of assessment in every setting could be advocated. Considerations of economy and the need to maintain co-operation in therapy mean that selection is necessary. Selection is influenced by:

(i) Certain assessments are crucial for certain problems, for instance, an individual interview with a family member who may be psychotic or depressed.

(ii) Assessment teams function better if they have routine methods. These give experience that enables behaviour to be compared and its significance to be assessed and also give confidence to team members.

(iii) If a particular therapy is envisaged assessment in that mode is usually indicated.

(iv) If the trust of family members is to be won:

(a) Information must not be sought without permission.

(b) The limits of confidentiality need to be established.

(c) A child/adolescent might be best seen before or with his parent.

(v) There is some evidence:

(a) That more families drop out of family therapy than therapy where the parents and referred child are seen separately (Shapiro & Budman, 1973).

(b) The first attendance of index child and parents is equally good whether the whole family or only the index child and his parents are asked to attend.

(c) That continued attendance is more likely if individual contacts follow a family assessment than if a family assessment follows individual interviews, with parent(s) and child.

It follows that if a family assessment and/or family therapy is intended, then first contact should be with the whole family. Individual assessment interviews with parent(s) and child, psychological testing, and neurological screening can follow; on another occasion, if necessary. Permission to contact other relevant informants such as teachers and GPs can be obtained at the first session.

If the child/adolescent has a severe disorder (psychosis or depression) which may merit immediate admission, or a disorder where individual assessment is crucial to diagnosis, a meeting with the child by himself will usually be necessary at the first contact. Family and individual interviews can, of course, follow one another on the same occasion.

2.3
Clinical assessment of the mentally handicapped child and his family

DEREK RICKS

To almost all parents early experience of their baby is a delight. The early fulfilment and enjoyment in prospect is tragically shattered by the realization that their child is mentally retarded. It cannot be too strongly emphasized how fundamental is the distress and sense of shame and helplessness such an event generates in parents, siblings, relatives, and, to varying degrees, in all those holding themselves responsible for helping such a family – including the doctor assessing the affected child. Professional satisfaction for doctors depends on being able not only to identify, but to some extent at least, ameliorate, the suffering with which their patients confront them. The retarded child and his family test this to the limit. The tragedy, compounded by the uncertainty of even small improvements, may arouse great concern and a deep sense of obligation which cannot apparently be met. In few fields of medicine is there a greater need for the clinician at the outset to recognize the manner and extent to which his own discomfort intrudes into his professional handling of the assessment. If he does not, he may conscientiously seek refuges all too readily available. He may resort to detailed investigations which have no practical consequences for the child's management. He may refer him to therapists to 'improve his functioning' in, for example, standing or talking, without admitting realistic limits to what can be expected. He may prescribe drugs to counteract behaviour he may well suspect to be situationally determined. Above all he may need to protect himself from sharing with the family the misery and anger that they feel. Since the purpose of assessing the retarded child is to elucidate his handicap, and how and to what extent it can be reduced, and since this will be an ongoing process, largely within his home and implemented by family members, then a crucial initial aim is to secure, as far as one can, their confidence and trust. However thorough or erudite the technical assessment of their child may be, it will be virtually valueless unless it equips the child's family to understand, accept, and work with his or her handicap. To achieve this, the doctor's primary aim must be to establish an honest dialogue for which the main prerequisite is to be honest with himself by recognizing his limits and coping with his own vulnerability (Woodmansey, 1971).

At the stage when the retarded child is referred to the psychiatrist for assessment, the origins of his handicap will usually already have been investigated and the findings conveyed to his parents. Apart from the obvious need to acquaint himself with these findings, the psychiatrist would be well advised to explore the parents' own understanding of this data. This implies no discredit to clinicians or departments previously involved but simply recognizes that parents need repeated opportunities to comprehend what they have been told has happened to their child – and the only way to find this out is initially to ask rather than tell them. In the same way, their view of their child's handicap, that is, what *they* regard as important in his disability, should be the starting point of the assessment with the aim of explaining as carefully as possible the connection between aetiology and handicap as they understand them. Parents need help to make their own practical sense out of their affected child, even to begin working effectively with him (see Ricks, chapter 1.4.1, p. 50).

The child should be observed together with his parents. This will provide behaviour pointers which will prove helpful for a subsequent, more detailed examination. At the same time the observations will clarify the parents' own priorities, whether these are a need for medical explanation, help with everyday management, or, rarely, concern for the future. With the multiple handicapped child a careful clinical examination is imperative, although it may need to be in stages; it may direct attention to other productive tests (Cavanagh, 1980) and it will confirm the assessor's level of concern simply by his taking pains and patience to complete it.

A major limitation of formal assessments in clinical surroundings is that, although signs may be elicited revealing pathology, and standardized tests may measure the degree of retardation (both of which are likely to be painfully self-evident to the family), such procedures rarely reveal what a child *can* do or will attempt spontaneously. Yet these are really the foundations on which to build, and will be elicited only in a familiar setting. Thus, no comprehensive assessment of the child is complete without a home visit; indeed the initial examination in the clinic acts as a prelude to such a visit, to be followed by a dialogue between professionals and the family on the child's developmental programme. Such a visit can reinforce, indeed establish, the credibility of a developmental programme earlier formulated in the clinic since it enables a sensitive, trained team to take stock of highly significant domestic variables. Relative accessibility of bathroom, lavatory, bedroom, and stairs dominate much of the everyday care of the dependent child; fencing, garden size, disposition of outside doors and available food cupboards that of the hyperactive child; the availability of separate rooms for siblings, the attitude of neighbours, the flexibility and overlap of working commitments are all practical issues which determine the feasibility of supposedly helpful advice emerging from the child's assessment.

If the assessment is to be more than a bureaucratic exercise then it should lay the foundations for future management, indicating as far as possible a sequence of stages and their likely duration towards preferably short term and modest objectives. In this way assessment continues into a service for the child and his family generating a working relationship and mutual respect between them and the assessing team for the testing years ahead.

2.4
Psychological testing
PADMAL DE SILVA

Psychological testing has an important role to play in the assessment of psychiatric patients, but this role varies with the nature of the problems presented. In the assessment of neurotic patients and those with personality disorder, this tends to be more limited than with certain others groups of patients, such as the mentally subnormal and those with, or suspected of, organic brain damage.

Testing of intelligence and specific abilities
With adult neuroses and personality disorders, formal intelligence testing is not normally required. There may, however, be cases where the psychiatrist feels that a patient's complaint, or other difficulties unravelled during the interview, may be related to – if not caused by – low intelligence. These would be appropriate to refer to a psychologist for formal testing of intelligence. For example, a housewife presenting with anxiety may turn out to have difficulties in managing the household expenses, or to find her weekly shopping a stressful experience. Although she is clearly not subnormal, it is possible that the difficulties arise from a mild degree of handicap; this could be either in general intelligence or a specific deficit such as very poor numerical ability. Formal intelligence testing, followed if necessary by special testing of arithmetical skills, should throw light on the nature of her problems.

Intelligence tests
There are several tests of intelligence for adults, the most widely used among them being the Wechsler Adult Intelligence Scale (Wechsler, 1955, 1958, 1981; see also Matarazzo, 1972). This test yields an overall Intelligence Quotient (IQ), and two separate IQs for verbal and performance (visuo-spatial) abilities. As in other intelligence tests, an IQ of 90–110 is considered to be average. A patient with a score of 80–90 is considered 'dull normal' and one with 70–80 'borderline subnormal', while scores below 70 are taken as indicative of subnormality. If our hypothetical patient's IQ happens to be in the 70–80 range, this would explain her difficulties in managing her expenses and shopping. The WAIS also gives separate scores (each with a mean of 10) on its sub-tests (for example, comprehension, arithmetic, vocabulary, block design), and a patient's specific difficulties may be assessed by examining the pattern of sub-test scores obtained.

When the need is for a quick general assessment of a patient's intelligence, Raven's Progressive Matrices and the Mill Hill Vocabulary Scale, which can be administered without the assistance of a psychologist, may be used (Raven, 1956, 1958; Raven, Court & Raven, 1978).

Specific abilities
Specific handicaps may be further explored with the aid of attainment tests of reading, spelling, arithmetic and so forth (see below). These are usually meant for children but, if handicap or low educational attainments are suspected, they may profitably be used with adults, as low individual scores will then reflect specific deficits.

Deterioration
Occasionally, the intelligence and attainment testing may show a level of functioning, in a middle-aged or elderly patient, which is quite low in comparison with the person's previous functioning as indicated by jobs held, examinations passed, and so on. Such a finding could be significant, as it could indicate some deterioration in the cognitive ability of the patient, thus suggesting an organic process.

Personality
Personality assessment is an area of psychological testing which used to be popular, but is rapidly declining in interest (Mischel, 1968). The evidence for the value of projective tests of personality is

unsatisfactory (Jensen, 1959). In the UK, the most widely used personality test is the Eysenck Personality Questionnaire, which is a paper and pencil test. This test, which is relatively easy to administer and score, yields three scores: psychoticism (tough-mindedness), extraversion/introversion, and neuroticism (emotionality) (Eysenck & Eysenck, 1975). Extreme scores in these dimensions, in relation to the age and sex norms that are available, can be of use in elucidating the overall picture of the patient, particularly in the case of a personality disorder. On the whole, however, personality testing of the conventional type (for example, projective, paper and pencil) adds little to what can be gained from clinical interviews and/or direct behavioural assessment (see below).

Other types of assessment

There are some other types of tests which are relevant in the assessment of neurotic patients. Specific instruments have been developed for the assessment of the nature, extent, and degree of certain disorders, and are a useful adjunct in assessment, especially in providing a quantified index that would help in monitoring therapeutic change. Among these the commonest are: the Wolpe-Lang Fear Survey Schedule (Wolpe & Lang, 1964), the Leyton Obsessional Inventory (Cooper, 1970), the Maudsley Obsessional Compulsive Inventory (Hodgson & Rachman, 1977; Rachman & Hodgson, 1980), the Beck Depression Inventory (Beck *et al.*, 1961), the Taylor Manifest Anxiety Scale (Taylor, 1953), and the Wolpe-Lazarus Assertiveness Scale (Wolpe & Lazarus, 1966).

Finally, psychologists also carry out, in appropriate circumstances, what has been described as 'functional analysis' or 'behavioural analysis' of problem behaviours (Kanfer & Saslow, 1969; Hersen & Bellack, 1976). When a clear analysis of the problem behaviour is desired, say, for example, in the case of a young woman who blushes excessively in certain social situations, such an approach can be invaluable. This type of analysis, based on close enquiry and – where needed – direct observation, would elucidate the antecedents of the behaviour in question, the nature of the behaviour itself, and the consequences of it. This would not only give a clear picture of the problem behaviour, but might also indicate ways in which a behaviourally-oriented treatment programme may be planned to modify it.

Assessment of children

In the assessment of disturbed children, psychological testing is of crucial importance. An accurate estimate of intellectual ability is invaluable, indeed essential, in understanding and describing the child's difficulties (for example Rutter, Shaffer & Sturge, 1975). The most widely used instrument for this is the Wechsler Intelligence Scale for Children, in its revised form (Wechsler, 1974, 1976). Equally important is the assessment of educational attainment and specific deficits. Several useful tests are available for this purpose. These include: the Neale Analysis of Reading Ability (Neale, 1966), the Schonell reading and writing tests (Schonell & Schonell, 1960), Vernon Graded Word Spelling Test (Vernon, 1977), Vernon–Miller Graded Arithmetic-Mathematics Test (Vernon & Miller, 1976), and the APU Arithmetic Test (Closs & Hutchins, 1976). In addition, specific problem behaviours, (for example, tantrums, aggressiveness, disruptive behaviour, tics) can be profitably investigated by direct behavioural assessment methods (see above).

The role of the psychologist

A note may be added, at this point, on the role of the psychologist in the assessment of psychiatric patients. The expertise the psychologist brings into this field is that of someone specifically trained to observe, assess and evaluate. The quantified data provided by the psychologist – as in intelligence testing – lend an objectivity which can usefully supplement the psychiatrist's clinical conclusions. There are also occasions when clinical evaluation conceals or distorts a person's true level of functioning, and psychological testing will help to minimize errors and inaccuracies. For example, the clinical assessment of a patient in the psychiatrist's interview may lead to the conclusion that the patient has a gross deficit – say, in concentration and memory. It is possible, however, that such a conclusion, based on the patient's subjective reports and the very limited sample of his performance in the interview situation, could be inaccurate. A systematic psychological test session could act as a useful corrective in such situations. Finally, in the case of patients whose treatment itself may be behavioural, the psychologist's preliminary analysis becomes an essential starting point for the therapy itself.

3
Principles of treatment in the neuroses and personality disorders

3.1
Methods of treatment

3.1.1
Psychotherapy
NANCY SWIFT

Psychotherapy is often defined as treatment by psychological means. Such a sparse definition, unpretentious by customary medical standards, has the disadvantage of being unenlightening, since the terms 'psychological treatment' and 'psychotherapy' are synonyms. If, however, as Aubrey Lewis (1956) and others have suggested, the expression 'psychological treatment' is taken to refer to those methods which primarily depend upon a direct and personal relationship between the patient and the therapist, and which rely on the capacity of that relationship to influence the patient in the direction of emotional health and a greater sense of well-being, then some progress towards a clearer conception of the nature of psychotherapy is achieved.

The personal influence of the doctor upon his patient is, of course, and always has been, an inescapable aspect of all healing procedures, from primitive and magical suggestions and rituals, through the activities of the temple priests of Aesculapius, down to the most technical and advanced techniques of modern medicine and surgery. Whether or not the physician or surgeon accepts the impact of his personality upon the response of his patient, there is no shadow of doubt that the sufferer himself is conscious of the need to respect and trust the person to whom he goes, in time of sickness or distress, and into whose hands he may have to put his life. This is manifest in the way in which ill people try to exercise choice in the matter of their doctors, and the more sophisticated they are the greater is that drive, so that doctors and nurses are the most selective of all when their time of need arises. It is also demonstrated in the simple language and behaviour of the people, from whom one so often hears: 'Well, no, I couldn't go to him (or her), or stay with him. I just haven't got any faith in him and anyway I don't like him'. Wisely the prophet of old proclaimed, 'Where there is no vision the people perish'. All medical treatments have a psychological facet and are influenced by the doctor–patient relationship, but the psychotherapies are dependent upon that powerful force, used within the particular body, or bodies, of theory which the therapist favours. There are many types of psychotherapy, which may be classified and examined, but there are certain features common to them all, as Jerome D. Frank (1963) has pointed out: there must be an individual who seeks help and perceives the need of it, an accepted, authoritative healer, and a structured procedure, usually in the form of planned interviews or treatment sessions, which are consistent and disciplined.

All psychotherapies have cognitive, emotional, and behavioural aspects. The overall goals of treatment are that the patient shall come to know about himself things of which he was hitherto unaware, or unclear, and shall undergo in the therapeutic encounter important, often intense, feelings which have the quality of illuminating emotional revelations, by nature inaccessible to the intellectual self. Finally, the goal is to achieve, through the interaction of these new insights, beneficial change in maladaptive personal reactions and behaviours.

There is a general, but mistaken tendency to equate psychotherapy with psycho-analysis. This is not surprising in view of the impact on psychological thought made by Freud and the various later analytic schools which, although widely divergent, nevertheless all took their original inspiration from that great man. However, there are many forms of treatment which are certainly psychological but which are not analytic or dynamic in the accepted sense. A useful way of distinguishing the main therapeutic approaches is to classify them into two groups which differ in method and goals. Jerome D. Frank (1963) distinguishes treatments which are directive from those which are evocative or, more familiarly in British terminology, dynamic.

Directive treatments

Directive treatments include all those methods which concern themselves with the symptom, or constellation of symptoms, which the patient presents but which do not address themselves in any depth to the personality of the sufferer. A rough analogy in general medical procedure would be the removal of a painful renal stone with impressive symptomatic relief but with inattention to the underlying metabolic disorder which brought about its development. However, relief from pain, whether it is physical or psychic, is always desirable, provided it does not mask a dangerous underlying pathology to the ultimate detriment of the patient. It must also be accepted in psychological, as it is in physical, medicine that it is sometimes the most that can be accomplished.

Treatments which make a direct assault on the patient's complaints and aim at ameliorating specific symptoms include supportive psychotherapy which amounts, in discussion, to sympathetic examination of the problems, explanation, and sometimes directive advice. It offers the patient an opportunity to ventilate his fears, angers, and frustrations to a concerned, but objective, listener who is both respected and authoritative. The patient is gratified by the attention paid to him, which must be concentrated, and he may be influenced by persuasion, advice, and cautious criticism in the condition of emotional arousal and accessibility which such a therapeutic encounter engenders. Supportive therapy is often coupled with special techniques such as suggestion (Karl Jaspers, 1963), challenge (Taylor, F. Kräupl, 1969), relaxation exercises (Barlow, Wilfred, 1973) and a wide range of behaviour procedures, including aversion therapies and gradual dehabituation (Gelder & Marks, 1966). Other interventions of a practical kind, usually undertaken by the social worker, include attempts to modify noxious environmental conditions such as poverty, family tension, lack of satisfactory occupation, or pressure of stressful and unduly demanding work conditions. The patient may, for a time, be removed, by his own consent, from an exhausting environment by short hospital admissions, so providing an ordered and protective atmosphere, or by the arrangement of a recuperative holiday, or attendance at a day hospital. These methods are used in almost all good general psychiatric practice and are often, and properly, combined with physical treatments, in particular, drug therapies. It would be as irrational to make control of symptoms the goal without at times calling upon the roomy resources of modern pharmacology, as to treat a slipped disc conservatively, without analgesics.

Dynamic psychotherapy

Dynamic psychotherapy is a much more radical procedure, both in concept and method. It is not so much concerned with the immediate problems as with the possible underlying psychopathology which brings about the disturbed responses and the symptom formation. Its goal is, for patient and therapist working together, to understand what has happened and is happening, both cognitively and emotionally, and thereby to correct, or more commonly ameliorate, the effects of the patient's distorted psychic development. Such distortions cripple the individual's experience of himself, and others, and often give rise to profound and personally unmanageable distress.

Within the phenomena of conscious functions are two areas which are accessible, the conscious and subconscious, or pre-conscious. The former comprises that material which is in the forefront of the mind at any particular moment of time, and the latter that material which can, by an effort of will, or an act of deliberate attention, be brought to awareness. Thus, whilst thinking of, or responding to, events in which one is presently engaged, it is possible to draw upon a vast store of memory of other events, feelings, and learned activity, which is not in immediate consciousness but which is available to recall. Such material may also erupt spontaneously, either elaborating or disturbing a current train of thought. The third area of psychological being, the unconscious mind, is widely postulated but not available to direct experience. Recognition of the importance of unconscious mental processes was the cornerstone upon which Freud (1971) built his psycho-analytic theories, and although other dynamic schools diverge in their concepts of the nature of the unconscious, they all view human experience and behaviour as being influenced by forces in the internal life of the individual of which he is not aware, nor able, without the use of special procedures, to become aware, and then only partially. When the unconscious material is in conflict with the dominant trends of conscious life, the individual is described, most vividly, by Karl Jaspers (1963) as being 'at war with his unconscious', sitting as it were on 'a smouldering volcano'. Such a state of affairs is experienced emotionally in terms of anger, despair, frustration, anxiety, inexplicable turmoil, and often deep loneliness, and is manifested in the whole gamut of the neuroses and sometimes in psychotic phenomena.

The psycho-analytic schools

The assumption that there exist unconscious mental processes was not first made by Freud. On the contrary, it was a concept actively preoccupying philosophers and psychologists before Freud was born (Lancelot Law Whyte, 1960), and certainly taught in schools and universities when he was a boy. Freud himself, in his early years, was probably not much influenced by the metaphysics of such men as Plato, Spinoza, Nietzsche, Schopenhauer, but he must have been exposed to the theories of Johann F. Herbart (1891, Eng. trans.), who died before Freud's birth and, later to those of William James and his followers, with their intense interest in consciousness and, particularly, subconscious or pre-conscious phenomena (James, 1912).

It was, however, Freud who introduced the revolutionary picture of the unconscious as a dynamic force playing an active part in mental life, rather than conceiving of it, as had his predecessors, as a reservoir of memories and ideas which had fallen, by inertia, out of awareness, although they had not become totally extinguished or wholly irrelevant. It was also his belief that certain emotional experiences, fantasies, and sometimes events were actively relegated to the unconscious because they were associated with powerful instinctual drives, unacceptable or frightening to the conscious socialized personality.

Before 1900 Freud had developed the concepts of repression, the means whereby threatening experiences were banished to the unconscious; resistance, the mechanism by which they were prevented from entering awareness; and transference, the powerful emotional relationship which sprang up between the patient and the analyst, at first astounding Freud but later seen by him as signifying buried feelings, and used by him, in the technique of interpretation, to release such feelings into consciousness, in the hope of diffusing their pathological influence.

However, he believed that so strong were the instinctual drives that, if the individual during the course of his personal development had not been able to diffuse them satisfactorily by acceptable integration into the entirety of his personality, they found expression by indirect means, such as abnormal character traits, clinical symptoms, or deviant behaviour. They could also reveal themselves in such phenomena as slips of the tongue, inexplicable emotional reactions, and, in symbolic form, in dreams. This concept of the dynamic unconscious, with all its implications, was the starting point of Freud's whole theory of psychopathology and with it came the birth of psycho-analysis.

The development of his thought and the influences upon him over the years is a long story, and is beautifully and faithfully chronicled by the most influential of all his British disciples, Dr Ernest Jones, in his biography of Freud (1954, 1955, 1957).

In an account such as this it is possible to refer only to the fundamental postulates upon which Freud built his theories. These are clearly defined in a small but invaluable book by J. A. C. Brown (1961) and can be briefly summarized:

(1) Human psychic life is profoundly influenced and sometimes dominated by unconscious drives, and associated fears.

(2) Human reactions are determined according to the principle of causality, an assumption upon which scientific procedure is, or certainly in Freud's time was, based. This means that he maintained that psychic events have a cause, but he accepted that there was not necessarily a single cause operative, leading him to the idea that human responses may be 'over-determined', that is, the final result of a number of converging causations.

(3) Human behaviour is directed towards the gratification of biologically determined drives, originally seen by him as primarily self-protective and sexual in nature, in accordance with the instinctual strivings towards self-preservation and procreation. He later expanded the sexual nature of 'libido' or 'Triebe' (instinct or drive) and embraced the notion of sublimation as a way whereby pure 'Triebe' could be subjected to civilizing influences, and be expressed in such feelings as love, friendship, and altruism.

(4) He saw personality as a potential which developed in accordance with the influence imposed upon the growing child by the milieu in which he matured; that is, he postulated that the developmental, or historical, approach was of intrinsic significance.

Freud worked, more or less, in isolation until about 1900. During the next ten years there gathered round him a number of outstanding men who were working in the fields of psychology and psychiatry and who were fired by his brilliant revolutionary concepts and his vision. During these years such men as Jung (1953) and Adler (1956) worked closely with Freud and their work became known and publicized widely (the first Journal of Psycho-analysis was published in 1909). These names are mentioned as being the best known of the many early adherents and the first, most determined, of the dissidents.

Both Jung and Adler came to disagree with Freud on fundamental issues of theory, too complex to be discussed in this short essay, and each developed his own school. Adler was a vigorous man of robust intellect and common sense who, while adhering to the importance of biological strivings, broke away from the primary interest in sexual drives and concerned himself more with the dichotomy of 'inferiority' and 'superiority' in human experience. His school of Individual Psychology has gradually ceased to have consistent influence but many of his ideas have been integrated into systems of later, more sociologically orientated, bodies of theory.

Jung, as much a philosopher and theologian as a brilliant psychologist, also became opposed to Freud on the issue of the central importance of sexuality. His work on psychological types was highly regarded, and words now in common usage, such as 'introvert', 'extrovert' and 'complex' were introduced by him. His further elaborate theories included the concepts of universal archetypes, the personal and collective unconscious, in which is stored the psychological heritage, not only of human life but all life, and his own conception of libido as the 'life force'. His thought has a powerfully mystical and religious aura, difficult for the scientifically minded to accept, but his school of Analytic Psychology still functions, and exponents of the methods based on his theories claim, and undoubtedly have, success in the analysis of certain patients, perhaps particularly the elderly, whatever significance that may have.

After the first world war psycho-analytic ideas spread widely into Britain and America, and attracted increasing attention from the general public. Gradually, rigid orthodoxy was replaced, in many places, by attitudes of thought which used many, but not all, of the Freudian concepts and methods. In Britain the so-called eclectic school sprang up, represented by such men as J. A. Hadfield (1950), Ian Suttie (1935) and W. H. R. Rivers (1920), who was a psychologist and distinguished anthropologist. In America G. Stanley Hall, primarily a child psychologist, translated Freud's General Introduction to Psychoanalysis in 1920, and thereafter the more sociologically orientated schools of such people as Karen Horney (1939),

Erich Fromm (1957) and Harry Stack Sullivan (1955) emerged.

Amongst those who came to Britain from the Continent were Freud himself (a refugee from Nazi persecution), his daughter, Anna, and Melanie Klein. Anna Freud (1966a,b), a true daughter of her father, but with her own outstanding brilliance, has devoted herself primarily to the analytic approach to childhood disturbances, and remains today a revered and authoritative leader of her school, which conforms, in essentials, to the theory of adult psycho-analysis.

Melanie Klein (1948), on the other hand, devoted herself to the study of very young children, depending on her observations of their play and behaviour for her theoretical understanding of the primitive emotional drives which motivate human reaction. Very briefly, she envisaged the young child as being caught between the primitive emotional need for security and love (that is 'good feelings') and, when denied these, reactions of aggression, rage, and despair (that is, 'bad feelings') which he sometimes incorporates into himself with disastrous results to his personal well-being. Melanie Klein saw this catastrophic conflict as the inevitable destiny of human experience, and believed that the only pathway to tranquil maturation lay in the early analysis of the dilemma. Thus, in her view, the only hope for humanity lay in the educative emotional experience of analysis for all young children, comparable to – though more essential than – their intellectual education. Her theories, though based on early reactions, are used today in the analysis of adults who, supposedly, bear the stigmata of their early conflicts, and her school flourishes alongside that of the orthodox Freudians, at the Institute of Psychoanalysis.

Group psychotherapy

In these forms of treatment – disregarding the variety of esoteric, cathartic, and overdramatic procedures which have attracted disciples on both sides of the Atlantic in recent years – selected patients meet regularly (either as out-patients or in in-patient therapeutic communities) with one or two trained group leaders. They proceed, as a body, to seek understanding, and some resolution, of their emotional difficulties. During the 1930s custodial care in mental hospitals had begun to yield to more personal contact between staff and patients. In the second world war some British psycho-analysts became interested in group interactions in the Forces, and the study of leader and follower roles among the men. Bion and

Rickman (1943) pioneered this work at the Northfield Military Hospital. A little earlier Bierer (1940) initiated the first therapeutic social club at Runwell Mental Hospital in 1938. This was followed by the establishment of such projects as the Roffey Park Rehabilitation Centres under Ling (1946), the self-governing community at the Cassel Hospital under Main (1946), and the Social Rehabilitation Unit at Belmont Hospital under Maxwell Jones (1957). In the early nineteen-forties S. H. Foulkes (1950) became an authority on the use of psycho-analytically orientated group therapy as a widely applicable psychotherapeutic procedure. Famous names and developments are too numerous to mention here, but an erudite and comprehensive account of the subject has been written by F. Kräupl Taylor (Taylor, 1958).

Techniques of individual treatment

Orthodox analysis as practised, in Britain, by the relatively few fully trained psycho-analysts is a long procedure. As such it is time-consuming and expensive. Analysts themselves may be trained psychiatrists, doctors, or lay persons, all of whom must undergo a personal training analysis and a long course of study and practical work, including the full analysis of at least two selected patients under intensive supervision. Acceptance at the centres for such treatment is not easy, since the personal suitability of the candidates is seen, rightly, to be of central importance. Apart from those who are taken on at the training centres, and treated for a token fee by analysts in training, patients must meet the expense of an analysis themselves. They are expected to see their therapist from three to five times a week, each session lasting fifty minutes, and must envisage attending for anything between two and four years. Since there can, of course, be no guarantee of a successful outcome this is no small undertaking, in terms of time, money, or commitment. The usual procedure is that the patient shall relax on a couch and say aloud whatever comes into his mind, however apparently irrelevant or even obscene. This is the technique of free association introduced by Freud and thought of by him as a pointer to unconscious material. It is curiously difficult to associate freely, since the habit of repression and censorship is in most people so well established. The analyst, out of direct vision, intervenes only with occasional interpretations, often particularly directed to the emotional reactions, either positive or negative, expressed towards himself, and also to dream material which the patient may produce.

Much more common than orthodox analysis is dynamically orientated psychotherapy, which either uses orthodox theory or is eclectic in approach. The procedure is much less rigorous. Interviews are usually conducted face to face, and may take place two or three times a week, or sometimes only once. The impact of the therapist upon the patient is, inevitably, more direct and components of personal influence and suggestion must creep into the encounters. There are various views on the desirability, or otherwise, of this. Rigid analysts deplore it, whereas many therapists see it as an inevitable part of the treatment relationship. It is of interest to recall the words of Aubrey Lewis (1956), not overtly sympathetic to the discipline of psychotherapy – essentially on theoretical grounds – but too wise to deny its value in skilled hands and for certain patients, 'Whatever rules the therapist follows, or whatever training he has undergone, he himself is more important than his method in benefiting his patients.' Individual psychotherapy is practised privately and is available to a limited degree in the Hospital Service. There it is mainly undertaken by psychiatrists in training, under consultant supervision, by dynamically trained social workers and nurses, and by some psychologists.

Selection of patients for individual psychotherapy

It is not beyond average clinical judgement to select patients who are likely to benefit from one or other of the directive therapies discussed earlier in this essay. It is more difficult to decide who is suitable for the more radical dynamic procedures. It must always be borne in mind that dynamic treatment can be profoundly disturbing to the individual, perhaps confronting him with intolerable insights, often depriving him of resistances by which he had managed uneasy, but just viable, adaptations, or fostering in him an introspective and hypochondriacal dependence on the therapist. Hence it may be dangerous. Economic factors are also a serious consideration, in both private and hospital practice, and only those patients who appear to have a good chance of benefit should be taken into treatment. In selecting such patients a few important criteria must be satisfied. The individual must reveal a certain degree of fortitude (ego strength); he must, by his history, show himself capable of persistence and commit-

ment; he must be apparent as a person capable of avoiding 'acting out' (that is, in actual behaviour demonstrating his disturbed feelings); and he must have sufficient intelligence to understand what is happening. This does not mean that he need be of superior intelligence, which sometimes, but not always, will allow him an impenetrable dimension of resistance. Finally there must be some indication that he is capable of rapport, or emotional contact, a judgement which is often dependent, initially, on the intuition of the assessor.

Selection of patients for group psychotherapy

These methods are particularly suitable for patients whose problems appear most clearly in relation to their social adaptations. Appropriate disorders include the social phobics, mild delinquents, the 'family inadequates', and various character disorders, in whom traits of greedy, demanding, self-gratification, alien to other aspects of the personality, produce manifest conflicts and neurotic symptoms. In the face of need to supply help for large numbers of people, who cannot afford to pay, the majority of hospital patients are treated in groups and selection cannot always conform to ideal criteria. In spite of this, for those who persist much relief is often obtained. Group therapy can also, in some centres, be obtained on a private basis.

In the present social climate, a wide range of individuals (trained and untrained) set themselves up as psychotherapists and practise widely, often in orthodox but sometimes in esoteric, ways, and there is no doubt that there are dangers inherent in the exercise of powerful influence by one person (a therapist) upon another (a suppliant) which should give rise to serious considerations. The 'ideal' psychotherapist is an individual of remarkable quality. He is a person capable of warmth and concern, but also of objectivity; he has learned to control his personal judgement values and emotional reactions without loss of sympathy; he has integrity, high intelligence, and the power of intense concentration. He is enlightened, mature, and stable; in the widest sense he is a being capable both of reason and of love. Ideal standards are rarely, if ever, realized, but the more of these attributes a therapist has, the wiser and better the work he, or she, is likely to do.

3.1.2
Behaviour therapy

M. G. GELDER

Behaviour therapy is the name for a group of psychological treatments which have three things in common. They are directed to symptoms and manifest behaviour, they are based on findings from experimental psychology, and they begin with a behavioural analysis of the patient's problems. Each of these points requires some qualification and some comment. Thus, to say that behaviour therapy is directed to symptoms and manifest behaviour may give too narrow an impression of its aims unless it is made clear that the word behaviour is being used in a very wide sense, which includes thoughts, emotions, expectations, and attitudes, as well as observable behaviour. Moreover, although the second characteristic of behaviour therapy, its basis in experimental psychology, is widely accepted, this also requires qualification. When it was new, behaviour therapy was often characterized as 'based on modern learning theory'. Today, few psychologists would wish to assert that there is a single coherent body of learning theory, and recognize instead a few established principles of learning. As well as these principles of learning, behaviour therapy is now based on cognitive and social psychology and increasingly on the observations made in the course of experiments with patients.

The third characteristic of behaviour therapy is that it begins with what is usually called a behavioural analysis of the patient's problems. Although it may seem a little odd to characterize a treatment by the assessment which precedes it, this analysis is in fact the most important common factor in the various forms of behaviour therapy. The analysis begins with a description of the patient's problems and a detailed account of the circumstances in which they increase or diminish. This is followed by the selection of techniques which are likely to modify these behaviours. Now in the present stage of development of behaviour therapy there is not a behavioural technique to match every behavioural problem. When there is not, the therapist must improvise and use any method which seems likely to help his patient, whether it is behavioural or not. It is in these circumstances that counselling and simple forms of directive psychotherapy are often used by behaviour therapists. They are right to use them but they cause unnecessary confusion if they insist that these borrowed techniques are part of behaviour therapy. It is better to think of behaviour therapy being accompanied by non-specific procedures, the latter overlapping those used in psychotherapy.

The range of procedures

There are so many behavioural procedures that some form of classification may be helpful. One useful distinction is between techniques which attempt to modify the link between the target behaviour and the stimuli which precede it, those which set out to change behaviour by altering its consequences, and those which provide training in behaviour which is under-developed. The account which follows serves merely to indicate the range of behavioural methods and to give examples.

The distinction between techniques which are directed to stimuli and those which attend to consequences is important because it reflects what was, until recently, a considerable difference between the practice of behaviour therapy in Britain and in North America. In this country, much attention has been given to desensitization and aversion therapy, both methods which are concerned with stimulus-response relationships. In the United States behaviour therapy grew more from work on operant conditioning and as a result has put more emphasis on the need to modify the consequences of behaviour. Recent findings have vindicated this second approach, but in a way which is somewhat different from that which was adumbrated by the original work in the operant tradition.

In the first group the most important techniques are aversion therapy and the 'deconditioning' methods – desensitization and flooding. These will not be described at length because they are gradually being superseded by other procedures, while a fourth method, covert sensitization, will also be dealt with in brief because its value has not yet been proven. *Desensitization,* developed by Wolpe, was the first practical behaviour therapy technique and it is a landmark in the development of the subject. The method is applied most easily to anxiety states and the first step is to question the patient carefully to determine the full range of stimuli which provoke anxiety and to arrange them in ascending order of severity. Patients are then encouraged either to encounter these stimuli in a carefully graded sequence, or to create them in imagination. In either case, anxiety is inhibited in some way, usually by relaxation exercises but occasionally with anxiolytic drugs. Treatment begins with the stimuli which produce least anxiety and it progresses up the hierarchy one step at a time. Wolpe (1958) provided excellent accounts of desensitization and the method is still widely employed although now gradually being replaced for many purposes by methods which will be described later in this section. In *flooding,* a very different method is used to break the link between the stimuli for anxiety and the response. Instead of a hierarchical approach, patients are encouraged to encounter the most potent stimuli from the start; and instead of attempting to minimize anxiety, it is deliberately encouraged to build up. Moreover, whereas in desensitization the encounters with the stimuli are brief and frequently repeated, in flooding a single encounter is prolonged to an hour or more at a time. Flooding has not been shown to give results which are superior to desensitization (Gelder *et al.,* 1973) and since it is considerably more distressing to the patient, it is gradually passing out of use. In *aversion therapy* an attempt is made to link unwanted behaviour with the response normally associated with aversive stimuli (usually mild electric shock). In this way it is hoped to make unwanted behaviour less likely to occur. The technique has been used most often for alcoholism and sexual deviations but, in both, its effects have proved to be short-lived. For this reason and because it is unpleasant for patients, it is now used infrequently. In *covert sensitization* the aims are similar to those in aversion therapy, but instead of using stimuli like electric shock, unpleasant mental imagery is manipulated. Thus, the patient might imagine a scene which causes disgust and associate this repeatedly with mental images con-nected with his fetishistic behaviour. By reversing the procedure, and imagining pleasant scenes, it is also said to be possible to increase the frequency of desired behaviour. However, although less unpleasant than aversion therapy, its value has still to be proven.

The second group of techniques contains the various methods of operant conditioning and response prevention. One method, *exposure treatment,* is included even though it shares some features with the first group because, although it attempts to modify stimulus response relations, it also pays considerable attention to the consequences of abnormal behaviour. Because it is in frequent use, exposure treatment will be described more fully in the next part of this section, but at this stage we are concerned only with its broad principles. The technique makes use of the common denominator of desensitization and flooding, namely exposure to situations which provoke anxiety. Research has shown that this exposure is most effective when carried out for long periods – an hour or more – and with anxiety kept at a moderate level (Johnston & Gath, 1973). In exposure treatment, attention is also given to the consequences of the abnormal behaviour, particularly the patient's own response to the first symptoms of anxiety (which can serve to magnify it) and the response of family members to the patient. *Operant conditioning* also falls into this second group but we shall meet it again in the third. The essential principle is that any behaviour which is persistent must be under reinforcement resulting from one or more of its consequences – otherwise it would fade away. Thus, if a schizophrenic or subnormal patient displays socially undesirable behaviour in a hospital ward, a search is made for unintentional social reinforcement by the ward staff, who may, unwittingly, be paying more attention to the patient when his behaviour is disturbed than when it is normal. The treatment attempts to alter the balance of the reinforcing consequences using techniques which are discussed further in the next section. Finally in this group we must mention *response prevention,* which finds its main use in the treatment of obsessional rituals. It will be described later and nothing more need be said at this stage.

Treatments in the third group are used when the patient lacks some socially desirable behaviour. The techniques which are employed to encourage such behaviour include operant conditioning, social skills training and some of the approaches to sexual disorders which have been incorporated into behaviour therapy from the work of Masters and Johnson (1970). *Operant conditioning* methods have been referred to already and the reader should have no difficulty in appreciating how they can be directed to encouraging desirable behaviour as well as to discouraging maladaptive habits. *Social skills training* derives from research in social psychology which seeks to explain non-verbal communication in the framework which has been used successfully to analyse motor skills. Patients' deficits in social skills are first identified by watching them in social encounters – for example, starting a conversation with a stranger or making a complaint. A combination of instruction, modelling, and role playing is then used to encourage appropriate behaviour, while the person is shown his own performance by using video recordings. The methods have been widely publicized and well-thought-out manuals have been prepared to guide the therapist (Trower, Bryant & Argyle, 1978). However, the evidence that they have useful and specific effects for psychiatric patients is still incomplete. The *methods for sexual disorders* devised by Masters & Johnson (1970) are now well known. Behaviour therapists have taken over the idea of teaching frigid or impotent patients forms of behaviour which can express tenderness without engendering anxiety. Such methods have also proved their value in the treatment of sexual deviations, where more progress can usually be made by attempting to encourage heterosexual behaviour than by efforts to suppress deviant sexual acts (Bancroft, 1974).

The reader will find a fuller account of some of these behavioural techniques in chapters 9.1, 9.2 and 9.3 on pages 335–6, 344, 349. He is also referred to one of the many comprehensive texts which are available (for example, Gambril, 1977; Garfield & Bergin, 1978).

Selection of patients

Whatever the method of behaviour therapy, certain general principles apply to the selection of patients. Three decisions should be made: whether treatment of any kind is required: if so, whether one of the techniques of behaviour therapy is likely to be the best method; and if it is, whether the patient can be motivated to carry it out. Both the first and last stages are often neglected. It is easy and at times rewarding, but a waste of scarce resources, to treat patients who will recover spontaneously. And much effort can come to nothing if treatment is offered to patients who drop out or take part half-heartedly. For these reasons it is most important that assessment is more than a decision that one or more of the behavioural techniques will fit the case. The first stage is therefore to assess the chances of spontaneous recovery, but also – and this is very important – to seek evidence for a concurrent depressive disorder. If significant depression is present, successful antidepressant treatment may lead to secondary amelioration of the behavioural disorder and remove the need for treatment.

The second stage of assessment is to consider whether effective behavioural techniques exist for the behaviour disorder. In general, *isolated phobias* respond readily to behaviour therapy, *agoraphobia* also does well, but the response of *social phobias* is less predictable. Generalized *anxiety states* are also responsive to relaxation or to anxiety management (see below) though it is not certain how far these effects are specific. *Obsessional rituals* usually respond well to response prevention but the methods for obsessional thoughts are of less certain value. *Hysterical symptoms* do not respond to specific procedures, although behaviour therapy can sometimes act as a useful medium for suggestion. The principles of behavioural analysis are also useful in such cases, particularly in formulating the part which family members are playing in reinforcing the hysterical behaviour (Bird, 1979). Until recently, behaviour therapy had nothing to contribute directly to the treatment of *depressive disorders*. Now cognitive-behavioural methods have been described and it has been claimed that they are as effective as antidepressants (Rush, Beck, Kovacs & Hollon, 1977). They are being evaluated at the time of writing but it is too early to make a definite judgement and the reader should refer to reviews appearing after this book is published.

Tics are one example of a number of less common symptoms which have been treated with behaviour therapy. Though several methods have been described (see Yates, 1970) there is no evidence that any form of behavioural treatment has a substantial and lasting effect. Both *sexual inadequacy* and *sexual deviations* have been treated with behaviour therapy. Sexual inadequacy is usually treated with a combination of methods to reduce anxiety about sexual matters and training in the techniques of sexual intercourse. Homosexual patients who wish to develop any capacities they have for heterosexual behaviour can often be helped by treatment similar to that used for sexual inadequacy. Aversive methods are not recommended. Marital problems have also been treated using principles derived from operant conditioning. They are described in chapter 3.1.3, on page 90.

Among other applications of behaviour therapy are methods to control eating in *obese patients,* alcohol intake in people with *drinking problems,* and *excessive smoking.* In general, these attempt to increase the patient's self-control by encouraging him to keep careful records of the behaviour and the circumstances in which he habitually loses control. At the same time steps are taken to improve motivation and to encourage the family to reinforce the patient's efforts. Finally, behavioural methods have been applied to *antisocial behaviour* and to the behaviour disorder of *schizophrenic* and *subnormal* patients. This may be through programmes of treatment devised for individuals – usually employing methods of operant conditioning – but at times it is by rearranging the organization of wards or whole institutions. In this section we are concerned only with broad principles of treatment, the reader who wishes to learn more of these methods is referred to the account by Garfield and Bergin (1978).

The third stage of assessment is concerned with the patient's motivation for treatment. It is now realized that this is of crucial importance in behaviour therapy, particularly as the methods which have been proved to be effective require considerable effort on the part of the patient, both in treatment and in the intervals between visits to the therapist. The questions which can be used to test the motivation of patients will be obvious enough to the clinician but, however careful the initial enquiry, some uncertainty often remains. For this reason it is usually wise to start with a trial of treatment offering only a small number of sessions of treatment in the first place and agreeing to a full course only if the patient co-operates fully with this first stage. None of the attempts by research workers to predict the outcome of behaviour therapy from variables measured at the beginning has so far been successful.

Principles of treatment illustrated in some commonly used methods

(i) *Exposure treatment for phobias*

This will be discussed at some length because it illustrates several general principles which apply equally to other techniques of behaviour therapy. Effective treatment for patients with severe phobias is now known to differ in an important way from the

treatment which is sufficient for minor phobias: much more depends on the patient's own efforts to overcome the symptoms in his daily life between visits to the therapist and correspondingly less on his response to treatment in the consulting room. As a result, considerable efforts have to be made to motivate patients and to make sure that they understand clearly what is required of them. Neither of these issues emerged clearly from studies of the treatment of minor phobias; they appeared only when clinical trials were carried out with patients. It seems to be generally true that although the techniques appropriate for serious disorders can be discovered by research with simpler problems, the manner in which they have to be applied can only be found out by studying patients.

The essential features of treatment are rather simple. The patient must enter the situations which provoke his fears and must learn not to leave them until fear has subsided. The situations should be chosen to provoke a moderate amount of anxiety and the patient must stay in them for a long time – about an hour seems best. Despite the successes obtained with Wolpe's methods of desensitization, it now appears that it is generally more effective to enter the real situation than it is to imagine it. That moderate anxiety levels are better than very high ones (such as those used in flooding) or very low ones (such as those used in desensitization), is probably because patients need to learn to master feelings of anxiety; and they cannot do this when there is too little anxiety or when there is too much. Anxiety can be reduced by the reassuring presence of the therapist, a relative, or a friend, but the high anxiety levels found at the beginning of treatment may require the use of an anxiolytic drug – a benzodiazepine is usually appropriate. Neither the support of other people nor the use of drugs should be continued for long because the patient must learn self-reliance. It is usual to supplement these simple steps with instructions in anxiety management and the patient must learn to use this both when he is in the situations which provoke fear and also immediately before he goes into them, for anxious anticipation is an important component of most phobic states.

It has been found best for the person treating the patient to act more as a teacher than as a therapist in the usual sense. He should make it clear to the patient that improvement depends largely on the effort he makes to overcome fear in his daily life between the visits to the therapist. Because instructions about behaviour therapy are rather complex, most patients find it helpful to receive an instruction booklet which can be studied at home. It is one of the problems of treatment that the practice which patients have to carry out is inevitably repetitive, sometimes frightening, and frequently monotonous. It is not surprising, therefore, that strenuous efforts have to be made to motivate patients. This can be done by treating patients in small groups in which they are encouraged to motivate each other. An alternative, which is often easier to arrange successfully, is to enlist another member of the family or a close friend to take a close interest in the treatment and share in its practical aspects. It seems possible that motivation is sustained most effectively by short courses of about five sessions of treatment followed by 'booster' sessions at three-monthly intervals until the disorder is controlled. There is also some evidence that, if patients are taught how to deal with problems in their everyday lives, agoraphobia improves gradually, presumably because they become progressively less anxious and gain in self-confidence (Jannoun *et al.*, 1980). In everyday practice, it is often appropriate to combine simple instruction in problem-solving with the other behavioural measures, particularly in the treatment of patients who worry about the upbringing of their children or their marital relationships. If the latter problems are serious, it may be necessary to employ a behavioural form of marital therapy (see chapter 3.1.3, page 90).

These simple measures, carried out persistently, produce good results in the majority of phobic states. In general, it is more important to ensure that the simple methods are practised regularly than it is to complicate treatment by adding to it procedures such as psychotherapy or marriage counselling. Nevertheless, if there are independent indications for either of these, they can be combined readily with exposure treatment for phobias.

(ii) *Response prevention and thought-stopping*

These methods are used for compulsive rituals and obsessional ideas. In response prevention, patients are encouraged to resist their rituals for several hours at a time. At the start of treatment, the patient may be able to do this only in the presence of the therapist or a nurse but he must learn gradually to do without this help. Contrary to the expectations of most patients, abstention, providing it is lengthy, does not worsen the distress but leads to a somewhat less severe urge to undertake the rituals. As the procedure is repeated many times, the rituals become progressively less frequent and less distressing, so

that response prevention can then be carried out in the presence of stimuli which normally provoke the rituals – for example, dirty hands increase washing rituals. This stage requires much further urging and reassurance and some therapists find it useful to demonstrate to the patient that the procedure can be carried out without distress by a normal person ('modelling'). Having practised in the presence of the therapist the patient must learn to practise on his own.

These simple procedures lead to good results in many patients with obsessional rituals and are, at present, the treatment of choice for the condition. They provide a further illustration of a principle which we have already noted: behavioural procedures should be as simple as possible and much effort should be made to ensure that they are persisted with. As in the treatment of phobias, it is sometimes helpful to combine behavioural treatment of obsessional symptoms with medication – in this case usually with a tricyclic antidepressant. Whether these drugs act by reducing the depressive mood changes which so often present in these patients, or whether they serve as long-acting anxiolytic agents is uncertain. In either case, antidepressants may have a use in combination with behaviour therapy for other neuroses which are resistant to behavioural measures alone.

Thought-stopping, another simple procedure, has been used for obsessional thoughts. In this treatment, patients learn to interrupt a train of obsessional thoughts with a sudden distracting stimulus. At first the therapist may shout 'stop', then the patient does so himself, then he 'speaks' the word silently to himself. Alternatively a sudden sensory stimulus can be used as the distraction e.g. the release of a stretched elastic band on the wrist. Many patients say they are helped by this training in distraction but there is insufficient evidence to judge how effective the methods really are. Whether or not it stands up to further evaluation, the method illustrates an important unsolved problem: are mental symptoms of neuroses modified better by attempting to alter associated behaviour (in this case rituals) or by attempting to modify them directly? It is a question to which we shall return, but first it is necessary to say something about cognitive therapy.

(iii) *Cognitive-behaviour therapy*

This is the name for a growing and important group of techniques which are concerned with changing cognitions, that is, recurrent ideas, attitudes and expectations. Since these are central to a large number of psychiatric problems, the importance of the aim cannot be disputed; the problem is how best to bring it about.

There is little doubt that cognitive changes follow successful treatment directed to overt behaviour. They are seen, for example, when agoraphobia is treated solely by exposure to feared situations or when obsessional rituals are treated by response prevention. It is much less certain whether cognitions can be changed directly – that is, whether attitudes and thoughts can be altered through verbal means rather than as a secondary effect of changing behaviour. There is probably no general answer to this question: it depends on the type of cognition and on the type and severity of the disorder. Thus Beck (1976) describes the use of verbal methods for altering the cognitions of the majority of depressed patients, but he advocates selected tasks (which he calls 'success experiences') for those who are most depressed. Equally, methods which are effective with the stereotyped thoughts of depressed patients may not alter obsessions.

Apart from the development of rational emotive therapy by Ellis (1962) the only cognitive treatment which has been worked out in any detail is that described by Beck (1976) for depression. Beck's treatment holds out considerable promise but at the time of writing it has not been tested thoroughly enough for it to be possible to assess its final place in treatment. It is considered further in the section on depressive disorders (see chap. 5.1.3, p. 207).

(iv) *Operant conditioning methods*

We have already noted that these are based on the simple idea that if behaviour persists, this must be because its consequences are reinforcing it. This central idea has been applied in many different ways. In a *token economy*, a whole ward, or a grouping of patients and staff within a ward, is the context of treatment. The patients are usually schizophrenic or subnormal, though the same principles have been applied to behavioural problems in people with disorders of personality. The aim of treatment is usually to modify social behaviour: to discourage socially unacceptable actions and to encourage those which are adaptive. Treatment begins with a careful search for any consequences of patients' behaviour which may give rise to reinforcement. For example, if nurses pay more attention to patients when they are noisy or difficult, they are unwittingly reinforcing that

behaviour. And if they dress patients who do not readily dress themselves, instead of encouraging their own efforts however imperfect, they are failing to reinforce adaptive behaviour. Much of the skill in operant conditioning treatments lies in identifying these contingencies of reinforcement, in making them clear to staff or to relatives, and in persuading these people to change what they do in a consistent way. The type of reinforcement which is used to encourage behaviour seems to matter less than the consistency with which it is given (Baker, Hall, Hutchinson & Bridge, 1977). Thus while some therapists employ tokens which can be exchanged for privileges, and others rely on verbal and social reinforcement, there are no striking differences between the two methods. Apart from consistency, the important point is that the patients do in fact find the 'reinforcers' rewarding.

Punishment has also been used in operant conditioning but it is difficult to arrange it in an ethical way. It is fortunate, therefore, that negative reinforcement has been shown to have only rather transitory effects. However, even the use of positive reinforcement is not free from ethical problems, for it is often necessary to withdraw something from the patient in order to give it back to him later as a reinforcer: for example, the patient may be told that he can use the hospital shop if he has earned tokens. Some programmes have gone further than this and have withdrawn visiting, magazines, weekend leave and so on, in order to manufacture reinforcers. It is not surprising that this practice has led to public concern; indeed, in the United States there have been rulings about the minimal rights of patients in hospitals and of offenders in penal institutions. These difficult issues should be discussed fully and openly with staff, patients, and relatives whenever the methods are used.

Operant conditioning procedures have also been used with individual patients. A common example is in the treatment of eating disorders, and the methods are discussed in more detail on p. 298 and pp. 304–5. With individual patients as with groups, problems arise about the way in which reinforcers have to be fashioned by withdrawing something from the patient – radio, magazines, visitors, and so on. However, with individual treatment the ethical problems are a little less difficult because it is easier to adapt treatment to each person's circumstances. Moreover, when neurotic or anorexic patients are treated, there is usually less ethical concern than with schizophrenics or subnormals because the former are more able to give informed consent to the procedures. Another growing application of operant principles is to the treatment of children, especially to those with autism. In such cases, staff or the parents are taught to ignore disturbed behaviour and to encourage normal social interchange either in a hospital ward, or in the child's home. As with schizophrenia or subnormality, behavioural treatment cannot effect the fundamental disorder of these children but it does sometimes reduce abnormal behaviour and may encourage the child to develop to the full his normal capacities.

Similar principles lie behind the method called contingency management, which can be illustrated by its use in marital problems. The essential feature is that each partner of the marriage lists those things which he or she most wants from the other, and states what he or she is willing to give in return. The partners then make a 'contract' to exchange these forms of behaviour. Put in this way, the method probably appears mechanistic and unlikely to improve the emotional state of a marriage. However, it need not be so in practice; indeed it often succeeds in reducing repeated quarrels and in giving the couple a constructive purpose which they can share. The method is described in more detail in chapter 3.1.3, page 90.

Conclusion

This section has been concerned with the principles of behaviour therapy. For more detail of the procedures used for specific disorders, the reader is referred to the sections of this handbook in which these conditions are considered, and to the reference works which were suggested on page 83. Our brief discussion of exposure treatment, response prevention, cognitive therapy, and operant methods has been intended to illustrate some general issues, and it may be helpful to summarize these at this point.

It is most important to carry out a thorough behavioural assessment before starting treatment. This assessment begins with a careful description of the disorder of behaviour for which the patient is seeking treatment and of the circumstances in which it occurs. Then we need to know what other behaviour disorders are associated with it, and what relation they appear to have to the primary disorder. We illustrated this with the 'fear of fear' which so often accompanied agoraphobic symptoms. Next, the factors which increase or decrease the behaviour must be examined more closely. What are the features

which are reinforcing the behaviour, are they internal to the patient or do they reside in the reactions of people around him? Last, but arguably most important, we must assess his motivation for treatment. Whenever the disorder is long-lasting, it is essential to find out why the patient has come at this particular time. Is he depressed and less able to cope with symptoms which he had learnt to live with? Has the patient with a sexual deviation been persuaded by his family or forced into treatment by the threat of legal proceedings? Is he prepared to work hard to overcome his problems or is he seeking an effortless solution? A determined attempt must be made to answer questions such as these which will throw light on the patient's motivation. But however searching the enquiry, doubt will often remain.

This brings us to two further general principles. The first is the value of trial periods of treatment to assess the patients' likely response to a full course of treatment. The second is the need to think not only of the procedures to be used but of the ways in which the patient is to be helped to persist in their application. We have noted already the value of engaging the interest and cooperation of the spouse or friend and the alternative of treating the patient in groups in which patients are encouraged to take a considerable interest in the progress of the other members.

In choosing the specific procedures the principle is clear: select a small number of simple and well tried procedures which match the main features of the behaviour disorder. Sometimes a single procedure will be enough – as it is in some agoraphobic patients – but often two or three will be needed, for example, exposure treatment with anxiety management and simple problem-solving methods directed to family difficulties. It may also be necessary to introduce drug treatment; schizophrenic patients treated by token economy methods certainly require concurrent neuroleptic medication to control positive symptoms, agoraphobic patients may need anxiolytic drugs to regulate anxiety in the early stages of treatment, and obsessional patients may need antidepressants. Simple counselling may also be appropriate and occasionally psychotherapy may be directed to wider problems of personal identity or social relationships. When this is needed it may be better to employ two therapists who keep in close touch with one another, because the therapeutic relationship needed for behavioural treatment, with its emphasis on self-help, is both less intense than that required for most forms of individual psychotherapy. There is however no absolute rule about this and there are cases in which the same person can achieve a relationship with his patient which is appropriate to both forms of treatment.

Having emphasized the need to combine a small number of carefully selected procedures to match the individual patient's problems, it is necessary to warn against complication for its own sake. As in the use of drugs, an unduly elaborate array of treatments often indicates that the therapist has not taken sufficient care in analysing his patient's problems. While combinations of behaviour therapies may not have the adverse effects which can follow drug interactions, they are wasteful and prevent the therapist from learning the value and limitations of the individual methods.

We have noted a shift of attention from external behaviour to mental symptoms (so-called cognitive methods). That cognitions must change cannot be disputed, but there is still much uncertainty about the relative merits for this purpose of cognitive and behavioural treatments. Whenever there is a behaviour disorder associated with the 'cognitive disorder' it is important to treat it. When this is done, the cognitions will often change as well – as they often do when obsessional rituals are treated. But when there is no obvious external behaviour to modify, as in some cases of obsessional neurosis or in mild depressive disorders, cognitive treatments have to be employed. However they must be regarded as less certain in their effects than the other methods

Do the same principles apply to behaviour therapy with children?

They do, but there are a few obvious ways in which they have to be modified. While specific techniques can be applied to particular behaviour disorders such as phobias and enuresis, the majority of problems require an approach which takes account of the reinforcement of the child's problems by other people and particularly by his parents. For this reason, the behaviour analysis must be closely concerned with the parent's response to the child and the treatment often relies heavily on operant conditioning principles. Similarly, it is as important in assessment to judge the motivation of the parents as it is to determine that of the child. Apart from these points however, all the issues which we have noted with the treatment with adults apply equally to children. The specific techniques are referred to more fully in chapter 3.3.1 on page 108.

3.1.3
Marital and family therapy
MICHAEL J. CROWE

Introduction

The practice of treating the problems of individuals by changing family interaction dates from the early 1950s, and Bowlby in England and Bell in the U.S.A. are credited with its introduction (Beels & Ferber, 1969). In family therapy the usual medical model of causation (aetiology, pathology, diagnosis) has to be supplemented by a model that takes into account the interaction of members of an active system: the symptom is a reaction to family stress, is reacted to by other family members, and is itself a form of communication. Von Bertalanffy (1966) and Bateson and colleagues (1956), working within systems theory, have developed concepts such as positive and negative feedback, balance, homeostasis, and perverse triangles to describe family interaction. In the most radical formulation, the patient is the 'ambassador' for the sick family, and the family as a whole is the entity to be treated. Put at its most conservative, most psychiatrists would agree that environmental factors can contribute to illness, that the family is part of the patient's environment, that environmental family factors can affect the patient's symptoms and that any change in the patient's symptomatology is likely to have family repercussions.

Systems theory

Although systems theory does not give rise to testable predictions, and is not in that sense a scientific theory, its use is probably indispensable to an understanding of family interaction and family therapy. In describing a natural group such as a family, it is unhelpful to say, for instance, that the daughter's depression is *caused* by the parents' marital problems or that the parents' marital problems are *caused* by the daughter's depression (although both statements may be partly true). It is more fruitful to describe the family in systems terms; for instance that there is *'enmeshment'* or a lack of *'boundary'* between parents and daughter, such that the daughter is over-involved in the parental problems, and vice versa. In talking of causation, the concept of *circularity* is useful, in that a stress in one part of the system (for instance the marital relationship) can be responded to by behaviour in another part of the system (a child being depressed) which either increases or decreases the marital problems (perhaps by causing a temporary lull in arguments while the parents deal with the child, or perhaps by intensifying the argument over who is responsible for the child's behaviour), which leads to a further change in the child's behaviour, and so forth. The chain of causality is thus seen to be circular and endless, until broken by separation or death. Behaviour within the system can be seen as having a *homeostatic* function (favouring the status quo) or a *morphogenic* function (favouring change): most repetitive behaviour which is responded to in a repetitive way is almost by definition homeostatic in its effect, and it is often the task of the therapist to discover what feared change is being resisted by the persistence of repetitive symptomatic behaviour. An example could be that the persistence of a daughter's depression could be seen as providing an enhanced nurturing role for her mother, who would otherwise be faced with an 'empty nest', and as allowing the continuation of a childish role for the daughter who is afraid of adult life.

Approaches to family therapy

There are a large number of more or less distinct approaches to family therapy (Madanes & Haley, 1977). One broad distinction that has some utility is between historically-based approaches, mostly dynamic and insight-orientated, and 'here and now' approaches which may be group-analytic, communication-orientated, strategic, structural or behavioural.

Of the psychodynamic approaches, Dicks (1967) and Ackerman (1966) used a fairly traditional psychoanalytic model, on which they skilfully grafted their techniques for conjoint work. While Dicks' marital

therapy was centered on traditional interpretations, Ackerman described a more challenging technique which he calls 'tickling the defences', and in which humour and teasing are used to change attitudes.

Paul and Grosser (1965) use a technique based on the process of mourning (see Parkes, 1972) in order to free family members from a pathological bereavement reaction which is postulated to be disturbing family relationships: often the symptom in another family member abates when this process (usually in one of the parents) is complete.

Byng-Hall (1979) and Pincus and Dare (1978) use a quite similar technique when family myths or secrets are found to be creating barriers or unrealistic expectations; insistence that myths and secrets are openly discussed in the family often alleviates problems.

Less obviously psychoanalytic, though still historical, are the approaches of Bowen (1966) and Bloch (1973). In Bowen's work, family members are sent to interview older relatives about the family's past, while Bloch advocates the construction of 'genograms', or family trees, in the conjoint family session. In both cases, understanding the 'system over time' helps the family to achieve insight into its present conflicts and thus to resolve them.

In the middle ground between present and past orientation are the approaches of Skynner (1976), Simon (1972) and Satir (1967), Skynner observes and understands family dynamics using group-analytic skills, but intervenes by challenge and side-taking in producing change. Simon uses 'family sculpting', a method in which during a therapy session, family members silently position each other in a kind of tableau to represent their relationships, both as a means of revealing emotional reactions and of inducing changed behaviour. Satir works directly on communication, verbal and non-verbal, with an eclectic approach to understanding the present and past feelings of the family, and thereby induces mutual empathy.

Strategic approaches have been advocated by Jackson and Weakland (1961) and reported by Haley (1976), Selvini Palazzoli and co-workers (1978) and Cade and Southgate (1979). From a pure systems theory background, they attempt to alter family homeostasis by such unbalancing techniques as positive connotation of symptoms or disruptive behaviour (for instance to say that a depressed son is 'sacrificing himself and his future to save the family'), setting 'ritual tasks' which will expose family collusion, and giving paradoxical tasks such as 'prescribing the

symptom' in such a way as to make the present situation untenable and to alter power structures in the
family. Past family influences are often taken into
account in setting tasks, although tasks arise mainly
from observations of family interaction in the conjoint session.

Structural family therapy (Minuchin, 1974)
concentrates more exclusively on present and future.
An analysis of the system in terms of boundaries,
alliances, hostility, power structure, flexibility, and
rigidity leads to therapy which includes crisis induction, side-taking, imposition of control, and a variety
of similar techniques designed to alter patterns of
interaction. This approach is particularly useful for
'enmeshed' families, such as when one of its members has anorexia nervosa, and for one-parent families with blurred generation boundaries.

Behavioural approaches (Crowe, 1978a) involve
simpler formulations of here and now interaction, in
terms of reward and punishment. In 'operant-
interpersonal' treatment (Stuart, 1969) couples are
encouraged to exchange rewarding behaviour (positive reinforcement) instead of complaining about each
other (negative reinforcement or punishment). In the
approach of communication training (Patterson &
Hops, 1972) couples are instructed in greater message-
transmitting efficiency. In the method of Alexander
and Parsons (1973), families are taught to communicate briefly, with immediate feedback, rather than in
monologues.

Operational aspects

Family therapy usually takes place in psychiatric or social work settings, and the whole nuclear
family is usually seen when the presenting patient is
a child, adolescent, or a young adult. Marital therapy
is also widely practised in these settings, and in the
somewhat similar approach of marriage guidance.
Behavioural work with young children and their
mothers, although related to family and marital therapy, will not be further discussed here. Sexual therapy, also related to marital therapy, will be discussed
in chapter 9.1 and 9.2.

Therapy often includes the whole family, but it
is also appropriate to work at times with only part of
the family (for example, the parents alone). Sessions
usually last between 1–1½ hours, most commonly
once a week (but with longer intervals in strategic
and group-analytic approaches). The number of visits varies from 3–6 in behavioural or group-analytic
work to 200 or more in psychodynamic approaches

and with families of schizophrenics. Co-therapy in
pairs is preferred by many psycho-dynamic therapists: behavioural and structural therapists usually
work alone, whereas strategic therapists often work
with several colleagues observing and advising
behind a one-way screen.

General indications

Problems treated by family therapy include
most child psychiatric disorders, such as neurosis,
conduct disorder, delinquency, school refusal, and
sibling rivalry: disorders in adolescence, such as
anorexia nervosa, depression, anxiety, phobias, and
behaviour disorder: problems in young adults, such
as addictions, criminality, depression, and anxiety:
and marital problems, such as morbid jealousy, violence, some forms of alcoholism, chronic depression,
sexual dysfunction, and simple marital disharmony.
Schizophrenia was one of the earliest problems
treated by family therapy (Wynne, 1965; Lidz *et al.*,
1963; Boszormenyi-Nagy & Framo, 1965). The position is still controversial: some workers such as Minuchin and Bowen advise against family therapy with
schizophrenics, whereas Selvini Palazzoli and co-
workers (1978) have produced encouraging case
reports in families with young 'schizophrenic' members, although there are some doubts as to whether
these patients are genuinely schizophrenic in the
sense that most psychiatrists use the term.

Outcome studies (marital therapy)

As with many forms of psychotherapy, there is
a dearth of controlled outcome studies. In the field of
marital therapy, earlier studies, reviewed by Gurman (1973) showed some evidence for the superiority
of various types of communication training (see
above) over control procedures. Azrin, Naster and
Jones (1973) showed, in an incompletely controlled
trial, that an operant-interpersonal approach involving the negotiation of behaviour exchange (Stuart,
1969) produced better results than 'cathartic counselling'. Liberman and colleagues (1976), using only
9 couples, showed a slight superiority for group
communication training over dynamically orientated
couple-group therapy. Crowe (1978b) showed that an
operant-interpersonal and generally directive
approach was superior to a 'supportive' control procedure, but that interpretative therapy was only marginally better than the control: at follow-up after 18
months these differences were maintained. Jacobson
(1977), using 20 volunteer couples, showed that

problem-solving and behaviour modification techniques were superior to no treatment, and the same author (Jacobson, 1978) using single case design in a series of disturbed couples, showed that specific interventions produced specific changes.

Outcome studies (family therapy)

The effectiveness of family therapy has been reviewed by DeWitt (1978). There is some evidence for the effectiveness of brief, eclectic, crisis-orientated family therapy in the work of Langsley, Flomenhaft and Machotka (1969). Three hundred families were studied, and against a control of in-patient psychiatric treatment, the out-patient family therapy group did equally well symptomatically, but returned to work more quickly and were less likely to be admitted to hospital during follow-up. Hendricks (1971) showed, in 85 narcotic addicts, that multifamily group therapy with hospitalization produced better results at follow-up after 12 months than hospitalization alone. Alexander and Parsons (1973) used communication training, which encouraged rapid interchange of views in the families of delinquents: the treated group showed significantly fewer court appearances than untreated controls or controls treated by other forms of family therapy. Lask and Matthew (1979) showed that brief family intervention with asthmatic children significantly enhanced the effects of conventional medical and individual treatment.

Conclusions

No firm conclusions can be drawn from these studies, or from the host of uncontrolled outcome studies not reviewed here. The indications are that at least the more focused treatment approaches have some value, compared to no treatment, individual treatment or more diffuse family treatment; and in the present state of knowledge it might safely be concluded that family and marital therapy are indicated for non-psychotic psychiatric patients (adult or child), living with a spouse or family with whom they have arguments, communication problems, or overinvolvement.

CASE EXAMPLE

The 'S' family were referred by their general practitioner with a complaint that their eldest daughter, Jean (aged 12) was showing difficult behaviour, including 'emotional coldness, difficulty in forming friendships, poor performance at school in spite of reasonable intelligence, and at times completely irrational behaviour'. Her brother Simon (aged 10) was described as pleasant and likeable, and her sister Carol (aged 9) as quiet, and suffering from poor co-ordination. The mother, in her late 30s, was an ex-nurse, who in her teens had, after her mother's death, devoted herself to her younger siblings. The father, in his early 40s, had been an only child, and had had a previous marriage. His ex-wife had subsequently had a daughter the same age as Jean, who had bullied Jean at school. Both parents had recently had surgical treatment, the mother a hysterectomy and rectal treatment, and the father treatment for perforated diverticulitis.

Three family interviews, by co-therapists with one-way screen supervision, were held over a period of a month, and a broadly strategic approach was used (see above). It emerged that Jean enjoyed jokes and play with her siblings, but that (as revealed by a family 'sculpt') she was more closely involved with the mother, both positively and negatively, than were her brother and sister. It was hypothesized that mother was insecure about the growing independence of Jean, and that her own 'lost' teenage had led to her being unable to enjoy herself apart from the family. On the first interview the family were reassured that the 'symptoms' were not serious, but on the second interview they returned to report that Jean had increased her teasing of her siblings and was eating bread on return from school and then rejecting her supper. The family interaction was analysed again, and it was concluded that Jean wanted to be independent but remain within the family: boarding-school was suggested by both Jean and the mother, but without any conclusion. At the end of the session, the children were congratulated on their sense of fun, and the parents on having such attractive children. It was suggested that the parents should go out for a meal together and that the children should help the parents to decide when and where to go.

On the third visit, the parents reported improvement in Jean's behaviour, with appropriate independence, developing friendships at school, and more co-operation with her parents. The parents had also been out for a meal and had taken the children with them. The therapists entered into a discussion with the parents about their interaction, while all three children played together quietly (a reinforcement of the parent–child boundary). At the end of the session, the father stated that he felt further treatment was unnecessary, but he agreed to write three months later to report progress. The family were given a paradoxical task to go home with, as follows. 'It is important for Jean to continue as she is, in the centre of the family stage, because this enables her parents to show their concern for the family. Mr and Mrs S. should continue to sacrifice themselves, partly in order to avoid some of the sadness they must feel about being unable to enjoy themselves as a couple. Simon should continue to have a full life outside the family, as his father did as a boy. Carol should continue to play for safety and not decide whether to be like Jean or Simon'.

At three months, father wrote to say that home life was 'definitely a little better, with signs of a better bond with Jean generally', but that his wife was 'a little tense whilst awaiting an operation'. In general, then, what was achieved was to re-label most of Jean's 'symptoms' as a wish to help her parents and also achieve some legitimate independence, and to increase the mutual support of the parents while accentuating the generation boundary.

3.1.4
Drug therapy and physical treatments

MALCOLM LADER

The neuroses comprise complex constellations of symptoms among which anxiety and depression are prominent. Drug and physical treatments for the neuroses are symptomatic, concentrating on complaints of anxiety and depression. Such treatments must be used realistically within the context of total patient management. Nevertheless, the symptomatic relief afforded is often substantial and this may provide the basis for the use of other forms of treatment which then have a greater chance of success.

In this section, principles of treatment will be emphasized with particular reference to the drugs used to assuage anxiety and to induce sleep. Antidepressive drugs and physical treatments such as abreaction and brain surgery will also be mentioned.

For millennia, man has used psychotropic agents to alter his mood and intellect and to lessen emotional symptoms. Alcohol, opium, and cannabis were supplemented more recently by bromides, paraldehyde, and chloral derivatives. This century the immensely successful barbiturates were introduced, followed by meprobamate in the 1950s and rapidly supplanted by the benzodiazepines in the last decade (Cohen, 1970). In many countries, the benzodiazepines are the most widely prescribed of all drugs (Blackwell, 1973). The antidepressive agents, tricyclics and monoamine oxidase inhibitors (MAOIs), first marketed 20 years ago represent a major class of medication.

Definitions

The term originally used for drugs to combat anxiety was 'sedative', but this now implies the induction of drowsiness and torpor, originally termed 'oversedation' and associated with the barbiturates. In its place the terms 'anxiolytic' or 'anti-anxiety agent' have been introduced with especial reference to the benzodiazepines. The term 'minor tranquillizer' does not do justice to the importance of these drugs in terms of usage or effects; 'tranquillizer' on its own is the usual lay term for these drugs. These drugs both calm and induce sleep, the distinction between these usages being artificial: anxiolytics in high dose will act as hypnotics; hypnotics in divided doses during the day will lessen anxiety.

Choice of drug

This comparison illustrates several important points regarding treatment. Thus:

(1) The benzodiazepines are more effective than the barbiturates. In scores of controlled comparisons, the majority show a distinct superiority for the benzodiazepines; some (usually with fixed dosage schedules) show little difference; only rare exceptions demonstrate any superiority for the barbiturates (Greenblatt & Shader, 1974).

(2) Twenty times the hypnotic dose of a barbiturate can result in coma and death. By contrast, overdose with the benzodiazepines is rarely, if ever, fatal in adults unless another drug or alcohol is taken simultaneously (Hollister, 1978).

(3) Unwanted effects tend to be milder and less common with the benzodiazepines.

(4) Dependence, psychological and physiological, can supervene with both barbiturates and benzodiazepines but seems less likely with the latter (Palmer, 1978).

(5) The barbiturates are notorious for inducing liver microsomal enzymes, thereby accelerating the metabolism of other drugs such as warfarin and steroids. Other psychotropic drugs such as chlorpromazine and amitriptyline may also be affected. Benzodiazepines do not do this.

For all these reasons, particularly (2), the barbiturates are obsolete and should not be prescribed *ab initio*.

Other drugs used include the antipsychotic agents in low dose which are often effective (Covington, 1975). However, while tardive dyskinesia remains a long-term possibility, such medication is best reserved for patients intolerant of benzodiazepines or predisposed to alcohol or tranquillizer abuse. The beta-adrenoceptor blocking agents are useful in patients with predominantly somatic symptoms, and antidepressives with sedative effects, such as amitriptyline and mianserin, in patients with symptoms of both anxiety and depression.

Benzodiazepines

Pharmacokinetics

Many of the currently available benzodiazepines are interrelated metabolically (Fig. 3.1.4.1). The key compound is N-desmethyldiazepam (nordiazepam), which has a long half-life (averaging over 80 hours) and thus persists in the body. Diazepam, medazepam, prazepam, clorazepate and to some extent chlordiazepoxide are converted to nordiazepam at a rate faster than it is metabolized. Consequently, after a few days' treatment the concentration of nordiazepam exceeds those of the administered drugs. Thus, all these drugs have long 'smooth' actions.

Temazepam and oxazepam (and lorazepam which is chlorinated oxazepam) are fairly swiftly metabolized by conjugation and excretion and have shorter durations of action (8–12 hours). Nitrazepam and flurazepam, widely-used hypnotics, are rela-

tively long-acting with persistent sedative actions the next day.

A few studies have examined the relationship between clinical response and plasma benzodiazepine concentrations: no consistent data have accrued.

Clinical efficacy

Hundreds of clinical trials, controlled and uncontrolled, have demonstrated the effectiveness of the benzodiazepines in lessening anxiety and inducing sleep. Although doubts have been expressed concerning the efficacy of these drugs and the deficiencies of almost all these trials have been pointed out (Solomon & Hart, 1978), the sheer bulk of clinical evidence attests to the usefulness of the symptomatic relief they provide. In my experience of treating chronically anxious patients referred to psychiatric hospital out-patient departments, the benzodiazepines about halve psychopathology scores rated either objectively (for example, the Hamilton Anxiety Scale) or by the patient (Lader, Bond & James, 1974). Nevertheless, those patients whose illnesses are acute derive less benefit from anxiolytic medication as their symptoms are more tolerable and less persistent. In general practice, the relief afforded by these drugs must be set against the dangers of long-term usage. Similar considerations apply to the antidepressives.

Fig. 3.1.4.1. Metabolic pathways of some benzodiazepines. (Nitrazepam, flurazepam and triazolam follow other metabolic pathways. Lorazepam is a chlorinated derivative of oxazepam, and is conjugated and excreted.)

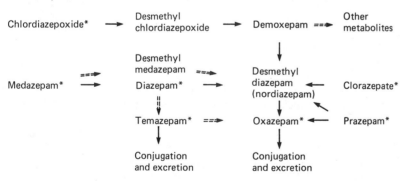

Clinical uses

The essential principle of drug treatment is to maximize the possibility of significant symptomatic relief by matching the patient's type of symptoms and pattern of illness to the type of drug (Rickels, Downing & Winokur, 1978). Both pharmacodynamic and pharmacokinetic considerations apply: that is, both the type of action and the speed of onset and length of action are important.

The most acute forms of anxiety are *panic attacks,* distressing both to patients and onlookers. Long-term medication may help reduce the frequency of attacks. If the attacks are predictable, the patient can take a short-acting benzodiazepine such as lorazepam an hour or so before entering the anxiety-provoking situation. Some patients find diazepam effective despite being long-acting. Either lorazepam or diazepam can be used to treat the panic attack; given orally or intravenously, they are rapidly absorbed and penetrate the brain.

Antidepressives, both tricyclics and MAOIs, have been advocated in the prevention of phobic anxiety. Behavioural methods of treatments have a better chance of success after symptomatic relief has been attained.

Acute stress responses are the commonest forms of anxiety state. They generally remit spontaneously and many patients do not even seek medical aid. Thus drug treatments are not generally indicated. The criterion for selecting those patients who do need drugs is that the anxiety is so severe that it interferes with his functioning at home, at work, in relationships with others, and in tackling his own emotional problems. Thus, for remission to be complete, the anxious individual must identify his problem, analyse it and take realistic steps either to obviate the stress or to minimize its impact on him. Anxiety impairs psychological functioning in all respects and high levels of anxiety may incapacitate the individual. Anxiety levels must be lowered and a benzodiazepine such as diazepam 10–30 mg/day is indicated (Dasberg & van Praag, 1974).

Chronic anxiety states are roughly of two types, those patients whose acute stress-related responses have not abated and those who have life-long abnormally anxious personalities. The former are usually seen by psychiatrists because the family doctor has despaired of helping his patient as the weeks of anxiety have lengthened into months and years of chronic anxiolytic medication. Despite drug treatment anxiety persists and secondary processes of conditioning, poor expectations and despair set in, maintaining the anxiety. Careful choice of drug and adjustment of dosage are needed. If anxiety levels are maintained at a constant high level, a long-acting benzodiazepine such as diazepam or clorazepate is usually appropriate. If anxiety levels fluctuate, the patient may prefer to take a short-acting compound as needed, oxazepam or lorazepam. Some patients like to have a background level of anxiolytic action upon which further sedation can be superimposed as necessary. Most patients can be trusted to co-operate in the choice and adjustment of their own medication and usually quickly determine the optimum dosage balance between symptom relief and minimal side-effects. Sometimes, despite the chronicity of the anxiety state, good symptomatic control for a few months is followed by resolution of the illness, almost as if a vicious circle had been broken.

In the chronic personality-bound anxiety state, full remission is unlikely and the patient is merely tided over acute exacerbations of a life-long disability. The hereditary element is often substantial with other members of the family affected. The patient is a chronic worrier; life is a great trial; each change in circumstance is a major upset; expectations are unreal and the patient deems himself a failure. Drug therapy is inevitably long-term but not necessarily constant. The criteria as to whether drug treatment be initiated are twofold: is the patient handicapped by his anxiety; is the patient definitely helped by anxiolytics? Because of the indefinite nature of treatment once instituted, placebo substitution is a legitimate ploy in establishing the true value of the drug treatment (with the patient's general consent but without his knowing the exact time). If the symptoms recrudesce within a week or so, the previous drug treatment was effective.

Yet another type of chronic patient has come to depend on his sick role as a defence against life's stresses. The administration of drugs reinforces the patient's invalidism. Indeed, some escalation of dosage may occur as the patient's personality type is often dependence-prone. Systematic planned, but firm, withdrawal with psychotherapeutic support and counselling is appropriate.

As mentioned earlier, patients with somatic symptoms such as palpitations, tremor, and gastrointestinal upset often respond well to beta-adrenoceptor antagonists such as propranolol. This can be combined with a benzodiazepine, the balance of the combination matching the emphasis of the patient's symptoms.

When the neurotic condition contains symptoms of depression as well as anxiety, similar considerations concerning antidepressive drug treatment apply. One important difference is that antidepressive medication is not as short-term a therapy as anxiolytic medication. That is, a trial of antidepressive medication should be for a minimum of 6 weeks. Furthermore, response of neurotic depressive symptoms is usually less gratifying than those in 'endogenous' depression.

Insomnia

Insomnia can be due to many physical and psychological factors (see volume 2, chapter 6). Anxiety of all degrees is a common cause of insomnia, the patient tossing and turning, mulling over his problems. Depressive reactions also tend to be associated with difficulty in falling asleep, but light, broken sleep is most common. The anti-anxiety and anti-depressive medications can be manipulated to capitalize on their secondary sedative properties. Thus, diazepam 10–30 mg can be given as one dose at night, and a sedative antidepressive such as amitriptyline, doxepin, or mianserin can also be administered once-nightly to depressives.

Nevertheless, some patients complain primarily of insomnia, especially at times of stress. In these circumstances a brief course of hypnotics may help tide the patient over. As daytime sedation is not needed, a short-acting benzodiazepine such as temazepam or triazolam is appropriate.

Duration of treatment

A stroke of the prescriber's pen starts a neurotic patient on a benzodiazepine or an antidepressive but it is difficult to discontinue such treatment unless prior measures are taken. First, the patient must be warned that his treatment will be of limited duration and that he must be prepared to discontinue the medication when this is appropriate. Secondly, drugs should be used as part of a general treatment and management plan utilizing social, behavioural, and psychotherapeutic techniques. Treatment should last a few weeks in the acute, milder states, longer in the more severe, chronic conditions. Long-term maintenance therapy may be needed in some cases but it should be embarked on as a definite option and not result by accident, with prescriptions renewed on a casual week-to-week basis.

Unwanted effects

These are listed in text-books of clinical pharmacology and therapeutics. Benzodiazepines have relatively few side-effects, drowsiness and ataxia being the commonest. Paradoxical aggressive outbursts may occur (Gaind & Jacoby, 1978). The antidepressives, both tricyclics and MAOIs, have many such effects, although the newer tricyclic/tetracyclic compounds are a definite improvement over the earlier drugs.

Patients should be warned about these possible unwanted effects. A judicious balance should be struck between raising excessive alarm in the patient and leaving him in ignorance of what to expect. One stratagem is to persuade him that such side-effects, providing they are tolerable, show that the drug is beginning to have an effect and that symptomatic relief will shortly ensue.

Most unwanted effects can be minimized by careful adjustment of dosage but some, especially with the tricyclic antidepressives, are inescapable concomitants of treatment. The danger is that patients will feel that the drugs are more trouble than they are worth and will fail to persist with them.

Overdoses

The problem of drug overdosage has increased year by year (Stewart *et al.*, 1974). The particular danger is that depressed patients with their greater likelihood of suicidal attempts are prescribed antidepressives, most of which are dangerous in overdosage, with marked cardiotoxicity. Some of the newer antidepressives such as mianserin and nomifensine seem much safer in this respect. The benzodiazepines are remarkably safe in overdosage and it is doubtful whether death can be induced in physically healthy adults by these drugs alone.

In the management of the patient, the best approach is to win the patient's confidence so that suicidal intent or thoughts are discussed. Prescribing no more than one week's supply of drugs at a time does not prevent the patient from hoarding his medication over a few weeks and lulls the doctor into a false sense of security.

Compliance

The patient's confidence must also be obtained to maximize his compliance with the treatment regimen. Perhaps up to a half of patients fail to take their medication as prescribed. Some take none at all but most take their tablets only when they feel the need for them, in anticipation of an anxious period or on a particularly miserable day. Careful explanation of the need for a *course* of treatment is essential. Some patients regard it as a sign of weakness in themselves to resort to medication. They believe that they should be able to conquer their symptoms by themselves, 'by pulling themselves together'. Much subsequent wasted effort can be avoided by careful questioning of the patient with regard to his attitude to taking medicines.

Other physical treatments

Considerations of space preclude detailed discussion of treatments such as drug-induced abreaction, electroconvulsive therapy, and psychosurgery. All are surrounded by mystique and controversy, the first because it is regarded by the naive as a 'truth drug' or 'lie detector', the second because inducing a fit seems barbarous, the last because deliberately causing irreversible damage to the brain offends some people.

Short-acting barbiturates such as amylobarbitone sodium and methohexitone sodium have three main uses: (1) an interview conducted under the influence of such a drug may reveal ideation, affect, and conflict not immediately apparent, especially in patients whose illnesses encompass much denial and dissociation; (2) the event precipitating hysterical conversion syndromes may be uncovered; (3) relaxation can be enhanced and accelerated during behavioural techniques such as systematic desensitization.

Electroconvulsive therapy has no place in the management of minor psychiatric conditions.

Psychosurgery should only be considered in the rare patient who has been severely ill for years after routine therapy, particularly drugs, given at usually adequate levels and usually sufficient periods have failed repeatedly to bring symptomatic relief. Full evaluation by an experienced multidisciplinary team is essential (Kelly, 1976).

Drugs in childhood

The use of drugs in childhood has been attended by some controversy especially with respect to stimulant drugs in the hyperkinetic syndrome. Antipsychotic medication has been used in childhood psychoses such as autism and antidepressives in depressed patients. Benzodiazepines are appropriate for incapacitating anxiety (Anders & Ciaranello, 1977).

Nevertheless, the drugs should be used carefully in low dosage for specific purposes for limited periods. Little is known of the effects of psychotropic drugs on the developing child but the widespread endocrine effects of the phenothiazines are an illustration that caution is necessary. The need for medication may be misconstrued by children and the taking of the tablets or elixir may become a focus for parent–child tensions. Also, both parent and child may come to believe that there is a pill for all life's problems. Both parents and child should be instructed in detail concerning the benefits and hazards of medication, the goals of treatment and when and why it will be discontinued.

3.2
Treatment settings

3.2.1
In-patient care and therapeutic communities

HENRY WALTON

Introduction

The development of the therapeutic community approach was part of the movement aiming to reform psychiatric hospitals to become a more humane and supportive environment for patients. The importance of the ward atmosphere came to be perceived more clearly from the study of mental hospitals by psychiatrists (Stanton & Schwartz, 1954), from the recognition that hospitalized psychotic patients responded and benefited from milieu therapy approaches (May & Simpson, 1980), from the investigations of sociologists (Goffman, 1968; Caudill, 1958), and from the clinical innovations of British psychiatrists after the Second World War.

The term 'therapeutic community' implies the systematic development of an intensive ward programme aimed to modify the behaviour of groups of patients in a psychiatric hospital setting. Principles include intensive group living, resocialization, therapeutic atmosphere, and active, planned patient-to-patient and patient-to-staff interaction. A therapeutic community depends on: the application of structured social processes; fostering of autonomy and responsibility on the part of patients; open awareness of and attention to staff attitudes; and the use of group and individual psychotherapy. Certain specific technical procedures constitute the method for bringing about and maintaining such an atmosphere, the chief of which is the holding of daily ward meetings. Other technical measures ensure that use is made of the therapeutic potential of all members of the treatment staff and that patients are given a major part in their own and their fellow patients' treatment. Social learning is a foremost treatment modality: the patient reproduces aspects of his problems in relationships involving fellow patients and staff members, which become the focus of exploration and potential change. The psychiatric ward is explicitly developed into a setting for promoting and investigating the personal relationships which patients evolve with each other and staff members, so that social learning can be fostered. The goal is that patients should receive treatment not only for their current psychiatric disorder, but also for their problems in living and the disturbances in their personal relationships which impair them as individuals and limit their existence. The therapeutic community is thus an in-patient unit which relies on social analysis and aims at social learning.

In the United States, H. S. Sullivan set up a special ward for treating schizophrenics at the Sheppard and Enoch Pratt Hospital in Maryland during 1929, reasoning that the patients would improve in an environment with healthy interpersonal relationships; he instructed the nursing aides how to talk and behave to patients, and held daily meetings with the aides. The concept of the therapeutic community was developed further before the Second World War, particularly for the treatment of patients with neuroses and personality disorders. Pioneering ventures in Britain include those of Dr Tom Main (1946) at Northfield Mental Hospital and Dr Maxwell Jones (1948) at Belmont (now Henderson) Hospital.

Interest has also developed in therapeutic communities in non-medical settings (Jensen, 1980), and in applying therapeutic community principles in out-patient settings at community centres and day hospitals. An association of therapeutic communities has been established to represent the staff of varying professional background in hospitals, approved schools, halfway houses, and the social services, with an interest in therapeutic community work (Hinshelwood & Manning, 1979).

Principles of ward management

Certain technical procedures are required to bring a therapeutic community into being in a ward setting and to maintain it, so as to enable patients to achieve appropriate and necessary change in behaviour and attitudes. The *ward atmosphere* is of critical importance. It has to be warm emotionally, encouraging, protective, lively and active, pleasant and interesting. To ensure such a facilitative climate is the responsibility of the staff team. Attention to the *communication network* is another primary responsibility. All staff members must be in possession of all relevant information about patients, relatives, and all else that is pertinent; all must know clearly the treatment plan for all patients, and every change or development in such plans; and all staff have the responsibility to ensure that they keep themselves aware of day-to-day events of relevance in the ward. *Patient government* requires that patients are provided with the appropriate information they need if they are to play an active and responsible part in their own treatment, by means such as regular administrative meetings, where they can discuss and participate in decisions about matters of ward organization and activities.

The number of patients treated at any one time should not exceed about 24, which seems to be the upper limit beyond which ward staff cannot keep in mind all the relevant biographical and other information generated about each patient from day to day. A recent writer has emphasized, 'The ideas of a therapeutic community can perhaps only be realized with a small autonomous unit . . .' (Lorentzen, 1981).

The staff

Generally the unit needs to be under the direction of a single senior psychiatrist; if more than one, the psychiatrists providing the clinical direction need to be very closely associated and to share a common outlook and purpose. In addition to the senior psychiatrist, the core team includes a senior nurse, a social worker, a clinical psychologist and an occupational therapist. These colleagues are the long-term staff, the culture-carriers who maintain the tradition and norms of that particular therapeutic community over time. Other staff who can be attached for a shorter term for training purposes are psychiatrists-in-training and nurses. In addition, because a unit of the type described is optimal for psychiatric training purposes, medical students and staff in training for all related professions can be attached for periods of weeks or months, provided that patients are adequately prepared for arrivals and departures. The training function can only be achieved satisfactorily if the clinical work is maintained at a high standard, and is evidently effective for the patients in the ward.

Ward and staff meetings

The main specialized technique is implemented when all patients and all staff on duty meet at least daily for a *ward meeting,* when group methods are the modality of treatment (Walton, 1974). These ward group-meetings are of the 'closed–open' type, patients entering as they are admitted and leaving on discharge. In this respect, ward group meetings are very different from small-group psychotherapy for out-patients. (Indeed, the procedures of the latter 'closed' form of group therapy are often mistakenly used in psychiatric wards, a practice that is misplaced and potentially harmful). The ward group meeting is a large one (Kreeger, 1975); moreover, the composition continually changes, as recovered patients are discharged from the ward and new ones admitted. One staff member conducts the daily session. The task of each session is to enable all patients to make themselves fully known to each other, and then to have their behaviour and current problems examined by the group as a whole. All members of staff should contribute as actively as is appropriate.

When treatment is particularly intensive, the practice may be to have a second 'informal' ward meeting in the afternoon; where nursing staff on night duty are sufficiently skilled, important unstructured meetings also take place in the evenings.

The *staff review session,* which has to be held each day immediately following the ward meeting as an essential accompaniment, allows staff members to explore and strive to understand the communications made by patients and staff in the ward meeting.

Special meetings are called whenever the need arises, and crisis meetings are held when a sudden unexpected event occurs (as when a patient admits to contemplating suicide, or attempts it, or when a patient who is not ready for discharge considers leaving the ward precipitately).

The treatment provided

Personality change, through replacement of maladaptive behaviour by new forms of relationship, is a therapeutic goal for the patients admitted to the therapeutic community. However, this will be promoted only if the general psychiatry practised in conjunction with the psychotherapeutic approach is of high standard; there is every reason why patients

should be given concurrent drug treatment, or other physical treatments, when any associated illness calls for such therapy.

The main clinical advantage of the therapeutic community is that the patient is provided with a setting in which treatment continues throughout the waking hours of each day. The behaviour of each patient is accessible for scrutiny by both staff members and by fellow-patients. The last point is crucially important: all patients are to regard themselves as in a treatment relationship to other patients, and the regimen fails if the philosophy of the unit does not promote such responsibility for one another among patients.

In addition to drug and other treatments mentioned above, individual psychotherapy is also provided. Each patient is assigned to a doctor. However, the provision of *individual psychotherapy* in a therapeutic community calls for an operation which many psychiatrists-in-training find onerous: the material elicited in each individual session needs to be conveyed to the team. Such sharing of information of course violates the confidentiality which traditionally characterizes individual out-patient psychotherapy: to disclose the patient's revelations in a way acceptable to the patient is a skilled procedure which requires care and supervised practice. Unless individual psychotherapeutic interviews are provided for patients, much critically important personal information will be kept secret, and the related sectors of the patient's personality will not become accessible. Furthermore, unless all members of the staff team are kept adequately informed about the content of individual interviews, their effectiveness will be impaired through incomplete knowledge about the patient. The potential conflict between individual and group therapeutic approaches is perhaps the most testing element in the therapeutic community, and a major cause of failure. Any disagreements among staff members need to be identified and discussed: the harm which occurs to patients when there are persisting covert disagreements among members of staff, well documented in traditional ward organization (Stanton & Schwartz, 1954), has to be avoided if the therapeutic community is to function.

The psychiatric social worker carries out *casework* with the relatives of all patients. Because patients can become greatly aroused emotionally, their relatives – such as parents or a spouse – will require support; in addition, the relatives assist therapy by providing important information, and by making themselves personally available to participate in the psychotherapeutic processes through which the patient passes.

The psychiatric nurses are naturally crucial in the clinical work undertaken, in that they are the most consistently in contact with the patients whom they support, encourage and often challenge psychotherapeutically, in addition to their other traditional psychiatric nursing interventions. The nursing staff can greatly catalyse ward interactions among patients, and ensure that proper social learning results for the patients concerned. Skilled members of nursing staff can also join patients during visiting times, and promote more frank and authentic encounters between them and their relatives who are central in their social adjustments. While separate professional activities have been indicated for staff of various categories, in a good unit extensive *role diffusion* occurs, and appropriately skilled nurses, for example, can also carry out individual psychotherapy or case work.

The *occupational therapy* programme is planned as an adjunct to the ward organization, using music, art, pottery, psychodrama, and poetry-reading. The sessions can be invaluable for patients limited in verbal communication: painting, especially, may release some patients from inhibitions in expressing themselves, and the pictures produced can be the focus of general discussion.

The therapeutic community, when it functions properly, provides intensive social learning for patients. They come to know each other very well. In the safe atmosphere which is essential for adequate treatment the patient can convey highly confidential personal information, which formerly was retained and concealed. Skeletons in cupboards may thus be revealed. At any time in a ward there may, for example, be an inhibited young man not succeeding in any of his occupational ventures because of low self-confidence and foreboding of failure; a suicidal housewife revealing that she had a prolonged incestuous relationship with an older brother during her childhood; a severely anorexic young woman, an only child of a mother who had her relatively late in life and was anxiously over-protective; a youngster who is emotionally distant from his stepfather and over-attached to his mother, and is unconfident and uncertain over his gender; and a single, mother-attached, socially inhibited alcoholic.

The totality of communications by all the patients, which constitutes the daily lived experience in which staff members share, is the clinical matrix in which patients come to grasp better their manner of relating to others, and the scope there is for change. The therapeutic community is a social laboratory, in which patients can safely expose their customary behaviour to the extent that it needs to be understood, and risk new behaviour which had seemed alien or inadmissible, and which, when successful, can be incorporated as new adaptive behaviour. All conflicts which arise can become the focus for social learning. Socially harmful behaviour can be reacted to by confrontation.

What is crucial for the staff to ensure is that the patients do not experience disasters. Their worst fears, which made them inhibit themselves or distort their social responses, must not come to pass. When a patient risks a major self-disclosure, and is then responded to by coldness or ostracism, he will adhere to self-destructive or self-defeating patterns of behaviour. Moreover, patients who are reacted to in a damaging way by fellow patients or staff members can be harmed psychologically, and the negative experience can make them profoundly wary of any subsequent offers of help, or block their way to fuller social efforts. For this reason, a therapeutic community has either to be effective or cease to function. A particular crisis can result when a pioneering consultant departs and a change of leadership occurs. Recently public steps were initiated to close Henderson Hospital, the original setting of Maxwell Jones' pioneering work, and only widespread protest led to this proposal being dropped.

There is a definite risk to patients when the provisions outlined are not met. On the other hand, when the necessary conditions can be provided, organization of a psychiatric in-patient unit as a therapeutic community can provide a humane and supportive environment for patients, and foster personality change. Close personal relationships between patients are not helpful after they are discharged from the ward; such protracted associations are often a substitute for, rather than a product of, increased maturity and autonomy.

When investigated, patients report that the benefits they gained from group meetings derived from the instillation of hope, the helpfulness of fellow-patients, the discovery that attributes considered as singular were in fact common to other patients, and the warmth and support of the group (Maxmen, 1973).

For staff the ward organization described can be challenging, rewarding and continually instructive. For the therapeutic community to fulfil its obligation fully, patients must be able to proceed to out-patient status: many in-patients can have necessary personality changes initiated, and be taken further by attending for out-patient interviews subsequently. In this out-patient phase of treatment, the unit can continue to contribute, augmenting the individual clinician's out-patient treatment. The patient might, from time to time, call on the ward and renew his contacts with members of staff and patients. Secondly, members of the ward staff, including nurses competent to do so, might undertake out-patient psychotherapy and thus preserve the continuity of patient care.

3.2.2
Day care
J. R. W. CHRISTIE BROWN

Introduction

The notion that admission as an in-patient to a psychiatric hospital can be harmful is not new, but it was one of the ideas behind the wave of change that has run through psychiatric thinking since the 1950s; at times, this idea has been recklessly and dangerously transformed into the belief that in-patient admission is inevitably harmful and this distortion has brought in its wake some of the damaging practices on the fringes of psychiatric work, as well as the spectacle of the disabled being turned out of hospital under the banner of rehabilitation to join the ranks of the destitute.

Curiously, there has been some sluggishness in building up day care, which occupies the valuable middle ground between in-patient and out-patient services. Part of the reason for this seems to be a certain rigidity of thinking which, almost from habit, sees nothing between the two administrative extremes and looks upon day care as something highly specialized.

A patient who is considered for admission presumably needs assessment, investigation, treatment or protection, or some combination of these which cannot be provided as an out-patient, but under what circumstances does such a patient need to sleep in the hospital? There can only be four reasons:

(1) If observations or tests are needed which have to be carried out at night as well as during the day.

(2) If the patient is so ill that specialized care is needed at night.

(3) If the patient is a danger to himself or others.

(4) If separation from his home environment is considered a necessary part of the treatment.

These are absolute reasons for admission but there are two partial reasons, the force of which varies from case to case. First, and quite frequently, patients may require admission simply because they have no worthwhile social support in the community and, secondly, distance of the home from the hospital demands admission. Where these various barriers do not operate, day care should always be considered as should its positive advantages. These are, first, that there is less disruption of the patient's contact with home, family and wider social environment, and secondly, some of the stigma of becoming a psychiatric patient is lessened and, indeed, some patients who refuse in-patient care may agree to being treated as day patients. Finally, the patient himself has less sense that his responsibility for running his own life and affairs is being taken over by others.

The development of day care in Britain

The first psychiatric day hospital was opened in Moscow in the 1930s (Beard, 1972) but it was not until 1948 that the first British day hospital was started in London (Bierer, 1951). The idea was, of course, not entirely new and small numbers of patients had been attending mental hospital wards on a daily basis for many years but the formal recognition of a new kind of service was followed by its fairly rapid spread in Britain, Canada, and the USA. By 1966 there were sixty-five day hospitals in England and Wales, admitting 1600 new patients every year. In the USA by 1966 Wilder and co-workers expressed the hope that two-thirds of all patients formerly cared for as in-patients would become day patients, and indeed such estimates spiralled upwards.

Particularly since the reorganization of local government in 1971, Social Service Departments have been providing day care in day centres. These differ from day hospitals in having no medical or nursing staff, and in fact quite often no trained staff at all, and yet have come to care for many of the most chronic and profoundly disabled psychiatric patients, the chronic schizophrenics. Of all day care provision about 75 per cent of places are in day hospitals and 25 per cent in day centres.

An interesting feature of day hospitals and to a lesser extent of day centres is the way in which dif-

ferent approaches have developed in different places. Some are run like conventional psychiatric units without beds, some on therapeutic community lines, some to provide work rehabilitation, and some to provide shelter and support. All day hospitals can usefully provide the same multidisciplinary staff team as an in-patient unit: the role of nursing staff is crucial and the senior nurse is often the lynch pin of the day hospital organization. In addition, the day hospital is a good base for the community nursing team with which a most fruitful liaison can be established. (See also chapter 3.4.1.)

Despite the expansion, and despite the theoretical advantages and the relative cheapness of day patient compared to in-patient care, the number of day places in England and Wales has fallen far short of the goals set by the Department of Health and Social Security, and the existing places are often under-used (Edwards, 1978).

The day care population

The patients in day hospitals are traditionally described as younger and more likely to suffer from neuroses and less likely to have organic disorder than in-patients. In a recent personal study comparing a day hospital and an admission ward serving the same London borough, it was found that on measures of social dislocation the groups were virtually identical, while in diagnostic terms there were more cases with organic disorders in the ward: neurotic illness was diagnosed in 19 per cent of the day hospital cases and 1 per cent of the in-patients, while the percentages for personality disorder were 8 per cent and 10 per cent respectively. Day hospitals, then, take patients in all diagnostic categories but many more with neurotic disorders than do in-patient wards.

The effectiveness of day care

Most of the studies providing a general evaluation of day care have been carried out in the USA, and it has been difficult for obvious reasons to assign patients at random to day care or in-patient treatment. Wilder and co-workers (1966) did succeed in random allocation of a group of acute psychiatric disorders and found day care as effective as in-patient care over a follow-up period of two years. Michaux and co-workers (1973) used the forced randomization produced by a catchment area boundary to compare 45 day patients with 54 matched in-patients and found that in-patient treatment gave quicker symptom relief while day treatment preserved social adjustment better. Other studies have produced similar findings.

A British study is that of Carney and colleagues (1970) who followed up 119 patients for at least one year after their discharge from a new urban day hospital and correlated general ratings of outcome with 26 clinical variables. Patients with a diagnosis of phobic anxiety state showed the greatest improvement, while those with a diagnosis of personality disorder did worst. A good outcome was also associated with longer duration of stay, living with a spouse, consultation with a psychologist, and being between 20 and 39 years old. The last two variables were probably related to the diagnosis of phobic anxiety state as patients with this diagnosis received behavioural treatment from a psychologist and fell into the age group in question. The majority of the phobic patients had previously received various combinations of in-patient and out-patient treatments with relatively less benefit and it seems that for this group day care was not only a successful way of organizing treatment but was superior to other methods.

The advantages of day care for patients with personality disorders and neuroses

The treatment of these patients is most commonly carried out on an out-patient basis but where more intensive measures are necessary, day care should always be considered before admission to an in-patient unit. As has been described, day hospitals can and do provide effective care for these patients and in addition in-patient units with special facilities can usually extend their services to day patients without difficulty and without the need for a designated day hospital, once the idea of doing so has occurred to the staff. Indeed, there are few investigations or treatments in the field of psychiatry that cannot be organized for suitable patients on a day basis. The advantages are obvious and yet often ignored. They have been outlined earlier but there are two which require further emphasis. First, the day patient remains significantly more firmly embedded in his social milieu and in family relationships than the in-patient and any attention that is required to these aspects of the patient's life is more easily given and the assistance of relatives in the treatment more easily harnessed. It follows, of course, that a slavish adherence to this advantage of day care is foolish in the case of patients who have suffered social breakdown, but day care then comes into its own during the process of social reconstruction. Secondly, in the field of personality disorder and the neuroses, and particularly in the case of the former, the psychiatrist has to make and work with extremely difficult judgements about the extent to which it is correct or useful to consider the patient as ill. An essential part of management is often a return to the patient of the responsibility for solving his own problems, a responsibility which has been handed over to some extent to those providing treatment when the person concerned is first identified as a patient. Such delicate transitions are much more easily handled in day care than in an in-patient unit.

3.3
Children, adolescents, the elderly, and the mentally handicapped

3.3.1
Principles of treatment specifically applicable to children and adolescents

LIONEL HERSOV

Introduction

Child psychiatric disorders are multifactorial in origin (see chapters 1 and 4) and present in different ways, depending on a child's and adolescent's age and stage of physical and emotional development and the interplay of constitutional, temperamental, family, and environmental factors. A variety of approaches to treatment is therefore needed including individual and group psychotherapy, family casework, family therapy, behaviour modification, drug therapy, in-patient and day-patient services, and consultation–liaison with paediatric services. Management using community resources includes placement in alternative families, consultation–liaison with child-care agencies, as well as with the staff of ordinary and special schools, and the use of special educational facilities, either day schools or boarding-schools, in conjunction with psychiatric supervision and treatment. All these forms of treatment are usually provided by a multidisciplinary team of psychiatrist, psychologist, social worker, and, in some instances, child psychotherapist, working in a hospital setting or in a community child guidance clinic.

Psychotherapy

The technical aspects of the psychiatric interview with children and their parents or the whole family are fully described (chapter 2.2). Family, social, and educational influences are then added to the individual appraisal of child and parents, and included in the overall assessment which leads to a dynamic formulation and strategy for treatment. Any of the approaches listed above can be used singly, as they often are in the more traditional settings. Modern practice combines several forms of treatment to gain the best effect. However, the principles embodied in a psychotherapeutic approach are inherent in most, if not all, of the treatments applied to psychiatrically disturbed children and adolescents and their families.

The methods of psychotherapy applied to adults are described earlier in this chapter (see chapter 3.1.1). The crucial importance of the personal relationship between patient and therapist and the psychological means of communication used are fully described by Frank (1979). This is especially so with children and adolescents. In treating younger children the use of symbolic objects in the form of toys and means of expression, such as drawing, painting, and modelling with clay and plasticine, is the medium of communication and exchange and therefore comparable to the exclusive use of words as a medium with adults. Play alone may be initially beneficial or sometimes therapeutic with children, but is not a psychotherapeutic procedure in itself, any more than is casual conversation with an adult. In some older children and adolescents verbal discussion alone can lead to a satisfactory diagnostic interview and become an effective means of communication in continuing with psychotherapy. The majority of children, and certainly younger children, are not at ease with words alone and need the medium of play to give voice to their feelings and display their fantasies. Normal children at play explore their feelings, increase their sense of excitement, attempt to understand a puzzling event by graphic representation, seek to confirm a hazy memory or, later, a memory of an event by making it more pleasant in fantasy (Millar, 1968). Many of these features are encountered and used in psychotherapy, so that toys available should lend themselves easily to the expression of feelings and ideas rather than constrain the children with a set of rules, as is the case with table games. Paints, plasticine, puppets, family doll figures, sand and water, houses and furniture, witch figures, wild animals, soldiers, small guns, airplanes, tanks, and target sets allow symbolic play to express fear and anger, feelings of loss, and the need for reparation. Most children and some younger adolescents will prefer a mixture of play and words to communicate with their therapist, so that a wide range of attractive play material should be available, preferably inexpensive and sturdy, and should be discarded or repaired or replaced when broken. The following illustrates symbolic play.

A 10-year-old boy suffering from separation anxiety symbolizes his fear of leaving home and mother using a doll's house in a sand-tray. The boy-doll figure is trapped in quicksand and dragged down to his death when he leaves the house, while his mother looks on helplessly.

Although there are obvious differences between children, adolescents, and adults in the technique, style, and medium of communication, the principles of psychotherapy with children have a great deal in common with those used in adults. One has to remember that most children do not come for treatment of their own accord but are brought by others, usually parents, who are worried about their slow development and their inappropriate behaviour at home, at school, or in the community. Some articulate children from middle and upper class backgrounds indicate their personal need for help with their intense anxieties, but they are uncommon. Shepherd and co-workers (1971) found that the major factor relating to referral to a child guidance clinic was the mother's personality, in that mothers who sought help with their children tended to be more depressed, anxious, easily upset by stresses, and perplexed and worried by their children's behaviour. Children come to psychiatrists with a variety of expectations, depending on what they have or have not been told about psychiatric assessment, their previous experiences with doctors and hospital staff, and the prejudices or knowledge of those other adults responsible for their education and care. They may be anxious or angry, silent and sullen, critical and mistrustful, or passive and uncommunicative. Children and youngsters like this are a test of the psychiatrist's skill, tolerance, and patience, and much hard work and many interviews are needed to gain the child's confidence and trust and establish a psychotherapeutic relationship. Important points in establishing and maintaining effective communication are the regularity, punctuality, privacy, and confidentiality of interviews, so that the child or youngster comes to feel that the psychiatrist is solely committed to the period spent with him/her whatever is done or said.

Reisman (1973) defines psychotherapy with children by what is *done* rather than by aims or goals as 'the communication of person-related understanding, respect and a wish to be of help'. He provides a useful outline of the main principles involved: (a) there should be careful assessment of the actual psychological processes responsible for the child's problems without necessarily adhering to any theoretical formulation (see chapter 2.2); (b) the child should be given ample opportunity (see chapter 2.2) to express feelings and beliefs in a situation which is deliberately structured to facilitate such communication; (c) the therapist should communicate his understanding of the child, his problems and his wish to be of help; (d) child and therapist should define their purpose or goal of their meetings at the onset and as psychotherapy progresses goals should be modified or new goals added; (e) the therapist makes clear what is ineffective or inappropriate about the child's behaviour and, in older children, the inconsistency of beliefs, actions, and feelings; (f) when dealing with inappropriate behaviour, which is mainly dependent on social interaction and relationships, the therapist may attempt to modify it by negotiation within the social system, or may step aside and focus directly on the system within the family or school (one could add in-patient hospital unit, children's home or other institution to the settings for focused intervention); (g) treatment should not be interminable but should be ended by negotiation when the therapist believes the advantages of ending outweigh the advantages of continuing even though the child may not be completely better.

This broad approach is in keeping with current practice in most child psychiatric and child guidance clinics and there is a continuing trend toward focused short-term therapy (Reid & Shyne, 1969, Rosenthal & Levine, 1971) in which the family is told the number of sessions planned from the outset. The treatment focus is explained early on and the issue of ending treatment kept in the forefront of meetings from the beginning. Active and even directive methods are used rather than non-directive type psychotherapy or long-term analytic psychotherapy. In general, there is an increasing trend to limit the use of psychotherapy to the specific disorders which are likely to respond rather than to use it indiscriminately as the only method of treatment. As a result, it is rarely used alone to treat autistic children or those with severe conduct disorders, and has its best results with children and adolescents with emotional and psychosomatic disorders.

Social casework

Parents of children and adolescents with psychiatric disorders often experience their own difficulties, which influence the way they bring up their children, respond to their developmental problems, or deal with the disordered behaviour and strong feelings they display at home or school. A parent who has experienced a deprived upbringing with or without physical abuse and neglect, and whose marriage is unstable or devoid of harmony and who lives in stressful circumstances of poverty, overcrowding, and lack of social support, often lacks confidence and self-esteem. Parents may be too depressed to take any active measures to deal with their child's problems or, while knowing what should be done, are unable to put their ideas into practice. In a therapeutic relationship with a social worker they can establish a sense of trust and stability which enables them to draw on their repertoire of coping skills to deal with the difficulties which might have been avoided or denied. This can be through the promotion of insight or self-understanding in those parents who can use these approaches or through direct techniques derived from the framework of learning theory (Sussenwein, 1977). Traditionally, social workers have preferred individual case-work which may continue in the family's own home as well as at a hospital or clinic. Working with family groups is now widely practised, and current child care legislation in the UK requires social workers to be able to deal directly with children and adolescents in a therapeutic as well as a supervising role. Social Service Departments now have statutory responsibility for abused and neglected children so that efforts are being made in the training of social workers to fill what has been up to now a glaring gap in their knowledge of child development and behaviour.

Family therapy

As mentioned above there is a trend toward psychiatric interviews in which all the family members are seen at the outset, usually by the psychiatrist or other members of the team, or by two 'co-therapists'. This may be for assessment only or may be followed by family therapy of which there are many styles and techniques of treatment as well as theoretical models (Skynner, 1969; Minuchin, 1974; Glick & Kessler, 1974; Haley, 1976; Dare, 1977).

There has been a stream of papers over the last 10 years but very few adequate studies of outcome of family therapy in spite of the wide-spread belief that it is an effective form of treatment (Lask, 1979). Indications for treatment are gradually being defined as well as attempts to establish family factors in certain psychosomatic disorders such as asthma (Lask & Kirk, 1979).

Systems-oriented family therapy (Minuchin, 1974) deals with present family functioning and how the problem or psychiatric disorder is being maintained rather than how it developed or was precipitated. The psychiatrist joins the family and takes part in its interactions during the assessment interview in order to understand the family's way of functioning and why it is necessary for one or more members of the family to be designated to provide the problem or display the symptoms. Stages of this process have been outlined (Barker, 1981) and there are many schemes for family assessment which include such factors as family structure, flexibility of function and capacity for change, 'resource' or sensitivity to the actions of family members ranging from the extreme of 'enmeshment' or over-sensitivity to change in family pattern, to 'disengagement' with little response to deviation from family pattern. The family is also assessed in its life context of social support and environmental stress in relation to the extended family, neighbours, school, and community. The stage of family development is also appraised by relating parents' own stage of personal and marital development to that of their children (Minuchin, 1974).

With this information in mind the therapist makes a family diagnosis which is a formulation or working hypothesis predicting certain changes if particular interventions are made. Family members are given tasks and the therapists may model appropriate behaviour for a family member or engage the family in role-playing, so allowing them to observe and alter their own and other members' behaviour. The skill appears to be in the therapist's sensitivity to communications within a family, ability to join a family on their own terms while retaining objectivity, and using his own personality and style of communication in empathic fashion. The term 'family homeostasis' has been coined to describe the balance of forces and patterns within families. Family therapy aims at altering fixed detrimental ways of relating and behaving so that movement can occur toward healthier and more effective development.

CASE ILLUSTRATION

A twelve-year-old girl, the daughter of well-established West-Indian-born parents, was referred as an emergency by the general practitioner for acute severe depression with suicidal ideas and gestures, and some mild paranoid beliefs. This had begun four months previously when she returned from school, burst into tears, complained that other children were teasing her, plotting against her, and telling lies about her. She cried all night, lost her appetite, but continued school attendance with constant and increasing complaints about feeling an 'outcast', even though her teacher had been contacted to intervene on her behalf. Menarche had begun two months before referral. The patient was described as intensely tearful, trembling, shaking, pulling her hair out. She complained that the whole class were swearing at her and expressed compulsive thoughts, 'I have lots of things on my mind, but I cannot say'. She asked her mother if she was going mad. Three days prior to attendance she ran out of her home threatening to smash windows and the parents bolted the door to contain her. The GP prescribed medication, but restlessness continued unabated and she locked herself in the bathroom, shook bottles of tablets, threatening to take them or jump out of the window.

The family consisted of father, aged 44 years, a warehouse manager, hardworking and stable with no history of psychiatric disorder; mother, aged 34 years, worked as a sales assistant. She suffered postnatal depression following the birth of her two daughters, requiring in-patient treatment for two months and ECT on both occasions. Six years before the present referral and four years after the last hospital admission she had a further depressive episode requiring two months in hospital. Since then she was prescribed continual medication and had mood swings with occasional periods of deeper depression. The patient's sister, aged 10 years, was described as happy and more outgoing than the patient, and therefore more 'troublesome' at home.

The patient's early development was apparently normal, but she spent her first few months in a psychiatric hospital with her mother who was undergoing treatment. She was described as 'bottling up her feelings' but an excellent pupil who had also complained of being 'bullied and beaten' at her primary school when she became quiet and depressed but recovered without active treatment.

At the initial assessment the patient appeared a tall, well-dressed, intelligent, articulate young teenager who talked normally and clearly, giving a good account of her feelings. She described herself as a split person, sometimes calm and in control, at others hysterical, screaming and crying, with suicidal thoughts about slashing her wrists, swallowing tablets, and taking poison. She felt guilty about this but could not control her feelings of depression and fight against them. She had lost confidence and hopes of an academic career and blamed other girls at school. She described the feelings of 'a barrier of hate against her at school.' There was no evidence of thought disorder, disorientation, or hallucinations.

The formulation was of an affective disorder with mild paranoid features, the illness being related to the mother's predisposition to depressive disorder. In addition, there appeared to be problems over communication within the family, centred on the stresses posed by the mother's previous psychiatric illnesses, her present state of chronic depression, and the upheaval caused by the patient's over-reaction to pressures at school. The decision was taken to use family therapy rather than medication with the aim of establishing boundaries between the parents as a couple and the children. It appeared that mother and eldest daughter (the patient) were overinvolved and resonating to each other's fears and mood swings. The father had been excluded and took no part in family discussions; the younger daughter had tended to be ignored and any attempts by her to discuss matters with her parents had been dismissed as 'troublesome'.

Seven family sessions took place with two therapists (psychiatrist and social worker). The strategy was to use a fairly directive approach to establish better boundaries between parents and children while encouraging communication between parents. The patient's depression and suicidal talk was interpreted as a way of keeping the parents from worrying about their own relationship problems by focusing on her disordered behaviour. By the fifth session the patient who formerly had been adamant about not returning to her old school agreed to a joint meeting between teachers, parents, and social worker. The meeting was successful, she returned to shool the next day, settled in well, and lost all manifestations of depression. A month later progress was maintained, she had made new friends, was reported to be enjoying school and due to go into the top group in the next academic year. The whole family atmosphere had greatly improved, with freer discussion of feelings and problems and a general air of cheerfulness and relaxation. Six months later she was still well settled in school, with no other problems.

Behavioural approaches

These methods of treatment have become increasingly popular over the last 20 years, not only for use by trained professionals such as psychiatrists and psychologists, but also by children's care-takers in institutional or hospital settings and by training parents to act as therapists for their children (McAuley & McAuley, 1977). The distinct steps in the behavioural approach are (a) the objective definition of the problem by enquiry about the frequency, severity and surrounding circumstances of the present behaviour, (b) setting up hypotheses to account for the problem with the aim of making predictions that if certain steps are taken the child's behaviour will be altered, (c) testing out these hypotheses by systematic observation and recording of the effects of the intervention, (d) assessing the outcome and relating it to the intervention (Yule, 1977). Direct observation plays an important part in behaviour modification techniques, both in discerning how the behaviour to be treated responds to physical and social stimuli and in leading to alterations in the behaviour itself by its consequences and effects. In simple contingency management, behaviour is modified by the use of rewards and punishments, but the more complex

techniques of desensitization, exposure, modelling and operant conditioning are also used in cases of phobias, school refusal and obsessional disorders (Yule, 1977).

CASE ILLUSTRATION

A six-year-old boy was referred for treatment of very frequent uncontrollable tempers when frustrated, controlling behaviour at home, reluctance to go to school, and unwillingness to eat school dinners. He was of very superior intelligence, already reading well above his age level, whereas both parents were relatively unintelligent, with limited interests. His mother had been treated several times in a psychiatric hospital for depressive disorder, and was on a heavy dose of maintenance medication. She could not withstand her son's demands and responded leniently, whereas the father was alternately furious and threatening or uninterested and unhelpful with the boy's behaviour. A behavioural approach was used to identify the situations in which the behaviour occurred, as well as details of the parents' inconsistent management which increased the frequency of problem behaviour. A point system of rewards for appropriate behaviour was followed by a 'time-out from reinforcement' programme to deal with temper tantrums. The removal of positive reinforcement for tantrum behaviour, either by removing the child from the source of reinforcement or removing the source of reward itself for a specified time period, had a powerful effect on the tantrums, which rapidly diminished and finally disappeared. The mother was able to cut down on her medication and finally stop it, and the family coped very well later with a move to a new town which involved change of home, work, schools and social relationships.

In-patient and day-patient hospital treatment

Children are admitted to hospital for treatment for a variety of reasons, usually because of such severe psychiatric disorder that treatment is impossible under other circumstances, for example, acutely psychotic or suicidal behaviour, severe anorexia nervosa, or because it is believed that a period of treatment in a therapeutic milieu will reduce tension in the home setting, allow work to be done with the family to restore an emotional steady state, and help the child or adolescent with sorting out his or her own intra-psychic and inter-personal problems. The whole range of treatments listed earlier can be employed singly or in combination, usually with the aim of returning the patient to the family (Holbrook, 1978). Hospital treatment is seen as a specialized and intensive treatment experience among a range of treatment facilities, which usually occurs only once, but may on occasions last quite some time, on average between three and six months.

The 'therapeutic milieu' of in-patient and day-patient treatment implies that the social, emotional, and physical environment and surroundings are themselves part of the process of treatment (Hersov & Bentovim, 1977). A setting is provided where different individual therapeutic strategies and experiences can be implemented for most, if not all, of the day. The experience and interaction goes beyond the daily routine and requires thoughtful concern about each child and adolescent's individual abilities, handicaps, needs, tolerance of stress, educational level, quality of interpersonal relationships, and social skills. The other patients provide a peer group which is very important for many of the children who have undergone in their own home or in schools faulty or inappropriate social learning experiences which have contributed to their psychiatric disorder and social handicaps. They can enter into the usual activities for their age group in the hospital school or as part of the daily programme. The aim is to help the child engage in all possible activities so that he/she can learn skills and master situations he/she may have avoided or in which he/she would usually display inappropriate or even antisocial behaviour. Group therapy may be of help to achieve this goal or where there are particular problems in social relationships.

Programmes of independence training or training in social assertiveness and social skills can be set up for immature and socially inexperienced children with emotional disorders, while those with conduct disorders will receive help aimed at improving impulse control and aggressiveness (Wilkinson, 1979). Remedial teaching for educational retardation is also available.

With pre-school children day hospital treatment allows therapy to be initiated and continued with parents and child together so avoiding unnecessary separations. The child can be examined, a neurodevelopmental and psychological assessment be carried out, and he can be observed in interaction with his own parents and siblings, other parents, and children and with members of staff. Parent groups are most effective for discussion of management problems with young children and inexperienced, immature mothers can be helped to add to their repertoire of parenting skills and replace limited inappropriate and rigid methods by more effective approaches. In some instances a whole family can be admitted to hospital so that family therapy and active skills training can be combined, and this can be very effective in certain cases of child abuse and neglect. However, the work that has been carried out in hospital must then be generalized to the home via home

visits and a continuation of the programme in the home setting. Not doing this invites failure, for parents may become quite competent in the supportive setting of a hospital unit but be unable to carry on as effectively once they have returned home.

Community services

Child guidance clinics usually function in close association with the school psychological services and health care services provided for school children. Although there may be differences in emphasis between hospital and community-based child and adolescent psychiatric clinics, the basic approach to problems is very similar. In a model system there would be close liaison between hospital and community services with access to the specialized range of hospital treatments when needed, but also with continuing supervision in school and community by the other services when the patient leaves hospital.

Social Services Departments deal with a large number of disturbed children either in their own homes or 'in care' and also have statutory responsibility for abused and neglected children, once they are notified. Liaison–consultation work with social services departments is an increasing part of psychiatric treatment for children and adolescents. It may take the form of assessments of children coming into 'care' or may provide support to staff groups in residential institutions such as children's homes. Special education in day and boarding schools for 'maladjusted' children under the 1944 Education Act has been a prominent feature of the services for children with psychiatric disorders. Psychiatric consultation and supervision is available in a number of these schools, and severely disturbed children are often placed there directly from home or after in-patient and day hospital treatment. There are dangers in using school services in such a way that the child becomes isolated from his most intimate relationships with family and friends, in the world outside the school. As with hospital units, boarding schools must try to function as an integral part of a wider community service even though this is often difficult and time-consuming.

There is an increasing trend toward providing 'alternative families' for emotionally disturbed children. The recognition of the fact that certain family circumstances are detrimental to healthy growth and development, while the need for a family to facilitate emotional and social development continues until early adulthood, means that a child might have to be removed from his own home and placed in another. The example that comes to mind is where severe physical abuse has occurred and here there is increasing use of foster families and adoption. Tizard (1977) has reviewed the studies on the efficacy of adoption and from her own research has concluded that there are many more advantages to be gained from placing children for adoption than from leaving them to grow up in children's homes or other institutions.

Drug treatment

There are specific indications for the use of drugs in child and adolescent disorders such as epilepsy, pervasive overactivity (see chapter 4.1.3), certain types of enuresis, and clearcut depressive disorders in older children and adolescents. Most often they are used to complement the other forms of treatment described in this section and therefore their effects are difficult to evaluate. Most studies of drug effects have been with the amphetamines, methylphenidate, the phenothiazines such as chlorpromazine, and with haloperidol. There is little evidence that benzodiazepines have any useful effects except in providing temporary relief in instances of acute and severe anxiety. In general, drugs can complement but cannot be a substitute for a behavioural and/or psychotherapeutic approach to children and youngsters and their families, for it is in this context that change usually is seen. However, there are drug treatments of established value in a limited range of disorders (see chapters 3.1.4 and 4), and possibly more to come as clinical research defines their indications and contraindications.

Conclusions

There has been a considerable change in treatment methods in child and adolescent psychiatry in the past 20 years. A range of methods is more often used than single treatment approaches, with an emphasis on consultation with community, educational, and social services. There is still a dearth of evaluation studies apart from those that have reviewed drug treatments. The most striking change is in the growth of family approaches to treatment.

3.3.2
Psychotherapy in the elderly
KLAUS BERGMANN

Introduction

There are formidable barriers to undertaking psychotherapy in older people. Foremost among these is the failure to recognize acute neurotic problems when they occur in the elderly. This is reflected in the low levels of hospital referrals, health insurance claims (in private office practice in the USA), and general practice psychotherapy for neurotic disorder in older people (Kessel & Shepherd, 1962; Shepherd & Gruenberg, 1957; Shepherd *et al*, 1966).

Another important barrier is that the psychoanalytic school, the foundation of practice for many psychotherapists, focuses on the problems of youth and early adulthood, especially in the areas of psychosexual development and socialization, so that maladaptive patterns to the stresses of later life are not considered a legitimate area of study. Even literature referring to psycho-analytic treatment at 'an advanced age' (Abraham, 1920) refers to patients who are 40 to 50 years of age.

Behind the problems already mentioned lies the lack of a theoretical approach to the dynamics of the relationship between therapist and the older patient; this is required for many reasons, not least in order to permit a structured approach to the therapy, one which goes beyond simple reassurance. Some descriptions of the use of psychoanalytic type of psychotherapy based on classical 'transference' models and focused on private office practice have been described (Blau & Berezin, 1975). A more specifically old-age orientated approach is outlined by Verwoerdt (1981) but still with the vocabulary and assumptions of classical psychoanalysis dangerously stretched to accommodate the latter end of life.

It is proposed in this account to focus on three questions which, it is hoped, will aid a dynamic approach to the psychotherapy of the elderly, more relevant to their life situation and needs. This will be considered under the following headings:

(1) Epidemiological and case-finding considerations
(2) Concepts of adjustment and aims of therapy
(3) A theoretical framework of the therapist/patient relationship in later life and specific dynamic issues of importance arising in the course of therapy.

Epidemiological considerations and case-finding

If neurotic disorder ameliorates or conversely if it becomes almost universal in old age then the question of selection of psychotherapy becomes irrelevant.

Epidemiological studies of prevalence (for example, those cited in Kay & Bergmann, 1980) suggest that the prevalence of neurotic and personality disorder of at least moderate severity is about 12 per cent in those aged over 65 years. A substantial proportion of these disorders appear to start after 60 years of age (Bergmann, 1971), and 5 per cent have a history of less than five years duration (Kay *et al.*, 1964a,b).

Cooper and Schwartz (1981) identified these patients by employing two out of three of the following criteria: clinical symptom scores, global severity ratings, and the presence of an ICD diagnosis. At least 12 per cent of his elderly random sample subjects rated as having 'clinical' issues.

Thus neurotic disorder is neither absent nor universally present and there is no *a priori* case for treating elderly neurotics differently.

Significant associations with recent bereavement, illness and discharge from hospital, loneliness, and the need for social services (Kay *et al.*, 1964b; Foster *et al.*, 1976; Bergmann, 1978) suggest that the patients' search for psychotherapeutic support may often be masked by exaggerated physical disability, inappropriate demands and social needs, unduly persistent disability following bereavement or loss, and complaints of loneliness in the absence of gross isolation. Further exploration of emotional

issues is often indicated when the above conditions obtain. Not uncommonly, for example, a person who had a myocardial infarction may develop a phobic anxiety state which gives rise to more disability than any residual myocardial ischaemia. In such cases, the patient's disability is frequently not recognized as being of neurotic origin.

Concepts of adjustment

In earlier life sexual adjustment, success at work, family relationships especially those connected with child rearing are important criteria of psychological integration. Erikson (1959), while recognizing these as important in the earlier stages of life, suggests that in old age the central issue is that of 'ego integrity versus despair'.

Those who work with older people recognize the intuitive validity of such an insight, but find some difficulty in translating it into more mundane terms. If, however, we consider the major stresses and challenges and try to formulate how they are adaptively met by successful, competent, and intact elderly people, a more concrete idea of what we mean by 'integrity' should emerge.

Some of the relevant issues on which a therapist has to focus will be discussed. They include coping with losses usually in the form of bereavement, but also of status, wealth, occupation, and self-image, due to ageing and ill-health. A process of mourning has to be gone through and new attachments made.

Impending death is an universal issue. A coherent personal philosophy is of importance in coping with this (Hinton, 1967) and many older people are still actively grappling with this issue.

The problems of dependence have to be faced; these include avoiding unnecessary dependence, and yet incorporating the necessary help to maintain life in the community. The older person is called on to evaluate a complex situation, and assesses with some subtlety the motivation and expectations of a variety of helpers.

Family relationships change; power passes to the next generation, but loving relationships must be maintained, the older person still giving and also obtaining support. Lifelong distortions in family dynamics may come to a critical stage.

Some elderly people also retain their dignity, interests, and capacities in the presence of chronic pain and discomfort, though the mechanisms whereby they do this while so many others succumb is not clear.

In formulating the aims of therapy, an important step is to review how the elderly person is facing the issues of adjustment and which aspects of life require help.

Theoretical framework and issues of therapy

The concept of transference neuroses undergoes considerable strain if applied to the therapeutic relationship with older patients, and Goldfarb (1967) noted the different properties of the 'attachment' of the older patient to the therapist; he suggests that the patient be permitted to employ the therapist as a substitute for a 'parent'. But to what purpose? The author in looking for an answer has found that the concept of Bowlby (1969) is important in providing a model. He points out that ethological evidence points to a need for maternal attachment in learning to cope adaptively with threats. He goes on to suggest that if such an attachment is impaired during a critical period adaptive reactions to external threats are impaired.

Old age *par excellence* can be seen as a period fraught with severe and frightening threats, and neurosis arising in this period as a maladaptive reaction to such threats. The elderly person, therefore, has to be helped to find adaptive coping mechanisms from a dependent position of attachment, and then gradually develop independence, detaching himself from the therapist. Some link may have to be maintained for a considerable period or transferred to another person or institution.

Major issues that can be tackled in therapy include the presence of abnormal mourning (Parkes, 1972), the need for a life review in adjusting to the approach of death (Butler, 1975) and the psychopathological effect of learned helplessness (Seligman, 1975). In old age many situations occur where elderly persons are left helpless and where whatever action they take cannot influence their environment, nor can they exert any power or influence over their fate.

The attitudes of caregivers, both professionals in institutions and families in the community, often unwittingly contribute to this situation. One example often seen is the cloying and unalloyed sweetness shown to old people, regardless of their behaviour or the content of what they say.

Behaviour therapy with its orientation towards current disability and manifest symptoms would appear to have a role in the treatment of maladaptive behaviour in older people. The appointment of psychologists to units which assess and treat elderly patients in day hospitals, out-patient departments, and domiciliary practice is likely to aid the exploration and expansion of available behavioural interventions. In a recent review of the behavioural aspects of geriatric psychology, Hussian (1981) considers a variety of techniques; cognitive therapy, social skills training, systematic desensitization, and graded exposure. These techniques and others are shown to be applicable to the older patient.

In conclusion, if the case for a psychotherapeutic approach to the elderly is accepted, and psychotropic drugs do not have a good track record with this group of patients, what is the setting in which this therapy should take place?

The care of older patients is undertaken by a multidisciplinary team in which nurses, doctors, social workers, psychologists, and occupational therapists are nearly always represented. The patient may make a significant attachment to any member of the team, and staffing of units for the elderly should be sufficiently generous to permit all professionals in this team to carry a number of cases for therapy. However, if the psychiatrist leading the team has not the knowledge nor the interest to encourage, supervise, and support other team members, little progress will be seen.

Special psychotherapy clinics for the elderly do not seem appropriate, but staffing levels and the dynamic orientation of the team caring for and assessing the psychiatrically ill older person should permit a psychotherapeutic approach within the structure of the present systems of health care delivery.

3.3.3
The principles of management of the mentally handicapped child and his family

JOHN CORBETT

A basic principle of treatment in child psychiatry is that the success of any intervention relies, to a large extent, on the child care skills and emotional adjustment and attitudes of the key individuals in the child's immediate environment. This derives from an understanding of children's dependence on adults, and for this reason, concurrent therapeutic work with families has become an integral part of therapy.

Mentally retarded children are more dependent and, in the severely retarded, this dependence is likely to persist throughout life; hence therapeutic work with parents assumes an even greater importance. The circle of significant individuals reaches beyond the nuclear family, particularly in the mentally retarded, and includes all personnel of the agencies involved in providing comprehensive care (Tarjan, 1977).

This does not mean that direct psychiatric intervention is required with all mentally retarded children or their families, and the majority make an adequate adjustment and have other priority needs. Much of the work of the psychiatrist in helping families with a handicapped member will necessarily be indirect, working with other members of the mental handicap team to provide the full range of services likely to be needed with consistency over a long period of time. Thus he may be involved with the paediatrician in counselling about the nature and extent of the handicap, with the social worker in helping families to deal with their reactions and attitudes, and with the social worker and community nurse in providing practical support and advice aimed directly at alleviation of the burden of care. The psychologist, nurse, and other specialist therapist or teacher may be involved in helping the parents to develop special skills, aimed at maximizing the child's potential and dealing with practical management problems, for example, difficult behaviour.

This calls for multiple skills and knowledge of the assessment of the handicapped person, particularly in a developmental context, familiarity with the role and special skills of the professionals concerned, and particularly an understanding of both the nature and extent of psychiatric disorders in the mentally retarded and the stresses imposed on families and others in caring for the handicapped child.

The stresses on families with a handicapped child, and their reactions, have been the subject of a number of comprehensive reviews (Wolfensberger, 1968; Carr, 1974; Willer *et al.*, 1978). Wolfensberger concludes that parents must cope with three major crises. The first is the initial shock on becoming aware of the diagnosis and the second is a value crisis which involves a re-fashioning by the parents of their hopes and expectations for the child. Thirdly, there is the reality crisis in which parents have to come to grips with day to day practical problems. Each of these crises may leave the family more vulnerable to further stress, for example institutionalization of the child, or to the normally occurring crises of family life. Over the years most families develop coping mechanisms for dealing with these stresses and therefore cannot be seen as static structures; they are individuals whose needs will vary considerably over time.

The first and possibly the most difficult crisis follows diagnosis. Most studies of family reactions to this event have concerned easily recognized groups, such as Down's syndrome or spina bifida, where the handicap has been apparent at birth. This probably involves less than half of the severely retarded, and depending on the severity of the retardation and the effectiveness of professional screening, the diagnosis may be delayed until school age.

Farber and Rykman (1965) suggest that the information most parents incorporate from the diagnosis is that the child is abnormal, deficient, permanently handicapped, or even inhuman. The most typical reaction is one of severe grief, similar to that of losing a family member, and the experience of mourning may be necessary before an adjustment can be made, yet unlike a death in the family, the birth of an abnormal baby means that the parents are constantly reminded of their sorrow by the child's continued presence.

Studies of the way in which parents are told of the diagnosis have been carried out by D'Arcy (1968), Berg and co-workers (1969) and Carr (1974) and agree in finding that more parents who were told early were satisfied than were those told later, and that if parents are told earlier, before loving attachments have been formed with the child, it does not necessarily lead to outright rejection. There is general agreement that the way in which parents are told is of utmost importance, as is the need for continued support and counselling during the early months after diagnosis.

Unless adequate coping mechanisms do develop there may be further inappropriate reactions, such as disorientation of family members, similar to that seen in families suffering from other crises (Hill, 1949) or denial or repression of the diagnosis and loss of self-esteem (Malvia, 1973). A common professional reaction to this crisis in the past was to advise institutionalization (MacKeith, 1973) in the belief that the presence of a mentally retarded child in the family will have long-term deleterious effects on the family, the marriage and on the siblings (San Martino & Newman, 1974). More recently the emphasis has been on providing families with support and services to enable the mentally handicapped child to experience the benefits of developing in a normal family environment.

Where the diagnosis is delayed, for example in the less severely handicapped, ambiguity may lead to the parents becoming suspicious of the diagnosis (Bryant & Hirschberg, 1961) and this longer-lasting coping mechanism may lead to ambivalent feelings towards the child which may be manifest in over-indulgent, over-protective or authoritarian attitudes towards child rearing (Schild, 1971).

It is not possible in this short account to review fully the effects of the mentally handicapped child on the family, which are complex, and the evidence for deleterious effects, for example on siblings, is conflicting (Gath, 1975). Skilled and continuous counselling, starting as soon as the diagnosis is made, may identify particularly vulnerable families and help them to meet the demands of the situation.

Ideally, in an effective community service, severely retarded children will be identified before they reach school age, and it should be possible to plan for most of the naturally occurring crises of family life. Services will include regular short-term care, appropriate residential care for more severely handicapped, particularly at times of crisis such as parental illness or death, and day care and special education for all children.

Over the past ten years there have been an increasing number of studies aimed at involving parents in the treatment of their children and the most common approach has involved the application of behaviour modification principles (O'Dell, 1974; Gath, 1979). Most studies have dealt with specific, easily recognizable behaviour disorders and have laid emphasis on teaching parents the principles of behaviour modification, and less attention has been paid to the problems of generalization and long-term maintenance of such programmes.

More recently greater emphasis has been placed on relating parent training to the needs and strengths of individual families and the importance of setting goals which can be realistically achieved without the risk of parents suffering further role failure and subsequent depression. Emphasis has also been placed on helping parents to teach their children skills which are developmentally appropriate (Revill & Blunden, 1979; Clements et al., 1980).

Psychiatric treatment of mildly retarded children will require many of the techniques used with children of normal intelligence, while with the severely retarded, more reliance will be placed on psychotherapeutic work with families, environmental manipulation, chemotherapy, and behaviour modification.

Treatment of mentally retarded children and their families will depend on many factors. Most important among these will be the degree of retardation; particularly the secondary handicaps of the child, both behavioural and physical, and also the coping mechanisms and dynamics of the family.

3.4
The therapeutic team

3.4.1
Nursing treatment

CHIRSTY GILLIES AND
GERALD F. M. RUSSELL

Introduction

Psychiatric patients are admitted to hospital for many different reasons, but the essential component of in-patient treatment is that of nursing care. Patients with neurotic or personality disorders are generally treated as out-patients in the first instance, but there are occasions when the degree of their disability, their need for intensive or specific treatments, or their social circumstances, require an in-patient regime. It is then that the nursing staff can exert a powerful therapeutic influence. It should be added that nursing skills are no longer confined to the ward setting but can also be applied effectively in day hospitals (see Christie Brown, chapter 3.2.2, p. 102). A role for the community nurse* may also emerge although at present she cares principally for the elderly and patients with chronic schizophrenia. In this contribution we shall concentrate on nursing treatment in the setting of the psychiatric ward.

While in the ward, the patient experiences the effects of living in a semi-closed community whose therapeutic potential is vitally influenced by the nursing staff. The sister (or charge nurse) plays a crucial part in determining the ward atmosphere which will reflect her skill and experience, her sensibility to the needs of her patients, and her efficiency as an

---

* Throughout this article we have attributed the female gender to the nurse. This is a matter of convention and in no way detracts from the equal status of male members of the nursing profession.

organizer and teacher of her staff. She will also act as a focal point of communication within the multidisciplinary therapeutic team. The way in which the ward milieu, reinforced by the use of therapeutic groups, contributes to improvements in patients including beneficial changes in personality, has been discussed by H. J. Walton in this chapter (3.2.1). In this section we shall confine ourselves to interactions between the individual nurse and her patient, and a consideration of specific nursing techniques and skills.

The interaction between the nurse and her patient

Writers who comment on the nature of nursing skills lay stress on the relationship that is established between the nurse and her patient.

> Nursing is one profession in which satisfaction, happiness, and success are dependent to a great extent on the skills a nurse has developed in providing good relationships . . . The success she experiences in her chosen field in her efforts to help other people will depend upon her ability to interact with them in a positive way. It will depend upon the interpersonal relationships she experiences and upon how she *uses* herself in these relationships. (Burton, 1965)

The personal qualities of the nurse are seen to be the means of implementing the therapeutic goals:

> The natural mothering qualities of warmth, compassion, support and acceptance, fundamental to all nursing care practices, are brought into harmony with other therapeutic measures and treatment aims. Much thought is necessary as the nurse works with the patient in building feelings of trust, in providing comfort, in offering support, reassurance, companionship, respect and acceptance. (Leininger, 1961)

These formulations contain laudable principles but the realities of nursing practice should be borne in mind. More often than not, the contacts between the nurse and her patient tend to be unobtrusive and indirect. As the nurse gains the patient's confidence she shows herself willing to listen to his problems, and expresses concern and understanding of his difficulties. These therapeutic contacts often take place before the development of a close one-to-one relationship. Indeed the nurse will often utilize seemingly casual contacts as a means of encouraging the beginnings of a therapeutic relationship. Perhaps because of her training, and her image with patients, the nurse is accepted as the person who is concerned with aspects of physical care such as dressing, serving food, or administering medicines. It may be while combing a patient's hair that she encourages the patient to talk about her emotional problems. Similarly, personal contact may begin by the nurse broaching a social conversation with the patient. The topics may be totally neutral at first (clothes, hair, food, television) but progress to enquiries about visitors, members of the family, and weekend leave at home. These conversations provide a gentle entrée into the more personal aspects of the patient's life, and convey to him the feeling that the nurse is interested in what happens to him outside the hospital.

A gradual and unobtrusive interaction between the nurse and her patients commends itself for a number of reasons. Patients may not, in the first instance, view the nurse as a member of staff concerned with the details, especially the intimate details, of their illnesses and private lives. They more readily accept the role of the doctor as the person who sets time aside specifically for this purpose, who elicits the necessary information in the privacy of his consulting room and who may provide treatment intensively during sessions of one hour or less. The efficacy of nursing care derives in no small measure from its continued influence, throughout the patient's waking hours and for the duration of his stay in hospital. Thus there is time to develop a therapeutic relationship gradually and capitalize on the more prolonged and often closer contact between nurse and patient.

The development of a therapeutic relationship may pose problems for the nurse herself. Most nurses are acutely aware of the risks of 'over-involvement' with patients. This concern is understandable in terms of the nurse often not being in full control of the maintenance or termination of the relationship (she may be moved to another ward), not receiving the necessary close supervision, or quite simply having to share her contacts equitably between several patients in the same ward. This is an added argument for commencing nursing treatment by means of unobtrusive interactions. In the event of a closer relationship developing between the nurse and her patient, she should use her skills to channel the relationship in a therapeutic direction, recognize the degree of her own emotional reactions, and seek guidance in how to deal effectively with excessive dependence or negative responses on the part of the patient.

The therapeutic team

Many of the factors which influence effective nursing treatment remain shrouded in mystery. Nurses often experience difficulty in conveying to others the methods they employ in the care of psychiatric patients. Similar difficulties are also experienced by medical colleagues. There may therefore be barriers to the clear exchange of views between nurses and doctors, barriers which need much effort on both sides if they are to be surmounted. In order to utilize the full therapeutic potential of nurses it is necessary for psychiatrists to enter into a more considered professional alliance with the nurses. It is this alliance which constitutes the central core of the ward-based therapeutic team. (In the case of the out-patient team the psychiatrist's closest professional colleague is usually the social worker.) The doctors on the team will endeavour to communicate their plan of treatment to the nurses and become receptive to their ideas. Much of the authority for day-to-day care of patients in the ward will be handed over to the nursing staff who will accept responsibility for trying to achieve realistic therapeutic goals. The key to success is clear communication and a mutual respect of colleagues' professional skills.

Patterns of interaction between nurses and psychiatric patients

Confirmation of the apparently weak theoretical basis for some aspects of nursing treatment has been received from the work of Altschul (1972) who investigated the frequency and extent of therapeutic relationships between nurses and patients on acute psychiatric wards. She provided operational criteria for establishing whether a therapeutic relationship had been established. Both patient and nurse were required to report that they perceived themselves as having experienced such a relationship with each other; there would be a mutual awareness that the nurse experienced interest, liking, and sympathy for the patient; this awareness would be communicated in a direct sort of way. Altschul observed patterns of nurse–patient interaction and the occurrence of therapeutic relationships on the psychiatric wards. Her interest in this study was based on her impression that whereas the nurse's training might emphasize the value of an 'intensive one-to-one relationship', this had little bearing on the practice of psychiatric

nursing as it occurred in the ward. Her study confirmed that a true therapeutic relationship was established with only a small proportion of the patients. When concentrating simply on interactions between a nurse and a patient, viz., observing the nurse's behaviour without making inferences about her attitudes, she found that many of the interactions could be viewed as aspects of physical care, but that the nurses simultaneously observed the patients and listened to what they had to say. Similarly, many interactions consisted of social conversations which nevertheless led to the nurses showing interest in their patients. Approximately 40 per cent of the interaction time was devoted to discussion of the patients' symptoms or psychological problems. Altschul concluded:

> It would seem that this kind of support and help was important to patients. Nurses gave it without any very high degree of conscious awareness of what they were doing or why they were doing it, but with a conviction that it was important. It seems likely that the time with patients in group activities, in social conversation or physical care was a necessary preliminary for psychological help given by nurses to be acceptable to the patient . . .

Furthermore it did not appear as if nurses followed any clear treatment ideologies or theoretical models. It was frequent for nurses to insist that all psychiatric nursing is 'common sense'. The patient's diagnosis appeared unimportant in influencing nurse–patient interactions. Opposing views were also evident: some nurses allowed withdrawn patients to remain solitary, others made special efforts to approach silent patients and establish personal contact. In spite of these contradictions, skilled nursing can be recognized as such:

> . . . the most skilled performances observed were not in the realm of relationships, but in some of the interactions. The perceptive and sensitive way in which some nurses responded to patients' distress without any verbalization on the part of the patient was remarkable. Some nurses succeeded admirably in utilizing what appeared initially trivial contacts. Their words and manner were just right to start the patient talking. Some nurses were able to interweave skilled interviewing techniques with physical care, some were able . . . to spot precisely the right moment for encouragement, or for remaining in the patients' company, in spite of

the patients' denials at the time that company was needed. (Altschul, 1972)

More specific nursing techniques and skills

So far the discussion has concentrated on principles of basic psychiatric nursing. We shall now look at a few examples of more specific nursing procedures adapted to different forms of neurotic disorder and disturbances of behaviour. They include the depressed and suicidal patient, hysterical behaviour, repeated self-injuries, and anorexia nervosa. Finally, we shall mention the role of the nurse in behavioural psychotherapy.

The depressed and suicidal patient

The nursing care of the depressed patient provides a good model of the nurse–patient relationship being built on the patient's needs for sympathy, attention to physical care, and coaxing from habitual withdrawal. He is encouraged to take care of his personal hygiene and dressing. Attention at mealtimes is important not only because the depressed patient neglects his food requirements, but also because these occasions provide opportunities for interaction with the nurse and other patients. Burr (1970) gives good advice:

> Remember there are ways of communicating with people other than by words. Give him your time and attention. It may be difficult to get any response from him at all, but if you can bring him just to sit in the same room with the others this is a start. Sit beside him when you can. Even if he doesn't answer when you speak he knows that you have chosen to be with him rather than any other patient. Putting your hand over his, or drawing his arm through yours as you sit or walk tells him of your concern. Use your eyes, your hands, your smile to show your sympathy.

The suicidal patient imposes the greatest responsibility on the nursing staff, for while he remains suicidal his life is in their hands. Constant supervision is essential. Modern nursing practice favours that the patient should be up and about, dressed and encouraged to mix with other patients in the ward, so avoiding the isolation which results from methods based on segregated supervision. The ambulatory method of supervision requires, however, that every member of the nursing team is alert to the danger of suicide. Scrupulous teamwork is essential, a nurse being within sight of the patient

and aware of his movements and activities every moment of the day and night. Observation is combined with the establishment of personal contacts. The patient is encouraged to talk about his depressive and hopeless feelings, including suicidal ideas, and the nurse explains that everyone on the ward team is concerned for his safety and welfare.

Patients with hysterical symptoms or behaviour

The nurse contributes to the treatment of conversion symptoms such as paralysis or blindness by reducing the patient's need to adopt an abnormal sick role. The nurse meets his need for attention and affection while discouraging him from relying on disabling symptoms as a means of arousing sympathy. Instead, he should be encouraged to talk about any underlying problems while the nurse expresses appropriate interest and sympathy. More nursing attention and other rewards are provided as the patient's behaviour improves. The tendency for some patients to 'play off' members of the staff against each other can be prevented by holding staff meetings at which the nurses may compare their reactions to individual patients in an honest fashion and agree to a general policy of management.

Self-injuries

Patients who repeatedly injure or mutilate themselves (for example, cutting their wrists) are likely to impose a severe burden on the nursing staff. They are given various diagnostic labels – hysteria, depression, or personality disorder (so-called borderline states, more recently). Their intention is not usually one of suicide, but to relieve mounting tension. This state may give way to one of depersonalization in which the patient may cut her wrists, often not feeling pain and with only a hazy recollection for the event.

The management of self-mutilating patients can be very difficult. Nursing and medical staff alike tend to react to these patients with mixed sensations of anger and sympathy, rejection, and excessive strictness. This clinical problem is also one which merits free discussion among members of the therapeutic team to reach agreement on a clear policy aimed at preventing further episodes. There should be a preliminary analysis of the behaviour, so as to identify the settings and precipitants of self-injuries. Treatment will vary according to the individual patient's needs. If the patient is an adolescent young woman it may be appropriate to nurse her in a part of the ward shared with more mature patients. Her care is allocated to more experienced nurses who will remain calm and non-rejecting even in the event of cutting episodes. Close nursing contact is desirable, not so much in order to maintain strict supervision but so as to detect the mounting tension and isolation which precedes episodes. In this event the patient is encouraged to discuss her feelings with the nurse who will encourage relaxation and may provide comforting physical contact by putting her arm round her shoulders (Simpson, 1976). Prevention of episodes is not secured by intensive restrictions which may have the paradoxical effect of increasing their frequency. Instead, the programme of structured and increasing activity is designed in collaboration with the occupational therapy staff. In some instances, after a sound therapeutic relationship has been established by an individual nurse, it may be appropriate for her to stipulate that certain rewarding aspects of the treatment regime are conditional on the cessation of self-injury.

Anorexia nervosa

The nursing treatment of the anorexic patient admitted to hospital is the most effective method of restoring her weight to normal. The technique is described in chapter 8.3 of this volume. Success depends on experienced nurses developing a relationship of trust with the patient. She is encouraged to hand over to the nurse the decisions about the intake of food and the weight to be gained. At the same time a basic degree of patient-supervision is necessary, especially at meal-times. The method is essentially one of nursing treatment although it can also be viewed as containing elements of re-education (Groen & Feldman-Toledano, 1966), psychotherapy and behavioural therapy (Russell, 1981).

The role of the nurse in behavioural psychotherapy

Methods of behaviour therapy have been applied to the management of selected adult neurotic patients with phobic or obsessional symptoms, sexual problems and deviation. Marks and co-workers (1977) have trained nurse-therapists in these methods so that they acquire a new clinical role as psychiatric nurses. The nurse-therapists focus on observable behaviour and the principles of behavioural therapy, but they act as case-managers and not merely as technicians. The emphasis of the treatment is on 'flexibility, pragmatism and interpersonal skills' (Bird *et al.*, 1979), rather than on exclusively behavioural methods. Thus the component clinical methods include interviewing skills, analysis of the patient's problems, the formulation of realistic treatment goals, as well as specific treatment methods such as gradual exposure to feared situations, response prevention, flooding, modelling, and social skills training. The nurses are also taught how to select suitable patients and appropriate methods of behavioural treatment. An analysis of the outcome of treatment for phobic symptoms showed that nurse therapists achieved a degree of success comparable to that of other professionals (psychiatrists, psychologists, and medical students). It would appear that the nurse-therapists owe their success to a specific form of training similar to that received by psychiatrists and psychologists. It could be argued that in this new role they do not rely very much on the 'traditional' or 'orthodox' methods of nursing care previously discussed in this section. Indeed, nurses were selected by Marks and co-workers (1977, 1978), rather than social workers or occupational therapists, on the grounds of availability of manpower and cost-effectiveness, and not by virtue of their basic professional training and experience. Thus the nurse-therapists may have acquired specific clinical skills, but they are not specifically those of psychiatric nursing. There is now clear evidence that nurse-therapy as described by Marks and his colleagues, provides a most useful extension of behavioural psychotherapy, with the additional benefit that the treatment can often be administered to outpatients.

Conclusions

Nowadays members of the various professions making up the multi-disciplinary team are asserting their independence within the team, while at the same time often and paradoxically rejecting their special treatment functions. Doctors express unease about prescribing, social workers about organizing placements, and psychologists about psychometric testing. They all want to be therapists. Nurses also run the risk of viewing traditional nursing as inimical to special methods of treatment. Such a development would be a great pity. It has been our aim in this section to stress the value of the traditional nursing methods, while recognizing the merit of analysing further the ways whereby nurses provide effective treatment for their patients.

3.4.2
The role of the psychologist in therapy
PADMAL DE SILVA

The role of the clinical psychologist in the field of mental health practice developed, historically, in two parallel directions: assessment of patients, and psychotherapy of various forms. The latter was confined largely to patients with neurotic disorders, and to those with specific problems such as sexual deviation and dysfunction. The therapeutic role of the psychologist has since changed both in form and in the areas of application. Since the mid-fifties, many practising psychologists have turned to behaviour therapy as their main mode of intervention, although some still practise psychotherapy. More recently, other forms of treatment have also been undertaken or developed and they include cognitive therapy, existential therapy and Gestalt therapy. The practice of these forms of treatment is not as yet widespread or well-established (for example, Beck *et al.*, 1979; see also Bellack & Hersen, 1980; Corsini, 1981; Mackay, 1975). Psychologists today treat a wider group of patients, for example, subnormal children and adults, chronic psychotic and geriatric patients, those with organic lesions, and children and adolescents with educational difficulties, in addition to those in the categories of neuroses and personality disorders.

Behaviour therapy
The predominant therapeutic role of the psychologist, however, is still with patients afflicted with a neurosis or, to a lesser degree, a personality disor-

der. It is easy to see why this has remained so with the advent and popularity of behaviour therapy. Behaviour therapy, being based on the methodology, findings, and assumptions of learning theory, is by its very nature most relevant to those areas of dysfunction where the presenting problem can be construed as an instance of wrong or maladaptive learning (for example, becoming anxious in the presence of a harmless object or animal), or of failure to learn (for example, not learning to respond discriminatively to different social cues). Most neurotic and personality disorders tend to fit this model; and it is no surprise that the most influential early writings in behaviour therapy dealt almost exclusively with these disorders (Wolpe, 1958; Eysenck & Rachman, 1965).

Role of the psychologist in behaviour therapy today
What is the role of the psychologist in the treatment of these patients today? Most practising clinical psychologists engage in behaviour therapy with patients (for example, phobics, obsessionals, addicts, those with sexual problems) directly. Much of this work is done in hospital and clinic settings as part of a psychiatric team, although more recently psychologists have also had patients referred directly to them, by doctors and other agencies. Most of this therapy is done on an individual basis, but there is an increasing tendency to use group-based therapy where relevant (for example, social skills training).

Though carrying out behaviour therapy with suitable patients is thus one of the major roles of the psychologist, it would be fallacious to argue that behaviour therapy is the field of psychologists alone. Psychiatrists, nurses, social workers, and other professionals are increasingly acquiring skills and experience in behavioural therapy (for example, Marks, Hallam, Connolly & Philpott, 1977). Despite this, however, there is a special role for the psychologist in behaviour therapy; the most obvious reason is that the psychologist, as someone whose main therapeutic skills are in this area, is expected to have more competence, greater interest, and more time to devote to such therapy than other members of the team. There are, in addition, other more specific reasons for this, which stem from certain special needs and considerations. Some of these are discussed below.

Special needs
Although the routine application of behaviour therapy techniques is a relatively simple matter (for

example, a straightforward graded exposure pro-gramme for a patient with a phobia of public trans-port), there is often the need to grapple with more complex problems where routine therapy sessions are inadequate. In such instances, proper application of behaviour therapy requires a frankly experimental approach, using the content and methodology of experimental psychology to evaluate the problems and identify the processes and mechanisms involved. The psychologist's basic training and approach as an experimentalist are clearly useful here. This experi-mental approach to therapy has indeed been argued by some as the main feature of behavioural treatment (Yates, 1970); in anything but simple and circum-scribed problems, such an approach is not only val-uable, but essential. Examples of the uses of this approach in the behavioural treatment of complex clinical cases are found, among others, in Eysenck (1976). At times this approach would lead to the development of entirely new treatment strategies (see Calhoun, Adams & Mitchell, 1974).

Related to the above, there are occasions when a treatment programme involves the use of special instrumentation for assessment or monitoring of tar-get responses, and at times as a major part of the therapy itself. The recent work on the uses of bio-feedback in the treatment of tension headaches, muscle tension, generalized anxiety, and other dis-orders provides examples of this (Yates, 1980). The psychophysiological recording and feedback tech-niques used in this context are usually part of the psychologist's repertoire, as an integral component of his training.

Therapy evaluation and design

A further role of the psychologist lies in the area of evaluation. The value of psychological testing in assessment has already been discussed (chap. 2.4). In therapy, there is an obvious need for proper baseline data, valid outcome measures, and a design which would enable one to conclude legitimately that observed changes are in fact the result of the inter-ventions carried out – and not due to spontaneous remission or extraneous factors. This need is partic-ularly great in behavioural therapy programmes, as ongoing monitoring of change would often dictate the need for newer strategies. Psychologists use for this purpose single-case research designs which enables them to evaluate the changes in individual patients over time. These include: (a) the reversal design (where a new factor – such as a reward con-tingent upon a given response – is introduced, and in a later phase withdrawn so as to assess whether the initial response is thereby diminished), (b) the multiple base-line design (where several variables are manipulated one at a time so that the effects can be ascertained unambiguously), (c) the changing crite-rion design (where the rate of a response required for a contingent reward would systematically vary), and (d) time-series analysis (where data over a period of time are analyzed for randomness or otherwise). These designs are fully discussed by Yule and Hems-ley (1977). Though it would be an exaggeration to maintain that such carefully-planned designs are essential in all instances of treatment, it is true that adherence to these methods would enhance the assessment of one's interventions, and in certain cases it is essential.

Training of others

Finally, a relatively recent but significant development ought to be mentioned: the teach-ing/advisory role that a clinical psychologist can use-fully play in the management of neurotic and other disorders. Training other professionals, such as nurses and teachers, in techniques of treatment and providing them with guidance has proved to be a valuable extension of the psychologist's role, wid-ening the range of patients who can be offered ther-apy. Such training and consultation has also been extended, quite effectively, to parents, peers, and other relatives, particularly in the treatment of child-hood neurotic and conduct disorders (O'Dell, 1974; Yule, 1974). This teaching role of the psychologist is not intended merely to save his time and effort but is increasingly being recognized as a necessary requirement, because the ultimate aim of all therapy is to foster adaptive behaviours of the patient to his natural environment.

Conclusion

There are several ways in which the psycholo-gist is expected to make a special contribution to the treatment of neurotic and personality disorders. The present discussion has been confined to behavioural treatment, which is the commonest form of therapy that psychologists practise today. Some of the com-ments made (especially those related to the need for treatment evaluation and design), would also be applicable to the other forms of therapy which psy-chologists undertake in managing these groups of patients.

3.4.3
Social services

MAVIS MACGUIRE

Within each local authority in England and Wales, the social service department is responsible for the provision of a variety of services, some defined by Acts of Parliament. Social workers are employed to carry out many of its functions and they may work in area offices in the community, in hospitals or child guidance units. In some areas they are also employed by education authorities, such as ILEA. In the treatment of adults and children with neurotic and personality disorders, the social worker may be involved in a number of ways.

Social service provision for children

The social worker is usually involved in treatment when it is considered that the child's difficulties indicate problems in the interaction between himself and one or both parents or when it is felt that the parents need help in coping with the particular demands of their child. Sometimes the problems in the relationship stem from the parents' own experience of deprivation. Not having experienced a close, positive relationship with their parents, they are unable to achieve this with their own child. In other situations, problems in the parent–child relationship result from the parents' neurotic difficulties. In the former situation, within the relationship established with the parents, the social worker will help them towards an understanding of the inappropriate aspects of their behaviour towards the child which arise from their own childhood experiences, so that

they may begin to modify them. In the latter situation, the social worker is more likely to provide long term support and the experience of a relationship in which concern and understanding of their needs are demonstrated.

As well as emotional support, practical help is given, aimed at enabling the parents to cope as effectively as possible. This may involve financial assistance or the services of a home help or peripatetic care worker who goes into the home to help parents at times of crisis. Social service departments also provide day nurseries, where pre-school children can be cared for on a daily basis. With this kind of support a mother may be able to cope better and her child benefits from being in a familiar and secure environment with other children. It may be, however, that despite the provision of various services the parents are unable to cope adequately with the child. This may be because of their own difficulties or because of the behavioural problems of the child, or a combination of the two. The child may then be voluntarily received into care by the social service department. Here the parents agree to the child being placed away from home, usually with foster-parents or in a small group home or larger children's home. As far as possible within the limits of the resources available, the needs of the child are considered in making the placements and the parents are encouraged to maintain contact. If the child is placed with foster-parents, the latter are visited regularly by the social worker from whom they receive support. This is particularly important where a child is exhibiting serious behavioural problems, since the placement may otherwise break down and the child will experience a series of unsuccessful placements which add to his difficulties and might make successful placement impossible. Such arrangements are usually short term, from a few weeks to six months, but may be longer when more permanent plans are made. In such a voluntary arrangement, the parents may ask to have the child returned to them at any time. If, however, a situation arises where it is felt by those involved with the child that he is in need of care and protection, the social worker on behalf of the social service department may apply to the magistrates' court to have the child's care transferred to them. Section 1 of the Children and Young Persons Act (1969) establishes the grounds on which such action may be taken, one or more of six possible conditions must be met, plus the requirement that the court must be satisfied that the child is in need of care or control, which he is unlikely to receive unless a specific order is made. These conditions are:

(1) that the child's development is being avoidably prevented or neglected, his health is being avoidably impaired or neglected, or he is being ill-treated
(2) similar conditions to (1) have been proved in respect of another child in the same home
(3) he is exposed to moral danger
(4) he is beyond the care and control of his parents
(5) he is not receiving efficient full-time education when of compulsory school age
(6) he is guilty of an offence other than homicide.

Such orders, which usually cease when the child is eighteen, are reviewed every six months by the social service department and may be revoked by the court following application by the social worker or by the parents and child. Placement for a child received into care in this way may be with foster-parents, in a group home or children's home or a community home if an offence has been committed. Instead of issuing a care order, the court may make a supervision order, when the child remains at home but under the supervision of a social worker or a probation officer. Although the particular needs of the child will be considered, limited resources and severe behavioural problems in the child sometimes mean that these needs are met in only a limited way.

Although adoption is more likely to be arranged at birth or soon afterwards, it may become a possibility for an older child in foster care. Sometimes the foster parents apply to adopt or the social worker may try to place a child with a suitable couple who have applied to adopt. Application may have been to the social service department or to a voluntary adoption society, perhaps one specializing in placing children with particular needs. Prospective adopters are carefully selected and the placement is supervised for at least three months. The Children's Act (1975) requires that each local authority provides a counselling service for those with problems relating to adoption.

Social service provision for adults

The social worker's involvement in the treatment of an adult with a neurotic or personality disorder is usually in situations where environmental stress of some kind is contributing to his difficulties. If the stress is within his family, the social worker works with the family or she may work directly with the patient, helping him to use the relevant resources in the community.

Where it is apparent that family conflicts contribute to the patient's illness, it may be decided to see the patient and his family together or the social worker may see one, or more, members while the patient sees the psychiatrist. Here the family is encouraged to look at the difficulties which they have in relating to one another, arising perhaps from their own earlier experiences. In some cases, the family needs help in understanding more about the patient's illness, so that they are more tolerant of his behaviour and make less demands on him. Sometimes a family feels a great sense of guilt that they are responsible for the patient's condition, which may express itself in depression or a hostile, defensive attitude towards those treating him. It is important that the social worker recognizes such feelings and demonstrates that she is not concerned to apportion blame. Work with a family may be primarily supportive, particularly where a patient has become chronically disabled by his illness. As a result he may make considerable emotional and practical demands on them and if they are to continue to support him they need an opportunity to express their feelings of despair, anger, or frustration to someone who they feel understands their difficulties. They may also require practical advice about the provision of various social services.

Among other stresses which may be identified are those related to finance, employment, accommodation, or those arising from social isolation. For some, financial problems arise when illness interferes with their ability to work and they are dependent on a lower income limited to social security benefits. If a patient is already experiencing difficulty in coping with his life, financial problems may become serious. Here the social worker is concerned to ensure that the patient is receiving all the benefits to which he is entitled, if necessary liaising with the social security offices concerned. It may be, however, that the patient's inability to deal with finances is part of a long-standing problem in managing his life. He may then be helped to gain more control over this aspect of his life, the social worker, perhaps, working out with him in detail his weekly budget and then supporting him in keeping to it.

Employment problems may be those of obtaining appropriate work or those which arise out of the work situation, such as an inability to cope with the stresses involved or with relationships with colleagues, particularly those in positions of authority. In the former situation, referral to the Disablement

Resettlement Officer may be made. He is employed by the Department of Employment to help with the work problems of the physically and mentally disabled and he can make direct contact with an employer explaining something of the patient's illness to him. Where it seems that assessment of a patient's particular abilities would help in placement in more suitable employment, he may recommend attendance at an Employment Rehabilitation Centre. The careers officer at the Youth Employment Office is available to help younger patients who are finding it difficult to make decisions about their future work. For a patient unable to cope with the demands of open employment, placement in a sheltered workshop, if available, may be made. Here in a supportive and relatively undemanding environment he can be involved in a regular work routine in the company of others. Day centres may also be considered and although these vary somewhat in nature, the patient is provided with a situation which has some similarities to a work one. He is required to attend daily for a set time, to undertake some practical tasks and perhaps light industrial work. It is a supportive environment which in some centres gives members the opportunity, through group discussion, to explore the difficulties which they have with particular tasks or in relationships with other members or staff, an understanding of which could help the patient cope better with a work situation in the future.

An important aspect of treatment may involve helping a patient with problems related to his housing situation. Most local authorities make some hostel provision for those who require this or will contribute to the maintenance of an individual in a hostel run by a voluntary organization, such as the Richmond Fellowship. Some hostels are specifically for those who have had psychiatric problems and offer a supportive environment for a limited period in which an individual can be encouraged to greater independence. Others aim, through group discussions with the residents, to help an individual during his stay towards a greater understanding of the difficulties he has in living with others. There are also hostels which specialize in particular problems such as drug addiction and alcoholism but these are still a scarce resource. Group homes in which small numbers of residents have their own bedsitting rooms, sharing other facilities, and with regular visits from a social worker, also offer residents a degree of support but some independence. In some local authority areas, fostering schemes are being developed, similar to those at present existing for children, where an individual is able to live as a member of a family. Where an older patient presents, perhaps living alone and socially isolated, accommodation in a warden-supported flat may be recommended.

For many who present with neurotic or personality disorders, problems of social isolation are often considerable. Since these often reflect difficulties in interpersonal relationships, making available the opportunity to meet others will not necessarily resolve the problem. With encouragement, however, some isolated individuals can benefit from attendance at social clubs which are provided in the community by local authorities or voluntary organizations for psychiatric patients. For the elderly there are also luncheon clubs which provide companionship and lunch for a small charge.

Proposals for prevention and treatment arising from research findings

The findings described in the section (1.2.2) contributed by Professors Brown and Cooper to chapter 1 have led to the following proposals for the prevention of disability due to neurotic disorders. Everything possible should be done to improve the living conditions of the most disadvantaged sections of the community through political and social action. Many life events which it is known can precipitate depressive disorder, such as loss of attachment figures, cannot be prevented, but attempts can be made to reduce the vulnerability of those known to be at greater risk. The available evidence of vulnerability factors suggests that social measures, such as improved family planning facilities, are of value, as is the use of cognitive theory in the therapeutic field, particularly for chronic depressive states (Beck, 1976). The therapist in the role of confidant may be able to improve the general coping skills of the individual by modifying his ideas about his world, thereby increasing his self-esteem (Brown & Harris, 1978).

Whatever forms of treatment are available, they will have little impact on large sections of those in need, unless medical and social care services reach them. This point becomes clear from a study in Camberwell, a metropolitan area with above average services available. Here only 10 per cent of depressed women identified in the survey had received psychiatric help and half the cases with onset in the year had received no treatment from their general practitioner for their condition (Brown & Harris, 1978).

Evaluative studies in this field suggest some

ways in which to improve the situation. Sainsbury and colleagues (1965) found that establishing psychiatric liaison with general practitioners brought more depressed patients and working class people to psychiatric services and Cooper and co-workers (1975) found a significant improvement in prognosis for chronic neurotic patients in a general practice where a social worker was attached as compared with the level of improvement in those with no such facility. Self-help groups may also be relevant here (Robinson, 1977) but evaluative studies are not yet available.

3.4.4
Occupational therapy
CHARLOTTE MUNDAY

Occupational therapy is a form of treatment where the patient is actively involved in his or her own cure and rehabilitation. The word 'occupational' should be interpreted as 'active involvement' rather than diversional – a common misunderstanding.

For patients with neuroses and personality disorders this active involvement is of primary importance and the potential of occupational therapy should be fully used as an aid to assessment and diagnosis and in all stages of treatment. Occupational therapy can be seen in broadly three overlapping categories as: (1) milieu therapy, (2) creative therapy, (3) functional rehabilitation.

Milieu therapy
Occupational therapy is a profession much concerned with seeing the patient as a person – a total entity – in relation to his or her own environment. The orientation is to think in terms of problems rather than symptoms and to aim towards independent living in the outside community. It is perhaps because of this orientation that occupational therapists are enthusiastic advocates of what D. H. Clark terms 'milieu' therapy (1964). This is the concept of the socio-cultural environment of the treatment unit being of prime importance in facilitating effective treatment. Milieu therapy recognizes the basic needs and inherent rights of the individual; it encourages communication and provides opportunities for those admitted for treatment to have a role other than that

of dependent patients. As occupational therapists usually instigate the daily activity programme for patients this view necessarily affects their planning and organization. Where the concept is not recognized and activities are planned on rigid, didactic lines, the 'primary rehabilitation aim' of helping the disabled person adjust to his continually changing environment may not be achieved. Ward meetings where all patients and staff can meet to discuss freely the daily problems of being together are seen as an integral part of milieu therapy. They are to be distinguished from psychotherapy groups but can nevertheless provide a motivating force for activities during the rest of the day (Mare & Kreeger, 1974).

Creative therapy

This is the use of the arts as creative media through which the patient relates to the therapist, himself, and others. It is a form of non-verbal communication and can be an expression of the unconscious. The forms most commonly used are painting, sculpture, dance, drama, writing, and music. (Westman, 1961; Jennings, 1975).

Most patients will say 'I can't paint, I can't act', and it must be made clear that creative therapies are not concerned with skills but with feelings. The anxious or depressed patient may not know why he is anxious and depressed and even if he expresses reasons this may not relieve his feelings. Medication may have helped but the patient has not felt in control of this intervention. However, by using paint spontaneously, for example, he is actively putting on paper his fantasies. In the act of painting these may appear as meaningless daubs but as the painter stands back from his work he can view it more objectively: he can discuss with the therapist how he felt as he painted and how different parts of the painting relate to each other, what they mean to him, and whether they connect with people or events in his life. Most important, the reasonable part of the person can look at the irrational part translated into a tangible form which he can preserve and look at again in sequence with his other paintings or art forms. The therapist's job is to help the patient identify with his own work and value it (Lyddiatt, 1970). This achieved, the patient has a way of gaining control of, or at least channelling, his otherwise overwhelming emotions. Equally with drama, forms like communication games and role playing can be used to examine feelings in a different setting.

The development of creative therapy has been influenced by psycho-analytic thought and the works of C. G. Jung (1934), by group psychotherapy developments (Bion, 1961, 1970; Foulkes & Anthony, 1957; Moreno, 1946, 1959, 1969; Rogers, 1965, 1973), and by humanist therapies (Lowen, 1958; Perls, 1969; Schulz, 1973). 'SCOPE' is an offshoot of the British Association of Occupational Therapists* which provides training and research into creative therapy methods, and there are separate therapy associations for art, music, and remedial drama.

Functional rehabilitation

Functional rehabilitation includes all activities of daily living and basic social skills necessary for survival in the community. These skills are often given priority in occupational therapy, but without the milieu and creative therapies they count for little. Most basic skills for the patients we are discussing return automatically when they are coming to terms with their irrational feelings. Lack of concentration, motivation, self-confidence, are all symptoms which improve when the fundamental malaise is attacked by appropriate measures. Detailed assessments on functioning in work and domestic situations can be made but observations concerning relationships and behaviour in diverse social settings are often more useful in diagnosis. Disablement Resettlement Officers will often confirm that the problem of placing the neurotic and personality-disordered patient in employment is not that of lack of skills but of unrealistic expectations and lack of motivation.

Having said this, providing facilities for activities such as cooking, typing, gardening, and woodwork can give patients the opportunity to find out for themselves their own strengths and weaknesses, as well as giving greater scope for interactions. Some classes, such as those teaching relaxation techniques or social skills, are useful. They may, for example, help the patient rehearse how to apply for a job and then learn how others see him. Establishing work routines is also important as a later stage of rehabilitation.

Occupational therapy activity programmes are planned as part of the general treatment programme in co-operation with the total treatment team and with short- and long-term aims for the individual patient (Bennett, 1977). Where there are flexible attitudes, all staff can be involved according to expertise and availability.

---

* The British Association of Occupational Therapists (20 Rede Place, London W2 4TU) will provide on request the addresses of 'SCOPE' and other 'Link Therapy' organizations.

3.4.5
Educational services

SULA WOLFF

Introduction

Schools as we know them, with age segregation and teaching based on the principle that, as they get older, children can master ideas and tasks of increasing complexity, began only in the seventeenth century. Compulsory education in the western world did not start until the nineteenth century, with the addition of scientific subjects to languages and religious teaching.

Pathogenic influences of school

School life on the whole enhances personality development and can protect vulnerable children. For some children, however, it has definite pathogenic consequences. Compulsory universal education at once identifies educationally handicapped children, among whom a major group is that of the mentally retarded. Prevalence rates of mental handicap are highest during the school years, many mildly subnormal people getting by within their families in early childhood and within the community after school-leaving age. Their low intelligence is most handicapping during the years of compulsory schooling, inducing in the children and their parents disappointment and a sense of failure. Such children are at high risk for emotional and conduct disorders.

School life can exert similar pathogenic influences on children of normal intelligence who for whatever reason have learning difficulties (chap. 4.2.2, pp. 168, 172–3). There are other children with unusual personality development: excessively shy and sensitive, unadaptable children, and children with schizoid personality traits (Wolff & Chick, 1980), for whom the school years of gregarious conformity are highly stressful. Moreover, even sociable children with good learning abilities can be stigmatized at school by other handicaps (physical or socio-cultural) which may require special educational arrangements. Such children too are at risk of secondary psychiatric disorders.

The organization and quality of school life

Compulsory schooling exposes handicaps not otherwise conspicuous. But the nature of the educational system itself and the administration and atmosphere of individual schools can either promote adaptive behaviour or, on the contrary, contribute to educational failure, psychiatric morbidity, and youthful delinquency. J. W. B. Douglas' longitudinal study of a national cohort of children (1964) demonstrated that academic streaming retarded the educational progress of duller children and also that primary school teachers, most of whom were women, underestimated the abilities, and were more critically sensitive to the behavioural difficulties, of boys and of socio-economically deprived children.

In their study of twelve London comprehensive secondary schools, Rutter and his colleagues (1979) demonstrated that differences in outcome, both scholastic and behavioural, were related, not to physical factors such as school size and the quality of buildings, but to the degree of academic emphasis, teacher behaviour during lessons, the amount of praise and incentives, good conditions for the children, and the extent to which pupils were given responsibility.

Therapeutic aspects of school life

It has been shown repeatedly that children display disturbed behaviour *either* at school *or* at home but rarely in both places (Rutter *et al.*, 1970). This is often a source of misunderstanding between teachers and parents. Much disturbed behaviour in childhood is situationally determined. A supportive family can compensate for school failure and many children under stress at home, thrive when good schooling provides them with interest and opportunity to discover their own competence. Psychiatrists frequently underestimate the satisfactions that come from successful learning.

A nine-year old, the last of five sons of a mother who had separated from her husband because of his heavy drinking and promiscuity, but who had previously been excessively dependent on him, was referred with a long list of aggressive and delinquent behaviours at home and in the neighbourhood. At 3 a hare lip was repaired; at 4 a corneal ulcer was treated; at 5 the terminal phalanx of an index finger was cut off by a chef he was helping at his mother's work. The mother was basically affectionate but offered no protective care, and her child rearing efforts consisted of warnings and inconsistent physical punishments. This boy of average ability was liked and given much protective care by his teacher at school. During his first psychiatric interview he said he enjoyed history and had got two stars at school for an illustrative picture. This was the one bright spot in his otherwise bleak and frightening existence. The therapeutic intervention in this case was to arrange admission to a residential school for maladjusted children.

The range of educational facilities for disturbed children in Britain

It is the duty of local educational authorities to provide all children with schooling according to their needs. The recent British statutory categories of handicapped pupils were the blind, the partially sighted, the deaf, the partially deaf, the educationally sub-normal (or mentally handicapped), the epileptic, the physically handicapped, pupils with speech defects, the maladjusted, and (in England only) delicate pupils. Yet multiple handicaps are common and there is no one-to-one relationship between the underlying nature of a child's handicap and the teaching methods best suited to his needs.

For these reasons the Warnock Committee on Special Educational Needs (Special Educational Needs, 1978) suggested abolishing statutory categories of handicap and instead identifying the individual educational needs of all children with special requirements and meeting these with a range of provisions in ordinary schools, special classes or units, and special day and residential schools. The report recommended an integrated special educational service for children of all ages, from the nursery stage to the stage of further education, and in all schools, including hospital schools and community homes (List D schools) for delinquent children and children in need of care or protection.

Among the important principles for teachers aiming to provide an emotionally helpful school environment for children are: (1) to have realistic expectations of a child's capabilities; (2) to respond positively to a child's achievements rather than negatively to his shortcomings; (3) to identify for all children, however handicapped, areas in which success

is possible; and (4) to enable all children, however intelligent, to work to the limits of their ability.

Other important issues in the management of educationally handicapped children are the choice between segregation and integration, and between day and residential schooling. Handicapped children often adapt better socially at school when segregated in special classes, for example for the physically handicapped or the maladjusted. On the other hand, such children are often socially ostracized and develop a sense of stigma in their own neighbourhood, and at times educational progress is less than optimal. Handicapped children in ordinary schools on the other hand may be under greater stress while at school, but are often socially better integrated in their own communities. Decisions often depend on the support the child can get from his family and, of course, also on the educational provisions available in his area.

Seriously disturbed children often benefit from the experience of increasing competence in non-emotional aspects of their lives, when to focus chiefly on their interpersonal relationships may be less rewarding. Residential schools tend to provide better opportunities for such experiences than children's homes and they also induce less stigma. Such schools help children to distance themselves from adverse home influences and to develop close relationships with adults who act as alternative role models, while attachments to parents and siblings are preserved during holidays and weekends.

Links between child psychiatric and educational services

School referrals

Teachers are second only to parents in how well they know a child. In about half the children referred to psychiatrists the problem was first noted at school. Whether the problem first manifests itself at school or at home is no indication as to where the underlying trouble lies. Children with difficulties first identified at school reach psychiatric clinics either because their parents seek out the family doctor or because the teachers turn to the school psychologist or the school doctor and he initiates the referral.

It will then be the task of the psychiatrist and his team to investigate the problem, obtain information about the child's educational functioning from the school psychologist, and, with the parents' full knowledge, convey to the school either directly or through the school doctor or psychologist the diagnosis, the aetiology of the child's difficulties, and how the school can help in the child's treatment.

Educational contribution to treatment

Sometimes child psychiatrists are the first to identify intellectual or educational retardation and will then alert the school psychologist or school doctor to the child's special educational needs.

Children with conduct disorders (especially aggressive, disruptive behaviour) often thrive when taught temporarily in small groups and some school phobics can make a graduated return to ordinary school through the 'half-way-house' of a small class. Many children with minor constitutional handicaps such as hyperkinesis or other constitutionally based personality difficulties flourish in small classes on a more long-term basis, whether these are officially classes for the maladjusted, for the delicate, or for children needing special remedial help. The intimacy possible in such small teaching units is often of great help both educationally and socially.

In the case of autistic children, child psychiatrists share the responsibility for ensuring that the existing special educational provisions, particularly adequate and systematic one-to-one teaching, are made available to the affected children. Often only child psychiatrists will make a confident diagnosis of autism.

School-based psychiatric treatment programmes

In the USA as well as in Britain many attempts have been made to give children deprived of a stimulating and secure family environment compensatory school experiences. 'Nurture classes' for young children, sometimes with their mothers, in primary schools, and a school-based counselling service for older children are examples.

A recent study into techniques for secondary prevention of psychiatric disorder in school children has shown that disturbed children do best when offered short-term school-based group psychotherapy, extra nurturing from classroom aides for young children and a behaviour modification approach from teachers for older children, rather than when a social work counselling service is set up for parents and teachers (Kolvin *et al.*, 1981).

3.5
Forensic aspects

3.5.1
Probation, prisons and Special Hospitals
JOHN GUNN

Penal systems are specific to each country and so this section will deal with only one system, the services available in England and Wales. This can be taken as illustrating a few general points, but it has to be remembered that even the Scottish system differs substantially. Penal systems are developed to correct, punish, and deter criminals, and sometimes they are used for preventive custody. Clearly they are not primarily designed for psychiatric care, nevertheless many people with personality problems and with mental illnesses do find their way into court and into the penal system.

Probation and after-care
In England and Wales there is an extensive service of trained social workers, employed by probation and after-care committees. These probation officers also act as after-care officers, parole officers, and prison welfare officers. They are available to courts to conduct social enquiries, to supervise and befriend offenders on probation, aftercare, and parole, and sometimes to support and supervise patients leaving mental hospitals.

There are three main ways in which psychiatrists and probation officers come into contact professionally. The first is when either the court via the probation officer, or the probation officer on his own behalf, requests a psychiatric report on a person who has broken the law. The second is when a patient is given a probation order with a condition of mental treatment. The third is when a patient on a restriction order is released from hospital by the Home Secretary, to be supervised by a probation officer and a doctor.

Dual management between a probation officer and a psychiatrist can yield rewarding results in suitable patients. These patients should, however, be carefully selected and prepared. A probation order with a condition of mental treatment, for example, is best reserved for serious offenders who are well motivated to have psychiatric treatment. It can be particularly useful in the management of patients who could legally fall into the 'psychopathic disorder' category of the Mental Health Act, but whom it would be clinically inappropriate to admit to hospital compulsorily.

The probation order with a condition of treatment is very flexible in that it is not confined to in-patient treatment and no particular type of psychiatric disorder has to be specified. Nevertheless it is not really suitable for the severely psychotic or for the severely subnormal, as consent and motivation are an integral part of the arrangements. No one can be forced to have probation and any prospective probationer has to agree, in court, to the order being made. It is vital therefore that before such an order is recommended to a court each party knows what his obligations and responsibilities are. The patient must actually want the treatment, know what it might entail, and accept that if he discharges himself from treatment, then he is liable to be taken back to court by the probation officer, for a breach of probation.

The psychiatrist and the probation officer must agree between themselves what type of management is to be offered, who will do what (the probation officer will usually want only a nominal involvement), what sanctions are to be applied if things go wrong and by whom (only the probation officer can charge the client with breach of probation). Courts are usually willing to allow this type of psychiatric order because it is for a specified period of time (up to 3 years) and there is some legal redress if the client abuses the arrangements. Such orders are probably most successful for patients who have serious behavioural problems or who have committed a serious offence (say violence, arson, sexual crimes) because in such cases everybody takes the order seriously and makes maximal effort. Imposing probation orders for trivial offences which could have been dealt with by a fine or by a conditional discharge brings about a disregard for such orders, as all parties tend to treat the whole matter light-heartedly.

The after-care licence arrangements for a patient on a restriction order (section 65) are usually carefully negotiated beforehand. Here the sanctions are with the Home Office, who can recall the patient to hospital if things go wrong; here again, the arrangements are usually taken very seriously as a previous offence has usually been committed.

Prisons

In spite of the fact that prisons are primarily designed to punish, the prison system in England and Wales (indeed in most countries) provides many psychiatric services. These are supplied mainly by the Prison Medical Service, but also by forensic consultants and by visiting psychotherapists.* The Prison Medical Service is separate from the National Health Service and employs both full-time and part-time doctors to provide medical care of a variety of prisoners. Most large prisons have their own hospitals, providing both in-patient and out-patient care; sometimes treatment as complex as abdominal surgery can be provided within a prison hospital. These services are staffed by the full-time prison doctors who can send patients out to NHS hospitals if necessary or call on NHS specialists to provide advice and/or treatment within the prison. A large proportion of the medical work load within a prison is psychiatric. A recent survey suggests that approximately one-third of all sentenced prisoners could be correctly classified as psychiatric cases (Gunn *et al.*, 1974) and there is concern about the increasing number of severely mentally ill people being sent to prison, (Orr, 1978). To assist with this work the Prison Department employs part-time visiting psychotherapists* on a sessional basis. There has also been a scheme, which is in process of being dismantled, whereby NHS consultant psychiatrists are employed half-time as visiting consultants at key prisons. Some prisons have no full-time medical staff; in them, medical care is provided by visiting local general practitioners. Such doctors can call on full-time prison doctors for assistance in difficult cases or have a prisoner transferred to a more intensively staffed prison.

One of the most demanding tasks undertaken by the Prison Medical Serice is the provision of psychiatric reports to courts. In 1978 they supplied 8962 such reports (Home Office, 1979). Courts in Britain have a tendency, if they suspect any psychiatric factors in a particular case, to remand into custody accused persons before trial and convicted offenders

---

* Visiting psychiatrists would be a better name.

before sentence in order to get a medical (or state of mind and health) report, and to obtain advice about fitness to plead, responsibility, and disposal. Unless there are security problems which the NHS cannot manage, remands into prison, in order to get a psychiatric opinion, are unnecessary, indeed unjust. More importantly such custodial remands do not lead to the best advice because prison doctors cannot speak for NHS colleagues. Furthermore, they cannot test an accused person in a treatment setting in order that, for example, a probation order with a condition of medical treatment can be recommended. This curious British anomaly of using prisons for psychiatric assesments can only be remedied by NHS psychiatrists accepting more responsibility for their patients, and developing closer links with local courts.

Besides routine psychiatric treatment and a court report service, the Prison Medical Service also offers a number of therapeutic communities. Some are purely for the management of difficult and disturbed prisoners. Others are for the treatment of men with disordered personalities – the best known of these facilities is Grendon prison near Aylesbury. Grendon is a remarkable institution in that men treated there are all volunteers serving ordinary sentences: no one can be sent there by a court. It is run on a group basis and has a doctor as governor. Men who spend a period at the prison seem to be considerably helped with their psychological problems (Gunn *et al.*, 1978). Whether it is appropriate that such a purely psychiatric facility should be within the prison system is debatable, what is indisputable is the importance of this particular experiment.

A major problem faced by any patient treated within the prison system is the disconnection between the NHS provisions and the prison medical arrangements. Many psychiatric services are less than enthusiastic about taking on prisoners as they leave gaol and it is very difficult for a prisoner to adapt to new faces and unfamiliar arrangements at this moment of great stress, when he has to try to fend for himself in a fairly hostile external environment.

Special Hospitals

In Britain there are five maximum security hospitals. These are Broadmoor, Rampton, Moss Side, and Park Lane (a hospital under construction and only partially operational) in England, and Carstairs in Scotland. The five serve the whole of the United Kingdom and admit patients considered too dangerous to be nursed in ordinary psychiatric hospitals.

The Special Hospitals are outside the regional structure of the National Health Service and are run directly by the Civil Service in the name of the Secretary of State for Health and Social Security in England or the Secretary of State for Scotland.

Although different in terms of the level of security provided and the way they are administered, the Special Hospitals are in other respects just like any other psychiatric hospital offering a wide range of psychiatric treatment, the patients being under the care of consultant psychiatrists. The biggest problems faced by the Special Hospitals are stigmatization and poor opportunities for rehabilitation. Public and professionals alike put patients who have been to a Special Hospital into an undesirable category. Many patients stay in these security institutions long after the need for strict control and supervision has passed. The Special Hospitals do not of course have out-patient clinics of their own and they therefore rely on ordinary NHS psychiatric services for rehabilitation and follow up. Recent research (Dell, 1980) has suggested that more of these patients would be taken into NHS facilities if the psychiatrists whose help is sought were willing to visit patients deemed ready for more open conditions, to see for themselves whether transfer is appropriate.

3.5.2
The Mental Health Act

P. T. d'ORBÁN

The guiding principle of the Mental Health Act (1959) was to allow psychiatric patients to be treated informally whenever possible. The Act contains powers for various forms of compulsory admission, but compulsion should be used only if the doctor is satisfied that four criteria are met:

(1) The patient suffers from a mental disorder (or, in the case of admission for observation, that there are strong reasons to suspect this).

(2) There is likely to be substantial benefit from treatment. Under Sec. 147 treatment includes nursing care and training (for example, for the mentally handicapped).

(3) The patient's judgement and insight are so impaired by his mental disorder that he is unable or unwilling to accept informal admission.

(4) Admission is necessary in the interest of the patient's health and safety or for the protection of others, and suitable care cannot be provided in other ways.

The reader is also referred to the Addendum on the Mental Health (Amendment) Act at the end of this section. The Addendum includes particular references to secs. 25, 26, 29, 30, 60, and 65.

Definitions of mental disorder and their legal implications

Sec. 4 of the Act defines four sub-categories of mental disorder:

(1) Mental illness (which is not further defined).

(2) Severe subnormality ('a state of arrested or incomplete development of the mind which includes subnormality of intelligence' where the patient is 'incapable of living an independent life or of guarding himself against serious exploitation').

(3) Subnormality ('which includes subnormality of intelligence . . . and requires or is susceptible to medical treatment or other special care or training').

(4) Psychopathic disorder ('a persistent disorder or disability of mind . . . which results in abnormally aggressive or seriously irresponsible conduct . . . and requires or is susceptible to medical treatment').

The Act is under review (DHSS *et al.*, 1978) and the Government White Paper recommends that 'subnormality' should be replaced by 'mental handicap' and its definition should include severe impairment of social functioning; psychopathic disorder should be retained but there must be a prospect of benefit from treatment.

The subcategories of mental disorder are legal definitions and equate only broadly with diagnostic concepts (Royal College of Psychiatrists, 1977). For admission for treatment (Sec. 26) and for offender-patients (Secs. 60, 72 and 73) the subcategory of mental disorder must be specified, but when admission is for emergency (Sec. 29) or for observation (Sec. 25) the subcategory of mental disorder is not required (and see Addendum). If a patient is classified as suffering from subnormality or psychopathic disorder, the following special provisions apply:

(1) He can only be admitted for treatment (Sec. 26) if aged under 21 and must be discharged on attaining the age of 25 (Sec. 44.1) unless the doctor in charge certifies that if released, he is likely to be a danger to himself or others (Sec. 44.2). These age limits do not apply to offender-patients (Secs. 60 and 72).

(2) If he absconds when aged over 21 he can be returned to hospital within 6 months; for others the period is 28 days (Sec. 40.3).

In cases of mental illness or severe subnormality:

(1) Magistrates Courts may make a Hospital Order without convicting the patient of a criminal offence (Sec. 60.2), but not in cases of subnormality or psychopathic disorder.

(2) Unsentenced prisoners can only be transferred to hospital if mentally ill or severely subnormal (Sec. 73).

If the White Paper's recommendations are implemented most of these distinctions will be abandoned.

Short-term powers of compulsion

Emergency admission (Sec. 29)

This section should only be used in emergencies. One medical recommendation is required (preferably by the general practitioner). The application for admission is made by an authorized social worker or by *any* relative. The section is effective for 72 hours during which a second medical recommendation complying with Sec. 25 can be made. (See addendum)

Admission for observation (Sec. 25) (and see Addendum)

This is the normal procedure and requires two medical recommendations. One of the doctors must be approved by a local health authority under Sec. 28; unless he previously knew the patient the second doctor should if practicable have such previous acquaintance. One of the doctors must not be on the staff of the hospital to which the patient is to be admitted (Sec. 28.3). They must have examined the patient either together or at an interval of not more than seven days (Sec. 28.1) and the patient must be admitted within 14 days of the last examination (Sec. 31.1). The application for admission is made either by the *nearest* relative (defined in Sec. 49) *or* by an authorized social worker. This section allows detention for up to 28 days, during which admission for treatment (Sec. 26) can be arranged unless the patient is discharged or remains in hospital informally.

Change from informal to compulsory status (Sec. 30) (and see Addendum)

This section provides temporary holding powers over an informal patient already in hospital who wishes to leave but is likely to harm himself or others, or who has to be restrained physically or by medication. It is implemented by the doctor in charge of the patient's treatment and is effective for three days, during which arrangements for Sec. 25 or (more usually) for Sec. 26. can be made.

Detention of publicly disturbed persons (Sec. 136)

The police are empowered to take a person believed to be suffering from mental disorder from a public place to a place of safety (in practice a police station or a hospital). The person may be detained there for up to 72 hours for psychiatric assessment and if necessary he can then be admitted informally or under compulsory powers.

Admission for treatment (Sec. 26)

The procedure is similar to that in Sec. 25 but the two medical recommendations must state the subcategory of mental disorder and agree on it, and the age limits apply for subnormality and psychopathic disorder. If the application for admission is made by a social worker he must if practicable consult the *nearest* relative, who can object (Sec. 27.2). A county court may override this objection and appoint another person or the social worker to act as the nearest relative (Sec. 52). Section 26 is effective for up to one year; it is then renewable for one year and thereafter at two-yearly intervals (Sec. 43) (for amendment see Addendum).

Admission of offenders

A criminal court may make a Hospital Order (Sec. 60) if the offence is otherwise punishable by imprisonment and there is no fixed penalty (as for murder). A hospital vacancy must be available within 28 days. Two medical recommendations are required and one of the doctors must be approved under Sec. 28. The subcategory of mental disorder must be specified but the age limits for subnormality and psychopathic disorder do not apply. The effect of the Order is similar to Sec. 26 except that the nearest relative cannot discharge the patient (Sec. 63.3). For protection of the public a crown court may make an additional Restriction Order (Sec. 65), usually without specific time-limit. Discharge, transfer, or leave can then be granted only with the Home Secretary's approval. Similar restrictions apply to sentenced prisoners (Sec. 72) and unsentenced prisoners (Sec. 73) transferred to hospital. Restricted patients are usually discharged conditionally (Sec. 66) which can ensure satisfactory aftercare and recall to hospital if necessary. (For amendments, see Addendum.)

Hospital Orders are most suitable for patients who would have required admission irrespective of their offence (Gunn, 1974). Over 80 per cent of these orders are made on the grounds of mental illness. Offenders suffering from neuroses or personality disorders who are motivated for treatment can often be helped more effectively as informal patients, with treatment as a condition of probation.

The management of neuroses, personality disorders and drug or alcohol dependence under the Act

Patients suffering from neuroses, personality disorders, or mild mental handicap may at times require temporary periods of formal admission, for example the potentially suicidal, the dangerously self-mutilating, or the patient with anorexia nervosa who is endangering her life. Often the need for compulsion in such cases is transient and Sec. 25 can be invoked to tide the patient over a crisis and ensure observation and care. However, if the patient requires treatment without consent, Sec. 26 should be implemented (Clarke, 1979) after discussion with the nearest relative and a second consultant opinion. Classifying such patients under the subcategories of mental disorder defined in Sec. 4 of the Act may give rise to difficulty but in practice the psychiatrist should be guided by the patient's current mental state and behaviour and the need to protect the patient. If he is a danger to himself and he meets the clinical criteria for compulsory admission outlined at the beginning of this section, his symptoms will justify his classification for the purposes of Sec. 26 as suffering from mental illness.

Similar considerations apply in cases of drug dependence and alcoholism. Although the Government White Paper (DHSS *et al.*, 1978) takes the view that drug dependence, alcoholism (and sexual deviation) should not *in themselves* be grounds for compulsion unless there is an associated mental disorder, in practice, decisions about compulsion are more complex and the psychiatrist should consider the overall clinical picture. The behaviour of the alcoholic or the addict may become so self-destructive that he seriously endangers his life, his health, and his social functioning. He may present a suicidal risk, destroy his family life, endanger others by his aggressive behaviour, or ruin his financial affairs. Evidence of depression and the risk of suicide or memory impairment due to organic deterioration will justify intervention, but in most cases the decision is less clear-cut. The psychiatrist will need to consider the risk the patient presents to himself or others and the likelihood of benefit from a period of compulsory admission. If the patient's insight and judgement are severely impaired by his dependence he may need at least temporary protection under compulsory powers and the possibility of admission under Sec. 25 should be considered. This will afford an opportunity for detoxification and the treatment of physical complications, and enable the patient to take a more sober stock of his situation which may lead to his co-operation in further treatment. It is debatable whether more prolonged detention is justified in patients who, despite short-term admission, continue on their self-destructive course. Nevertheless, Sec. 26 should be considered where there is a prospect of benefit from continued treatment and the patient's mental state is so impaired by his dependence that his symptoms merit description as mental illness.

Addendum: the Mental Health (Amendment) Act

The Mental Health (Amendment) Act was passed in October 1982 and most of its provisions will be implemented on 30th September 1983. The most important provisions are the establishment of a Mental Health Act Commission which will exercise general protective functions in respect of detained patients, and legislation relating to consent to treatment. A number of amendments have also been made to the sections of the Mental Health Act previously referred to. Subnormality and severe subnormality are now termed mental impairment and severe mental impairment. Mental impairment is 'a state of arrested or incomplete development of mind which includes significant impairment of intelligence and social functioning and is associated with abnormally aggressive or seriously irresponsible conduct'. Patients with mental impairment or psychopathic disorder can be detained only if treatment 'is likely to alleviate or prevent deterioration' of the patient's condition. Patients cannot be detained by reason only of sexual deviancy or dependence on alcohol or drugs (there must be an associated mental disorder). The age limits for detention of non-offenders have been abolished. Under section 29 the *nearest* instead of *any* relative must be the applicant for admission. Section 25 is now admission for assessment and can include treatment. Patients admitted for assessment may appeal against detention to a Mental Health Tribunal within fourteen days of admission. Under section 30 a Registered Mental Nurse can detain an informal patient for up to six hours until a doctor can sign the application for compulsory admission. Detention under section 26 and section 60 is now effective for six months and is renewable for six months and thereafter at yearly intervals. Restriction orders under section 65 will now be made only for the protection of the public from serious harm. Mental Health Review Tribunals chaired by a judge will have the power to discharge restricted patients. Courts may remand a person charged with an imprisonable offence to hospital for treatment or for assessment and reports, and interim hospital orders (lasting up to six months) can be made after conviction to see whether a section 60 order is appropriate.

PART II
Disorders specific to childhood

4
Disorders specific to childhood

4.1
The pre-school child

4.1.1
Disorders of early childhood

NAOMI RICHMAN

There is increasing interest in infant behaviour and in factors affecting early parent–child relationships; research findings in these areas suggest a number of ways in which disorders of both early and later childhood might be prevented.

Isolated difficulties are common in young children, for instance approximately 15 per cent of one-year-olds wake regularly at night, and behaviour difficulties frequently follow such stresses as hospitalization, birth of a sib, being in a car accident, or sudden and prolonged separations. Many of these disturbances are likely to be transient or unimportant in terms of the child's overall progress. The decision on whether a disorder exists requiring further investigation or that the difficulties lie within the normal limits of variation expected in a child of that age, depends on a number of factors.

(1) The extent, severity and persistence of behavioural difficulties described by parents. It is important to appreciate that even single manifestations can be extremely distressing to the family, for example, sleep disturbances, and may have serious import, for example, language delay.

(2) Evidence of impaired development whether in physical, general intellectual, or language development, or in the sphere of social and emotional relationships.

(3) Evidence of markedly disturbed relationships within the family, such as violence, neglect,

gross family disharmony, or more subtle factors such as parental over-involvement.

(4) The amount of concern or distress shown by the parents even if the problems seem trivial. First, distressing symptoms may in themselves affect relationships adversely; secondly, child abuse or other impaired parent–child relationships, serious parental mental illness, or marital conflict, may all present with frequent but apparently trivial complaints about a child. It is also important to remember that parents are usually good judges of their child's progress, and their persistent concern about developmental progress more often than not reflects a real problem. It follows that diagnosis of disorder does not necessarily imply that the child has a psychiatric disturbance, but only that the child is a focus of family distress or parental anxiety (Richman, 1977b); adequate assessment must include both the child's developmental status and the interaction of the child with the family.

Classification of disorder in early childhood

Clinically most disorders in early childhood do not fall into well-defined syndromes, clearly distinguished by aetiological factors, course, and response to specific treatment; the majority would probably be classified as adaptation or adjustment reactions. A descriptive scheme is given below of the problems commonly presenting to clinicians (Wolff, 1961b). It does not contain mutually exclusive categories, as several conditions frequently occur in combination. For instance, eating difficulties can be associated with autism, failure to thrive, and with problems of control.

(1) *Behaviour difficulties*
    (a) tempers, unmanageability, running away.
    (b) over-activity, restlessness, and distractibility.
    (c) emotional difficulties such as irritability, apathy, fearfulness, unhappiness, obsessional, or ritualistic behaviour.
    (d) sphincter control problems, eating and sleeping difficulties, habits.
(2) *Relationship difficulties*
    Excessive dependence and attention seeking; withdrawal; inability to play with other children because of aggressiveness; indiscriminate friendliness; jealousy of siblings.
(3) *Developmental problems*
    Language delay or general delay in development.

(4) *Failure to thrive and child abuse*
(5) *Autism, childhood psychosis*

Aetiology
Family factors

The factors associated with behaviour disorder in the pre-school child are similar to those found in older children – an interaction between factors in the family, the environment, and within the child himself. Interest has focused particularly on maternal depression since this appears to be particularly high in mothers of young children and likely to affect the mother's ability to cope with her responsibilities (see chapter 5.1.4). Of at least equal importance are social stress and poor family relationships as expressed in an unhappy, unsupportive marriage, or extreme criticism and lack of warmth and acceptance of the child (Wolff, 1961a; Richman, 1977a).

Extremely destructive and uncontrolled behaviour including lighting fires, brought *Sam* to the clinic aged 3½. The parents' covert encouragement of Sam's wildness deflected attempts to resolve their own fierce marriage conflict. On the other hand fear of assertive behaviour and pressure for achievement by Jim's father led to the four-year-old boy becoming over-controlled and unassertive. His bland behaviour and presenting symptom of severe constipation were the only signs he showed that he found this pressure too much.

Developmental status

Children with behaviour difficulties score lower on neuro-developmental and language tests than do controls. Language delay is particularly associated with behaviour problems, and over half the children with language delay may be expected to have behaviour difficulties, compared with about one-fifth in the general population.

Prematurity and physical handicap

Premature children or those with physical handicap are a vulnerable group. Need for special care in the neonatal period can lead to great anxiety in the parents, lack of adequate contact with the baby, and difficulties in establishing a loving relationship. Inability to accept the handicap, persisting feelings of rejection or marked anxiety may then compound the already considerable difficulties of coping with the child's physical problem (see sections on infant problems and child abuse: pp. 182–3 and 411–44).

Three-year-old *Jane* had epilepsy and was mildly retarded. She was brought to the clinic for refusing medication and kicking and beating her mother, whose guilt about the handicap made her incapable of controlling her daughter.

Environmental conditions

Poor environmental conditions may be more significant because of their direct effects on the parents, and act only indirectly on the child. Low income, isolation, poor housing, large families, and lack of play facilities make it more difficult for parents to cope with young children (Richman, 1977a).

Interactions between the above factors are shown by *Martin*, the eighth of nine children. At four he had delayed speech and a severe behaviour problem, being completely out of control, particularly jealous of his younger sister, throwing her nappies on the fire and violently hitting her. The family lived in an overcrowded council house and were short of money; the parents were not getting on well, and the mother was depressed.

Awareness of these aetiological factors highlights the stresses involved in bringing up young children and the need to examine critically possibilities about sharing child care within the family, providing adequate money, housing and pre-school facilities and enabling women to go out to work if they so wish.

Prevalence of disorder

Individual symptoms like fears show developmental age and sex trends in their occurrence. Very young children do not show fear of strange objects but these and loud noises cause fear in the toddler. Later, fears of imaginary witches and monsters develop, and nightmares and anxieties peak at the age of four to six years.

Isolated problems, like nightmares or night terrors, are so common that on their own they cannot be taken as indicators of disorder. For instance habits such as thumb-sucking and rocking when going off to sleep are usually comfort behaviours. However a child who spends prolonged periods of the day rocking, headbanging, or masturbating should be viewed with concern as possibly retarded, grossly neglected, or understimulated. If the habit is being reinforced by undue parental attention it may also be extinguished by attending to more appropriate behaviours. If children who only show impaired functioning in a number of areas are considered, it is estimated that approximately 7 per cent of pre-school children have marked behaviour problems and another 15 per cent milder problems. Overall rates of behavioural difficulty do not differ between the sexes, but boys show more developmental and maturational problems with higher rates of problems of

sphincter control, restlessness, and language or general developmental delay (Richman *et al.*, 1975).

Assessment of the child presenting with a behaviour problem must cover all aspects of the child's emotional and physical development and family and social environment. The following areas should be considered:

(1) The child's emotional status, ability to relate to others within and outside the family, independence and activities appropriate to age.
(2) Relationships between family members. Attitudes to the index child and why this particular child has been referred for treatment.
(3) Psychiatric status and emotional difficulties in other family members.
(4) The family's social and economic situation.
(5) Physical and neuro-developmental status of the child. Particular attention should be paid to height and weight and to the child's language ability; delay in language development should prompt consideration of possible deafness.

Dawn lived with her mother, stepfather, and six sibs. At three she had severe tempers, only a few words, and was socially withdrawn. Only after repeated efforts by her mother to get her examined was high tone deafness discovered.

Infant problems

Parent's abilities to cope with their infant's demands depend on their social situation and the resources they can draw on. Those who have had poor parenting, early bereavement or separations, and inadequate substitute care may be less able to give adequate care themselves (see p. 411–14). Maternal depression, occurring more commonly during the puerperium (see chap. 5.14 and vol. 2, chap. 5), or the advent of an unwanted child may reduce coping abilities.

Frequently parents who could just about manage an easy child find a difficult one too much to cope with.

Maureen, an only child, was referred at fourteen months because she was unresponsive and difficult to manage. She seemed to lack affection and reject physical contact from birth and the parents felt she had a poor emotional attachment to them. She was one of a premature twin birth (birth weight – 4 lb), her twin brother dying at 24 hours. She was in an incubator for the first six weeks of life and her mother who had previous episodes of depression did not visit her for two weeks as she was so depressed after the twin brother's death. Maureen had been slow in development, cried and screamed a lot, and was only just beginning to play and show pleasure. At interview it was noticeable that Maureen and her mother did not interact at all, whereas her father was more responsive to her needs and gestures. She made eye contact with strangers and responded playfully for short periods, only after much coaxing. It was felt that Maureen had shown developmental problems and marked difficulties in relating, and that her mother had had particular difficulty in coping with her lack of responsiveness so that a mutually rejecting situation had been set up.

Maureen's case illustrates the fact that an infant or young child is not a passive partner in the parent–child relationship. There is evidence that from birth the infant's individual characteristics are contributing to the parent–child interaction. Children vary in many characteristics such as amount of crying, and ease of soothing. Those children who are irritable, moody, irregular in their eating and sleeping habits, slow to adapt to new things, are more likely to develop behaviour problems later. Whatever biological substrate predisposes to these variations in behaviour it is clear that right from birth complex interactions develop between adult and child; as in Maureen's case, it is important to identify factors which might hinder or promote a good beginning. These could have included encouragement to have early and regular contact with the premature baby, plus support for the mother in coping with her grief over the dead twin and with the early problems of relating to Maureen and accepting her slow development.

Child abuse

Cases of child abuse are one end of a continuum of inadequate care ranging from neglect and deprivation to actual physical abuse (non-accidental injury). The definition of abuse is somewhat arbitrary and is now tending to have wider limits including sexual abuse, but it is generally applied to cases where actual bodily harm is inflicted on a child. The commonest injuries are bites, bruises, lacerations, and fractures of the skull or other bones; scalds and burns – often caused by cigarettes; whiplash head injuries due to shaking and leading to fundal or cerebral haemorrhage or subdural haematoma; and cases of poisoning are not unknown (Baldwin & Oliver, 1975, Rogers *et al.*, 1976). Other children may present with failure to thrive following neglect and inadequate food intake (see later: eating problems and failure to thrive).

Neurological handicap and retardation often occur in abused children and it is sometimes impossible to decide whether these were caused by the injury or were contributory factors in its occurrence. Children under three are most likely to come to notice

as cases of non-accidental injury, possibly because they are more demanding as well as more vulnerable; whereas shaking a four-year-old may not be as harmful, in a baby it can cause a cerebral haemorrhage (Lynch, 1978). A high proportion of abused children show emotional difficulties and problems in social relations. They are described as showing 'frozen watchfulness' as they sit apart silent and still, unable to participate in playing with other children. It is estimated that the rate of severe abuse ranges between 1 and 3 per 1000 for the under fives, with a death rate of about 1 per 10000 (Baldwin & Oliver, 1975).

Why do certain children get abused?

It is true that if one child in a family is abused the others are also at risk of injury, but certain children do seem more at risk of becoming victims in predisposed families. Amongst those factors implicated in this increased risk are several which appear to make it difficult for a parent to establish an easy relationship with the child from the beginning. Predictors of child abuse include young parents, illegitimacy, an abnormal pregnancy including an unwanted child, an abnormal labour or delivery, physical handicap and congenital abnormalities, neonatal separation and need for special care, other mother–child separations in the first six months, and illness in the mother or child in the first year (Lynch, 1978). Abusing parents are likely to have been deprived or abused as children themselves, to lack social support, and to be under stress. The initial behaviour of a mother with her baby seems to be a sensitive indicator of risk of abuse; her unresponsiveness and inability to care for the baby are likely to cause concern to nursing staff on the ward, and this concern should lead to more detailed assessment of the family.

Knowledge of the factors predictive of child abuse makes it possible to identify at birth those children at risk and by intensive support reduce the incidence of the problem. Alertness to the possibility of abuse is essential if families and children are to receive help in time; it is only too easy for professionals to be incredulous or deceived. Even when recognized, the legal, social, and psychiatric complexities present formidable problems of management. In the majority of cases, abused children are taken 'into care', as it is unsafe to leave them with their parents. Where they are returned home intensive work is required to support the family and try to improve parenting abilities.

John at three was referred as being out of control; the family had been moved to a ground floor flat in case he jumped out of the top floor. His younger sister was in intensive care at birth, had recurrent bronchitis, and had been severely burned in obscure circumstances for which the mother blamed John. The father was frequently away for work reasons, did not accept responsibility for the children and there were violent rows between the parents. The mother was depressed and neglectful of both children. Help consisted of weekly visits by the NSPCC male worker who saw the parents together and weekly attendance at a day centre for the mother and two children. Here they could be provided with a nurturing environment and the mother was helped to carry out a specific programme of child care, whilst her ambivalent feelings towards her children were explored in case work.

Eating problems and failure to thrive

Many toddlers develop food fads; presenting a varied diet early on, although helpful, is not necessarily preventive. Mealtimes easily become a battle and a means for gaining attention and control by refusing food. A calm approach, with the minimum of attention to not eating and appropriate attention at other times, will, it may be hoped, deal with most difficulties.

However if 'failure to thrive' develops, defined as height or weight below the third percentile, this is a serious problem which requires careful evaluation with *simultaneous* physical and psychiatric investigation. Height and weight curves over the child's lifetime can provide useful clues.

There is no clear evidence that in the absence of physical illness children will fail to thrive if they have adequate food intake. Inadequate food intake may result from actual deprivation or merely neglect, from emotional disturbance in the child, often associated with vomiting, or from impaired parent–child relationships. If management advice is not successful it will be necessary to admit the child and parent to hospital for assessment and an attempt to improve food intake. Sometimes these are extremely difficult problems, as with Ann who at four years weighed only as much as an eighteen-month-old.

She had possetted and regurgitated since early infancy and continued to vomit and refuse food. She had been an unwanted child and it was difficult to enlist the co-operation of the parents, who were extremely defensive and hostile to offers of help. *Ann* eventually responded to a carefully controlled eating programme, which the parents were able

to carry out efficiently although remaining detached emotionally.

Sleeping problems

These occur in about one-fifth of children. They include difficulties over going to bed or settling to sleep, waking at night (especially common in one- to two-year-olds), nightmares and night terrors, and wishing to sleep with the parents. In probably about one-third of children the sleep problem is part of a generalized behaviour difficulty for which help may be required.

Treatment specifically aimed at the sleep begins with simple management advice, for example, being firm about taking the child back to his own room or altering sleeping conditions with a night-light or moving in with a sib. More detailed management programmes aim at removing factors which maintain the sleep difficulty, for instance gradually reducing the amount of attention given when a child wakes.

Sedatives may not affect a child's sleep pattern permanently but as a last resort can tide the family over a difficult period. If used, the dose must be adequate, otherwise the child will be half drugged and more upset. Young children often require surprisingly high doses. Trimeprazine tartrate (vallergan forte) 30–60 mg, and possibly promethazine hydrochloride (Phenergan) 10–40 mg appear to be effective. Their administration should be closely supervised, with very short courses at intervals rather than prolonged use. Night terrors respond specifically to small doses of diazepam (2–5 mg).

Prognosis

Behavioural difficulties in young children should not be dismissed lightly, they are currently distressing and a considerable proportion are likely to continue into school age.

An epidemiological study of three-year-old children compared a group with behaviour problems and a similar group matched for sex and social class without problems. At four years over 60 per cent of the former and 10 per cent of the latter had behaviour difficulties. At eight years these figures were 62 per cent and 22 per cent respectively with twice as many marked problems (28 per cent) in the original behaviour problem group compared with the original control group (11 per cent). School and learning difficulties were also more common in the former group; for instance 25 per cent were receiving special educational help in school, compared with 10 per cent of the control group (Richman *et al.*, 1982). Boys were more likely to have persisting problems compared with girls – 73 per cent and 48 per cent respectively, and to have developed conduct disorders, whereas in the girls whose problems persisted these were more often neurotic in character (Richman *et al.*, 1982).

Other factors associated with poorer outcome are family disharmony, low IQ or definite evidence of brain pathology, and having been 'in care' (Wolff, 1961b). This last is probably due to a combination of family and social factors which necessitate periods of care, and the sometimes unsatisfactory nature of the care institutions. Children under the age of two when first 'in care', or those who have long or frequent periods of 'care' are most at risk (Wolkind & Rutter, 1973). Children identified as having been abused have a particularly poor prognosis, presumably because they remain in a hostile and unaccepting family. The chance of being physically damaged again is low, but social adjustment is often poor with low self-esteem, social isolation, and difficulties in school. These children are also less likely to do well if placed away from home compared with other children 'in care' (Lynch, 1978).

Principles of management of disorders in early childhood

Treatment depends on the diagnostic formulation of the severity of the problem, associated factors, and possibilities of changes. As yet few studies have actually been carried out on the effectiveness of treatment in the young child.

(1) Environmental changes: these may be helpful although difficult to organize or evaluate; for instance, several parents report dramatic improvement in sleep problems after moving from an overcrowded house or a tower block.

(2) Provision of facilities: these can lead to new social relations and experiences and may relieve the stress between parent and child sufficiently to allow change to occur. An extremely hyperactive boy could not get to playgroup because his mother was agoraphobic. This was organized with the help of the local playgroup leader and was the beginning of change for both him and his mother who also attended a group. In general, groups can play an important supportive and preventive role for parents of young children, and there are an increasing number of self help groups.

(3) General management advice: this is often desperately sought by parents.

Jane was very attention seeking, did not play independently, and presented tremendous difficulties over eating and sleeping; she was much more difficult with her mother than with her father. Discussion with the parents focused on the following areas:
The mother's unwillingness to draw limits because she felt children should be allowed freedom; the way in which the father undermined the mother's authority and her feelings of inadequacy compared with her husband; the parents need to agree on decisions.

(4) Specific management advice using behavioural techniques: a preliminary detailed history may give a new perspective on the parents repertoire of handling skills which changes their handling for the better without specific advice. This detailed history is the first stage in using behavioural techniques in management, and can be applied to a wide variety of problems such as eating and sleeping difficulties, tempers, headbanging, wetting, soiling and constipation. The history can often usefully be supplemented by a diary kept by the parents of the target behaviours, thus providing a base line and sometimes showing specific contingencies which are maintaining the behaviour. Problems of control may be particularly responsive to behavioural techniques.

A base line of *Tom*'s severe tempers was first recorded by his parents over a two week period. The parents were then advised to use a 'time out' procedure whenever he had a temper, that is, to take him out of the room for five minutes and ignore his screaming. They were also advised to reward good behaviour i.e. paying particular attention to him and rewarding him with praise whenever he did things which they had asked him to do. The frequency of tempers decreased rapidly with only one relapse following a visit of rather indulgent grandparents.

(5) Specialized day centres may be used for particularly difficult problems. Attendance at the day centre provides support for the family, new models of behaviour for both parents and children and the possibility of advising the parents on structured behavioural programmes for coping with their children's difficulties; it also enables those children and parents who have particular difficulty in separating to do this gradually.

(6) Drugs, are of limited use in the pre-school child apart from their use in sleep difficulties and with the overactive child (see above and chap. 4.1.3 of this volume).

(7) Various forms of individual and family therapy concentrating on family relationships.

4.1.2
Speech and language disorders of childhood in children of average intelligence

ISRAEL KOLVIN

A common question in general practice and paediatrics concerns the long-term consequences of delayed development of speech and language in the early years of life (Fundudis *et al.*, 1979). Formerly, the most frequently held view was that most young children with speech and language problems would eventually develop normally. Recent research reveals that this may be a rather optimistic view – it is more likely to be true of children without major mental and physical handicaps. Two allied clinical questions remain: first, which children will eventually develop normally; second, what is the differential diagnosis in the case of those who do not?

In a brief chapter there is no space to discuss theoretical aspects of the development of speech and language, particularly new psycholinguistic concepts or the rules of grammar and language competence (Chomsky, 1957, 1965; Menyuk & Looney, 1972) which are competently surveyed elsewhere in the psycholinguistic literature. The focus will be on those types of disorders which present in clinical settings, such as deafness, specific developmental speech/ language disorders, and elective mutism. Apart from considerations of classification and prevalence, it will not include those disorders associated with mental handicap, brain damage, or infantile autism which are fully dealt with in chapter 4, and in volumes 2 and 3.

Classification

One of the more useful functional clinical classifications is that of Ingram (1959a, 1959b, and 1972) who describes three main categories of speech and language disorders: primary, secondary, and developmental. Modifications of this classification have been developed by other workers (Fundudis *et al.*, 1979).

Primary. These are disorders of speech sound production which occur in dysarthria or with cleft palate. In these conditions there is either demonstrable dysfunction or structural abnormality of tongue, lips, teeth, or palate.

Secondary. These are disorders of speech sound production secondary to other diseases or environmental factors. These include: marked intellectual impairment; demonstrable neurological disorders, and cerebral palsy; deafness; specific psychiatric syndromes, such as infantile autism and elective mutism; acquired dysphasia and the effects of an adverse psychosocial environment.

Developmental speech/language disorders (syndrome). This is a descriptive label for retardation of speech/language development in children who are otherwise apparently normal.

In addition to the above classification a distinction needs to be made between speech and language. For the purposes of a brief chapter, speech can be simply defined as the articulatory skill associated with the production of word sound and spoken language.

Language is a cognitive skill which utilizes a system of symbols (Lewis, 1968) and whose main purpose is communication; it has various forms such as spoken, written, gesture and sign (Rutter, 1972).

Prevalence

The rates of retardation of speech and language reported in population studies are a function of the definition employed. In Newcastle upon Tyne, Morley (1965) reported that 5.7 per cent of 944 children were not using two- to three-word phrases at three years; according to Fundudis and co-workers (1979), 4 per cent of 3300 three-year-old children failed to use three or more words strung together to make some sort of sense. Stevenson and Richman (1976) studied expressive language delay at the same age, but their criterion when standardized tests could not be used consisted of inability to speak in three-word phrases. They report a rate of 3.1 per cent of 705 children.

It is impossible to provide an accurate estimate of prevalence of rarer conditions when studying a relatively small population of children (Fundudis *et al.*, 1979). The following, therefore, is only a rough guide to the prevalence rate of the different types of conditions associated with speech and language disorders.

Mental handicap. Ingram (1972) reports that the single most common cause of slow speech development in paediatric clinics is mental handicap. If this is defined as an IQ of less than 70, then over 2.5 per cent of the child population is likely to be affected, with over half of these children showing severe language or articulation defects, or both (Rutter & Mittler, 1972).

Deafness. This is one of the major causes of delay in speech and language development (Morley, 1965). About 2 in 1000 children have deafness severe enough to merit the use of hearing aids (Reed, 1970).

Infantile autism. A rate of 2–4 in 10000 children has been described by Lotter (1966) in his Middlesex survey.

Elective mutism. In their population study, Fundudis and colleagues (1979) report a prevalence rate of 0.8 in 1000 at the age of 7–8 years, and therefore conclude that it is as rare a syndrome as infantile autism. However, the frequency is dependent on the age under scrutiny and whether the condition is broadly or narrowly defined.

Severe dysphasia. Serious and persisting language disorder has been estimated as occurring in 0.7 in 1000 children in Scotland (Ingram, 1963) and in 0.4 in 1000 in Newcastle (Fundudis *et al.*, 1979). Again, the condition would seem to be as rare as infantile autism.

Dysarthria. The rate is approximately 1 in 1000 births (Morley, 1965).

Developmental speech/language disorder syndrome. Newcastle research shows that this occurs in 33 in 1000 children of school age (Fundudis *et al.*, 1979). It is likely that the population studied is similar to that described by Stevenson and Richman (1976) as showing expressive language delay: it is not surpris-

ing, therefore, that the latter report a similar rate of 31 in 1000.

Types of disorder
Specific developmental speech/language disorder syndrome

In the past it was assumed that if a child had an isolated delay in speech development and was not obviously abnormal in other ways he would usually grow out of it. This is the basis of the specific speech/language disorder syndrome. In this sense the syndrome may be considered to represent an extreme variation in normal development (Rutter & Yule, 1970). The salient features have been described by Ingram (1972): it affects apparently physically healthy children with normal hearing and average intelligence, coming from normal home backgrounds. Other commonly reported features include a family history of slow speech development; an excess of close relatives who have ambidexterity or left-handedness or who previously had difficulties in the early stages of learning to read and write (McCready, 1962; Brain, 1965); and a high ratio of males to females. Others assert that the course of the condition may be influenced by environmental factors (Tizard, 1964).

Ingram's view is that the syndrome comprises a heterogeneous group of articulatory and language disorders in which speech development may not only be delayed but deviant as well. Nevertheless, he finds it useful to regard it as a spectrum of clinical disorder which range from mild to very severe.

The mildest are the dyslalias, which are simply delays in development of articulation giving rise to 'retardation of acquisition of word sounds but with normal language' (Ingram, 1972). Most authorities consider that these are commonly developmental mispronunciations which usually have little predictive importance for later cognitive or linguistic development.

The moderate developmental speech/language disorders are the developmental expressive dysphasias. The affected children have greater degrees of retardation of word sound acquisition, impaired development of and often deviant spoken language, and impaired comprehension of speech.

The severe developmental speech/language disorders are serious disorders of language comprehension. The affected children have greater degrees of retardation of word sound acquisition, impaired developmental and often deviant spoken language, and impaired comprehension. One report claims that this form is not only equally common in boys and girls but that partial high-tone hearing impairment may accompany it (Rutter, 1972).

More recent research has shown that, as a group, speech-retarded children have shorter gestational ages and lower birth weights than controls and are less frequently first-born (Fundudis *et al.*, 1979). Early reports of left-handedness or mixed laterality in developmental speech/language disorders (Orton, 1934, 1937) have not been consistently confirmed (Rutter & Yule, 1970) and this is particularly true in the case of population studies (Rutter & Yule, 1970; Fundudis *et al.*, 1979).

Modern epidemiological research reveals that the rate of problem behaviour in 3-year-old children with language delay is four times that in a random sample of children (Stevenson & Richman, 1978). Furthermore, 50 per cent of the language delay group were also retarded in their non-verbal abilities (Stevenson & Richman, 1976, 1978). However, the predictive value of such early assessments is not great and the crucial question that remains is, how many children with language delay at three years will catch up in their cognitive and language ability and lose their behavioural disturbance?

One in five of the Newcastle cohort who were previously speech retarded were found at school age to have serious language, intellectual, or physical handicaps and to have been labelled a 'pathological deviant' group. If this extreme group is set aside we are left with a residual group of speech-retarded children. There are firm grounds for believing that this group of children with serious speech retardation is very similar in speech and language development to the children with language delay described by Stevenson and Richman (1976) and both of these groups consist mainly of children with moderate or severe developmental speech/language disorders. The Newcastle research can, therefore, be used to answer some of the questions about outcome posed in this section. A high percentage of the residual speech-retarded children group still had significant cognitive and educational impairment, poor language development, including poor expressive language skills, and more restricted type of language expression (as defined by Bernstein, 1962). In addition, the prognosis in terms of behaviour is likewise poor. An important finding was that speech delay is a better predictor of impaired verbal intelligence than of performance intelligence. Furthermore, combined delay of speech and walking significantly predicts poor

cognitive and language development, less educational achievement, behavioural problems, and also introversion and social withdrawal (Fundudis *et al.*, 1979).

Acquired dysphasia

This consists of a loss of acquired language functions (Ingram, 1972). Hence, a birth-injured child cannot be described as having lost language functions, but more accurately as showing retardation of development of speech and language. In a child aged two to three years there is likely to be an impediment of language and thereafter slowing of speech.

Psychological mutism

This has two forms: traumatic and elective mutism.

Traumatic mutism has an acute onset following a psychological or physical shock or injury. Some consider it to be a hysterical phenomenon and the literature suggests that it is common, but a clinical survey does not corroborate this (Kolvin & Fundudis, 1981).

Elective mutism is the term coined by Tramer (1934) to describe a fascinating condition where talking is confined to a familiar situation and to a small group of intimates. This, too, is a rare condition and is distinguished from the excessive shyness that occurs relatively frequently in reception classes in schools (Wright, 1968; Brown & Lloyd, 1975), by its severity and its persistence. Earlier accounts were usually anecdotal but recent studies of more representative series of cases indicate that such accounts are often misleading: more girls than boys are affected, which is unusual for childhood disorders (Wright, 1968; Kolvin & Fundudis, 1981); furthermore, elective mute children are born significantly early in the sibship. There is evidence of slow or uneven development compared with controls, including delay in the beginning of speech, excess of developmental mispronunciations, EEG immaturity, and associated problems of speech, bowel and bladder function (Kolvin & Fundudis, 1981), poorer non-verbal intelligence, and a high rate of associated behavioural problems.

With regard to aetiology, some workers suggest that mutism may be secondary to some biologically based symptoms – for instance, some children avoid speaking because they are teased when they mispronounce words (Rutter, 1977). On the other hand, the literature is also replete with single or small-group studies postulating psycho-dynamic bases such as faulty mother–child relationships (Parker *et al.*, 1960), family neurosis (Browne *et al.*, 1963) or psychological trauma in infancy (Salfield, 1950). In the recent Newcastle study, personality problems of parents, particularly those concerning social relationships, proved common. In addition, more than double the number of parents of elective mute children attended psychiatric clinics than did those of the control children.

Finally, follow-up reveals that elective mutism is a more intractable disorder than most of the other non-organic, non-psychotic psychiatric disorders of childhood, with less than 50 per cent subsequently improving (Kolvin & Fundudis, 1981).

Deafness

Both because of its rarity and because the deaf infant sporadically babbles, deafness may remain unsuspected in early infancy. Subsequently, parents may be alerted because of a poor expressive response to sudden meaningful noises, or the condition may be detected using developmental screening tests from about 9 months of age. Likely causes of profound deafness can be identified by careful history and include such conditions as serious post-natal middle-ear infections and neonatal hyperbilirubinaemia. In contrast, epidemiological studies usually do not reveal an excess of social and family pathology in families of deaf children (Fundudis *et al.*, 1979).

In a short review it is possible only to touch on some of the complex theoretical issues concerning speech, language, and intellectual development of deaf children (Moores, 1972; Meadow, 1975). In profoundly deaf children the development/acquisition of speech and language is different from that of children with normal hearing, but may also differ for different deaf groups according to the modes of communication used by those taking care of them. The difficulties of language acquisition which deaf children encounter cover not only more superficial language skills, such as spoken language, but also include inner language abilities (Meadow, 1975). On the other hand, there is evidence that the rules of language learned by deaf children in their earlier years are similar to those of hearing children (Fundudis *et al.*, 1979).

The literature provides much evidence that childhood deafness hampers the development of language and verbal abilities, but not necessarily that of non-verbal abilities (Wiley, 1971; Fundudis *et al.*,

1979). However, this comparatively poorer performance on cognitive tasks appears to improve with age and appropriate stimulation. In addition, there is evidence that the academic achievements, particularly progress in reading, of deaf children are poorer than those of hearing children (US Office of Demographic Studies, 1973; Conrad, 1977). Some consider that these cognitive and educational impairments are more an indictment of the educational system than an inevitable consequence of deafness (Vernon, 1976). Surprisingly, deaf children of deaf parents often show better linguistic development than deaf children of hearing parents – which seems to favour an early introduction of non-verbal methods of communication.

Research findings usually report that hearing children are better adjusted socially and behaviourally than deaf children: in the case of profoundly deaf children, antisocial disturbance often reveals itself in school (Fundudis *et al.*, 1979). Furthermore, deaf children raised in families where other members are deaf often prove better adjusted than those raised in families where other members are not deaf (Myklebust, 1964).

Organic brain damage may cause deafness and contribute to the poorer intellectual and educational performance of such children. However, there is no way of estimating the extent of this contribution.

Social influences

While some workers emphasize the biological determinants of speech and language, others stress the importance of psychosocial influences. Chomsky (1969) postulates the presence of an innate language acquisition device which determines the deep-seated properties of organization and structure which are found in all human languages. Lenneberg (1967), too, argues that the emergence of speech is most easily accounted for by maturational changes which are only moderately affected by abnormal factors in the child's environment. He and others (Critchley, 1967) have pointed out that children of deaf parents were found to babble appropriately and to develop speech adequately, despite being brought up in a grossly abnormal linguistic environment.

Environmental stimulation (Irwin, 1960; Routh, 1969) and interchange, particularly with adults, facilitates progress in vocalization and language development in the early years (Cazden, 1966; Brown *et al.*, 1969). The converse is also true, in that it has been shown that speech and language may be adversely affected, as may verbal intelligence, in those situations which reflect an impoverished social environment, as in those institutions where there is inadequate emphasis on the quality and intensity of stimulation (Brodbeck & Irwin, 1946; Tizard, 1970) in large families and in the case of multiple births. However, even serious impoverishment of the social environment appears to give rise to only moderate degrees of impaired vocalization (Provence & Lipton, 1962), speech delay and language retardation, with the retardation being confined mainly to language expression (rather than to comprehension (Klaus and Gray, 1968)), and retardation of educational performance.

On the basis of the above brief review, it would seem that those more moderate theories which stress interaction of innate factors and social influences are likely to have more general validity (Bruner *et al.,* 1966). We can conclude that adverse social factors must be very unusual to seriously impede the emergence of speech in a normal infant.

Assessment

In the assessment of children with speech and language problems a preliminary formulation and differential diagnosis can usually be made on the basis of relatively simple assessment. The main areas of inquiry include biographical information; observation of the child during interview; assessment of hearing, speech, and language; a study of the child's play and capacity for imitation; cognitive ability; social and behavioural functioning; and, finally, neurological assessment.

Biographical information

This may provide information not only about psychosocial influences, but also about relevant physical factors, such as cerebral insults, history of clumsiness, and so forth.

Observation

This constitutes an integral part of all other forms of assessment. Most clinicians, even while gathering biographical information, will use observation to determine whether the young utilize clues from parents, or display the clumsiness of gait typical of the child with cerebral palsy.

Hearing

This should always be assessed, with the clinician checking whether the child responds to a wide range of auditory stimuli, including responses to sudden or unusual noises and a variety of domestic noises in the absence of visual or gestural clues. Where there are any doubts, expert assessment is indicated, which may include audiometry or even EEG audiometry and other specialized techniques.

Speech and language in its various forms

Speech may be delayed, or articulation skills deviant. For instance, articulation may be defective in deafness, immature in mental retardation and developmental speech/language disorders, defective and immature in autism and variably disordered in elective mutism. The articulation defect in dysarthria is characteristic.

Language can be assessed in a number of modalities, for example, spoken, sign (manual), or written. Language comprehension can be tested by assessing the child's ability to understand simple commands both *with* and *without* the provision of visual and gestural clues. Careful observation will indicate by what means the child is trying to understand his environment. Evidence of language *production* can be obtained from the way the child communicates through gesture, mime and conversation (Rutter, 1977). 'Inner language', which reflects an understanding of a symbolic code can be indirectly assessed by observing whether there is a meaningful use of objects and by constructiveness and creativity in play.

In *profound deafness* the child does not attend to, or respond to, auditory stimuli, but will extensively use gesture, attempt conversation when older, and may be constructive in his play. In many respects the child with the most severe form of a *developmental speech/language disorder* will show a similar pattern and, indeed, there may only be limited evidence of inner language, but usually there will be evidence of normal hearing. In milder forms of development delay there is usually no suggestion of deafness but rather a lack of understanding of verbal but not non-verbal communication and usually there is reasonable evidence of inner language. The younger *autistic child* may not respond meaningfully to auditory stimuli, and, indeed, may tend not to respond to any form of verbal or non-verbal communication. There is little indirect evidence of language either in terms of gesture, mime, imitation or play. In *mental handicap* there is usually no evidence of deafness, but rather of limited language abilities and usually a delay in development of articulation, together with other evidence of slowness of development.

Constructive play and imitation

Evidence of constructive play reflects the presence of inner language and augurs well for the growth of language in general. Gestural imitation and play constitutes a form of communication which is impaired in infantile autism and in severe language retardation.

Cognitive ability

Parental reports of the child's social abilities and play, combined with clinical observation, provide only a rough guide to the child's cognitive level. However, clinical impressions can be most deceptive and need to be validated by careful psychometric assessment of both non-verbal intellectual skills and language performance. A wide range of tests are now available, which limit the amount of spoken instruction, and measure performance rather than verbal abilities and a wide range of language skills (Mittler, 1972). Even if formal testing is not possible, a social maturity scale, which employs evidence from the mother or the person taking care of the child, may be profitably employed to provide a crude estimate of intellectual level.

Social and general behaviour

Accounts from parents complemented by direct observation may provide useful information about the basis of the speech delay – the manifold social and behavioural abnormalities of autism; the absence of startle to loud noises or alerting to domestic noises – or those reflecting social behaviour of peers, such as occur in the young deaf; and the social withdrawal of the electively mute.

Neurological assessment

If the clinician is not experienced in neurological examination of the child, important signs may be missed. Collaboration with a paediatrician or paediatric neurologist will usually ensure identification of relevant physical anomalies.

4.1.3
Hyperkinetic syndrome

ERIC A. TAYLOR

Definition

Over-activity is a complaint frequently voiced about normal children. When the mothers and the teachers of children selected at random have been asked about them in research studies, some 30 per cent of the children are described as over-active. Much more rigorous definition is therefore needed than the impression of a single adult.

The *hyperkinetic syndrome* consists of severe over-activity which is not specific to any one situation; a very short attention span; and extreme distractability. Social disinhibition and impulsiveness are frequent concomitants. Defiant, destructive, or aggressive behaviour is often associated, but commonly appears only after the other features have impaired social development. The onset is usually in the first five years of life; parents frequently recall restlessness and inattention as being continuously present from the first few months.

Prevalence

The condition is uncommon, being diagnosed in around 1.5 per cent of children assessed in the children's department of a psychiatric hospital. Milder degrees of restlessness, however, are very common. In some parts of the world, notably North America, the diagnosis of 'hyperactivity' is applied to many children with this milder pattern, and accordingly 4 per cent to 10 per cent of all children can be seen as affected (Safer & Allen, 1976). However, in this sense of the term there is very great overlap with the other problems of conduct disorder, and the symptom of over-activity alone does not have any specific implications for aetiology (Sandberg *et al.,* 1978).

Causes

Hyperkinesis is very much more common in children with neuroepileptic disorders than in the general population, and particularly so in intellectually retarded children. (Rutter *et al.,* 1970). Temporal lobe epilepsy may well be specifically associated (Ounsted, 1955). None the less, the majority of children with pervasive over-activity does not show evidence of brain damage. Conversely, children with brain damage are vulnerable to the whole range of psychiatric disorder and not to hyperkinesis only. When unequivocal brain damage is present, then it is probably the deciding factor in the development of severe inattention and pervasive over-activity. Social disinhibition is particularly closely associated with the results of brain damage (Brown *et al.,* 1981).

It is much less clear how far a biological cause can be invoked for hyperkinetic children without definite brain damage. The early onset and the lack of specificity to particular environments suggest a constitutional basis; and in some cases it is best seen as an extreme form of temperamental deviation. Extensive North American research (Cantwell, 1977) has produced some evidence of minor degrees of muscular incoordination and neurophysiological dysfunction. The significance of these is not yet known; and diagnostic imprecision renders it very hard to know to which groups of children such findings should properly apply. One must not generalize from restless American children to the uncommon but severe problem of hyperkinetic syndrome as considered here.

It is very probable that some psychological factors can also lead to marked inattention and to restless over-activity. Tizard and Rees (1975) showed that the environment of an institutional children's home can lead to a deficit in attention which can be reversed (at least in part) by adoption into a family. Shaffer and colleagues (1974) demonstrated that inattention and restlessness were associated with conduct disorder rather than with brain damage.

Clinical features

An excess of physical movement is not the only implication of 'over-activity'. Indeed, many children so described are notable only for the inappropriate-

ness of their actions, not for the frequency. Vigorous but well-directed play is not evidence of over-activity; rather the criterion is of chaotic, undirected behaviour especially manifest in situations where orderliness is required, such as the classroom and the dining table.

There is a natural, if vague, connection between undirected activity and poor concentration. In fact, 'attention' is a complex set of processes and its development is not a simple progression from breadth and distractability to a narrow focus (Taylor, 1980). An important line of development is that from random exploration of the world, guided by external features of the environment, to logical and systematic sampling of information. Impaired concentration is therefore revealed in a disorderly and impulsive choice of what is relevant and an inability to sustain concentration on a task for more than a very small number of minutes. Impairment of learning is the rule where attention is severely disordered.

Reckless impulsiveness can be of major importance in its own right. It may endanger the child by leading to accidents. Further, an accident-prone child may require a degree of supervision from parents that exacerbates the strains in relationships.

CASE HISTORY

Ian was born with congenital agenesis of the cranial nerve nuclei and in consequence underwent numerous hospital admissions in his first year of life, in all of which he was accompanied by his single mother. Hospital records from the age of 1 year indicated that he was exceptionally active, exploratory and boisterous to the point of uncontrollability. His mother became isolated and, eventually, depressed; the requirement for unending vigilance was a major stress upon her. She cared for him closely until the age of 6 years, when he started at school and was at once identified as a very difficult classroom problem and 'a whirlwind of activity'. His first class could not cope with his throwing things around and pinching other children; his second school arranged for psychiatric referral at the age of 7 years. He was then noted to have very limited concentration, changed activities about every 15 seconds, and persisted in tasks introduced by the examiner for no longer than 10 seconds at a time. In spite of this his IQ was above average. He was overfriendly, and physically affectionate to strangers; although not overtly sad, he thought himself 'rubbish'. He broke a basket and several toys in his assessment, but was always cheerfully responsive to adult directions (for a few seconds), and was generally liked. Treatment with methylphenidate was followed by a marked increase in time spent on tasks given by others, and his teacher then introduced a programme of behaviour modification. His behaviour was then acceptable, he made good progress in learning to read, and after 3 months medication was discontinued. Progress was maintained over 18 months; but he has continued to be impulsive in his behaviour, and has had no close friends.

Management

The problems of hyperkinesis are various, and so must management be. We have seen that 'over-activity' may often be a misnomer for defiant, disruptive behaviour. This is best seen as a form of conduct disorder, and its management is considered in that section (chap. 4.1.1). Similarly, 'over-activity' may be invoked as an explanatory concept for children who are failing academically, and the section on learning disorders considers management here (chap. 4.2.2).

However, the impairment of the ability to attend can be so great as to compromise any lines of management that are based on learning. Under these circumstances, a trial of drug treatment is indicated. The first choice will usually be methylphenidate in a dosage of 0.25 to 0.75 mg/kg, or another stimulant, such as dextroamphetamine or pemoline.

The value of stimulant medication has been investigated in many placebo-controlled trials (Barkley, 1977). The results are unequivocal, that over the course of a trial (usually 6 to 12 weeks) the active drug causes an improvement in behaviour problems according to teachers' and parents' ratings and an improvement in performance on certain laboratory tests related to cognition: especially tests of reaction time, of motor control, and of sustained attention to repetitive tasks. These effects are not paradoxical, but similar to those seen in normal adults (Weiss & Laties, 1962) and intelligent children (Rapoport *et al.*, 1978).

There are, however, known and suspected hazards associated with these drugs. Diminution in appetite and sleep are frequent central effects, and growth retardation may be a consequence of continued medication. Dysphoria is frequent. Allergic effects and psychotic reactions have occasionally been reported. Stimulants can be abused, both by children seeking a euphoric experience and by parents seeking control of their children. To set against this there is very little evidence of long-term efficacy, nor knowledge of the effects on psychological development. It should also be noted that the evidence on efficacy is derived largely from trials conducted on mildly affected children who would, in the UK, be diagnosed for the most part as suffering from 'conduct disorder'. The more severe the problem, the less likely it is that stimulants will be helpful. Phenothiazine drugs and haloperidol can control wildly overactive behaviour when stimulants fail; but they are likely to produce a worsening of concentration and an impairment of learning. Low-dose haloperidol (0.02 to 0.08 mg/kg body weight) is to be preferred; high-dose regimes are hazardous and likely to be of only transient efficacy. Tricyclic antidepressants have an action rather similar to that of stimulants.

Drug treatment should therefore be given to a child only as a monitored trial, preferably with a placebo control. Monitoring must focus on the target symptom, since different behaviours show different dose-response relationships (Sprague & Sleator, 1975), and a high dose of stimulants which controls disruptive behaviour may actually worsen a central problem of attention deficit. They must also be combined with other modes of intervention.

Counselling to parents can, first of all give information and remove the guilt and sense of inadequacy experienced by many. Most parents can learn the techniques of behaviour modification; these should not be seen only as a form of symptom control, but as a major educational tool for the instilling of behaviour patterns important to the overall development of the child. The stress of care may lead to problems within the parent or the family that can usefully be managed by conjoint family psychotherapy or by the methods of case work with parents. However, the presence of hyperkinesis is not *per se* an indication for psychotherapy and is unlikely to respond to it. Families may well be helped by the opportunity for short periods of residential care. It is possible for this to be provided in smaller, more informal children's homes rather than exclusively in hospitals. Spells of in-patient treatment enable methods of handling hyperkinesis to be worked out for that child, allow training of specific skills, and can be very helpful in controlling complications, such as aggressive behaviour.

Classroom management may well need to take account of detailed advice from the assessment of such a child. Both teachers and parents can learn to teach a reflective strategy to problem-solving but it has not yet been shown that either this or systematic teaching of perseverance at a task is effective.

Prognosis

Studies which have followed the course of children diagnosed as hyperactive give contradictory and inconsistent results (Shaffer & Greenhill, 1979). This is, of course, only to be expected when the diagnosis is made in so many different ways. The broadly conceived North American diagnosis appears to have some important implications for adult personality. Whether or not over-activity persists, social adjustment remains impaired in adolescence (Mendelson *et al.*, 1971); and the over-active will become more restless adults, likely to have failed in school (Weiss *et al.*, 1971, 1979). Personality disorder of an impulsive or immature type is the likeliest psychiatric diagnosis to be applied to this group. However, it is not at all clear that this course is any different from that associated with conduct disorder generally.

A more gloomy outcome in adult life was suggested by a follow-up of children who had been diagnosed at a paediatric neurology clinic (Menkes *et al.*, 1967). Only half of the 14 cases were self-supporting; four were 'psychotic' and in hospital and two were retarded. Theoretical formulations of schizophrenic psychopathology which stress the role of cognitive abnormalities would argue that a high rate of schizophrenia will be found among those with seriously impaired attention; little evidence yet supports the contention, but there is a notable lack of information on the outcome of the severely hyperkinetic. However, severe and refractory hyperkinesis must carry a poor prognosis for social adjustment. Diminished restlessness at puberty may occur, sometimes to the point of apathy; but it is by no means inevitable and substantial problems can persist. Hyperkinetic behaviour among the intellectually retarded remains a major reason for long-term hospital admission.

4.1.4
Disturbances of toilet function

ERIC A. TAYLOR

Toilet training

Human beings did not evolve to use lavatories. The toilet training which children receive from their parents is an early demand for self-control, and can be the setting for increased autonomy and also for angry confrontation. Delay in the acquisition of continence, and breakdown of established continence, are common problems with substantial psychiatric implications. Successful training requires an intact neuromuscular apparatus and its coordination; an adequate teaching of the behaviour required; understanding of the social demands; and the will to comply with them. Problems in all these areas, as will be seen, are found in some groups of children who wet or soil.

Much emphasis has in the past been given to deviant training practices by parents. Undue harshness and excessive laxness have both been blamed, as has the pattern of overprotection which encourages regression in the child. Certainly great differences in practice exist between different cultures, which are reflected in the average age at which children become clean and dry. In the non-industrialized societies of the undeveloped world, training is usually early. The society of the Digo, for example (deVries & deVries, 1977) expects night and day continence by the age of 6 months. In cultures where the constraints of the nappy and the water closet dictate a less responsive and more demanding approach by the training parent, toilet training tends to be late. It is not clear, however, that such large differences are paralleled by major differences in the prevalence of enuresis and encopresis. A relaxed and delayed approach, for example, has been reported by Brazelton (1962) to lead to an extremely low prevalence of enuresis; yet a similar approach has been invoked by Kaffman & Elizur (1977) to account for the rather high prevalence of enuresis in Israeli children living in kibbutzim. It may be that deviations in toilet training are of less importance in themselves than as markers to a disturbed relationship between child and caretaker.

It is unlikely that training practices have in themselves major implications for the development of adult personality. Studies such as that of Hetherington and Brackbill (1963) have failed to document a link between early training and 'anal' traits of character. Nevertheless, the disorders of excretion to be considered below can give rise to pervasive problems of social adjustment and can be adversely affected by emotional upset.

Nocturnal enuresis

Bedwetting at night is much more common than the other disorders of excretory function. At the age of 7 years, about 7 per cent of boys and 3 per cent of girls are enuretic at least once a week. It should seldom be regarded as a problem requiring intervention before the age of 6 years.

Causes. Bedwetting is frequently an isolated problem, without other signs of psychiatric disorder. Indeed, boys of 7 who are enuretic are no more likely than their contemporaries to be deviant in their behaviour. On the other hand, girls of 7, like older boys, are substantially more likely to be judged as psychiatrically disordered if they are also enuretic. It is not proven that this is because psychiatric disorder causes enuresis: though disordered children are more likely to develop enuresis, this may be because both conditions have associated factors in common (Rutter *et al*, 1973). Reading delay and low IQ are also more common in the enuretic. In addition, enuresis causes shame and rejection and is therefore a potent cause of behaviour problems: children whose enuresis is successfully treated will often become happier and more self-confident (Baker, 1969). There are probably multiple causes. A genetic contribution is implied by the finding (Bakwin, 1973) that monozygotic twins display a higher degree of concordance than do dizygotic twins. It is, however, much less

clear just what is inherited. Structural abnormality of the urinary tract is only rarely encountered; urinary tract infection is more commonly a result than a cause of wetting. Functional abnormalities of the base plate of the bladder have been observed in some children. Some enuretic children have a pattern of voiding urine at quite small bladder volumes; in the daytime this is shown by the sudden onset of an urgent need to micturate.

Wetting can occur in any stage of orthodox sleep, but is uncommon in paradoxical sleep. In some children there is a clear relationship with external stress; in most there is not. It is possible (Douglas, 1973) – but not established – that stress around the third year of life prevents dryness being achieved then or later. Living in an institution (even a kibbutz) is associated with high rates of enuresis. No single pattern of family interaction or mode of toilet training has been established as a basis for bedwetting; in individual cases, however, the symptom may be an important part of an abnormality in relationships. This will, of course, be more frequent in the very small fraction of enuretic children who are presented for psychiatric treatment.

Management. The above considerations imply that assessment of the symptom of enuresis should always include consideration of the child's emotional and cognitive development. The strengths and weaknesses of family life also need to be taken into account in planning feasible treatment; this becomes particularly important when the failure of standard treatments is the reason for referral.

The urine should be cultured; antibiotic treatment, if it is successful in sterilizing infected urine has sometimes led to the acquisition of continence. No other urological investigation is required for the majority of children, who are incontinent only at night and who show no abnormality on physical examination. Assessment should also include a period of record keeping for about 3 weeks, with particular attention to noting and rewarding dry nights. A star chart is often used for this, and many children become dry with no further intervention.

The first line of treatment should usually be the use of an enuresis alarm. This device (whose use is described in detail by Dische, 1973) sounds a buzzer and wakes the child as soon as urine begins to soak through his sheet. He should then micturate voluntarily, completely and immediately into a suitable receptacle. Any delay in waking reduces the efficacy of treatment, suggesting that a learning process takes place. It needs to be carefully explained to families, and an early opportunity must be taken of monitoring progress and smoothing out technical problems. Under these circumstances, around 80 per cent of treated children become dry; usually over the course of a period up to 3 months. Failure may stem from the child's not waking at the buzzer (when a louder alarm or the parent's waking may be required as mediators) from technical failures or false alarms, and from lack of co-operation (when the reasons should be carefully sought). Furthermore, about a third of successfully treated children relapse when they stop using the alarm. The number of children relapsing can be reduced by a period of overlearning, during which the alarm continues to be used and a fluid load is given at bedtime. The presence of emotional disorder is no contra-indication to this treatment; the substitution of other symptoms for the wetting need not be expected. On the contrary, coexistent emotional disorder is likely to be improved by treating the wetting.

Tricyclic antidepressants are another established treatment. They reduce the frequency of bedwetting in about 85 per cent of children, and in 30 per cent they stop it completely (Shaffer, 1977). They are effective in low dosage (for example 10 to 50 mg of imipramine taken at night) within a week; but relapse is the rule when they are stopped. Their mode of action is therefore clearly different from their antidepressant action, and probably represents an unidentified effect on the central nervous system (Shaffer *et al.*, 1979). They are chiefly useful when urgent treatment is required or when social conditions make the alarm impracticable. They are very dangerous in overdose, causing the deaths of several children each year; and must therefore be considered a secondary treatment.

Psychotherapy alone is not an adequate treatment for enuresis (Werry & Cohrssen, 1965); but it may of course be indicated on other grounds. Sometimes, as we have noted, it will be necessary for family attitudes to be changed before the nocturnal alarm can be given an adequate trial.

Behaviour therapists have evolved several techniques for teaching continence, mentioned under 'diurnal enuresis' below. These techniques can also be used at night, with regular waking of the child followed by rewards for dryness and procedures such as overcorrection and positive practice of appropriate micturition if the child is wet. They offer real hope

for those resistant to other treatments, but are not easy to use and may make hospital admission advisable.

Prognosis. Most enuretic children are never presented for treatment and most recover spontaneously (Miller *et al.*, 1960). However, persistence into adult life is not rare and is a serious obstacle to the adjustment to independent life. The frequency of adult enuresis was brought forcibly to professional notice by the high prevalence among army recruits in the mass conscription of the Second World War; when figures of around 1 per cent for male recruits between 17 and 27 were typically found (Thorne, 1943; Levine, 1943). Michaels (1955) has argued extensively that there is a rather specific association between persistent enuresis and a particular form of ill-balanced personality characterized by delinquency, impulsiveness, and lack of controls: 'persistent enuresis was seen as the prototype of the expression of deficient inhibitory tendencies as revealed in the persistent delinquent or psychopathic personality'. A somewhat higher prevalence of night-time wetting has indeed been found in delinquents than in the general population. The study of adult enuretics, however, (Dominian, 1961; Stalker & Band, 1946) argues neither that they are much different from juvenile enuretics, nor that they show any single pattern of psychiatric disorder. The persistence of enuresis can be seen as non-specific evidence of psychological vulnerability, and as a contributing cause to psychiatric ill-health; it does not bear witness to any one pattern of personality organization.

Diurnal enuresis

Regular wetting by day is much less common than at night; but it has been found in approximately 1 per cent of all seven-year-olds (de Jonge, 1973) and 17 per cent of nocturnally enuretic seven-year-olds (Hallgren, 1956). By contrast with the other disorders of toilet behaviour, it is more common in girls than boys. It can be considered as an abnormality after the age of four years has been reached. It has attracted many fewer studies than the other disorders, and conclusions are accordingly more tentative (Berg, 1979).

Causes. Diurnal enuresis may well be more closely associated than nocturnal enuresis with symptoms of psychiatric disorder (Hallgren, 1956). It is, of course, more likely to be apparent to a child's contemporaries and so to stigmatize him; and it may be more irritating to parents. It is not necessarily the result of a specific stress, as it is usually present continuously from infancy; but stress during a critical period of development remains a possibility.

The 'unstable bladder' (which contracts, at relatively low volumes, before it is fully distended) has already been noted as a possible factor in nocturnal enuresis. The results – urgency of micturition, and perhaps frequency as well – are particularly associated with the pattern of daytime wetting (Berg, Fielding & Meadow, 1977). Attempts at direct modification of this pattern of voiding have so far been therapeutically unrewarding, but are not fully explored. It is doubtful whether it is caused by local urological factors (Yeates, 1973); and indeed it might be caused by the psychological consequences of chronic stress – perhaps interacting with a genetically determined overresponsiveness of bladder musculature. The high prevalence of enuresis in the families of the diurnally enuretic (Hallgren, 1957) would be compatible with a genetic contribution to aetiology.

Mental retardation is an important association of enuresis (often in conjunction with encopresis), and can indeed impair the recognition of social demands as well as the ability to comply with them.

Management. Full psychiatric assessment of the child and his close environment is indicated. The pattern of voiding should be noted over a period, and specificity to one situation may point to alterable stress. Culture of the urine demonstrates bacteria in about 50 per cent of afflicted girls, probably as a consequence of frequent wetting. Difficulty in the actual process of micturition, and incontinence on sudden exertion (including laughing and crying) suggest a need for further urological investigation. The functional bladder capacity can readily be determined by giving a fluid load after voiding, encouraging as long a wait as possible before further voiding, and measuring the volume of urine passed.

Treatments have been very little evaluated. It has been demonstrated that a programme of intensive training using the methods of behaviour modification (Foxx & Azrin, 1973) can be rapidly effective in young children and children whose enuresis stems from mental retardation. The techniques offer some promise for the treatment of diurnal enuresis generally. It is also possible to teach children to increase their functional bladder capacity by progressively delaying micturition after a fluid load.

Psychotherapeutic involvement is not usually focused on the symptom of wetting as such. Even when there is a definite improvement in the child's general mental state, the symptom of wetting very often persists. It is, however, justifiable to sustain an optimistic attitude in view of the strong natural tendency to recovery.

Finally, when treatment for nocturnal enuresis is effective, daytime wetting is sometimes helped as well. This is by no means invariable (Berg, 1979) but can justify a trial of imipramine for this unpleasant and poorly understood symptom.

Faecal soiling

The deposition of faeces in inappropriate places is usually regarded as an abnormality after the fourth birthday. It is found in about 1.5 per cent of 7-year-old children; with increasing age the prevalence steadily falls, and it is decidedly uncommon beyond the age of 16. Boys are more frequently affected than girls. The term 'encopresis' is usually applied only to those children who have no organic reason for the symptom. In practice, however, both organic and psychological factors are very often present together; both need treatment and a rigid distinction is misleading.

Causes. There are many causes, and it is therefore important to recognize different patterns of soiling. (a) *Incontinence of fluid faeces* can result from diarrhoea, often due to physical causes but also occurring for psychological reasons (Wender *et al.*, 1976). (b) *Retention with overflow* is the commonest pattern of incontinence in the general population. Severe constipation leads to anal incompetence and faeces (usually liquid) leak out. The constipation may result from local pathology such as a painful fissure or an abnormal segment of rectum; but can also be the result of psychological factors, such as anxiety centred on toileting or a battle between parent and child. (c) *Passage of formed stools* inappropriately is the pattern most commonly referred to psychiatrists, and often the hardest form to treat. Developmental delay is sometimes a factor: low intelligence, physical clumsiness, and delay in language development are all known to be associated (Bemporad *et al.*, 1971). Low social class, on the other hand, is *not* associated either with the symptom or with any particular pattern of soiling (Olatawura, 1973; Stein & Susser, 1967). Emotional disorder in the child is frequent, but not invariable. Family disharmony, disturbed relationships between parents and child, and marital problems are all more common than in normal families; and a harsh, coercive style of toilet training has been suggested as an antecedent cause by studies based on retrospective recall (Pinkerton, 1958).

With such a complicated set of causes, it would be helpful further to classify the pattern of soiling with formed stools. Anthony (1957) argued for the distinction between *continuous* and *discontinuous*: those with discontinuous soiling have had a period of continence as testimony to their having learned to control defaecation. Hersov (1977) distinguishes between those soiling in their underclothes (as evidence of diminished control) and those depositing faeces elsewhere (perhaps more emotionally determined). The classifications overlap.

Rowland was referred at the age of 10 years after extensive physical investigation had revealed no physical cause of his twice-daily soiling. He had never achieved a period free from this, but until the age of 8 years the only symptom had been the presence of formed faeces in his pants. After that age he became increasingly quiet and withdrawn, avoided his previous friends, and took to wrapping his faeces in paper or leaving them about the house, on the mantelpiece, in the oven, and in the freezer. His parents, both professionally successful and with no other children, had high hygienic standards and were seriously distressed but avoided all mention of the soiling at home; they found him smilingly compliant in other respects but somewhat unspontaneous. In conjoint meetings with a psychiatrist, all three rapidly changed from excessive politeness to strong verbal attacks on each other, chiefly about father's frequent absences from home, mother's frequent nagging, and Rowland's 'dirtiness', perceived as ingratitude. All felt that family life was much less strained as a result of the changes they made, and Rowland became sociable again and made several friends at a railway club. The pattern of soiling reverted to deposition in his underpants. However, it was only after 10 months of regular sessions that he rather suddenly stopped all soiling, and it was not clear that this improvement was associated with the treatment given.

Management. The initial stages of history taking should therefore establish the pattern of soiling and the likely reasons for the problem. Abdominal and rectal examination should seek local pathology, particularly the presence of marked constipation. If this is present, it will require physical treatment if control is to be regained. This will usually start with an enema, and proceed rapidly to maintenance treatment, for example, with lactulose or with the combination of dioctyl sodium sulphosuccinate as stool softener and senna laxatives; normal diet and adequate hydration will need to be achieved. In paediatric practice this regime alone often seems effective (Coekin & Gairdner, 1960); but for patients seen in psychiatric practice other measures will normally be needed. Assessment will accordingly include detailed attention to the patterns of family interaction and to the mental state of the child.

There are effective behavioural techniques for training bowel function; their use is not confined only to those with a predominantly 'untrained' pattern. It is important to teach appropriate defaecation as well as reducing the actual behaviour of soiling. Star charts often succeed alone. Stars are given for successful defaecation in the lavatory and for periods without soiling; they can act as tokens and lead to a tangible reward.

More complex methods are sometimes useful. Regular checks on cleanliness (with consistent, clear, warm feedback) can be preferable to a daily interrogation. Some children have been helped by direct teaching of correct elimination. For instance, a therapist can model to the child how to defaecate, and then reward him for successively closer approximations. Furthermore, the strategy of relaxing immediately before defaecation can be effectively taught. Overcorrection and positive practice procedures may be more effective responses to an act of incontinence than punishment. Some children need to learn and rehearse how to excuse themselves from class or play. Some children respond to the call to stool with an anxious rush that increases their likelihood of soiling; they may be helped by learning to contract the pelvic floor voluntarily until the urgency has diminished.

These techniques nearly always have to be combined with some components of the psychotherapeutic approach. Listening, advice, and reassurance are always indicated. The therapist's demonstration of acceptance of the child and understanding of the symptom is a major part in developing trust; his optimism can be salutary for a despairing family. Some of the behavioural techniques described probably act in part by enabling some modification of family relationships, and in particular by diminishing a vicious cycle of rejection, punishment and shame. Conjoint family counselling has much to recommend it, not only as an adjunct enabling other treatments to be applied but also as the most direct form of modifying essential components of the clinical picture.

Prognosis. Persistence into adult life is not unknown, but is decidedly uncommon (Bellman, 1966). It is sufficiently rare that series of adult encopretics have not been reported; and therefore theoretical accounts of persistent encopresis as a factor in personality development are not appropriate. Nonetheless, the distress and stigma are sufficiently great for it to be considered a barrier to the attainment of independence and emotional order.

4.2
The school child

4.2.1
School non-attendance
IAN BERG

School Refusal
Definition

A disorder characterized by severe reluctance or complete refusal to attend school, emotional upset at the prospect of having to go there and staying home when not at school with the knowledge of the parents.

Prevalence

Population studies (Rutter *et al.*, 1970; Miller *et al.*, 1971; Rutter *et al.*, 1976) and investigations of clinic samples (Kahn & Nursten, 1962; Chazan, 1962; Smith, 1970) have shown that school refusal occurs in about 5 per cent of psychiatrically disturbed children, in a smaller proportion at the primary school stage and a larger one in early adolesence.

Aetiology

Boys and girls are equally affected. There is no social class bias (Berg *et al.*, 1969). Intelligence and educational achievement do not deviate from what would otherwise be expected (Berg *et al.*, 1975). Family size and the proportion of only children are normal. School refusers tend to be younger than their brothers and sisters when there are more then two children in the family (Berg *et al.*, 1972). There is no tendency for them to come from broken homes (Hersov, 1960a, b). A fifth of mothers are psychiatrically disturbed (Berg *et al.*, 1974 a) but this is similar to other kinds of disorders in childhood (Rutter, 1966).

Any child of school age can be affected but the condition is most often reported in young teenagers in Britain (Kahn, 1958; Morgan, 1959; Hersov, 1960a, b; Berg, 1970) and in younger children in the USA (Waldfogel *et al.*, 1957; Eisenberg, 1958).

Dependency and overprotection. School refusers tend to be unduly reliant on their mothers and to stay home excessively (Berg, 1974; Berg & McGuire, 1971). Their mothers are inclined to be overprotective, that is to condone or actively encourage dependency, (Berg & McGuire, 1974). The term 'school phobia' which is often used interchangeably with that of 'school refusal' was first applied to children who were unduly dependent on their mothers and who consequently reacted to threats that would otherwise be seen as trivial, by developing 'separation anxiety' (Johnson, *et al.*, 1941). There is still a tendency to presume that excessive attachment to and reliance on the mother always underlies school refusal (Waller & Eisenberg, 1980; Gittelman-Klein & Klein, 1980), although, in fact, the problem sometimes occurs without obvious fears of leaving home and mother (Hersov 1960a, b; Smith, 1970).

Alternative explanations. There is as yet little evidence that most children with school refusal are suffering from a depressive disorder (Hersov, 1976) even though school refusal may rarely be the first sign of a manic-depressive psychosis (Berg *et al.*, 1974c). Although refusal to go to school can come 'out of the blue', with the emotional disturbance connected with going to school as the only evidence of a neurotic disorder, the majority of cases have additional emotional problems (Warren, 1948; Hersov, 1960a, b; Berg, 1970). An attempt to show that school refusal is due to excessive wilfulness in the child (Berg & Collins, 1974) was unsuccessful. The inability of parents to stand up to a degree of assertiveness that other mothers and fathers can cope with is perhaps a more likely explanation of some cases. Neurotic tendencies would appear to be an important aetiological factor in the development of school refusal.

Staying home excessively, and limited social contacts which are features of school refusal and help to account for it, might be due to living with parents who have similar tendencies. However, it has not in fact been found that families of children with school refusal are any different from others of a similar background in the way in which they live their lives (Berg *et al.*, 1981). The fact that about a third of school refusers have had difficulties for many years (Coolidge *et al.*, 1957; Berg *et al.*, 1969; Baker & Wills, 1978) suggests that a sizeable proportion of cases come from the 5 per cent of children in normal school who are chronically reluctant to attend (Moore, 1966; Mitchell & Shepherd, 1980).

Onset

There is often a gradual development of symptoms over a period of several weeks with manifestations of emotional upset occurring when it is time to go to school. Complete refusal to attend eventually occurs in most instances. However, the problem may sometimes come on quite suddenly (Hersov, 1960a, b).

Precipitating factors

Change of school, especially from the small intimate primary school to the large impersonal secondary school, often appears to bring on school refusal. Absence because of illness or holidays can precipitate onset. Unusually stressful events in school may sometimes precede the development of symptoms (Smith, 1970).

Symptoms

Obvious fear of going to school with reluctance or refusal to go is a common feature. Occasionally misery, tearfulness and apathy are more apparent. Sometimes tempers, irritability, moodiness, and resistiveness predominate. There may be concern about some aspect of school life such as lessons, games, children, or teachers; there may be worries that a parent may become ill or die, or alternatively leave the family whilst they are at school. Quite often there is a marked fear of attending school and of leaving home without any particular concern being identified. Physical symptoms which appear to be manifestations of anxiety are frequent. They include abdominal pain, anorexia, vomiting, headaches, frequency of micturition, and diarrhoea. All these symptoms are clearly related to having to attend school, occurring at a time when the child is expected to go there. School refusal may masquerade as an illness such as 'colitis' or may complicate a genuine physical disease leading to more time off school than is really necessary, a circumstance which has been called the 'masquerade syndrome' (Waller & Eisenberg, 1980).

Obsessional symptoms sometimes occur. Pains, weakness, or attacks suggesting hysterical manifestations are occasionally reported (Warren, 1948; Hersov, 1960b; Smith, 1970). There may be marked depressive features. Overdoses occasionally occur and very rarely, successful suicide has been reported (Reporter, 1979). Whatever the previous degree of dependency on mother, many children with school refusal stay home excessively once it has started. They often express fears of meeting people from their school or of being seen to be out in public when off school. Conduct disorders are rarely associated with school refusal (Hersov, 1960a). It is perhaps a reflection of their lack of antisocial tendencies that school refusers stay at home when not at school and show 'homebound school absence' (Waller & Eisenberg, 1980). They presumably see themselves 'at home ill' rather than 'out truanting'. Some school refusers have no obvious difficulties there when they can be got into school, others appear distressed, and some run home during the day.

Severity

All degrees of severity occur, from transient reluctance to attend school with no previous problem and very little associated disturbance to persistent refusal in a housebound severely neurotic child with a long history of similar difficulties.

Outcome

In primary school children, follow-up studies, after 3, 10, and 20 years respectively, have shown that although return to normal school attendance is usually achieved, persisting neurotic disturbances are found in as many as half the cases, causing marked limitations in adjustment in about a fifth (Rodriguez et al., 1959; Coolidge et al., 1964; Waller & Eisenberg, 1980). Similar investigations of affected teenagers have revealed that although a half to two-thirds return to school (Hersov, 1960a, b), about a third still have severe neurotic symptoms and social impairment, and another third retain less disabling manifestations of emotional disturbance three years later (Berg et al., 1976). Agoraphobia affecting adults may be preceded by school refusal in childhood (Tyrer & Tyrer, 1974, Berg et al., 1974b).

Management

General principles. The restoration of regular attendance is of importance since it relieves the presenting symptom and removes the cause of emotional problems created by being off school. However, much of the later disability which follow-up

studies have shown seems to be a consequence of associated neurotic disturbance. It would thus appear essential to try to reduce this as far as possible, using the appropriate methods which are described elsewhere in this book, if later difficulties are to be averted.

Initial assessment. A full psychiatric history should be taken from child and parents. It is important to establish the nature and extent of the emotional disturbance and any factors in the family, school, or peer group which may be aggravating the condition. An initial contact with the school that the youngster should be attending and any community agency, such as the Educational Welfare Service, involved in dealing with the problem is to be recommended. In addition to getting relevant information, it may be possible to arrange for the relief of some stressful circumstance, by the teachers taking action when there has been intimidation or by excusing the child from some particularly threatening activity, such as games and showers, or from a lesson which the child feels unable to participate in, for the time being.

Early return. There is wide support for the view that energetic efforts should be made to secure an early return to school (Klein, 1945; Eisenberg, 1958, Kennedy, 1965, Leventhal et al., 1967; Lassers et al., 1973). It is usually possible to achieve this without too much trouble in children under the age of 11 (Rodriguez et al., 1959). Young adolescents are more difficult to get back. It may be difficult to convince teachers, educational welfare officers, and even family doctors that the best way of helping is to apparently add to an obviously disturbed child's problems by increasing the pressures to attend school. Yet that is exactly what is usually required. It is helpful if a parent or a professional person concerned with the child can provide an escort every morning to go to school for as long as is necessary. The fact is that children with school refusal do need a lot of practical assistance to get back. In school, some toleration of tearfulness or strangeness may be necessary to settle a child into class.

Medication. A controlled trial of imipramine in the USA has suggested that the initial response to treatment in school refusal is improved by administering this drug in doses of at least 150 mg a day (Gittelman-Klein & Klein, 1980). Unfortunately an equally well-conducted trial in Britain has not confirmed that clomipramine, a closely related antidepressant, is of value in the management of this problem (Berney *et al.*, 1981). It may be that a minor tranquillizer or sedative at night would help to reduce emotional upset and facilitate an early return to school. Many children with school refusal seen by child psychiatrists have received some such medication from their family doctors without obvious benefit.

Co-operation of parents. Parents sometimes find it difficult to accept that school refusal is a psychological problem which is best overcome by facing the aversive situation and not running away from it. They may side with the child in feeling that the main fault lies with the school or alternatively that some physical illness is responsible for the symptoms. Some mothers find it difficult to leave their children when they are obviously upset and in a stressful situation. They may be worried in case the child comes to some harm, for example in trying to escape from a car taking him to school. The establishment of a regular contact between a member of the clinical team, psychiatrist, psychologist or social worker, and the family is important, so that these issues can be discussed and hopefully resolved. It may need to be arranged on a weekly basis or even more frequently in the early stages of treatment. It has been suggested that a short period of respite from pressure to go to school may permit the child and parents to become more relaxed (Cameron, 1978). Very occasionally there is such a lack of parental co-operation in treatment that it is necessary to ask the Educational Welfare Authorities to remind parents of their legal responsibility to ensure their child attends school (Rodriguez *et al.*, 1959).

Change of environment. In itself, transfer to a new school rarely solves the problem of school refusal. However, when it appears that another school would be more appropriate for a variety of reasons such as the attitudes of teachers, educational demands made on the pupils, or their situation, a move can be arranged before return is attempted. When attempts at getting a school refuser back to a normal day school from home fail, attendance at a special educational establishment or a hospital psychiatric day unit, where daily transport is usually provided, may be achieved. When these efforts do not meet with success either, a residential placement should be considered. A hospital psychiatric in-patient unit has the advantage of providing treatment for associated neurotic symptoms, can help the child to mix better with others, become more self-confident, and overcome

phobic inhibitions such as those connected with travelling (Berg & Fielding, 1978). Weekends may be spent at home and after a few months attempts to go back to day school may be started again with more hope of success. Occasionally a boarding school is required.

Specific forms of therapy. Individual psychotherapy with the child has been recommended in the treatment of school phobia. Family therapy has also been put forward as a useful remedy (Lewis, 1980). Unfortunately neither have been shown to be effective by evaluation studies, possibly because of the difficulties in saying exactly what the treatment consists of. The situation is more hopeful in this regard when behavioural treatments are considered, since what is done can be more easily specified. There is now a sizeable literature on the employment of various kinds of behaviour therapy in school refusal. Desensitization in real life seems most promising as far as the child is concerned. Operant techniques can also be employed and may be used to bolster parental decisions and reduce factors which encourage the child to remain at home (Yule *et al.*, 1980). These methods can be nicely combined with the more general clinical approach as described here.

ILLUSTRATIVE CASE HISTORIES

Suzanne, a physically mature 12-year-old, was referred because of a hair-pulling habit. She was the only child of middle-class parents. Her mother suffered from depressive symptoms. It came to light that six months before, on being transferred to secondary school, she had refused to attend, complaining that she was unable to make friends. Her father escorted her to school every morning and was able to get her there using a lot of persuasion. The problem lasted about six weeks and then completely resolved.

David, aged 10, became increasingly tense and worried in the last year of primary school. He complained of weakness in the legs and felt the need to ask his mother to look after herself when he was at school. He had suffered from a severe physical illness at the age of 3 and his mother felt that this had made him closer to her than the two other children. Getting him to school became increasingly difficult and medical advice was sought. It emerged that the class teacher was being unusually severe with the children in his class. The father, who was himself a teacher by profession, was able to convince the form teacher that some of his methods were too harsh. A few weeks later David appeared relaxed and cheerful. He was attending school normally.

Jennifer, aged 14, was one of identical twins. The father had left the mother two years before and was receiving treatment in a psychiatric hospital. The girls had found him a rigid, eccentric, domineering person. The mother was nearly twenty years younger than he was. Over a period of two months Jennifer became increasingly worried about being away from her mother. She complained of abdominal pain and diarrhoea. It was called 'colitis' and treated with medication by a surgeon. Meanwhile she missed a great deal of school and stayed home practically all the time. She was clinging to her mother and could not bear to be out of her sight. She finally refused to go to school altogether. She found mathematics difficult and said the maths teacher's attitude towards her was reminiscent of that of her father. Efforts to get her back failed but with a great deal of effort she was persuaded to attend a hospital unit for adolescents as a day patient. After three months and with the help of staff taking her at first, she returned to another school from home. She was by now in the same class as her sister which had not been the case before and she was nearer her mother's place of work. Six months later she appeared to be completely recovered.

Judith was first seen when she was 12. She had always been reluctant to attend school. Getting her there was proving increasingly difficult as she got older. There were severe emotional difficulties between her parents and she was concerned that her mother would leave. She had always been very anxious, moody, miserable, and tearful. She mixed poorly. A period of out-patient treatment lasting several months produced little improvement and she was admitted to an adolescent psychiatric in-patient unit. Although she relaxed there, made friends, and became obviously less upset, she remained house-bound when she was at home and could not be got back to day school. A place at an independent boarding school for boys and girls was arranged and she stayed there until the age of 16, having out-patient psychiatric treatment all the time. When around the age of 19, she was at home, not working, and appeared to be agoraphobic.

Truancy

Definition
Truancy is characterized by staying away from school without adequate reason, and by the absence of features indicative of school refusal. Although this is how the term truancy is often used, an alternative narrower definition may be preferred, in which case the feature of attempts to conceal absence from parents should be included.

Prevalence
Regular unjustifiable absence from school is a common problem in Britain and affects about one per cent of primary school children and increases in prevalence during the secondary school years, so that as many as 10 per cent can be away at any one time, especially in the last two years of compulsory schooling which ends at age 16 (Fogelman *et al.*, 1980). If the narrower definition of truancy is used a smaller proportion of children will then be identified, but even then it is a common problem.

Aetiology
More boys are affected than girls, but the sex difference in prevalence is not very great. Children from families in the lower social strata of society are predominantly affected. Truancy occurs more frequently in children who are under-achieving educationally. There is good evidence that, at least in boys, truancy is usually one symptom of a conduct disorder, so that antisocial behaviour of all kinds is commonly associated. Affected youngsters tend to come from families characterized by marital discord, criminality, and adverse social circumstances (Hersov, 1960a,b; Farrington, 1980). Causes of truancy are also to be found in the characteristics of the school attended (Reynolds *et al.*, 1980) and the wider social and cultural environment, especially that associated with the peer group (Fogelman *et al.*, 1980).

Clinical features
The severity of truancy varies greatly, between occasional days off school and persistent absence over months or years. The circumstances in which it occurs also vary considerably. In cases covered by the narrower definition, there is often an elaborate pretence by the youngsters to keep their parents from finding out that they are away from school. The day is spent roaming the streets or spending time where there is little likelihood of discovery. When the parents do discover that their children are truanting they are likely to seek help from a medical, social, or educational agency. However, in cases covered by the wider definition parents often appear to have accepted the child's absence and may even seek to justify it (Galloway, 1980). Many truants spend the day at home when they should be at school (Belson, 1975). Antisocial behaviour, such as stealing, destructiveness, and aggressiveness, which is associated with truancy may result in the child being prosecuted for delinquency and brought before the juvenile court. When they do go to school, disruptiveness, fighting, and other antisocial conduct often complicates their educational backwardness. Emotional upset in truancy is usually conspicuous by its absence and in particular, there are no difficulties about leaving the mother at home, travelling about, or venturing into strange situations. However, an excess of other neurotic symptoms has been reported (Tennent, 1969; Farrington, 1980; Berg *et al.*, 1978a). Truancy may involve one child who goes off alone, or may be a group activity.

Outcome
Persistent and severe truancy, broadly defined, is an important predictor of antisocial conduct in early adult life. Follow-up studies in both the United Kingdom (Farrington, 1980) and North America

(Robins, 1978) have indicated this. However, despite the strength of the relationship between truancy and deviant behaviour after leaving school, it must be borne in mind that many truants appear to become well-adjusted adults who manage to avoid getting into trouble with the law.

Management

Truancy is not usually dealt with primarily as a clinical problem. Truants are identified by schools and attempts are then made by teachers and educational welfare officers to improve attendance. Other social workers, perhaps if they are already involved with the child's family, may help. In a small proportion, when unjustifiable absence is severe and persistent, parents and/or child may be taken to court, since truancy is against the law. It has been shown that juvenile court magistrates can help to get truants brought before them under care proceedings back to school, and keep them out of trouble in other ways, by repeatedly adjourning the proceedings and reviewing the case about once a month (Berg *et al.*, 1978b).

However, many children with antisocial problems, including truancy, are referred to child psychiatric clinics (Gath *et al.*, 1972). It is sometimes possible to arrange a placement in a special class which is able to cope with any disruptiveness, can help with educational retardation, and may even provide transport to be sure the child gets there. This may serve as a useful expedient to overcome truancy (Galloway, 1980). Conduct disorders when present also require treatment. Return to normal school may sometimes be achieved by making arrangements with the educational welfare service to escort a child there for a few days to facilitate the process of settling back in. Behavioural psychotherapy has been employed to get truants back to school (Herbert, 1978).

ILLUSTRATIVE CASE HISTORIES

June, a lively 14-year-old-girl, was away from school for over six months without her parents being aware of the fact. She set off every morning and returned home every evening as though she was attending school normally. Surprisingly, it took all this time before an educational welfare officer called and brought the matter into the open. It turned out that she had spent most of the time when not at school in a café frequented by truants. Although somewhat devious and wilful, once she returned to school it was clear that she did not have a conduct disorder. She was popular with other young people and able to cope well with school work. There was a good home life and concerned parents. However, about the time she had begun to truant, her father, who worked as a lorry driver, had spent a lot of time away from home and there had been a temporary marital problem which had caused a family upset. Liaison with school kept her mother informed of any further absence. Support in the form of interviews with a child psychiatrist was arranged on a monthly basis. With one or two lapses June returned to school and continued to attend regularly. A year later she was planning on starting at a college of further education.

Gary, a 12-year-old, was seen after he had been put on an interim care order by a juvenile court for failure to attend school and had consequently spent three weeks in a local authority assessment centre. The father worked as a fitter. The parents were in their forties and provided a good home. Gary, the youngest of four, had been taking time off school for about two years despite efforts on the part of the educational welfare officers and his parents to ensure attendance. He wandered around the neighbourhood, usually on his own, when off school. He had not been in trouble for delinquent behaviour. At home he had severe tempers, was aggressive to his brother and sisters and refused to co-operate with his parents. He was of low average intelligence and backward in his schoolwork. His ability to get on with other children was limited. The school attendance improved after his stay at the assessment centre and he became much more manageable at home. Once school attendance was satisfactory his parents stopped bringing him to see the child psychiatrist.

John was seen while waiting to go to court. He was only 10 years old. Despite his tender age he had already been involved in a large number of criminal offences including burglaries, breaking into cars, and shoplifting. This was nearly always with the same group of children including his younger brother. The latest in a long line of such misdemeanours had resulted in a fire causing hundreds of thousands of pounds worth of damage. School attendance had been very poor for several years. The father was unemployed. He had been in prison a number of times. The mother worked in the evenings as a barmaid. She had also been in jail for theft. The parents had been separated on numerous occasions and their five children had spent some time in care as a consequence. John was chatty and talked about his exploits quite freely. He was of low average intelligence and hardly able to read at all. It was considered that he had a severe conduct disorder. A care order was subsequently made by the juvenile court and he was placed in a childrens' home.

4.2.2
Learning disorders
GERALD F. M. RUSSELL

Definition

The expression 'learning disorders' will be applied to a number of circumscribed handicaps that may be experienced by children during the course of their development and may persist into adulthood. The child's ability to learn specific skills is impaired in comparison with other children similar in age and general intellectual capacity. The word 'learning' is used here in its everyday sense of increasing knowledge or developing new skills as a result of instruction, usually provided at school. Learning disorders comprise mainly difficulty in learning to read, write, or perform arithmetic. There is no implied failure of learning in other senses of the word such as acquiring general knowledge or practical skills, recalling previous experiences, or developing new responses as a result of experiences.

The main varieties of learning disorder will be described in turn:

(a) Difficulty in learning to read (developmental dyslexia), always combined with impaired learning of spelling

(b) Difficulty in learning arithmetic (developmental dysalculia)

Other learning problems will be mentioned as part of these main disabilities.

Learning disorders may be multiple, but even in these instances the child's disabilities fall short of the general lowering of intellectual capacity known as mental handicap which is dicussed in chapter 4.2.3

of this volume. The more specific learning disorders should also be distinguished from an overall reduction in scholastic progress resulting from psychosocial stress.

Developmental dyslexia
Synonym: Specific reading retardation

The terms 'specific reading retardation', 'developmental dyslexia' and 'specific spelling difficulty' have been adopted in the International Classification of Diseases in its ninth revision (WHO, 1978).

History and terminology

In 1896 an English general practitioner, Pringle Morgan (1896), described a 14-year-old boy, named Percy, as an example of *congenital word blindness*:

> His great difficulty has been – and is now – his inability to learn to read . . . He has been at school or under tutors since he was 7 years old, and the greatest efforts have been made to teach him to read, but in spite of this laborious and persistent training, he can only with difficulty spell out words of one syllable . . . The schoolmaster who has taught him for some years says that he would be the smartest lad in the school if the instruction were entirely oral.

Pringle Morgan later disclosed that his choice of the name 'word-blindness' was the result of reading an article on 'word-blindness and visual memory' in the *Lancet* in 1895 by James Hinshelwood (1895), a Glaswegian eye surgeon. He had described a 58-year-old schoolmaster who had suddenly lost his ability to read, presumably as a result of a cerebrovascular accident. His central visual acuity was unimpaired but he had developed a right lateral homonymous hemianopia. Hinshelwood deduced that loss of reading could result from a lesion of the 'visual word centre' in the left angular gyrus or its connections with both occipital lobes. He also concluded that the loss of reading was due to an impaired visual memory and a 'blindness' for words. Pringle Morgan presumed that his patient Percy's problem was similar, and as it had been present from an early age he named it congenital word blindness. We can see, therefore, why this first description of a learning disorder of reading favoured an explanation which relied on the neurological substrate of language. Already the term dyslexia had been introduced in Germany, meaning a partial impairment of reading. Hinshelwood (1917) himself proposed that milder cases of reading disorder in children should be called examples of 'congenital dyslexia'. In 1926, Samuel Orton, an American neurologist, proposed that the term strephosymbolia ('twisted symbols') was more appropriate than 'congenital word-blindness'. His reason was that these children tended to muddle the order of the letters that were recalled during attempts to read and spell (Orton, 1937). He is best remembered for his view that the underlying cause of the confusion in recognition and recall of words was an interference between oppositely-oriented memory traces in the dominant and non-dominant cerebral hemispheres. He also believed that this interference was the likely reason for the reversal of letters often noted in the reading and writing of these children. Today, the name of strephosymbolia has not survived, but Orton's ideas are still with us. In Britain, Critchley (1964) made a valuable contribution in identifying the disorder he named 'developmental dyslexia' and providing a detailed account of its clinical features.

Prevalence rates

There is considerable variation (1 per cent to 25 per cent) in the frequency of reading disorders reported in different countries (Klasen, 1972). This is partly due to differences in the expected standards of reading and attainment, but is mainly the result of failure to define carefully the type of reading disorder being considered. Rutter and Yule (1975) overcame these objections by applying the epidemiological method to defined populations of school children. They distinguished between reading difficulties which could be accounted for by the child's overall reduction in intellectual ability and those which were not so explained. By means of a multiple regression analysis, they derived the reading level which was to be expected from the child's age and intelligence level. If the child's actual reading age fell markedly below that predicted (for example, by 28 months or more), he was considered to fall within the category of specific reading retardation. It was found that the prevalence rates for this category ranged from 3.7 per cent among 9- and 10-year-old children in a rural community (the Isle of Wight), to 6 per cent among 10-year-old children in London. These results were significantly higher than would be expected if reading ability were merely distributed along a normal distribution curve. The concept of specific reading retardation is closely related to that of developmental dyslexia, as defined below (p. 169), and the terms will

be considered as interchangeable throughout this account.

Causes of dyslexia

A delay in learning to read may be due to any of a variety of obvious causes such as a general low intelligence, a brain injury, or defects of vision or hearing, including high-frequency deafness. Deleterious factors within the family may include a lack of the necessary emotional or physical support, insufficient encouragement to learn from lessons at school, or a difference between the languages spoken at home and taught in school. Most obvious of all is a failure to read because the child has missed a great deal of schooling as a result of illness, frequent moves of the family, school refusal, or truancy.

The diagnosis of developmental dyslexia is, however, only made in children in whom the more obvious causes do not apply, or are insufficient to account for the learning disorder. The cause of the dyslexia is thus essentially unknown apart from a partial role of heredity for which there is much evidence. This evidence is derived mainly from family studies but also from twin studies. Hallgren (1950) found that among the first-degree relatives of 116 dyslexic children, 41 per cent had a reading disorder. Of the children 80 per cent had one parent with dyslexia, 3 per cent had both parents dyslexic and only 17 per cent had unaffected parents. In a smaller but more thorough study, Finucci and co-workers (1976) found that 45 per cent of first-degree relatives had a reading disability. As in Hallgren's study, only a small and similar proportion of the children had neither parent affected (3 out of 16). In a review of twin studies, 17 pairs of monozygotic twins were all concordant for reading disability, whereas only 12 out of 34 pairs of dizygotic twins were concordant (Zerbin-Rudin, 1967). A further point of interest from epidemiological and genetic studies is the much higher frequency of reading disability among males than females (usually 3:1). In spite of compelling evidence that genetic factors predispose to dyslexia, the precise mechanism of the genetic effects remains in doubt. Hallgren favoured a single autosomal dominant gene, whereas Finucci and co-workers thought that there was equal support for a polygenic and a dominant mode of transmission. The predominance of dyslexic males is not considered to be due to a simple sex-linked inheritance. Hypotheses include a sex-controlled inheritance or non-genetic factors (Hallgren), a lower threshold for expression in males of a polygenic inheritance or a sex-modified expression of a single genetic mutant (Finucci *et al.*, 1976).

Not only are we largely ignorant of the basic causes of dyslexia but there is even uncertainty about the nature of the cognitive deficits that prevent learning to read with normal ease. We have seen that the early investigators thought they knew the nature of the underlying defects, and postulated faulty visual perception and memory (Hinshelwood, 1917), or confusion between the memory traces from the two cerebral hemispheres (Orton). In fact, these earlier views have become discredited (Vellutino, 1979).

Recent research by educational psychologists and linguists has stressed that the reading process is dependent on the ability to analyse the sound structure of spoken words into their component units (phonemes), and to blend them in creating the sounds of syllables as the basic units of reading (Elkonin, 1963, 1973; Mattingly, 1972; Shankweiler & Liberman, 1976). The historical analysis of the development of writing over the course of some 3500 years supports this view (Russell, 1982a). It reveals that scripts gradually evolved from pictograms to hieroglyphs or cuneiform symbols and eventually became alphabets. The progressive development toward a perfected script in general depended on its becoming increasingly phonetic. This process is likely to have been adaptive to human cognitive and linguistic abilities and thus would facilitate the encoding of spoken language on to the written cypher. Universal literacy became attainable once writing had evolved into a highly phonetic script. This same process may, however, have been maladaptive for a minority of would-be readers. These are the children who do not have ready access to the benefits of highly phonetic writing because they lack the specific cognitive and linguistic skills needed to process spoken sounds for purposes of reading and writing. Experimental studies of children and young adults with reading disorders have supported a general defect in verbal processing (Bradley & Bryant, 1978; Russell, 1982b), and impairment of phoneme segmentation (Liberman *et al.*, 1974), or difficulty in transposing spoken and written units of language ('grapheme and phoneme' conversion) (Snowling, 1980).

Clinical features

The commonest mode of presentation is for the child to be found lagging behind his peers in learning to read at school. The age at which this discovery is made ranges from 6 to 9, varying with the severity of the disorder, and especially with the perceptiveness of the parents and teachers. An earlier age of detection is more likely if the parents have been alerted by a prior delay in speech. For example, speech may have remained infantile with defects of articulation until the age of 5 or 6. Problems in learning to spell and write are likely to be noticed at the same time as the reading disability, or soon after. In children who have mixed learning disorders, difficulties with calculation are usually noticed at a later age, commonly 7 to 10.

CLINICAL CASE HISTORY

Robin's parents first sought help when he was aged 8: learning to read and spell had been painfully slow. His mother recalled that when Robin was 3½ his grandmother was often annoyed by her inability to understand his speech which was poorly pronounced. By the time he started school at 5, however, this had improved so much that it elicited no special comment from his teachers. From the age of 9 considerable efforts were made to help Robin with reading at his own school and at the Word-Blind Centre in London. The teachers reported that he tended to be disobedient and aggressive with other children. This disturbed behaviour was not noticed at home, but there he was liable to cry easily and become frustrated with his reading. There had been other learning problems: for long he had been unable to tie his shoelaces and he could not tell the time till he was 10½. At 12½ he was referred to the Royal Free Hospital because of generally slow progress and newly-observed difficulties in learning arithmetic: he was unable to count the change given for his purchases in shops. Robin was found to be a friendly and relaxed boy. He read in a slow and halting manner making several mistakes, for example reading 'was' instead of 'as', and 'excellent' instead of 'exciting'. Examples of his spelling were *hows* for 'house'; *larph* for 'laugh' and *hospel* for 'hospital'. There were only minor errors of speech: for example, the word 'hospital' was first pronounced 'hostipal' and then spontaneously corrected. He could perform simple addition and subtraction but this was slow, as he had to count on his fingers. The only multiplication table he knew was the two-times table. He could tell his right hand from his left, but muddled the points of the compass.

Further enquiry revealed that the father was a poor speller and had been a 'late developer'; the mother also found spelling difficult. Testing on the Wechsler Intelligence Test for Children gave a Verbal IQ of 122 and a Performance IQ of 117. The results of serial measures of reading age (Schonell) and spelling age (Schonell Graded Word Spelling Test) were as follows, including a later result:

Actual age	Reading age	Spelling age
9	7.4	6.5
12½	8.6	7.6
19½	14.1	10.7

Robin passed only two 0 level examinations when aged 15½. He left school but after an interval he returned to studying, this time at a college of further education. By the age of 19 he had passed 6 additional 0 level examinations but had again failed in English language. His arithmetic had improved markedly and he was preparing himself for a career in engineering, having enrolled at a technical college. In his view he had mastered the reading problem but his spelling was still 'hopeless'.

This case history illustrates the principal clinical features of dyslexia. The difficulty in learning to read is sustained over several years, and is not merely an initial delay, soon to be overcome. Indeed, there may be an increasing gap between the reading level achieved by the dyslexic child and that of his peers, especially if he has received no remedial teaching. As a result, he is unable to derive much pleasure from books for long, or only from those that are at a very simple level or largely illustrated. In later years the disadvantage of poor reading takes a further toll, because learning of all school subjects becomes increasingly dependent on the written word. The child's laborious difficulties with English are often perplexing to parents and teachers, for they are manifestly not due to a low intelligence or any other obvious explanation. The discrepancy is most evident in the intelligent child whose reading ability may be well below that of a less intelligent peer. Dyslexia can, however, be recognized in the child whose intelligence is below average, for his reading will be very low, below that computed after allowing for his low IQ.

The dyslexic child is prone to some common reading errors. He may recognize the first letter or two of a word and guess incorrectly the remainder (beagle instead of beguile, champagne instead of campaign); or he may muddle the order of the letters (for example, pots for tops). Attempts at phonetic reading are often laboured: a polysyllabic word may be recognized only after the teacher has helped to break it up into its component syllables by uncovering one syllable at a time.

The dyslexic child's writing and spelling are always worse even than his reading. Some children will learn to print letters neatly, only to highlight the gross spelling errors. Often the script is quite incomprehensible, even to the child himself. He has special difficulty in distinguishing the spelling of homophones (for example, right, write, rite, wright); or in writing words with phonetic ambiguities (for example, laugh, cough, colonel, pneumonia). Polysyllabic words are shortened, whole syllables or essential vowels being omitted. Letter reversals (b for d, p for q, b for p) are common and so are letter transposi-

tions (saw for was). Inevitably, written schoolwork fails to do justice to the child's factual knowledge of a subject and his slowness in writing is a further disadvantage.

Additional problems are often associated with dyslexia. There may have been an earlier delay in the development of speech which may have remained infantile in form for several years, with the persistence of baby-talk including made-up words. Words are mispronounced, sounds such as f, s, and th being particularly difficult. The sequence of consonants may be altered (for example, hostipal for hospital). Learning to tell the time is often delayed. Most constantly found are signs of a confusion between the right and left sides of the child's own body and of outer space. He will thus hesitate when asked to raise his left hand, or point to the right hand of the examiner facing him. Often he can only guess when asked to indicate the east and west points of the compass. This spatial confusion may persist into adult life.

A learning disorder in arithmetic is also present in a much higher proportion of dyslexic children than was originally thought. The clinical features of dyscalculia will be described below, but it should be mentioned now that it is often associated with visuo-spatial and constructional disturbances. For example, the child may be unable to draw a clock face with the hands set at a specified time; or he may find it difficult to copy a three-dimensional drawing of a cube, or arrange matchsticks in the shape of a star.

Not surprisingly the dyslexic child often reacts to his difficulties at school by becoming emotionally disturbed and sensitive about his failures. He feels envious about a younger sibling who overtakes him in reading. He may reveal this in aggressive acts or outbursts of temper. More frankly antisocial forms of behaviour may extend beyond the home into the school. Frequent antisocial activity has been reported among children with reading disability (Rutter et al., 1967).

Diagnostic criteria of dyslexia

It is sometimes said, rather unfairly, that there is 'no precise operational definition' for developmental dyslexia (*Bullock Report*, 1975). If this judgement were applied to other disorders described in this *Handbook*, few diagnostic categories indeed would survive. One reason for quibbling about the recognition of dyslexia may be the undoubted difficulty of reaching a diagnosis when a young child first presents, before there has been time to establish that he is handicapped by a persistent learning disorder. To establish this, it is desirable to make serial observations, proving that specific learning remains impaired over a long period. Otherwise, it is necessary to make 'cross-sectional' observations on the child and reach a conclusion from discrepancies between his attainments in different spheres. Thus we are dependent on a clinical judgement, but one which is nevertheless entirely valid. The following diagnostic criteria are presented, depending on circumstances.

(1) If a longitudinal study is possible, serial observations reveal that

(i) the child persistently lags behind his peers in learning to read. Thus, measures of reading age remain significantly below the chronological age. This discrepancy may be modest at a younger age (for example, below the age of 9 it may not be more than 18 months) but tends to increase later (to 2 years or more).

(ii) the learning disorder is relatively selective for reading and spelling, but it may be multiple and include difficulties in learning arithmetic; overall ability remains unimpaired.

(2) If serial observations are not yet available, the criteria listed below may be the only ones that can be met at the initial assessment:

(i) the child's reading attainment falls below the level which would be expected from his age and intelligence level. This can be computed by means of the statistical technique of regression analysis (Yule, 1967). Thus the measured reading age will fall below the predicted reading age by 18 months or more.

(ii) There is always an impairment of spelling ability exceeding the disability in reading. Thus spelling age is even lower than reading age.

(iii) There is no evident basis for difficulties in learning, such as deafness, blindness, cerebral injury, social deprivation, emotional disturbance, poor educational opportunity, or mental handicap.

(3) Although not essential diagnositc criteria, the following may support the diagnosis when present:

(i) The detection of additional disorders of learning such as the inability to distinguish between right and left, or an arithmetical disorder (together with a defective performance of visuo-spatial and constructional tasks).

(ii) A history of developmental delays especially retarded speech.

(iii) A positive family history of learning disorders (reading, spelling or arithmetic) in first-degree relatives.

Developmental dyscalculia

Synonym

The terms 'specific arithmetical retardation' and 'dyscalculia' have been adopted in the ninth revision of the International Classification of Diseases (WHO, 1978).

Diagnostic criteria

Criteria may be put forward for the diagnosis of developmental dyscalculia similar to those adopted for developmental dyslexia.

(1) There will be evidence of a persistent difficulty in learning arithmetical skills, out of keeping with the child's age and level of intelligence, not accounted for by obvious cerebral disease, and relatively resistant to standard methods of teaching.

(2) The learning disorder is relatively selective, although it may, in some children, coexist with dyslexia.

(3) When the child is first seen without the benefit of previous assessments, the clinician has to rely on establishing a discrepancy between the child's actual level of arithmetical ability on the one hand and that to be expected from his age and IQ on the other. There may also be evidence of poor performance with visuo-spatial and constructional tasks, or a poor score on tests of rote memory.

History

The term 'acalculia' was proposed by Henschen (1919) to describe a 'disturbance of calculation produced by a focal lesion of the brain'. In 1924 Gerstmann described the syndrome which was to be named after him: a set of four disturbances – acalculia, right-left confusion, finger agnosia and agraphia – associated with one another and resulting from disease of the dominant parietal lobe. Guttmann in 1937 described children whose ability to learn how to calculate was impaired. He borrowed Henschen's term 'acalculia' and pointed out their similarity to children with 'congenital reading disability'.

Causes of developmental dyscalculia

Convenience is the main reason for writing a separate section on developmental dyscalculia, but it should be questioned whether it is distinct from developmental dyslexia. Clinical experience teaches that the two learning disorders frequently coexist in the same child although their severity may differ. Occasionally a subject will complain of a significant arithmetical disability but without any trace of developmental dyslexia or even minor spelling problems. Moreover, there is evidence that the principal cognitive deficits underlying the reduced calculating ability differ from those leading to a reading disorder. In particular, a defect of rote memory for meaningless material is closely associated with the dyscalculic subjects' inability to memorize multiplication tables (Slade & Russell, 1971), whereas the dyslexic's impaired reading depends probably on defective processing of spoken sounds. Landsdown (1978) has suggested that several cognitive factors contribute to impaired mathematical performance, including poor spatial ability. He points out that no study so far has systematically identified or described children with specific arithmetical difficulties. Our knowledge regarding the frequency of developmental dyscalculia as defined earlier is also very limited. There are no genetic studies comparable to those on developmental dyslexia.

Clinical features

A child between the ages of 7 and 10 may be noted to be experiencing undue difficulty in learning arithmetic, in comparison with his ease of learning other school subjects, and in spite of a normal intelligence. Such a problem is usually neglected, however, unless it is associated with a reading and spelling disorder, when concern and remedial help are usually directed at the latter. Thus many dyscalculic subjects present themselves only in adulthood.

CLINICAL CASE HISTORY

A 42-year-old lady came forward in response to a letter in the *Sunday Times* asking for dyscalculic subjects to volunteer for testing. She recalled that her early schooldays had been trouble-free, and she proved to be a quick reader and speller. From the age of 7, however, she was caned by unsympathetic teachers for not knowing her sums. At the age of 12 she felt humiliated when she was relegated for a day to a junior class to learn her 7-times table. She found that she could retain the table for only one or two hours and then forgot it. She left school at the first opportunity when aged 14 to take up factory work. She was rejected by nursing schools because of her poor arithmetic. She eventually found congenial work as a telephonist, but she had to write down telephone numbers because she could not remember them. She gradually acquired greater responsibility and became a trainer of telephonists. Full IQ on the WAIS was 109. Reading and spelling were of a high standard. She performed simple additions on her fingers. She only knew the 2, 3, 5 and 9 times tables, and for other multiplications added the multiplicand the requisite number of times.

A dyscalculic child will encounter difficulties in counting money during shopping transactions, but will eventually learn to give the exact money needed to pay for a single purchase. His main problems arise at school when attempting to learn arithmetic. He finds the four basic steps extremely difficult, with subtraction harder than addition, and multiplication and division hardest of all. He devises methods to compensate for his difficulties, by breaking down arithmetical problems into simpler stages or using a dotting system. For example, he may multiply 6×9 by producing 6 sets of 9 dots on paper and laboriously counting their total number.

The most characteristic feature is a failure to memorize multiplication tables beyond the 3-times table (Slade & Russell, 1971). This failure is paralleled by a poor performance on tests of rote memory, for example the 'letter-tables' test designed by Slade and Russell (1971). Faults of misalignment in written work are also common, so that long multiplication and division are exercises doomed to failure. Reversals of numbers may also occur (31 written for 13). With persistence some of the basic steps can eventually be learned, but there is frequently an obstinate failure to master the principles of the decimal system (for example, one-hundredth is the same as 0.01) or even simple fractions.

Associated with dyscalculia is often a poor performance on visuo-spatial and constructional tasks, for example, drawing a clock-face with the hands set at a given time, copying a three-dimensional drawing of a cube (see Figure 4.2.2.1), or assembling 8 matchsticks in the shape of a four-pointed star.

Management of learning disorders with emphasis on dyslexia

Principles

The dyslexic child and his family require a skilful and attentive form of general management, dependent mainly on appropriate remedial teaching. Even though there is no specific approach to treatment or teaching, the results of a general programme of management are usually gratifying. An early diagnosis and a precise assessment are essential if the dyslexic child is to be saved from complicating emotional disturbances, if the parents are to be spared the fear that their child might be mentally defective, and if the optimum results are to be obtained from remedial teaching. Teachers and educational authorities play a central part in the remedial programme but the general practitioner, psychiatrist, and clinical psychologist also have important contributions to make. The treatment and progress of the child require to be monitored over the course of several years and it is therefore essential that this team-work should be efficiently established and maintained throughout. The advice contained in this section is addressed to the clinician, so as to guide him in his approach to the child, his family, and his teachers.

The dyslexic child and his family

It will be necessary to explain to the child's parents that his reading difficulties are likely to engender distress and frustration which may give rise to emotional disturbances or outbursts of aggressive behaviour. They should be encouraged to show understanding and encouragement, without harbouring unreasonable expectations for his progress at school. The dyslexic child requires particular sympathy and affection in the event of a younger sibling progressing effortlessly with his own reading and thus overtaking his older brother.

With parents who set little store on scholastic achievement, there is a risk that the child's problems may go unnoticed and neglected. In their case it may be necessary to assume a great deal of responsibility in providing the optimum education and an environment best suited for learning. It may therefore be appropriate to recommend a suitable boarding-school, with teachers experienced in the problems of reading disorders. Often, however, the converse is the case and the parents react with undue anxiety to their child's slow progress with reading. This may be compounded with inappropriate feelings of self-

Fig. 4.2.2.1. Performance on visuo-spatial and constructional tasks in a 9½-year-old dyslexic boy.

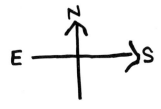

Points of the compass

Two attempts to place the hands of the clock at 9.45.

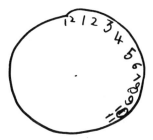

First attempt

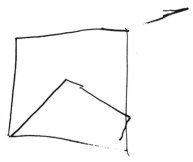

Copy of cube.
Patient said: "It's a bit wonky."

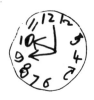

Second attempt

blame if there is a family history of reading disorders. These emotions may be projected on to the educational authorities and the parents may make unrealistic demands on them and the teaching staff. They may even proceed to litigation with the object of securing state support for the education of their child at an expensive private school. We have seen that it may indeed be appropriate to send a dyslexic child to a suitable boarding school, but the advantages and disadvantages for the individual child must be carefully weighed up. It is obviously desirable that parents and teachers should avoid being at loggerheads with each other and that a mutual understanding of each other's problems should be established. The clinician can play a useful role in acting as a diplomatic mediator. It is, moreover, appropriate to explore the possibility of the child's mother, or father, supplementing the teaching at school by listening to the child read at home and by assisting him with written homework. Some of the best remedial teaching can thus be provided by solicitous parents, the criteria being patience and sympathy rather than any specific training in teaching. An important aim is to counter the child's prevalent expectation that his efforts will lead to failure. Admittedly it is only a minority of parents who have the emotional strength to undertake what may be an arduous task. It is nevertheless useful to put this suggestion to one of the parents, for it may serve the purpose of demonstrating that the teacher's task is not an easy one, and he too deserves his share of understanding.

The school and educational authorities

A minority of teachers are unduly suspicious about the concept of dyslexia. They misinterpret the theoretical discussions about the nature of dyslexia into sweeping generalizations. For example, the following utterance has been cited as coming from an educator: 'dyslexia is only found in middle-class areas where parents won't admit their child is too dim to learn to read' (Finlayson, 1973). Thus it is important to be aware of the educational controversies surrounding learning disorders. The clinician must show tact towards the dyslexic child's teachers, and recognize that the main burden of treatment has to be borne by them, often for several years. It is best therefore when reporting the diagnostic findings to the school to state plainly the nature of the child's learning difficulties and to give the results of psychological testing. If the teachers can be convinced that the child's level of reading is below that to be expected

from his level of intelligence, they will more readily appreciate the need for additional teaching, notwithstanding shortages of staff and genuine difficulties. Criticism of the school or the teachers is seldom appropriate. If they are voiced by the parents, they should be interpreted as expressions of anxiety and transmitted in that form rather than as criticism.

It has been indicated that we lack specific methods for the teaching of dyslexic children. Nevertheless, there is a growing body of opinion that the old-fashioned method of phonic teaching is more likely to help the disabled reader than the look-and-say method. Chall (1967) explains that the child beginning to read requires a 'code-emphasis method', one that emphasizes learning of the printed code for the spoken language. Williams (1980) goes further in recommending an instructional programme with explicit training in phoneme analysis and blending, and letter-sound decoding. She stresses that this instruction should be contained within a comprehensive reading programme. The dyslexic child remains at the beginner's stage of reading for longer than the normal child and needs a greater and more persistent effort on the part of his teachers. The experienced teacher may, by trial and error, discover which approach best suits the individual child. Combining illustrations with the printed word serves the dual purpose of resorting to multiple channels for learning and maintaining the child's attention. Individual teaching greatly facilitates the process of advancing at the child's own pace and providing him with the reward of encouragement each time he is successful.

Even less is known about specific methods of improving the dyscalculic child's arithmetical weakness. The same general principles apply – sympathy, individual attention, and encouragement by praise for success. Learning multiplication tables is such a formidable hurdle, and yet is so basic to many calculations, that it is advisable to provide the child with a chart of the ×2 to ×10 tables so that he can at least make some progress with other arithmetical problems. By dint of practice, some of the tables will eventually be retained. This is preferable to a total reliance on a calculator, although this instrument will be useful later on as a means of bypassing residual arithmetical deficits.

In Britain remedial facilities for dyslexic children still fall short of ideal, but considerable advances have been made over the past 15 years. The approach of the Department of Education and Science is outlined in a Report of the Advisory Committee on Handicapped Children (*Children with Specific Reading Difficulties*, 1972). They recommend that remedial teaching should be tailor-made to the individual child. Skilled help should be based on a warm and encouraging approach. Most children with reading difficulties are best taught in their regular primary and secondary schools, otherwise they may miss learning from the general curriculum. Most schools nowadays endeavour to provide this remedial help, if not on a one-to-one basis, then at least for a small group of children taught by a teacher experienced in reading disorders. Some areas have remedial education centres where children attend, preferably on a part-time basis: others employ peripatetic teachers who give additional reading lessons in the child's own home. It is important to extend the additional teaching during secondary education and beyond, for the reading disability may persist, and help with spelling is always required. Unreasonable scholastic stresses should be avoided, and it is best to forego the learning of foreign languages. To facilitate general learning, emphasis is given on oral methods of teaching and on educational programmes on television. Colleges of further education are particularly helpful in providing an adolescent with an opportunity to extend his education and so compensate for earlier difficulties due to delayed reading.

It is often at the late adolescent stage that the former dyslexic can approach examinations at an appropriate level, including 0 level and even A level examinations. He can now read his textbooks with sufficient understanding and make more rapid progress. The clinician should offer his help in certifying to the examining bodies that the candidate is or was dyslexic, for they are usually ready to make appropriate concessions, with an extension of the time period given for written answers to questions, and allowances for spelling errors. Examining bodies understandably cannot make these concessions for tests in English language, and it is in this subject that a dyslexic adolescent has often the greatest difficulty in passing the 0 level examination. Dyslexia may persist into adulthood and is an important cause of adult illiteracy in countries where educational opportunities for normal children are good. The recent campaign for adult literacy has achieved significant success in encouraging adults to enrol with local authorities where voluntary tutors come forward to provide aid with reading. The BBC has also broadcast special programmes. A list of voluntary organizations prepared to provide help is included in the publication, *Adult Literacy* (1976).

Follow-up and prognosis

The poor prognosis of children with specific reading retardation who receive no remedial teaching has been stressed by Rutter and co-workers (1970). There is growing evidence, however, that with skilled and persistent remedial teaching a much higher level of reading attainment can be achieved. Most dyslexics nevertheless continue to have serious difficulties with spelling. Defects of calculation often persist into adult life. It is likely that the limits of therapeutic success will be pushed further with a better understanding of the cognitive deficits underlying the learning disorders and a wider availability of remedial teaching.

4.2.3
Psychiatric, social, and educational aspects of mental retardation in childhood

ANN GATH

Definition

Mental retardation implies a failure in cognitive functioning with problems in coping with everyday life. The most useful working definition is that in official use by the American Association for Mental Deficiency (AAMD) devised by Heber (1961) in which mental retardation is defined as 'subaverage general intellectual functioning which originated during the development period and is associated with impairment in adaptive behaviour'. This definition immediately calls for two further definitions. In general, subaverage or below average intelligence is commonly defined as an intelligence quotient, as measured on intelligence tests, of *below* 70. This is more than two standard deviations below the mean. However, there are many problems in testing intelligence of which racial, cultural, and sex differences in performance on the tests are the most common. Intelligence tests measure the ability of children to do well at school, bear close correlation to success in exams, but are much less accurate at predicting ability to cope in the ordinary working world. The cultural and racial problems in testing have given rise to the situation in which disproportionate numbers of immigrant children may be labelled as retarded.

The American definition of retardation includes the concept of adaptive behaviour as well as that of intelligence as measured on intelligence tests. Adaptive behaviour is defined as standards of personal independence and social responsibility expected in a person's age and cultural group. This goes some way to rectify the problems that arise through making a diagnosis of retardation from intelligence tests alone. However, measures of adaptive behaviour, particularly the Adaptive Behaviour Scale devised by the American Association for Mental Deficiency (Lambert *et al.*, 1974) are still not standardized for countries other than the United States and there is still inadequate information on their use with children brought up in their own homes rather than in institutions. However, despite these difficulties the American definition of mental retardation is a step ahead of the British definition of 'severe subnormality' which is based on the Mental Health Act, 1959, and is 'a state of arrested or incomplete development of mind which includes subnormality of intelligence and is of such a nature and degree that the patient is incapable of leading an independent life or of guarding himself against serious exploitation, or will be incapable when of an age to do so'. The last part of this is particularly difficult to apply in childhood. Overall, somewhere between two and three per cent of all children fall into the group with IQs, as measured on tests, of below 70. This comparatively large group can be divided into two subgroups which overlap but do have some important distinctions. The two groups, well defined and described by Edgerton (1979), are clinical retardation and socio-cultural retardation.

Types of mental retardation

Clinical retardation can usually be attributed to some medical cause. The intelligence quotient is usually less than 50 but there are many exceptions to this. The diagnosis can be made early, largely because there are accompanying organic deficits which may be neurological, metabolic, or physiological. The cause of the retardation is thus often determined. In parents of children with clinical retardation there is no social class bias. The group is made up of 20 to 25 per cent of all retarded children and the majority of children in ESN(S) – Educationally Sub Normal (Severe) – schools in Great Britain and TMR (Trainable Mentally Retarded) classes in the United States. Examples of clinical retardation include Down's syndrome (mongolism, trisomy 21) which is the most common single cause of clinical retardation. There are other less common chromosomal abnormalities. Amongst the clinically retarded are also the very large number of genetic disorders either inherited as autosomal recessives or, less frequently, as sex-linked disorders. Many of these are inborn errors of metabolism due to enzyme failure resulting from the genetic defect.

Their course and prognosis varies. Some can be diagnosed early, such as in phenylketonuria, the child put on the appropriate diet, and mental retardation prevented. In other cases retardation is noted and the offending metabolite identified by urine chromatography and other techniques but little can be done to ameliorate the disorder. In the conditions due to autosomal recessives there may be a history of consanguinity, such as first cousin marriage, which greatly increases the chance of an autosomal recessive making its appearance. First-cousin marriages are more likely to occur amongst culturally deprived and isolated people. Other causes of retardation are due to infection *in utero* such as toxoplasmosis; placental insufficiency producing poor nutrition of the foetus resulting from heavy smoking by the mother, toxaemia; birth injury and injury during early infancy, insults to the brain from trauma, including child abuse; infection, particularly meningitis, and encephalitis; seizures producing prolonged anoxia; and, extreme cases of malnutrition.

Social cultural retardaton is usually mild, the intelligence quotient being between 55 and 69. The diagnosis is often not made before school entry, and after the youngsters concerned have left school they may never again come to the notice of medical, social, or educational authorities. It has been said that the diagnosis of socio-cultural retardation is a result of the school system. This point of view is arguable. In socio-cultural retardation, physical handicaps are rare and most medical investigations are negative. However, in contrast to clinical retardation the parents are economically, socially, and educationally disadvantaged to a much greater degree. Socio-cultural retardation comprises most of children attending the Educationally Subnormal (Moderate) (ESN(M)) schools in the UK, or the EMR (Educable Mentally Retarded) classes in the United States.

There is however, considerable overlap between the two groups. Poor antenatal care is more likely to produce complications of pregnancy and birth. Mothers who are socially or economically disadvantaged are less likely to make good use of even the best antenatal care and in areas of social deprivation there are often poor medical facilities. There are areas in the United States, usually isolated in mountainous regions, where there are small pockets of population

with little contact with the outside world. In a relatively small country like the UK there are also areas where people are suspicious of outsiders, commonly marry blood relatives, have a high incidence of inherited disease and a high proportion of children requiring special education.

There is also a considerable overlap in IQ measures. Many children with clinical retardation showing obvious signs of a medical syndrome have IQs above 50. In a group of Down's syndrome children followed from birth, two children had IQs of above 75, and a significant proportion of over 50. Some educational authorities make it a policy not to have children with Down's syndrome or other obvious clinical retardation in the ESN(M) schools. This is clearly unjust, as the children, on testing, are capable of competing on equal terms with children in ESN(M) schools, if not in some ordinary primary reception classes. However, it is common to find considerable hostility expressed by the parents of the children with socio-cultural retardation towards the children with obvious clinical syndromes. Some parents of the clinically retarded are concerned about their children mixing with the socially deprived but this concern is less frequently voiced.

Parents learn that their child is retarded early on when there are obvious abnormal physical signs. Most parents of children with socio-cultural retardation do not know or do not appreciate the child's problems in learning until the child fails to cope with ordinary school life.

Impact on the parents of the news of retardation

A young child may be diagnosed as mentally retarded early in life. There are two ways in which the problem comes to light before development has proceeded far. Either there is recognition of a syndrome with a high likelihood of mental retardation or there are delayed milestones. In some cases, particularly when the milestones are delayed but there is no clear medical diagnosis, the paediatricians may fear making a wrong diagnosis and may delay until they are absolutely sure. The delay can perhaps mean that there is more time for normal child and family relationships to develop. However, there is certainly much more doubt and anxiety and the parents may resort to 'shopping around' to look for further medical opinions. However, if the delay is deliberate the parents feel cheated and lose trust, often never to regain it in any other doctor. In every parent group and in many an individual consultation, parents describe how they were told the news. Time has often distorted their recollection of the original happening. However, it is clear from various studies that have been made (Carr, 1970) that, on the whole, parents are most satisfied if told as soon as the paediatrician or obstetrician has any doubt about the child. There is no evidence to support the notion that mother and child must be allowed to 'bond' before the child's obvious abnormality is discussed with the parents. Many maladaptive responses lasting throughout the child's life date from the way the breaking of the news of the handicap has been handled. Parents are different and have different responses to bad news of this sort.

Effects on parents having a mentally retarded child may be summed up as first *grief* (Drotar *et al.*, 1975) and second, *a burden of care* (Tizard & Grad, 1961). Certainly the burden of care has been made significantly less heavy by the improvement in services over the past 10 years. This improvement was largely the result of parental demand and parental pressure groups. Just, imaginative, and sufficient provision of services, such as appropriate schooling, relief care, informed advice on practical problems, and the provision of incontinence aids and special push-chairs, greatly decrease the burden on parents, and enable children to live in the community.

Grief at the birth of a child who is unable to match the ordinary everyday dreams that every parent has about an expected child is universal. Many parents still show some evidence of this grief eight or even twenty years after the birth of the child. As in grief following other losses, such as death of a child or spouse, there are several stages. First is the stage of shock in which parents describe themselves as being numbed and unable to comprehend what is happening to them. It is important for those explaining the problems to parents to realize that this stage takes place and that what they said to the parents at this time may not be remembered clearly. The second stage is denial and a parent may feel that the doctor was mistaken, the child only looks odd because he looks like an unprepossessing relative, or that somehow a cure will be found, or the child will grow out of it. It is perhaps particularly common for the grandparents to become fixed in the stage of denial. The next stage is that of sadness and anger, which is perhaps the most noticeable of the stages. The anger may well be directed to the person who told the parents of the condition giving rise to mental retarda-

tion. Here the psychiatrist can be of considerable help to his paediatric colleagues to explain projection of hostile feelings and to support, particularly those junior doctors who may have to cope with emotionally fraught situations alone. Towards the end are the two more positive stages, one of adaptation in which the reality is faced and finally that of reorganization which may very well be of positive growth through the experience. Not infrequently there are problems in getting through certain stages and each of the parents may get stuck at different stages. One parent may be still in a stage of denial and the other in the stage of anger. One parent may be actively working towards adaptation while the other is still immersed in sadness.

There is little evidence that parental health is permanently marred by the presence of a child with mental retardation in the family. Early studies have often been uncontrolled or have compared institutionalized samples with non-institutionalized cases where there is no support or services available at all. Approximately a third of mothers giving birth to a Down's syndrome child are clinically depressed in the 18-month period after the birth (Gath, 1977). This, however, was not significantly different from the numbers of mothers of normal babies who were depressed and there is a very similar proportion of depression found in other young mothers raising children in less than ideal circumstances, such as those in urban areas with many social problems (Brown & Harris, 1978) or even mothers of perfectly normal twins. In some studies there is a suggestion that families with a mentally retarded child are more likely to report psychiatric symptoms than children with physical handicaps but are probably less likely to have psychiatric difficulties than the parents of emotionally disturbed children. However, the most serious effect on the parents of having a retarded child is that on the relationship that exists between them. In a study of Down's syndrome, nearly a third of the marriages were classified as poor with high hostility and little evidence of warmth. They included three families in the group of thirty that broke down irretrievably during the first eighteen months after the birth of a Down's syndrome child. This finding is similar to those found in conditions such as autism and also in some physical conditions, such as spina bifida. The effect seems to be part of the original grief rather than due to the burden of care. In the families who kept a Down's syndrome child at home there was a less than expected rate of divorce and separation but this was balanced by the very high divorce and separation rate in the families of children of the same age who were in the institutions serving the same area. Thus, when the family is sufficiently secure to embark on keeping a retarded child at home it is possible that the shared task binds them together. Indeed, many parents say that they have been brought closer.

Prevalence of mental retardation in children

The classic epidemiological study of children aged 9 to 11 years on the Isle of Wight (Rutter, Tizard & Whitmore , 1970) showed that 2.53 per cent of the children had a score on the Wechsler Intelligence Scale (WISC) which was at least two standard deviations below the mean score for the whole group, corresponding to an intelligence quotient of below 70. Edgerton (1979) estimates that three out of every hundred children born will be diagnosed as mentally retarded at some time in their lives. Severe retardation corresponding to an IQ of below 50 was estimated on the Isle of Wight using a wider age group (Rutter, Graham & Yule, 1970) of all school age children and a prevalence was found of 3.1 per thousand. Other investigators have found prevalence rates of 3.61 per thousand in children aged 10 to 14 in Middlesex (Goodman & Tizard, 1962), 3.64 and 3.84 in youngsters aged 15 to 19 in Salford and Wessex respectively (Kushlick, 1961, 1964; Susser & Kushlick, 1961). In his study in Camberwell, Corbett (1976) found 140 children with an IQ below 50 in a population of 170 thousand. In that particular area there is a high incidence of other social problems.

Psychiatric disorder and mental retardation

Despite the scarcity of reports of well designed research, there appears to be little doubt that psychiatric disorders do become more common with decreasing levels of intellectual functioning (Rutter, 1971; Corbett, 1976). In the Isle of Wight study 50 per cent of the severely retarded children were judged to have a psychiatric disorder as compared with 6.6 per cent of children in the normal range. Rutter clearly demonstrates from the Isle of Wight data that psychiatric disorder is associated with relatively low IQ over the whole range of intellectual functioning, thus children of average intelligence have a higher rate of disorder than those of superior intelligence and those of borderline ability a higher rate than those of average intelligence. Individual items of deviant behaviour – such as misery, fighting, and poor concentra-

tion, show the same slope in incidence across the intellectual range.

Philips and Williams (1975) found that only 13 per cent of the retarded children seen at the Langley Porter Neuropsychiatric Institute had no psychiatric disorder. Despite the efforts of the research team to get children with no behaviour or emotional problems referred to them for assessment, there is a likelihood that the sample was biased as there is an understandable tendency to refer children with difficulties to a psychiatric department. Chess and Hassibi (1970) have reported a study of 52 children aged between 5 and 11 years 11 months, with mental ages of between 4 and 6 and IQ scores of 50 to 75, all living with their families. They found no psychiatric disorder in 21 (40 per cent) of these children, judging that the behaviour could be accounted for by the fact of retardation alone. In Boston children, again all living at home aged between 3 and 6 years and attending local nursery schools, Webster (1970) found none who were 'simply retarded'. He states 'Even those retarded children who showed the best emotional development were not comparable to non-retarded children of the same mental age'. Webster describes in detail the 'primary psycho-pathology' of mental retardation found in those he rated as having mild emotional disturbance, being 56 out of his 159 subjects (35 per cent). He discusses Chess and Hassibi's (1970) findings and attempts to reconcile them with his own, concluding that the difference lay more in semantics than in conflicting data.

A child of 10 with an IQ of 50 is not comparable to a 5-year-old of average intelligence. The retarded child may be able to perform on a test with an overall score roughly equal to the total achievement of the younger child but he may be socially much more advanced and yet far slower in picking up new skills.

Michael, a 7-year-old with an IQ of 50 was observed clearing the table after lunch at school. He sorted the plates and cutlery with an efficiency exceeding that of any pre-school child. On the other hand, his conversation at table had been monotonous, lacking the enquiry and variety of most 3-year-olds. Similarly, he was skilled in putting together jigsaws he had been practising for months but took much longer than a normal, younger child to adapt to a new task and learn what was required of him in different situations.

The features of Webster's (1970) 'primary psycho-pathology' of mental retardation include repetitiousness, inflexibility, and simplicity of emotional life, all clearly seen in children such as Michael. Chess (1977) suggests that these behavioural features and monotony of play indicate merely a lack of ideas, which is an essential part of the picture of mental retardation. It was also stressed that well organized adaptive behaviour can exist side by side with repetitiveness and inflexibility in the retarded child whereas in the child of normal intelligence these features are much more likely to be associated with other aberrant behaviour or emotions.

Impulsive behaviour was considered by both Webster (1970) and Chess and Hassibi (1970) to be part of a more serious behaviour problem in the retarded child. Yet minor degrees of impulsive behaviour have been found almost invariably, even in the best adjusted of a group of children with Down's syndrome studied by the present author.

Rebecca is a happy 9-year-old girl with Down's syndrome. She has an IQ of 75 and fits well into her local primary school, as does her 7-year-old normal sister. Rebecca has learnt to read, has self-care skills equal to other children of her age and has well socialized behaviour adjusting easily to a variety of situations. Yet despite having learned and practiced road drill, Rebecca forgets it instantly when distracted by the sight of a relative or friend on the other side of the road, and serious injury has been prevented only by the prompt action of the younger sister. Similar stories were told of the other otherwise well adjusted children in the group.

Classification of behaviour and emotional disorders has proved difficult in children with mental retardation. The range of disorders is similar to that found in children of average intelligence. As in the general population of children of the same age, neurotic and conduct disorders were the most common, followed by the mixed disorders with both emotional and antisocial features. However, certain disorders and certain items of behaviour are more common in the severely retarded group. In particular, children with profound language and communication problems were found to have a high incidence of the hyperkinetic syndrome and of childhood psychosis. Over-activity may be age-related, particularly in retarded autistic children who are extremely over-active between the ages of 5 and 10 and may swing to the opposite extreme and be very low in activity in adolescence. Stereotyped repetitive movements are much more common in retarded children but rare in children whose intelligence lies within the normal range. The relative preponderance of childhood psychosis is evident in Philips and Williams' study (1975) of 100 mentally retarded children in which 38 had

psychotic symptoms. The three most common symptoms were aggression, problems in social relationships, and developmental delay. Hyperactivity was noted in 39 of the 100 children but this study found no relationship between hyperactivity and psychosis or brain damage, nor was there a higher frequency of hyperactivity in comparison with the group of children of normal intelligence (Philips & Williams, 1977).

Chess, (1977) in her study of 52 children found reactive behaviour disorder in 18, neurotic behaviour disorder in 1, cerebral dysfunction in 11, and psychosis in 1. Reactive behaviour disorder could be explained by retardation together with environmental stress, and differed from neurotic behaviour disorder where the symptoms persisted after removal of the stress. Cerebral dysfunction showed a clear relation to neurological malfunction, and psychosis to severe symptoms. The children in Chess's group were in the milder range of IQ between 50 and 70 and she describes them as having favourable life situations.

Rutter (1971) emphasizes the importance of disordered brain function in the genesis of behaviour disorders, particularly in the severely retarded child. Over the whole intellectual range, brain lesions above the brain stem are associated with increased vulnerability to psychiatric disorder (Rutter, Graham & Yule, 1970, Seidel, Chadwick & Rutter, 1975). The association of behaviour problems with epilepsy and the improvement in psychiatric status after surgical removal of the malfunctioning hemisphere are quoted in support of the argument. However, organic brain damage alone cannot account for the increased incidence of psychiatric disorder in the retarded population, because of the high rate of psychiatric disorder in retarded children with no evidence of neurological damage and because retarded brain-damaged children are more likely to have psychiatric disorder than brain-damaged children in the normal intellectual range. In Chess's group those with behaviour disorders due to neurological damage showed no improvement at the three-year follow-up, in contrast to the reactive disorder group, the majority of whom improved although some went on to more serious psychiatric disorder (Chess, 1977). The importance of temperament is emphasized by this follow-up study as the intellectually retarded child with a difficult temperament is even more vulnerable from the psychiatric point of view, than is a similar child of normal intelligence.

No psychiatric syndrome is characteristic of any one medical diagnosis to which the retardation could be attributed. Webster (1970) found the children with Down's syndrome, referred to as 'mongoloid' and with metabolic disorder to have mild emotional problems and to escape serious disturbance. Much has been written about the characteristic Down's syndrome temperament but the extensive review of research on this theme by Gibson (1978) leads to the conclusion that there is considerable variation of personality and temperament.

Autism occurs in association with all types of medical diagnosis and brain damage but Webster (1970) noted its absence in his group of Down's (mongoloid) children. Only 2 children in more than four hundred with Down's syndrome known to the author have symptoms producing a clinical picture compatible with the diagnosis of autism. Chess and co-workers (1978) noted a particularly high incidence of autism in their series of children with congenital rubella, 18 or 7.4 per cent as compared with an expected rate of 0.7 per 10 000 of the population.

Social rejection can be seen as contributing to the development of psychiatric disorder in both the mild retarded and the more severely affected. Less able children are more often rejected by their peers in normal schools and the children who go to special schools have less opportunity of making friends in the locality. When they do, they may be tolerated only temporarily until the game becomes too complex or their companions tire of their less stimulating company.

The susceptibility of children with particular problems in language development to autism and the hyperkinetic syndrome has already been referred to. Other workers have found that aggressive behaviour is more common in the language-disabled group. This finding has been attributed to poor ego development by Webster (1970) but can be seen as also indicating a deficit in non-verbal communication as the child fails to learn in play, the signals for limiting aggression.

Children who have been brought up in institutions do not develop cognitively as well as those brought up at home and also have a higher incidence of behaviour disorder which cannot be accounted for by a bias towards admission of children because of their behaviour problems. Poor quality institutional care (Oswin, 1978) produces deprivation which can be both emotional and sensory. However, relative deprivation also exists in the home and the child himself contributes to it. The placid quiet child who initiates little interaction with his parents can be at a disadvantage as compared with the more demanding or even more ill child (Webster, 1970). The opposite extreme, the inconsolable screaming child, also gets less rewarding parental attention.

Although all children, retarded or not, are susceptible to the social and family influence on emotional development, there is little information from research available about the social and family background in most studies of retarded children. Over-infantilization, which does imply some warmth and affection from the family, can prevent more adaptive behaviour developing. Recently the author was asked by a parent how he could give up the habit of a piggy-back ritual each evening. His son was now 12 and proving too heavy for a frail 60-year-old parson to carry. Infantilization carries with it the denial of physical development. Occasionally, habits acceptable in a young child are not tolerable in adolescents. Webster (1970) quotes a 7-year-old girl becoming erotically stimulated by hugging games in bed with her father. A similar case is that of a psychotic boy who enjoyed feeling different fabrics particularly nylon but, by the time he was 8, his hands straying up ladies' skirts could be seen in quite a different light.

Treatment of behaviour disorders in the retarded child

Treatment of behaviour disorders is more difficult than in normal children. However, a positive line can be taken, once accepted, but a significant number are reactive to environmental circumstances and can improve. Mentally retarded children need the same high degree of expertise as do normal children in investigating their difficulties and in establishing social and family factors in the environment, assessing particular difficulties, such as relatively greater handicaps in language, as well as in the diagnosis of any medical condition underlying the retardation itself. Too hasty a resort to removal of the child from home or to psychopharmacology, should be resisted. Hospitalization is rarely in the interests of the child and even short temporary admissions can produce reactive emotional disorder in these very vulnerable children that can exceed the original difficulty. The literature on drug therapy for mentally retarded children is sparse and the studies poorly controlled. Chlorpromazine, thioridazine, and haloperidol are all useful in controlling very severe behaviour disturbances, but they also produce side effects especially the extrapyramidal disturbances. Haloperidol in particular presents difficulties, as the side-effects can be severe in even very small doses in children. The minor tranquillizers, chlordiazepoxide and diazepam are of doubtful use in retarded children and diazepam is also needed to be kept in reserve for the treatment of status epilepticus. Anticonvulsants are useful in controlling epilepsy, but not behaviour. Methylphenidate has some role in the treatment of hyperkinetic syndrome but, for the more minor degrees of hyperactivity complained of in the school situation, the use of caffeine in the form of a cup of black coffee can be effective in producing somewhat more acceptable behaviour.

Attention to management in the home and in the school is often more fruitful than chasing the behaviour with a battery of psychopharmacological weapons. Clear instructions, often complemented by signing, by means of the Paget-Gorman Sign System (Paget-Gorman Sign System) or Makaton sign language (Walker, 1980), can help retarded children, particularly with language impairment, to develop acceptable modes of behaviour. Consistency within the home and the school is important, and so joint meetings involving parents, teachers, and therapists are advised. More formal behaviour modification is indicated for specific problems of behaviour. Unfortunately, modern design of homes and of school with open plan arrangements makes handling of the behaviourally deviant retarded child more difficult. Freedom from distraction is required for learning and a safe 'time out' place is invaluable for sorting out aberrant behaviour before it becomes unmanageable. Once the position of admission into hospital is reached the prognosis is not good but some success can be achieved if work on the problem behaviour in hospital is followed by the therapists moving into the home to allow generalization of what improvement has occurred. All too often treatment of behaviour disorders, if effective at all in the hospital, is followed by relapse on discharge with resulting deep disappointment and a feeling of futility in the parents.

Special education
Children who are unable to manage at ordinary schools attend special schools for the educationally subnormal (ESN). There are two types, ESN(M), mild (EMR in America), and ESN(S), severe (TMR in America). The two types can be on the same campus, merged as one or entirely separate. Both types emphasize social training and, particularly in ESN(S) schools, active participation by parents. The practical emphasis is illustrated by the occurrence of toilet training in the reception class and by work experience and the teaching of domestic skills in the school-leaving class.

A wide range of intellectual deficit is catered for. Where there are separate schools the overlap is considerable and there may be misfits as well as parental resentment at the recommendation. There are sometimes prolonged and bitter battles between parents and educational authorities, which are often at the expense of the child. Flexibility is desirable and a child should be placed according to his needs and not because of a label, as recommended in the Warnock Report (1978). Problems arise when parents put more value on reading and formal education than on the fostering of independence. Local educational authorities provoke problems when they put children into rigid categories or allow expectations to remain low.

4.2.4
Psychiatric, social, and educational aspects of physical handicap in childhood

ANN GATH

All children have to learn to adapt to the changing demands of their environment as they grow older. When physical disorder distorts the developmental process, the child has more to cope with as he comes to terms with the real world around him. 'Handicap' can be defined as this additional set of problems which are secondary to the disease process itself (Tavormina *et al.*, 1976).

Physical abnormality and the process of development

Both congenital malformation and acquired disease in childhood can interfere with development. Where there is an obvious physical deformity, such as in the case of severe spina bifida or cerebral palsy, a child may never acquire the necessary skills to walk, to be continent, or to keep himself fed and clean, and is therefore totally dependent on the care of others, particularly his mother. Such a severe degree of handicap may also occur after initial normal development from a disease occurring later in childhood, as after poliomyelitis or a traumatic head injury. The impact of a congenital abnormality is different from that of a permanent injury to a previously normal child.

Disease can interfere with growth. Small stature is one of the complications of congenital heart disease and of chronic infection, as in fibrocystic disease affecting the lungs. Many children resent being

small, but excessive height, as in pituitary malfunctioning, can also be an encumbrance. The most common cause of 'physical handicap' in school is obesity, more often due to faulty family eating habits than to emotional difficulties or a medical condition.

Sexual development may be delayed as a result of chronic disorder but emotional problems associated with sexual awareness are more common if there is a sense of physical inadequacy.

As he grows, a child also develops intellectually and emotionally. It is necessary to see a child in the context of his home and at school or in the neighbourhood before coming to a judgment on his general well-being. The degree of handicap experienced by the child is a sum total of the impact of the disease or malformation on him, on his family and on his activities in the community, particularly at school. Like all children, the child with a handicap has to negotiate the ordinary developmental hurdles of growing up.

The demands of treatment

The effect of any illness or any longstanding medical problem in childhood is due not only to the direct effect on the pathological process but also to the effect of the treatment, if any, given to the child.

Diabetes in childhood affects hitherto healthy children and is compatible with an essentially normal life. However, the child is on a metabolic tightrope and the treatment demands daily injections, even twice daily injections in adolescence, routine urine testing, and adherence to a diet. Some children are distressed every day by their injections but the majority very quickly master injecting themselves and take in their stride the necessary routine of syringe, urine testing, and diet. A few, particularly in early adolescence, resent the restrictions and may rebel even to the extent of running away from home and, it appears naively, from the diabetes. This rebellion is shortlived and almost invariably followed by diabetic pre-coma or even coma which requires energetic medical treatment. There are undesirable side effects of the insulin treatment of which hypoglycaemic attacks are the most alarming. However, less extreme fluctuations of blood sugar may produce mood swings or difficulties in perception, adding to the child's difficulties.

The treatment of acute leukaemia is still more demanding and unpleasant for the child, with consequent distress to him and to his parents (Broadbent, 1980). Repeated hospital visits with regular sternal punctures to obtain specimens of marrow may be a source of fear to a child whose emotional equilibrium becomes disturbed for several days before each appointment. Medication can be unpleasant to take, cause ulcers, and have other side effects on mood and behaviour. Radiation to the skull may produce nausea but some children who have behaved stoically throughout the ordeals of blood-taking, sternal punctures, and other distressing experiences are finally deeply distressed by the loss of the hair and the necessity of wearing a wig. The threat to life, less obvious in diabetes, is more acute in leukaemia, which despite improved five-year survival rates still spells out death to most parents.

In contrast, certain orthopaedic conditions are clearly benign, with few parents fearing lasting incapacity and certainly not death. Such a condition is Perthes disease, osteo-chondritis of the head of the femur. The direct effect of the pathological process is an increased risk of arthritis in later years, a threat not taken too seriously by the typical nine-year-old boy with the condition. He strongly resents the demands of the treatment which means immobilization of an otherwise healthy child. Behaviour problems have been found as a frequent occurrence in children with this condition, and can lead to tension within the family, particularly with brothers and sisters. However, the benign nature of the condition means that most parents are not unduly worried and can use their ordinary skills to cope with what is usually a temporary upset in the family.

A chronic illness often necessitates many hospital visits. Multiple admissions in early childhood are associated with behaviour problems (Douglas, 1975; Quinton & Rutter, 1976). The difficulties are exacerbated in families with social disadvantages and problems with transport, substitute care of other children, and the financial consequences. Rural families with a chronically sick child are particularly prone to fatigue and financial strain as a result of treatment at a distant medical centre, (Satterwhite, 1978). In Burton's (1975) detailed study of fibrocystic disease, the families had the combined burden of existing social problems and the added demands of the hospital visits for treatment or when a child was admitted. Encounters with the hospital were particularly distressing to parents and frightening to younger children, when one child in the family had already died of fibrocystic disease, which is inherited through recessive genes.

Parental reactions to physical disorder

Most of the research on families of chronically ill or congenitally abnormal children have centred on the mothers rather than the fathers. To some degree this has been justified by the very large part that mothers play in the lives of their sick children in contrast to their husbands. Mothers of asthmatic children made most of the decisions about child management without referring to their husbands who rarely took such responsibility (Reddihough *et al.*, 1977). A similar disparity of parental responsibility was also noticed in the families of haemophiliac boys (Agle, 1964) but in this sex-linked condition, the overinvolvement of the mother could be seen as an attempt to compensate for her part in the transmission of the disease. Few of the studies reported on parents made any attempt to interview fathers, an exception being Freeman's (1977) study of deaf children.

Many studies of parental reaction to chronic illness in children are poorly designed, with inadequate controls and doubtful measures of parental attitudes. Subjective comments on guilty feelings are common. From a number of studies of congenital heart disease, there seems to be some evidence that the effect on the mother is not related to the severity of the disease. Considerable difficulties in mother – child relationships were found when there was no actual heart disease (Landtman *et al.*, 1968). Normal attitudes were shown by the majority of mothers whose children had to undergo cardiac surgery and those who had been over-protective became more positive in their attitude after surgery.

As in mental retardation, parents are understandably shocked and distressed when first told of the physical abnormality or long standing disorder. Some conditions interfere with mother – child relationship early in life. These include all those that necessitate separation at birth and admission to a special care baby unit, which may make it difficult for the mother to get to know her child and feel he is truly hers (Richards, 1978).

Conditions producing difficulties in feeding such as cleft lip/palate, pyloric stenosis, and cyanotic heart disease all upset the normal development of attachment and may be associated with difficulties in mother – child relationships in the future.

Parents may well be the first to realize that something is wrong with a child. Instead of having the shock of bad news being broken to them, they will have instead the equally traumatic experience of not being able to get the doctor to accept that there is a problem needing investigation. Precious time, especially that needed for the best results from early treatment, as in the case of deaf children (Rapin, 1978), is lost because investigations are delayed. In addition, a bad relationship at this time with a medical practitioner can have lasting consequences, to the detriment of the child.

There are few studies of treatment aimed at helping parents of chronically ill children. Parent groups are run at many hospitals and there are now a large number of associations, usually concerned with a particular condition. The parents lose their feeling of isolation and are helped by co-operating in fighting for better treatment facilities or in raising money for research or holidays for the children. The hospital or clinic-based groups discuss topics that are similar to those mentioned by groups of parents of mentally handicapped children. They want to know how to be 'fair', how to discipline the sick or handicapped child, and how to treat the normal brothers and sisters. They talk about how they were given the news of their child's illness or abnormality. Later they discuss the implications of this news for them as individuals, as married couples and as members of larger groups. The parents are eager for facts, to know about new treatment and about what hope there is for the future. Only after several meetings will the most disturbing question come up with those families who know that their child's life is threatened. Death is difficult to talk about, particularly in relation to children but once the taboo is broken, the parents can be of considerable help to each other (Heffron *et al.*, 1973). However, not all parents join groups and many will drop out (Churven, 1977). It is clear therefore that individual contact with families must continue at the same time as groups are held. In the last decade family therapy has come into prominence. It is a technique which may be useful for the problem families who show the extremes of overprotection on one hand and non-acceptance on the other, as noticed in parents of asthmatics (Pinkerton, 1967), poliomyelitis victims (Davis, 1963) and thalidomide-damaged children (Roskies, 1972). Theories of family functioning based on the work of Minuchin have been used to study and treat 'brittle' diabetics, asthmatics, and anorexic patients (Minuchin *et al.*, 1975) and families of children with haemophilia (Paquay-Weinstock *et al.*, 1979).

Marital disharmony as a result of the strain of caring for a chronically ill child has been frequently referred to in earlier studies which emphasise the stress placed on the 'handicapped family'. Spina bifida was thought to have a devastating effect on the marital relationship (Tew *et al.*, 1974). Other recent studies have not found an increased rate of separation and divorce in families of deaf children (Freeman, 1977) or of adolescents with spina bifida (Dorner, 1975).

Brothers and sisters of the sick or disabled child

Even a mild and transient illness in one child in a family will affect the relationship between siblings. It is common for the healthy ones to be concerned and caring at first and then if the illness persists, to become somewhat envious of the privileges given to the sick one. This natural course of events has been described in a book on families of children who contracted poliomyelitis (Davis, 1963). In the first phase of the illness, the victim was acutely ill and in hospital and the parents were in considerable distress. At this time, the brothers and sisters were full of solicitude and would bring even their treasured possessions as gifts for the child. They expressed their remorse for any previous wrongdoing or injustice that they had dealt the sick child in the years before. Throughout the period in the hospital, the parents indulged the child with poliomyelitis by giving him many, even daily, presents and by relaxing discipline. After discharge from hospital, the healthy brothers and sisters were initially delighted to have the sick child back but they quickly became intolerant of the special treatment. Gradually discipline had to be reinforced and the habit of giving presents abandoned. In time, the brothers and sisters would forget the promises they had made at the time of the acute illness and revert to the same pattern of quarrelling as they had had before poliomyelitis struck.

Very helpless children are less likely to be resented than the child well able to exploit the advantages of illness or incapacity. Victims of severe head injury in childhood were treated with concern and sometimes persistent remorse by the healthy brothers and sisters, who behaved quite differently from the eventually resentful siblings of some of the children with Perthes disease, who had reacted to their immobilization in plaster casts by becoming tyrannical. In general, children older than the sick child are likely to be protective while younger ones are more often jealous and demand attention in other ways. Few difficulties with siblings are reported in chronic conditions that are compatible with an apparently normal life and do not have recurrent crises. In a recent study of diabetic children, emotional or behavioural difficulties in siblings were not common.

However, where there is a threat of death, parents frequently express great anxiety in handling both their normal children and the one they are expecting to lose. In most cases those older children can share their parents' concern and identify with them in their distress rather than competing with the dying child for attention. In the families of the children with fibrocystic disease, there are recurrent crises, when the child is acutely ill and needs hospital admission. A previous experience of death means that all the children are afraid that each admission of the sick child could well be the last.

Guy aged seven has a sister Tracey aged four with fibrocystic disease. Tracy has had many admissions to the hospital and the parents have been told that her expectation of life is brief. Every time Tracey develops an infection, Guy becomes very anxious and, if she is admitted, his behaviour deteriorates, particularly at school, with distractability, temper tantrums, and aggression to other children. When seen by himself, it was clear that he knew that Tracey was likely to die. He shared his parents' concern and spent considerable effort trying to invent a magic cure for his sister. He could not express his anxiety in terms other than uncontrollable behaviour.

The effects on brothers and sisters are mediated through the parents' reaction to the problem of chronic illness in the child. The other children will suffer if the parents' relationship becomes strained and they begin to quarrel. In some cases children also suffer because they are expected to excel in order to compensate for the sick or imperfect one, which places too heavy a burden of expectation upon them. When a child dies, the parents' behaviour towards the surviving children can alter. Parents tend to over-protect the children they have left but occasionally they may reject the living, comparing them unfavourably with the one who died.

There are few systematic studies of the siblings of chronically ill children. Where the families of sick and healthy children are closely matched for total sibling size and the social class, few differences can be found. On the other hand, crippling conditions are particularly likely to affect the whole family in areas of social deprivation, as in the study of spina bifida in South Wales (Tew *et al.*, 1974) or of fibrocystic disease in Northern Ireland (Burton, 1975). One

study found that brothers and sisters of children with visible problems treated by plastic surgery were more likely to show signs of general disturbance on the behavioural check list than were siblings of children with invisible but potentially more dangerous conditions such as haematological disorders or congenital heart disease (Lavigne & Ryan, 1979).

The effect of physical disorder on the child himself

Most early research has emphasized the problems of physical disorder and suggested that long-standing illness is usually associated with deviance in psychological and social adjustment of children. As with parents, the research has been designed to search for areas of weakness rather than strengths and to use questionnaires of doubtful validity. Observations of children attending an out-patient clinic in which they frequently have to wait a long time or have some unpleasant thing done to them bears little relation to what the child is like at home with his family or at school with his peers.

Even very minor physical anomalies have been found to be associated with an increase in psychiatric disorders in childhood. Sandberg (1976) studied children with congenital malformations and found a high rate of disorder, 49 per cent which included developmental deviations, mental retardation, and psychoneurotic disorder. Some of the abnormalities were indicative of more severe abnormalities of brain development. Steg and Rapoport (1975) found a high number of minor anomalies in boys with learning difficulties and boys with severe behaviour disorders or psychosis as compared with others from a paediatric ward or psychiatric outpatients. A sex difference was found by Halverson and Victor (1976), as boys with minor anomalies were likely to be hyperactive and girls 'quiet, shy, timid, mean, and uncoordinated'. In Sandberg's (1976) study, the children with malformations and those in her control group did not differ in the incidence of antisocial behaviour at school, which was 10 per cent. The high incidence of reported problems at home reflects some disturbance of maternal attitude towards children with physical abnormalities, particularly the visible ones.

Cleft lip is one such abnormality that is very striking at birth but can be modified considerably by plastic surgery. In an early study on congenitally abnormal children, it was noted that children with cleft lip were unusually quiet and compliant, a comment echoed by the parents (Gath, 1972). This observation is supported by those of Richman and Harper (1978) who found children with cleft lip and those with cerebral palsy to be more inhibited than control children and to have lower educational achievement.

Psychiatric disorder in the physically ill child is more common where there is clear evidence of brain damage. This was demonstrated in the Isle of Wight study (Rutter, Tizard & Whitmore, 1970), by the more detailed study at the same time of neurologically abnormal children (Rutter, Graham & Yule, 1970) and a more recent study of crippled children in London (Seidel, Chadwick & Rutter, 1975). The behaviour disorder is associated with brain malfunction and this is also the explanation for the disorder associated with those minor anomalies indicating deviant embryological development in the first trimester of life.

However, it is clear that chronic illness, abnormal appearance, or physical disability make children more vulnerable to stress and to development of psychiatric disorders, particularly if reared in an unsupporting or even hostile environment. A higher than expected rate of disturbance has been found in children suffering from diabetes (Swift, Seidman & Stein, 1967), asthma (Werry, 1972) and hearing deficit (Bakwin & Bakwin, 1972). The incidence of psychiatric disorder does not appear to be related to severity (Offord & Aponte, 1967) and is no less common where the parents erroneously believe that there is a heart condition (Landtman, Valanne & Aukee, 1968). No specific psychiatric disorder is related to the presence of a chronic medical problem. Some children, usually those with over-protective mothers, become withdrawn, timid, and miserable.

Such a boy was *Peter,* a ten-year-old diabetic, whose mother was an outspoken woman who had succeeded in frightening most of the medical and nursing staff with whom Peter had had to come in contact. Peter was allowed to do very little for himself but he became very upset if his mother tried to give him his injection. He became more socially isolated, did badly at school which he finally refused to attend. A short period away from home at a special hostel did much to restore Peter's self-confidence. Family therapy involving Peter, his mother, his timid father, and the two robust siblings helped to improve relationships sufficiently to allow Peter to return home.

Another probably temperamentally different child reacts in an opposite way by rebelling and appearing to fight against the infirmity. As mentioned above, rebellion against the diabetic regime is risky and may even be fatal. 'Dare devil' deliberate risk-taking behaviour is described in haemophiliac boys (Agle, 1964).

A similar reaction was seen in *Miles,* a fourteen-year-old boy who had muscular dystrophy and was well aware of the outcome. Miles was furious when he realized that his increasing difficulties in getting around his school had been noticed and that he was to transfer to a school for the physically handicapped. He committed a number of spectacular robberies which became the talk of his small town. On remand, he was still extremely angry but his mood improved when a place was found in a school which had no stairs and he received an encouraging letter from a well-known legless hero.

Although the incidence of psychiatric problems may be higher than in a normal population, it is important to remember that most children with even severe physical problems do very well. Mattsson and Gross (1966) commented on the good adaptation of most of the young haemophiliacs they studied. The majority of children in a group of seventy-six diabetics were happy youngsters enjoying a wide range of activities as well as school life (Gath, Smith & Baum, 1980).

In some conditions, such as haemophilia, there appears to be an improvement in the physical state in later childhood and this precedes a change from passive dependence on the parent to a healthy and active independence. Unfortunately, other conditions such as diabetes can become more difficult to control in adolescence thus complicating still further a vulnerable child's life.

The school life of the child with a chronic medical problem

School attendance can be severely disrupted by recurrent illness, admission to hospital or even regular out-patient appointments. Diabetic children had lower attendance rates than had other children in their class but the difference was not large (Gath, Smith & Baum, 1980). Children with fibrocystic disease may have to miss school because of illness but they retain a considerable enthusiasm for going to school because they are pleased to be part of the group of ordinary children. Teaching in paediatric wards helps to fill the gaps in learning as well as to provide a normal structure for the day and sometimes a helpful distraction from painful procedures.

As is pointed out in the report on Special Educational Needs (Warnock Report, 1978), there is no simple relationship between the degree of physical impairment and educational handicap. Some severely disabled children can manage well in ordinary schools (Welbourn, 1975). Other larger establishments where the children move from place to place all day are found too stressful for all but the most robust.

Boarding schools specializing in one form of disability were in vogue thirty years ago and it was sometimes advocated that children should board from even as young an age as four years. Recently, special units for physically disabled, for deaf, or for language-impaired children are found attached to normal schools. The child thus gets specialized teaching without losing his place in the family or the community.

Treatment

Treatment for emotional or behavioural problems associated with chronic disease or malforma-tion should be based on full co-operation with the family, the paediatrician treating the child, and the school. In some cases, full explanation of the condition and its practical implications can make a major difference to the child's life at school. In others, where the family relationships are constricting the child's life, family therapy is a useful mode of treatment. In later adolescence, the youngster, with a chronic disorder affecting his life expectancy or, his chance of marriage or of having a child himself, may need considerable time spent with him on an individual basis. By no means do all families with a handicapped child of any sort need a psychiatrist but much pain can be avoided if the child psychiatrist is an integral member of the team treating children and is easily available to parents and ward staff.

PART III
Neurotic states, sexual disorders, and drug dependence

5
Minor affective disorders

5.1
Depressive syndromes

5.1.1
Minor depressive syndromes in childhood

PHILIP GRAHAM

Introduction

Although it is generally agreed that depressive and sometimes hypomanic disorders do occur, even though with great rarity in the pre-pubertal period (Anthony & Scott, 1960), the validity of the concept of a depressive disorder in childhood is a matter of controversy (Gittelman-Klein, 1977). In the following section the assumption is made for reasons of clarity that minor depressive syndromes do exist in childhood as reasonably well defined entities, but the reader should bear in mind that this approach cannot, as yet, be fully justified on the basis of available evidence.

Incidence and prevalence

Transient disturbances of mood, such as relatively brief episodes of sadness and unhappiness, are very common in children. They are readily observed by parents and teachers and admitted to by children with increasing frequency as they get older. In the total population study reported by Rutter and co-workers (1970) 11 per cent of boys and 13 per cent of girls living on the Isle of Wight were reported by their parents, and 11 per cent of boys and 8 per cent of girls by their teachers, to 'often appear miserable, unhappy, tearful or distressed'. In discussion of their feelings, a high proportion of children over about the age of nine or ten years will describe their experience of sadness. Usually, this is attributed to boredom and is described as occurring especially when the child feels he has too little to do. Albert and Beck (1975) studied a sample of 63 normal children in 6th and 7th grade (aged twelve to thirteen years) and found 29 per cent agreeing to feelings of sadness, 48 per cent a sense of failure, and 33 per cent at least occasional thoughts of harming themselves.

Transient mood disturbances are of no pathological significance in themselves, but they occur more frequently in children who show handicapping psychiatric conditions especially emotional and antisocial disorders. Thus, in the study of Rutter and co-workers (1970), 26 per cent of boys with antisocial and 24 per cent of children with neurotic disorders were reported by their parents to appear 'often miserable and unhappy' and so forth. The mood changes shown by children with psychiatric disorders are different in duration, intensity, and quality from those shown by children without such disorders. They are likely to be longer in duration ('ordinary' sadness and misery lasting usually no more than a few hours) and to be more unpleasant in quality. Further, the boredom to which the mood change is attributed is itself more likely to be identifiable as a pathological response. The child may lack the physical or mental energy to engage in activity or the boredom may be enforced by the inability of the child to maintain social relationships with other children or by parental insistence on activities which the child finds too difficult, unenjoyable or unrewarding. Finally the mood change in the disturbed child is more likely to be attributed by him to circumstances other than boredom – for example, to distressing family relationships, parental illness, separation from a friend, a death in the family, or failure in school.

Most children with emotional disorders show a mixture of anxiety, irritability, and somatic symptoms such as headache and stomachache. Prolonged unhappiness is usually not a prominent feature. In a minority of children of primary school age (five to eleven years) however, depressive symptomatology is prominent, and in early adolescence the proportion of children showing pure depressive disorders increases until, by late adolescence, depressive conditions form a substantial proportion of the total picture of psychiatric disorder. In the Isle of Wight study (Rutter *et al.*, 1970) the rate of depressive disorders was within the region of 0.1 per cent to 0.2 per cent in ten- and eleven-year-old children and rose to 0.5 per cent in fourteen-year-olds, with a further 1.1 per cent showing mixed affective disorders characterized by both anxiety and depression. However, the fig-

ures provided by Albert and Beck (1975) and cited above, suggest that in the United States rates in the general population may be higher. Further confirmatory evidence for this suggestion is provided by Petti's finding (1978) that a significant proportion of children in an in-patient unit could, according to him, be diagnosed as depressed. In the UK a lower proportion of in-patients would be given this diagnosis, and there is a need for a cross-national study using uniform criteria to examine this issue.

The increase in rate of depressive disorders with age is accompanied by a change in sex ratio. While in younger children boys and girls are affected in roughly equal numbers, by mid-adolescence affected girls outnumber boys by 2 or 3 to 1 and, of course, in adults epidemiological studies reveal that the predominance of females is maintained. In the absence of longitudinal studies, the reasons for this change in sex ratio are unclear, but it is likely that both physiological and sociocultural factors are relevant.

Increasing age also brings with it a more clearly defined depressive syndrome. With the onset of adolescence depressed mood is more commonly accompanied by feelings of guilt, expressions of self-blame, insomnia, and appetite disturbance (either over-eating or anorexia), together with self-destructive thoughts and activity. Adolescents find it easier to voice these feelings of distress than do younger children and this may be one reason why their symptomatology appears more clear-cut, but it is also probable that in younger children depressive experience is less well defined.

Aetiology
Aetiological features of special relevance to emotional disorders of childhood are discussed in some detail in chapter 1.3.1 and 1.3.2, and here discussion of aetiology will be limited to issues of particular relevance to depressive symptomatology.

(a) *Genetic factors.* Evidence for the importance of genetic factors in the production either of depressive symptomatology in emotional disorders or of the pure depressive disorders of childhood is thin. There is no particular tendency for the parents of children with depressive symptomatology to have had psychiatric disorder (Rutter 1966). The evidence regarding children of parents with affective disorder is less clear-cut. McKnew and co-workers (1979) studied 30 five- to fifteen-year-old children of 14 consecutive patients with a diagnosis of bipolar or unipolar affective disorder and found a high incidence of depressive symptoms, with 9 of the children showing significant depression at two separate interviews. However, the study was uncontrolled and needs replication.

(b) *Temperament*. Thomas and Chess (1977) have suggested that children with a particular style of behaviour characterized especially by withdrawal, high adaptability, and low intensity of emotional expression are likely, when disturbed, to show emotional disorders rather than other types of problems. It is uncertain whether a particular personality type predisposes to depressive symptomatology.

(c) *Febrile illness*. Lack of energy and mild depression of mood are quite common after febrile illnesses. In a small minority of children, much more severe depressive reactions occur and these may be prolonged and handicapping. Physical investigations are usually non-contributory and the mechanisms involved (for example, transient encephalitis, immunological deficiency, psychological reaction to stress) are in general not clarified.

(d) *Stress*. Systematic studies such as those reported by Brown and Harris (1978) of vulnerability and life stress in depressed adults have not been carried out amongst populations of depressed children, although there is evidence for life-events as contributory factors in the diseases of children more generally (Heisel *et al.*, 1973). However, Caplan and Douglas (1969) have demonstrated that child psychiatric clinic attenders with depressed mood have more commonly previously sustained a parental loss than disturbed children without such mood disturbance. It is probable that, as with depressed adults, the onset of depression is commonly precipitated by an experience involving disappointment or loss, and that children with a previous experience of loss or repeated rejection are especially likely to suffer depressive symptoms when stressed in this way.

Clinical features

The manifestations of depressive symptomatology vary with the age of the child.

Pre-school

From the first few weeks of life infants can be observed to be affected by loss, and sometimes their response bears close resemblance to a depressive state. Heinicke and Wertheimer (1965) described the behaviour of 10 children aged thirteen months to thirty-two months who were admitted to a residential nursery and separated from their parents. The

behaviour of the children varied, but some, after initial angry protest, spent a good deal of time rocking and fitfully crying, became relatively immobile, refused food, and slept poorly. Regressive behaviour with loss of bladder control was common. Similar behaviour has been observed in young children admitted to hospital without their parents. Such responses cannot be regarded as pathological – normal children must be expected to behave in this way when separated from their parents into unfamiliar surroundings and cared for by people they have never met before. Any pathology that exists is present in the society which permits such unnatural separations.

Sometimes, however, a similar pattern of behaviour can be seen in children living in families who have apparently not sustained such traumatic separations. Typically, the child involved is aged between one and two years and is referred to a paediatrician because of failure to thrive, often accompanied by non-specific diarrhoea (O'Callaghan & Hull, 1978). Psychological investigation reveals a fretful, insecure, depressed child. The social background is usually stressful with many of the features common to other psychological disturbances occurring in the pre-school period (see chapter 4.1.1). The failure to thrive is most commonly due to inadequate food intake (Whitten *et al.*, 1969) arising from parental ignorance or neglect, or from food refusal occurring in the context of a disturbed mother – child relationship, but has also been attributed to psychological factors.

Middle childhood

During this period, as already stated, emotional disorders are common, but their symptomatology is usually dominated by anxious rather than depressive manifestations (see below). A minority of children, however, do present with listlessness and lack of energy. They may complain unduly of boredom and show a disinclination to mix socially with their friends. At school they may show a lack of application to their work, with inattention, daydreaming, and lack of concentration. Sometimes, they may refuse to go to school because of apathy and inertia (see chapter 4.2.1). Appetite is rarely affected, but there may be difficulty in getting off to sleep. Headache and stomach-ache are sometimes present and, indeed, are likely to provide a reason for medical referral. When such a constellation of symptoms represents a change in the child's behaviour it is reasonable to regard the child as showing an emotional disorder of depressive type. Kovacs and Beck (1977) have usefully summarized criteria for the presence of clinical depression in children of this age group.

Adolescence

In older children and teenagers depressive conditions begin to resemble more closely those occurring in adults. The adolescent, to begin with, is more likely to perceive himself as suffering. Whereas younger children rarely complain of depression but are noted to be so by their parents and teachers, teenagers are much more likely to complain of their feelings. As part of their depressive symptoms they may experience a sense of futility and aimlessness in their lives. Bodily preoccupation with hypochondriasis is common at this age, and a teenager may present to the doctor with concern about the shape of his nose or the size of his penis. Self-blame and guilt are commonly accompanied by feelings of hopelessness and of the uselessness of existence. Suicidal thoughts (see below) are common. Many of these symptoms are not specific to depressive syndromes in adolescence and may form part of a schizophrenic, schizo-affective, or obsessional illness.

Parasuicide and suicide in childhood and adolescence

Kreitman (1977) defines parasuicide as a non-fatal act in which an individual deliberately causes self-injury or ingests a substance in excess of any prescribed or generally recognized therapeutic dosage. He prefers the term 'parasuicide' to 'attempted suicide' because the latter implies a motivation of self-destruction which is often absent (see below).

Threats of suicide are not uncommon even in young children. A six-year-old may, in a temper, thwarted for example in a desire to stay up to watch a TV programme, say that he is going to kill himself. Such threats can best be seen as angry responses calculated to produce the maximum distress and disturbance in those, usually one or other parent, to whom they are directed. Repeated threats of this type occurring in older children well capable of harming themselves must, however, be taken seriously and call for careful investigation. The rate of parasuicide has increased rapidly in the United Kingdom and this increase has occurred particularly sharply amongst the young. Admissions to the Edinburgh Poisoning Centre rose over tenfold in fifteen- to nineteen-year-old boys and over threefold in girls of the same age between 1963 and 1974 (Kreitman, 1977). A proportion of such acts, probably about a third, occur as part of depressive states, the remainder arising largely out of situational crises in which the youngster takes an overdose as one way out of an intolerable situation which allows him both to communicate his anger or distress and to legitimize his requirement for comfort and nurturance.

By contrast, suicide rates have not risen significantly over this period in the United Kingdom although they have risen in many other countries. Shaffer (1974) found no cases of completed suicide below the age of twelve years in a study of the UK extending over seven years. National United Kingdom figures remain tiny up to the age of fifteen years when a significant rise occurs. Shaffer found that children who had committed suicide had often shown previous antisocial behavior and the final act was often precipitated by a disciplinary crisis. A family history of depression and suicidal behaviour was common.

Management and treatment
Relief of stress

The assessment procedure involving the identification of a depressive state in a child will usually, though not always, have resulted in the recognition of stresses acting upon that child. First approaches to management should logically attempt the relief of such stresses. Thus, a child who is failing in school because of a specific difficulty in reading may be recommended for remedial help. A father who, because of work involvement, sees little of his son, who consequently feels rejected and unwanted, can be encouraged to find more time to spend with his offspring. A fat, depressed girl teased at school because of her appearance can be put on a diet at the same time as the school is contacted to enquire whether any action is possible over the teasing. Such straightforward measures are always worthwhile, even though they will by no means always be effective on their own.

Improvement of communication

Communication can be faulty at two main levels. A child may be unaware of the reasons for his feelings. A boy stealing to buy sweets so that he can bribe other children to be friendly with him may well not realize that his stealing is preceded by feelings of loneliness and despair. A teenage girl may not be aware that her feelings of depression arise from her incapacity to express her anger with her mother who is frustrating her wish to embark on heterosexual relationships. The development of awareness of the reasons for the presence of unpleasant affect may be enhanced by individual psychotherapy or counselling. In younger children communication with the therapist may occur best through the medium of play or drawing, whereas older children and adolescents can participate in verbal psychotherapy (see chapter 3.3.1 and 8.9). Secondly, communication between family members can be faulty. The assessment procedure usually provides good opportunity for sharing communication between family members, but more formal family therapy sessions may be necessary. The depressed child may, for example, be carrying more than his share of grief for a loss which the whole family has sustained and discussion of feelings of mourning experienced by other family members may release the depressed child from his inappropriate burden.

Enhancement of self-esteem

It has been suggested (Beck, 1967) that the central features of depression lie in the individual's negative view of himself, of the world about him, and of his future. For the child, the first of these seems of especial importance, and it is to the enhancement of self-esteem that the therapist should direct particular attention. During the assessment it is important to communicate warmth and concern, together with a sense of involvement with the problem, so that the child feels he matters and that his problems are of significance. Subsequently it is important to maintain a hopeful attitude towards the future and to look for ways in which to take a more positive approach to the child in question. Depressed children often appear unattractive and they may be rejected by their family and friends. Such rejection may not be obvious, either to the family or to the therapist, and further, during a period of depression, a child's need for affection and concern may be greater than that of his sibs, so that the usual equal distribution of parental time and solicitude may fail to meet the child's needs. Emphasis on the depressed child's positive qualities and the provision of opportunity to exercise his interests are both likely to be helpful in the relief of depression. Any suggestion which enables a child to gain greater control of his environment, for example, the undertaking of a journey by

himself on public transport, is similarly likely to enhance self-esteem.

Physical methods of treatment

There is no evidence that the first response of the doctor making a diagnosis of depressive disorder in a child should be the prescription of antidepressants. Various claims have been made, for example, by Frommer (1968), that specific antidepressants are indicated for different types of depressive reaction, but in general there is a lack of adequately controlled studies to support these contentions. An authoritative group set up to consider the place of antidepressants and treatment concluded that it would be premature to make recommendations in the absence of a clear-cut syndrome (Rapoport, 1977). Nevertheless, the evidence from studies that have attempted some degree of control, for example, Weinberg and co-workers (1973) and extrapolation from adult work, suggest that if other measures are ineffective and the child remains significantly handicapped by depressive symptomatology, it is reasonable to institute drug therapy. Imipramine in anergic, depressed children, and amitryptiline in agitated, depressed children would seem the drugs of choice and should be prescribed in the dosage recommended for children. For example, a twelve-year-old of average build might receive up to 75 mg daily of either drug.

Very occasionally, children approaching puberty and others in early puberty develop unipolar or bipolar affective illnesses of adult type. In these cases, the use of lithium (Youngerman & Canino, 1978) may be indicated especially for preventive purposes and this is described elsewhere (see volume 3).

Prognosis

The absence of a clear-cut distinction between depressive syndromes and emotional disorder of other types means that adequate information regarding the outcome of depressive states in childhood is lacking. Nevertheless, it seems likely from outcome studies of emotional disorders in general (Graham & Rutter, 1973) that about 50 per cent of such disturbances have cleared up within three or four years. Longer-term follow-up studies (Robins, 1966) suggest that the prognosis is such that the depressed child has no special predisposition to develop psychiatric disorder in adulthood (see chapter 1.3.2), though if he does develop such a disorder, it is likely to be of a similar type.

5.1.2
Personality disorders in adults predisposing to minor depressive reactions

DAVID GOLDBERG

Psychiatrists have long known that there is no particular personality type which is a necessary precondition for minor depression to occur, and have therefore asked whether particular sorts of abnormal personality are at greater risk of developing illness under stress, or whether particular personality traits increase the risk of depressive illness. Recent research in England and the United States (Brown & Harris, 1978; Hurry *et al.*, 1980; Weissman & Myers, 1978) has indicated that only a small proportion of depressive illnesses are actually treated by the psychiatric services, so that it is possible that the idea that abnormal personalities are at greater risk of depressive illness is simply a reflection of the greater likelihood of those with such abnormalities being referred for a psychiatric opinion. Most of the research to be reviewed in this section is based upon patients who have been referred to the psychiatric services, and it is therefore open to the objection that positive findings may tell us more about the factors which determine who receives treatment than about vulnerability to depression. Moreover, most of the reviewed studies are concerned with patients who later develop severe depressive illnesses, whereas the present contribution is mainly concerned with minor depressive reactions. The reader must bear in mind the impossibility of drawing sharp lines of demarcation between predispositions to depressive illnesses of varying grades of severity (See chap. 5.1.3, pp. 199–200).

The depressive personality

Kraepelin referred to a persistent sense of gloom as the hallmark of a depressive disposition, and this was considerably elaborated by Kurt Schneider in his description of a 'depressive psychopath'. It will be recalled that Schneider did not make the distinction between abnormal personality and minor neurotic illness which is familiar to Anglo-Saxon psychiatry, since he wished to confine the notion of illness to those with 'morbid changes' in their body. He anticipated the dethronement of 'neurosis' urged recently in the United States:

> the expression is really out of date and now discredited by facts. It is also psychotherapeutically harmful since it gives the patient a false picture of himself and his condition. A patient may announce that he has a neurosis; in reality he has no neurosis but he is a neurotic. Psychotherapeutic procedure requires the patient to see that he must take some responsibility for himself, a responsibility which having a neurosis seems to remove from him. (Kurt Schneider, 1950)

Schneider therefore makes no real distinction between minor affective disorder and abnormal personality; both are within the same universe, so that his model has difficulty in accounting for the fact that individuals whose premorbid personalities are within normal limits may develop affective illness under stress. Most of the German classifications of abnormal personality reviewed by Schneider suffer from this disadvantage: it is impossible to test whether there is an association between abnormalities of personality and liability to affective illness if the terms are defined in such a way that anyone who suffers from the latter is assumed to be an example of the former.

In his description of depressive psychopathy Schneider emphasized the pessimism and lack of capacity for enjoyment. 'They have little heart for their own purposes and are deeply distrustful. They are distracted by daily worries, hypochondriacal fears, self-analysis, doubt over life itself . . . (they are) very conscious of their duty but find little pleasure in doing it and any relaxation seems vaguely threatening to them.'

Writing from an entirely different perspective, psycho-analysts have produced broadly similar descriptions, which typically emphasize the low self-esteem of such patients. This low self-esteem is related in turn to failure to resolve early emotional problems with the mother: thus, Klein and Fairbairn described a depressive phase in infancy, while Jacobson related a deprivation of love in infancy to the angry or guilty inner conviction of the impossibility of ever achieving adequate love. Later writers enlarged this model to take account of those swamped by a surfeit of love. Thus Bonime (1966):

the depressive character develops in an environment in which the normal needs of a child for solicitous parents are unfulfilled; a milieu in which he is manipulated (often by aggrandisement) used, pushed, squelched, instead of having his realistic desires reasonably respected, and reasonably nurtured. He may be doted on, ignored, competed with, abused, but whatever form of neglect, oppression, oversolicitous confinement, or overt exploitation, the depressive is in reality deprived of a decently parented childhood. Much of the depressive's psychodynamics involves his dealings with this problem of an unrealised childhood. He personality achieves its dynamic form as the expression of practices developed for dealing with depriving and manipulative parental individuals. He fights against tyranny, against withheld affection, against derogation and against manipulative oversolicitude. He begins very early to develop the depressive practices – the elusive, withholding, punitive, demanding, seductive, angry manipulative personality – the depressive personality.

Bonime follows Schneider in relating depressive illness to long-standing personality traits: depression is seen as a *practice*:

the depressive is an extremely manipulative individual who, by helplessness, sadness, seductiveness, and other means, manoeuvers people towards the fulfilment of demands for various forms of emotionally comforting response . . . he does not define his demands, which may be enormous, but somehow subtly creates vacuum into which the giver is sucked. (Bonime, 1966)

From here it is a short step to a view which relates such manipulativeness to the need to maintain self-esteem, and sees this as a manifestation of the 'oral character':

Depression prone people are inordinately and almost exclusively dependent on narcissistic supplies derived directly or indirectly from other people for the maintenance of their self-esteem. Their frustration tolerance is low, and they employ various techniques – submissive, manipulative, coercive, piteous, demanding, and placating – to maintain their desperately needed but essentially ambivalent relationships with the external or internalised objects of their demands. (Chodoff, 1972)

It seems likely that many people who do not develop depressive illnesses need the good opinions of others to maintain their self-esteem, but they manage to remain liked by others without resorting to coercive techniques such as 'manipulativeness'. However, no one has so far demonstrated that those who use manipulative techniques are at greater risk of developing depressive illness.

The concept of the oral character is derived from Freudian theory, and the relationship between it and depression was articulated by Abraham (1924). The two basic oral functions – incorporation of food and biting – are seen as prototypes for the character traits that are thought to be related to the oral character, and the orally-fixated depressive exhibits an excessive amount of behaviour centred around the mouth and gut, partly due to constitutional factors and partly due to severe narcissistic disappointment with the mother in the pre-oedipal period. Mendelson (1967) related pleasurable stimulation of the mouth zone to general feelings of security, warmth, and nourishment.

Empirical support for these theoretical formulations is not very impressive. Although it is possible to produce measurements of 'orality' by factor analytic technique, it is not possible to relate such traits to mouth habits, such as chewing, finger-nail biting, and smoking (Gottheil & Stone, 1968); and measures of orality based on non-purposive mouth movements in children do not correlate with depressive tendencies as measured by the childrens' teachers (Blum & Miller, 1952). However, for many analysts the 'oral character' has lost its original connotations rooted in normal development, and means no more than an exaggeration of needs for affection and support with traits expressing excessive dependency: Chodoff (1972) thus defines orality as being measured by the degree to which a person's self-esteem is maintained more or less exclusively by the approval and support of others, and concludes that it carries with it a potential for developing a severe affective illness.

Grinker (1961) has pointed out that dynamic

formulations of depression are usually highly stereo-typed and vary little from patient to patient: 'an unfortunate by-product of focusing on the dynamics of depression has been the underemphasis on sound clinical observations and adequate description of these and other mental patients'. However plausible descriptions of the depressive character may seem, they are no substitute for an actual demonstration that particular antecedent variables increase the risk of the development of depressive illness.

Furthermore, all such theories tend to assume that the universe of patients with depressive illness is contained within the larger universe of those with depressive personalities, yet this model is so far unsupported by evidence.

The neurasthenic personality

The term was introduced by Beard (1880) to connote an irritable weakness. Such individuals are easily fatigued, and readily respond to minor stress by experiencing discomforts and pains. Janet (1908) was later to describe 'psychasthenia' as being due to a diminution in psychic energy, and to relate this to the experience of obsessional symptoms and phobias. Gruhle (1935) related psychasthenia to low self-esteem, self-distrust, and anxiety states; while neurasthenia was related to gloominess, constitutional depression, and hypochondriasis.

In Schneider's typology 'asthenic psychopaths' readily experience 'psychic inadequacy' and weakness, and are especially likely to become introspective about their bodily functions. 'Once the body has become the object of a fixed conscious interest, the normal smooth-running unconscious activity of the organism is interfered with and disturbance follows.' Such personalities are said to be liable to frequent depressions: 'these tend to rise spontaneously from the emotional depths of the personality or from a miscellany of bodily discomforts and this may bring on an increased depressive reaction. At other times an anxious reactive hypochondria is predominant'.

Since the concept of 'psychic inadequacy' is peculiarly reminiscent of the idea of psychopathic inferiority based upon degeneracy, interest in the concept of neurasthenia has waned since the Second World War. The term has been reserved for those non-specific disorders in which fatigue and exhaustion are prominent features and which tend to follow episodes of glandular fever, infectious hepatitis, or influenza. However, the work of Imboden and his colleagues (1961) used a prospective design to show that those most at risk of developing post-influenzal depression have abnormal scores on an MMPI scale measuring depression and the CMI when these were administered several months before the episode of influenza. A thirty-year follow-up study of 115 patients with personality disorders was reported by Tolle (1968) who showed that when patients originally diagnosed as asthenics were confronted with life crises 70 per cent of them responded with depressive episodes. Lundquist (1973) used the term asthenic personality in his study of alcoholics and showed that they were 'strongly inclined towards tension, depressive states and anxiety'.

There have been remarkably few systematic studies of asthenic personality. However, Standage (1979) has shown that it can be reliably diagnosed (Cohen's Kappa = 0.86); while Andrews, Kiloh, and Kehoe (1978) have confirmed this and have identified items of life history and psychometric tests which correlate with it. Condensation of these items by means of principal components analysis showed that two factors – anxiety proneness and inability to cope with stress – together defined the disorder. Eysenck's 'neuroticism' was highly loaded on the first of these factors, and correlated +0.35 with 'asthenic personality' in the raw data.

None of the studies reported so far provides conclusive evidence for supposing that asthenic personalities are at greater risk of depressive illness, since it is quite possible that such personalities are more likely to receive psychiatric care. If it were true that those with asthenic personalities were selectively referred, while those with relatively normal personalities were treated in primary care settings, then this would explain the clinical impression that many psychiatrists have that such personalities increase vulnerability to depressive illness. The research which conclusively demonstrates the importance of asthenic traits in increasing the vulnerability to psychiatric illness is that of Hagnell (1966), who carried out a prospective study of mental disorder over a period of 10 years in a total population of 2550 inhabitants in an area near Lund, Sweden. This population had been studied ten years earlier by Essen-Moller and his colleagues (Essen-Moller, 1956), who had carried out a full psychiatric evaluation on each inhabitant. Those who complained of habitual feelings of tension, fatigue, and nervousness in the original survey were said to display 'asthenia', and this was classified as 'early' if it took its onset in childhood, and 'late' if it took its onset in adult life. 'Late asthenia' was the only personality variable measured by Essen-Moller which was associated with a significantly higher expectancy of mental disorder developing over the next ten years in both men and women in Hagnell's study. For women only, early asthenia was also associated with an increased expectancy (Hagnell, 1966, table 32). It is not possible to use Hagnell's data to relate antecedent personality variables to the expectancy of developing depressive illnesses, since his data are not broken down by diagnosis. However, his study supports the view that those who develop minor 'asthenic' symptoms in early life are thereafter at greater risk of developing psychiatric illness and this finding is independent of the tendency of the individual to seek medical care for his symptoms.

The hysterical personality

The fact that introverted neurotic individuals are referred to as 'dysthymics' has tended to distract attention from the fact that extraverted neurotics – Eysenck's 'hysterics' – are also liable to develop depression in appropriate circumstances. It is a clinical commonplace that depression tends to accentuate the 'hysterical' personality features, so that such patients often appear more histrionic and manipulative than they do when well. Lazare and Klerman (1978) have described 'hysterical' depressions in 45 per cent of a series of depressed female in-patients who were shown to have certain behavioural patterns which distinguished them from non-hysterical depressives, and to have illnesses which were judged to be less severe. This group may represent the effect that Eysenck's extraversion, or Foulds's (1965) 'hysteroid personality' has on the epiphenomena of depression.

In terms of Sjöbring's classification of personality, 'subsolidity' refers to a cluster of traits that are thought to be associated with 'hysteric-primitive' reactions under stress. Hirschfeld and Klerman (1979) have administered Eysenck's MPI, the Mark-Nyman (Nyman, 1956) temperament scale and the Lazare-Klerman-Armor (Lazare *et al.*, 1966) trait scales to a population of depressed patients and shown a personality dimension which appears to correspond to the hysterical personality: extraverted and neurotic on the MPI, subsolid on the Mark-Nyman, and 'hysteria' on the last scale. (The same authors showed that Sjöbring's 'subvalidity' – which was intended as a measure of neurasthenia – appeared on the same dimension as 'oral personality' on the Lazar-Klerman-Armor scale, and 'dysthymic' on the Eysenck person-

ality inventory. The correlation between 'oral personality' and dysthymia has been demonstrated by Paykel and Prusoff (1973).)

However, although such studies provide compelling evidence that minor depressive reactions are not confined to those with 'dysthymic' or neurasthenic personalities, they cannot be used to show that hysterical traits increase the risk of minor depression in the general population. Hagnell's (1966) study bears directly on this problem in that ratings of personality using Sjöbring's classification of normal variants had been made on an entire population, and none of them, in contrast with Essen-Moller's asthenic symptoms could be related to a greater liability to mental illness over the next ten years. Thus personality variables may determine the form of a mental disorder if an individual breaks down, but they do not increase liability to breakdown. In Birnbaum's terminology, they are pathoplastic rather than pathogenic.

Eysenck's 'neuroticism' (N) (Eysenck, 1959) is perhaps the obvious candidate for the personality dimension which should be related to an increased vulnerability to develop neurotic symptoms under stress, but there is no direct evidence that it does so. Within the restricted universe of identified psychiatric patients however, Perris (1966) has shown that patients with reactive depression have higher 'N' scores than either bipolar depressives or normals; and Weissman, Prusoff and Klerman (1978) have shown that 'N' was the most important predictor of long-term outcome in a group of 150 female depressives. The problem with this particular scale is that it is an uneasy amalgam of longstanding traits and symptoms of illness: even when precautions are taken to minimize the effects of the latter it is a relatively unstable measure in depressed patients that tends to fall with clinical improvement (Hirschfeld & Klerman, 1979).

The importance of low self-esteem as an antecedent of depression

Low self-esteem is postulated as an antecedent of depressive illness by theorists writing from a wide variety of standpoints.

Gruhle (1935) saw self-esteem as one of seven basic psychic characteristics and held that low self-esteem was an antecedent of psychasthenia. Mendelson (1967) views neurotic depression as a manifestation of a breakdown in self-esteem, and reviews the diverse determinants of self-esteem from a largely psycho-analytic viewpoint. Positive self-esteem is ascribed to early parental influences and childhood experiences, and it is pointed out that negative aspects of the self-image tend to be repressed during periods of healthy adjustment. Decreased self-esteem can be traced back to Freud's formulation of the lost love object, while self-doubt and pessimism are component parts of the 'oral personality' already described. Foulds (1976) related states of depression to the personality measure of intropunitiveness, and draws attention to a 'deep underlying shame or a potentially catastrophic lowering of self-esteem'.

Cognitive theories of depression depend on a 'cognitive triad of negative views of self, one's surroundings and one's future (Beck 1974). An individual's self-concepts are clusters of attitudes derived from personal experience, identification with significant others, and attitudes of others towards him. Realistic self-concepts are thought to facilitate healthy adjustment, while those that deviate from reality make the individual vulnerable to psychological disorders. Negative judgements from others may reinforce negative attitudes towards the self, and if a cycle is set up negative concepts may become an enduring feature of an individual's cognitive organization. Such negative self-concepts may be latent during periods of healthy adjustment, but become activated by certain adverse life situations and result in a depressive illness. Thus, a broken marriage may activate the idea of irreversible loss that followed the death of a mother in childhood; a physical disease may activate the idea that life can never be happy; or failing an examination or losing a job may activate earlier self-concepts of inferiority or worthlessness.

Similarly, Brown and Harris (1978) writing from a sociological perspective, implicate self-esteem as a major variable determining whether a provoking agent will release a depressive illness, and identify low intimacy with husband and loss of mother before the age of 11 as 'vulnerability factors' related to low self-esteem. Foulds (1976) writes that 'self-esteem, like happiness, is not something to be sought consciously and directly, but is more appropriately a by-product of the successful exercise of social and perhaps occupational skills. Successful artists, craftsmen, parents, lovers and friends all have in common a deep concern for something other than themselves'.

5.1.3
Depressive reactions in adults

DAVID GOLDBERG

Introduction

The WHO Glossary (1978) gives 'depressive reaction' as an inclusion term for 'Neurotic depression' (300.4), which is defined as 'a neurotic disorder characterised by disproportionate depression which has usually recognisably ensued on a distressing experience; . . . there is often preoccupation with the psychic trauma which preceded the illness, e.g. loss of cherished person or possession. Anxiety is also frequently present and mixed states of anxiety and depression should be included here . . .'

This is an unsatisfactory definition. It is unhelpful to declare that those who suffer from minor affective illnesses are, by definition, neurotic; and we have seen in the previous section that there is in any case little evidence to support this assertion. Furthermore, many psychiatrists use this code for those minor depressive disorders which have not followed 'a distressing experience' and in which there is no 'preoccupation with psychic trauma'. Finally, it is often very difficult to say that depression following bereavement is 'disproportionate', although it is often relatively easy to say that a depressive syndrome following bereavement is persistent and impairing a patient's ability to function normally.

In practice, 'depressive reactions' refer to those depressive states which fall short of the diagnostic requirements for 'Affective psychoses' (296) but which are persistent and which are frequently accompanied by other features which distinguish them from transient mood swings experienced by most people in response to the vicissitudes of everyday life.

Slater and Roth (1977) neatly avoid the problems associated with the official definition, and state

The most notable feature is the mood change itself. The patient feels unhappy, unfit to cope with day-to-day affairs or to face the future, which seems a gloomy one. Lack of energy, difficulties in concentration, early and excessive fatigue and other neurasthenic symptoms are frequent. An endless circle of unpleasant thoughts goes round in his head, and he finds it difficult unaided to throw himself out of his preoccupations. Although his judgement of the future and of his own affairs is impaired by his consistent gloom, there is no tendency toward the formation of outspoken delusions.

Depressive reactions may therefore be defined as persistent states of pathological depression which is itself an intense, exaggerated form of sadness accompanied by symptoms such as anorexia, fatigue, insomnia, loss of sexual drive, loss of motivation, anhedonia, indecisiveness, and a negative self-concept. The diagnosis will therefore only be made where there is reason to suspect a disorder of psycho-biological equilibrium which goes well beyond a mood swing which is unaccompanied by other phenomena.

The distinction between depressive reactions and subclinical disorders

Since there is an unbroken continuum between those with minor, transient mood disorders on the one hand and those with profound melancholia on the other, the dividing line between 'normality' and 'illness' is arbitrary, but must take account of duration and extent of symptoms.

For example, a 'minor depression' according to the Research Diagnostic Criteria of Spitzer, Endicott and Robins (1978) must have a relatively persistent depressed mood which dominates the clinical picture or is coequal with anxiety; there must not be abnormalities which would allow more differentiated diagnoses to be made; the disorder must have lasted one week for a 'probable' or more than two weeks for a 'definite' diagnosis; and there must be at least two other symptoms from a list of 16 common depressive phenomena given to the rater.

The requirements for a 'Catego' diagnosis of neurotic depression are depressed mood with or without anxiety, together with 'certain other important symptoms' which permit a syndromal diagnosis. For example, depressed mood on its own is regarded as 'below threshold' according to Wing's 'Index of Definition', but depressed mood together with 10 or more 'non-specific neurotic symptoms' will qualify for a 'threshold disorder'. (Wing *et al.*, 1978; and see volume 3, chapter 16).

Beck (1967) carried out an intensive study of 966 psychiatric patients, and found the following 19 symptoms were between two and ten times as common among depressed as among non-depressed patients:

Emotional: sadness or apathy; crying spells; self-dislike; loss of gratification; loss of feelings of affection; loss of sense of humour.

Cognitive: negative self-concept; negative expectations; exaggerated view of problems; attribution of blame to self.

Motivational: increased dependency; loss of motivation; avoidance; indecisiveness; suicidal wishes.

Physical and vegetative: loss of appetite; sleep disturbance; fatiguability; loss of sexual interest.

The nosological status of depressive reactions

Opinion is divided between those who regard depressive reactions as a homogeneous clinical entity, and those who regard them as a residual classification to account for those depressive states which fall short of the requirement for a more elaborate diagnosis. Naturally, the homogeneity of a sample of depressive reactions depends on the decision rules that are used to establish the diagnosis: if it is diagnosed by exclusion of psychotic depression then the available evidence suggests that the remaining depressive states are heterogeneous.

Foulds (1973) argued that psychiatric illnesses are arranged in a hierarchy, with psychotic illnesses at the apex of the hierarchy, and 'dysthymic states' at the bottom: the relationship between the levels is said to be an inclusive one, so that patients with psychotic depression will also have symptoms of 'dysthymic states'. 'Dysthymic states' refer to emotional deviations from an individual's normal self, and include states of anxiety, depression, or elation. Surtees and Kendell (1979) have confirmed that this is so for over 90 per cent of patients with depression, although it is often untrue for patients with schizophrenia or mania. In an earlier paper, Kendell (1976) argues that the concept of 'endogenous/psychotic' depression is more soundly based than reactive/neurotic depression, and that the available evidence suggests that the latter are a heterogeneous group of depressive disorders. Kiloh and co-workers (1972) suggested that whereas the former was a disease entity with a biological basis, the latter was 'a diffuse entity encompassing some of the ways in which the patient utilises his defense mechanisms to cope with his own neuroticism and concurrent environmental stress'.

Several investigators have suggested rough groupings of such depressive illnesses. Paykel (1971) used cluster analysis to derive four groups of depressive illnesses, of which one corresponded to the classic descriptions of psychotic depression; the second was a group with mixed anxiety-depression, a high incidence of previous illnesses and high 'neuroticism' scores; the third group comprised depressives with a considerable element of hostility; while his fourth group contained young patients whose relatively mild illnesses developed on a background of personality disorder. The first three of these groups are very similar to those reported in an earlier study by Overall and co-workers (1966).

Incidence and prevalence

Weissman and Myers (1978) have recently shown that depressive symptoms as measured by self-report inventories are widely distributed among random community samples: between 10 per cent and 16 per cent of men, and 20 per cent and 24 percent of women, have high scores at a particular time. It is usual for more sophisticated measures of psychiatric case identification to report lower rates than these; thus Henderson and co-workers (1979) using the Present State Examination reports a prevalence of depression of 2.6 per cent for males, and 6.7 per cent for females in Canberra. These figures are remarkably similar to the 3.9 per cent for males and 7.4 per cent for females, reported by Wing (1980) in Camberwell. Both these investigators have grouped all depressive illnesses together, but in the latter study the illnesses were almost exclusively depressive reactions. Brown and Harris (1978), reported a somewhat higher figure for depression among Camberwell women; if borderline cases are ignored, the rate for depression was 14.8 per cent, of whom rather more than half had an onset in the previous year, so that the annual inception rate was 7.8 per cent. The latter figure is very much higher than the inception rates for depression reported by Hagnell (1966), possibly because the Camberwell investigators used a more

structured interview and only expected their subjects to remember their health over the previous year, thus ensuring a more complete inclusion of cases. Dr. Hagnell used a less structured approach and endeavoured to collect information concerning the previous ten years: the decennial inception rate for depression was 0.92 per cent for males, and 2.8 per cent for females.

Aetiology

There is no evidence that genetic factors make a specific contribution to the aetiology of reactive depression. Stenstedt (1966) showed that the expectancy of mental disorders among the relatives of probands with 'neurotic depression' was no different from that found among controls, and Bornstein and colleagues (1973) showed that those developing depression following bereavement do not have an increased expectancy of depression among first-degree relatives. Price (1968) studied 24 twin pairs in which the proband was suffering from reactive depression, and found no similar cases among the co-twins. Psychiatric illnesses other than reactive depression were found among 38 per cent of the MZ and 25 per cent of the DZ twins. Shields (1971) has shown that although there is disagreement between various twin studies about whether there is a higher MZ concordance for 'neuroticism' and 'psychoneurotic complaints' there is general agreement that traits variously described as 'self-confident', 'active', 'vigorous', and 'surgency' are strongly determined by genetic factors. The latter finding is of especial interest since such traits are the obverse of the neurasthenic traits described in the previous section (see chap. 5.1.2), and we have seen that those with neurasthenic traits are at higher risk of becoming ill. It is also worth noting that there is some evidence that genetic factors are important in anxiety states (Slater and Cowie, 1971; and see chap. 1.2.3, pp. 26–27), and that these states merge inextricably with depressive reactions among cases seen in community settings. Goldberg (1979) has shown that patients seen in primary care settings with minor disorders (mainly states of mixed anxiety-depression) have an increased expectancy of mental illness among their first degree relatives over normal controls. However, it seems likely that a general susceptibility to anxious and neurasthenic traits may be inherited rather than a specific predisposition to depressive reactions. In the previous chapter we have also seen that the available evidence suggests that premorbid personality type exerts a pathoplastic rather than a pathogenic effect on minor depressive illnesses (see chap. 5.1.2, pp. 197).

From a clinical standpoint, the three groups of factors which need to be considered in relation to the aetiology of a particular depressive reaction are loss events, physical illness, and stressful social circumstances. Although bereavement on its own produces a fairly clear-cut clinical syndrome, it must be appreciated that the various factors typically occur in combination with one another, with symptoms gradually developing in response to each factor until the individual reaches a state of depression which is unresponsive to normal homeostatic mechanisms.

Physical illness commonly makes a strong contribution to the development of depressive illness, and this is by no means confined to infections which are commonly followed by depressive syndromes, such as influenza, glandular fever, and infectious hepatitis. A common sequence is for a physical illness to take its onset during an episode of relatively mild dysphoric symptoms, and to be followed by a marked exacerbation of depressive phenomena. There would appear to be nothing specific about such physical illnesses, although it is true to say that they are commonly infective in nature. The first case example illustrates such a sequence.

Mrs A was a 47-year-old housewife coming to her family doctor for treatment of obesity. The family had to leave Yorkshire 18 months earlier because of her husband's job, and she had felt distressed at leaving a familiar environment and tense and unhappy in her London house. Two weeks after arriving she developed shingles, which was followed by post-herpetic neuralgia which only gradually cleared up. Her father's death six months earlier had 'nearly broken her heart', since they had been very close. Her mother developed carcinoma of the uterus shortly afterwards. The patient's husband worked longer hours in his new job and she saw much less of him. She felt tense and worried all the time, and ruminated about her father and wept continually. She began to avoid going out, feeling that people were looking at her, and talking about her behind her back. Gradually, her feelings became 'dead and numb'. Nothing worried her any more, because she 'no longer had feelings'. She blamed herself for being like this, and felt guilty and inferior to others. 'I'm letting people down, and not pulling my weight.' She asked her husband if there was anything wrong with her, since people seemed to look at her when they went out. In the week before her consultation her teenage daughter reported an illegitimate pregnancy but 'I'm too numb for it to matter'. She was treated with antidepressants and supportive psychotherapy and made a complete recovery which she attributed to the tablets and her faith in her doctor. 'He said he would get me right, and he did.' The vision of her father, which had been with her continually, had faded at six month follow-up. She

had become secretary of a voluntary organization, and felt better than she had done for years.

The first point to make about this case is that by no means all loss events involve bereavement: this patient also suffered loss of a familiar environment and the threatened future loss of her mother. The second point is that her physical illness took its onset when she was already experiencing dysphoric symptoms, and added severe neuralgic pain to her previous symptoms. This may well have increased her vulnerability to the severe depressive illness which followed her father's death. Finally, it should be noted that sensitive ideas of reference are quite commonly experienced by depressed patients although they usually do not mention them unless asked, for fear of being thought 'mad'.

The third group of factors – stressful social circumstances – are protean in their manifestations. Unsatisfactory living conditions, chronic illness in close relatives, and poor interpersonal relationships are recurring themes in individual case histories. As the next case history demonstrates, such factors interact with the factors already mentioned:

Mr B was a 43-year-old insurance agent, presenting to his family doctor with dyspepsia and depression. His wife had developed multiple sclerosis 14 years earlier, and at about the same time he had injured his back and had to give up his job as a master carpenter. His wife's disease had been slowly progressive, with incontinence for the past eight years, and paraplegia for the past seven. He divided his time between nursing her and keeping up with his job, but the latter had suffered for the previous two years. His wife nagged him continually, and was described as demanding and ungrateful. His usual backache had become worse twelve months before consultation, and he noticed a flatulent dyspepsia: for three months before his consultation he had been sleeping poorly and had developed symptoms of depression and anxiety. He experienced repeated episodes of severe sadness with listlessness and a feeling of constant tension. He ruminated continually about his wife, and would feel very guilty because of his angry thoughts that she should have committed suicide. At times he had periods of total despair.

His family doctor arranged a short period of hospital care for Mrs B and treated Mr B with antidepressants, advice on her management, and supportive psychotherapy. At six-month follow-up, he was greatly improved, although still clinically mildly depressed. 'I've pushed things aside, I've got to push on to the bitter end.' He had turned down a place in a permanent nursing home for his wife, because a relative had died there and it 'had memories'. He had taken his wife for a short holiday abroad, and was now solicitous about his wife's occasional suicidal ideas. She was no longer so critical of him: 'we come from a long line of kidders'. He still had occasional bouts of sadness, but they did not last so long and he no longer brooded about her so much: 'I have no feelings about the future – I can't have.'

In this case, the loss experiences are represented by the serious nature of his wife's illness and having to give up his job. The stressful social circumstances are the changes in his own life forced by his wife's illness with a gradual deterioration in interpersonal relationships in the years that were to follow. The exacerbation in his usual backache may possibly have been related to mechanical stress since he had to lift her, but his flatulent dyspepsia sounded functional, and was probably related to emotional stress. Once more, the addition of physical pain in the form of backache and dyspepsia caused a great deterioration in his mood state, so that by the time he sought help he had a marked depressive illness. It is noteworthy that this depression was susceptible to treatment despite the intractable nature of the environmental stress.

Recent research findings fit fairly well with these clinical impressions. The early studies showing an increased rate of stressful life-events before onset of depression (Paykel *et al.*, 1969; Brown *et al.*, 1973) have been followed by more detailed studies showing that the excess of life-events before depressive illnesses is largely accounted for by 'exit events'. Jacobs and colleagues (1974) describe such events as those which involve departures from the subject's social field, such as death, divorce, or family members leaving home; and they also implicate a variety of other events, such as interpersonal arguments. Brown and Harris (1978), in their study of Camberwell women, argue that the only life-events which have a causal role in the aetiology of depression are those involving long-term threat focused on the woman herself and that most of these 'severe' events involve loss. However, it is possible to develop depression without such an event; just as it is possible to experience such events and not become depressed. In the Brown and Harris study, for example, severe threat had been experienced in the previous 38 weeks by only 68 per cent of the onset cases of depression, and in 25 per cent of the 'normal' women. The investigators went on to show that their depressed women had a rate for 'major life difficulties' which was 3.3 times higher than the expectancy in that population. Eighty-three percent of the onset cases had *either* major difficulties *or* 'severe' life-events immediately prior to the onset of their depression, and these were termed 'provoking agents' for episodes of depression. However, since only a fifth of

women with such provoking agents present actually become depressed, it is necessary to invoke other factors to explain their vulnerability to depression. Four such factors were found: the absence of an intimate, confiding relationship with husband or boyfriend; unemployment; the presence of more than three children below the age of 14 at home; and loss of mother before the woman reached the age of eleven. It is argued that these factors are related to the long-term level of self-esteem among the women, and that the provoking agents exert their effects by causing a state of hopelessness and thus a catastrophic lowering of self-esteem eventuating in a clinical depression.

Brown and Harris did not attempt to measure the premorbid personality of their women, so that it is not known whether the 'subvalid' or 'neurasthenic' personality described in the previous section makes an additional contribution to their model, or whether such personality traits correlate with the presence of the vulnerability factors examined in their study.

Clinical features of depressive reactions

The clinical features of depression are dependent upon the age, sex, personality, and culture of the affected individuals. For example, self-cutting behaviour in the setting of depressed mood is more likely in younger patients with hysterical personality traits; crying is more frequent among depressed women than among depressed men; and it seems likely that depressive syndromes with predominantly neurasthenic symptoms are related to asthenic traits in the pre-morbid personality.

It must not be thought that only those with abnormal pre-morbid personalities are at risk of developing depressive reactions; indeed, Kerr and colleagues (1970) showed that those with such illnesses were similar to the general population in terms of extraversion, and had lower neuroticism scores. The form of depressive reaction which undoubtedly occurs in those with normal pre-morbid personality is that following bereavement, and this will be described separately, since it has some distinctive features and is perhaps the simplest form of such an illness.

Depressive reactions following bereavement

This illness is in many ways a good example of a depressive reaction as defined by WHO, in that it follows a psychic trauma and there is typically preoccupation with the lost person. Controlled studies have shown that bereavement is followed by an increased incidence of depressive and neurasthenic symptoms, including anorexia and weight loss, fatigue, poor sleep, indecisiveness, and poor concentration (Maddison, 1968; Parkes & Brown, 1972). A study by Clayton and her colleagues (1971) showed that a triad of depressed mood, disturbed sleep and crying was seen in more than half of their bereaved subjects, and just over a third met the St. Louis criteria for depression one month after the death. Depression following bereavement was as common among men as among women, but was more common among those who did not have children living nearby whom they considered close (Clayton *et al.*, 1971). A follow-up study (Bornstein *et al.*, 1973) showed that 15 per cent were still depressed 13 months after bereavement, and this group also reported four physical symptoms more commonly than the non-depressed group (general poor health; dizziness; blurred vision; and chest pain).

However, there are a number of interesting differences between depressive reactions following bereavement and other depressive illnesses. As Freud (1917) pointed out, there is typically no disturbance of self-esteem in the depression which may follow bereavement.

Depressive reactions to bereavement typically proceed through a series of stages (Parkes, 1970). The most frequent immediate reaction is a state of numbness which is sometimes preceded by a brief period of distress. Episodes of tearfulness are common during this stage, and there may be panic attacks. About five to seven days after death there is a sharp increase in affective symptoms, often with intense pining for the lost person. Preoccupation with thoughts of the deceased is described by Parkes as 'a central and pathognomic feature of grief. Without it grief cannot truly be said to have occurred and when present it is a sure sign that a person is grieving'. These experiences tend to be accompanied by crying, and a tendency to concentrate on aspects of the environment which are associated with the lost person: in extreme form there may even be searching behaviour.

There are wide variations between individuals in the time course of events. Parkes describes a group of widows who were severely disturbed in the first week and thereafter gradually improved over the next three months; a group with a moderate distress in the first week, more in the second, and thereafter a decline; while a third group expressed little or no

distress in the first two weeks but a steady increase therafter so that most were depressed by the end of the third month. He observes that for the whole group there was a significant negative correlation between overall distress in the first week and that in the third month.

Mrs C was a 78-year-old housekeeper whose husband had died when she was a young woman, and who had looked after her employer, Mr. D, for 48 years until his death six months before her consultation with her general practitioner. She had nursed Mr D in his last illness, and his death was the greatest grief in her life. They had cared for the garden and greenhouse together, and she would rub embrocation into his back after his wife had gone to bed. She wept a good deal after his death, and spent much of her time painfully preoccupied with thoughts of Mr D. She had difficulty getting to sleep and felt constantly tired, and developed irritability with Mrs D that was quite unlike her. Later she began to feel guilty because she had not realized that Mr D was so ill, and had not done even more for him while he was alive. She worried about her ability to care for Mrs D in the future and sought medical help for her feelings of depression. She was treated with antidepressants and supportive psychotherapy, and was symptom-free six months later. She attributed her improvement to the tablets and to the passage of time, and getting it into her mind that she has to do things on her own that they had done together before. 'Being north country we don't like to speak of our feelings: but talking to the doctor about them did help a lot'.

Perhaps because the depression following bereavement is so readily 'understandable' there is no increase in the rate of use of psychiatric services, although there is an increased rate of visits to family doctors and a corresponding increase in prescriptions for sedatives and tranquillizers. Most bereaved people do not seek professional help, but work out their own ways for dealing with their stress experiences.

The case examples given earlier in the chapter will have served to illustrate that the majority of depressive reactions do not conform to this simple pattern. Although there are innumerable combinations of the various symptoms, they may be considered in greater detail under the headings proposed by Beck (1967) that were given at the onset.

Emotional changes

In the early stages of a depressive illness the individual may notice that he no longer derives pleasure from life: this *anhedonia* may precede the experience of sadness and unhappiness. The central feature of a depressive reaction must necessarily be such a mood change, with any cognitive* changes being derived from it. Thus Lewis (1956) writes: 'The mood is one of grief and misery, looking in every direction for material to feed on. The past supplies peccadilloes or graver lapses; what is wretched in the present is dwelt on inordinately; the future is foreseen as hopeless ruin'. The sadness is commonly accompanied by crying spells, although some patients report that they feel like crying but are unable to do so. Sense of humour is often lost in that, although the patient still sees the point of a joke, he no longer finds it funny. Similarly, there may be a diminution in feelings of affection for those close to the patient. Feelings of anxiety and irritability are common in minor depressive illness but not themselves diagnostic of it: the relationship between the two will be considered later.

Cognitive changes*

These include feelings of self-dislike and self-blame with an exaggerated assessment of problems, and feelings of hopelessness concerning the future. It is always essential to explore the patient's self-concept in the assessment of depression; asking how the patient compares himself with others, and whether he blames himself for his present state. Depressed women may complain that they are ugly, or say that they find their bodies repulsive. Finally, there may be difficulties in making decisions, either, because of a lack of confidence in one's ability to make the right decisions or because of subjective difficulty thinking through the consequences of alternative plans of action.

Motivational changes

It is here that the overlap between depressive and neurasthenic syndromes is most evident. Low energy, fatigue, apathy, and inability to concentrate is seen in both conditions; but whereas the depressed mood is presumably secondary to the neurasthenic symptoms in the syndromes which follow attacks of systemic disease such as influenza or brucellosis, a mood change may also have effects upon motivation. Depressed patients tend to escape responsibility and to avoid demanding tasks. They may do this because their usual tasks seem boring or meaningless, or because they lack confidence to make the right deci-

*In this chapter the expression 'cognitive changes' refers to changes in thinking which are secondary to an alteration of mood and reflect its quality. The expression differs therefore from 'cognitive state' (see vol. 2) which includes the functions of orientation, attention and concentration, memory, general information, intelligence and so forth.

sions. They are often said to be 'dependent' because they become willing to allow others to take over responsibility for giving them guidance.

Neurovegetative changes

These include disturbances in appetite, sleep rhythmn, libido, energy level, and posture. Depressed mood may influence the way the patient speaks, walks and sits. In minor depressive illnesses an increased appetite with a consequent gain in weight is almost as common as anorexia and weight loss. There is a diminution of sexual interest and a reduction in energy level. Sleep is hard to come by, light, and unrefreshing. Emotional energy no longer flows outward to the world of other people and events, and the patient becomes lost in miserable self-absorption with his own discomforts. In this way the patient often presents to his doctor with headache, backache, or other pain, and the doctor may be so distracted by these physical symptoms that the depressive syndrome of which they are part passes unrecognized.

The relationship between anxiety and depression

There is no longer any doubt that there is a strong correlation between the symptom of anxiety and that of depression (Carroll et al., 1973; Goldberg et al., 1976; Wing, 1980) and that depressed mood is a common secondary phenomenon in anxiety states, just as anxiety and tension are commonly seen in patients with depressive reactions (Klerman, 1977; Roth et al., 1972). There is still disagreement between those who regard the various minor affective disorders as overlapping syndromes which merge inextricably with one another (Ey, 1963; Lewis, 1956) and those who regard anxiety states and depressive syndromes as fundamentally different syndromes (Roth et al., 1972).

Protagonists of the former view concede that pure cases of reactive depression, anxiety states and hypomanic syndromes occur, but consider that there is so much overlap between the syndromes that fastidious discriminations between them are futile.

Furthermore, if one studies minor affective disorders in a primary care setting, mixtures of anxiety and depression are more common than either pure depression syndromes or typical anxiety states (Goldberg & Huxley, 1980). Roth and his colleagues (1972) have argued that depressions are distinct from anxiety states in a study in which they carried out a principal components analysis on a group of patients admitted to hospital with diagnoses of either depression or anxiety states. The investigators found that their first component accounted for 14 per cent of the total variance, with items traditionally associated with anxiety clustered at the end, and items suggesting depression clustered at the other. However, since the latter items included early waking, diurnal variation of mood, psychomotor retardation, delusions, and hypomanic episodes, it seems likely that this dimension reflects major depression versus other affective disorders rather than depressive reactions versus anxiety state. Although these data are often held to justify a distinction between depressive illness and anxiety states, they would appear to be irrelevant to the present problem. Downing and Rickels (1974) used discriminant function techniques to distinguish between those minor affective disorders that had been selected for anxiolytic drugs and those selected for antidepressant drugs in trials carried out in a primary care setting. Anxiety and depression dominated the symptom profiles of all patients, but in the trials of anxiolytic drugs anxiety tended to be more severe, while the reverse held true for the antidepressants. Insomnia was the only symptom which increased the discrimination between the two groups beyond that obtained by considering only the ratings of anxiety or depression; it is worth emphasizing that phobia-obsessions, somatic over-concern, somatic symptom formation and appetite disturbance score did not differ significantly between the groups, or contribute in any way to the discriminant function separating the groups. There seems no doubt that there is a substantial overlap between the syndromes of anxiety state and depressive reaction, and the available evidence does not support a separatist model. It seems reasonable to confine the diagnosis of anxiety states to those minor affective disorders where any depression is either very much less than anxiety-related symptoms, or is clearly secondary to such symptoms. The diagnosis of depressive reaction will be made in all those cases where there is significant depressive symptom formation, irrespective of the severity of anxiety-related symptomatology.

Management and treatment

Provided that the patient can be prevented from committing suicide, the majority of depressive reactions presenting to doctors will improve, either because of, or despite, the treatment offered. We will therefore first consider the management of the suicidal patient, and then go on to consider various aspects of treatment.

Suicidal threats

It is not true that 'those who talk about suicide never do it': a substantial majority of those who commit suicide have communicated their intentions to others beforehand (Robins *et al.*, 1959; Schneidman & Farberon, 1957), and approximately 10 per cent of those who attempt suicide will eventually carry it out (Kessel, 1971; Schmidt *et al.*, 1954). The assessment of suicidal risk therefore becomes an important matter for the clinician.

Before considering the details of the patient's clinical state, some general points deserve mention. The risk of suicide is greater with advancing age, where there is a previous history of attempted suicide or a family history of suicide, where there is associated alcoholism or drug addiction, and is somewhat greater for men than for women. Social isolation, unemployment, and sudden financial difficulties will all increase the risk. It is important to make a thorough assessment of the severity of the patient's depression, since the risk is particularly high where psychotic depressive phenomena are present. It is important to elicit the patient's beliefs about his physical health: the risk is increased when a previously healthy man develops a serious physical disease, just as it is in the presence of delusional ideas about health.

One should next establish the extent to which the patient has been preoccupied with ideas of suicide, and whether any concrete steps have been actually carried out. Has the patient decided when, where, and how? A serious view should be taken of plans which involve a painful method such as hanging or swallowing disinfectant; or one which is likely to be successful, such as shooting or jumping from a high building. Have materials been specially obtained? If the patient intends to take an overdose, has he handled the bottle, or tipped the tablets out and looked at them? If it turns out that some of these events have occurred, then what has so far prevented the patient from carrying out his plans? If the patient is to be allowed to go home, one must consider the environment to which he will return. Has the patient anyone with whom he can confide? Will he be under surveillance from others? Is he prepared to give an undertaking that he will not harm himself before his next appointment?

There is no evidence that asking about suicide

increases the likelihood of an attempt: on the contrary, many patients report relief of feelings of anxiety and guilt after they have had such a discussion. It would be quite impracticable if all those who had contemplated suicide were referred to psychiatrists: the assessment of risk must be part of the skill of every family doctor, and patients should only be referred if there is doubt about the assessment or if the risk is judged to be real.

Non-specific aspects of treatment

It is worth asking why patients who receive placebos in double-blind drug trials of depressive reactions treated in community settings do as well as they do. It is likely that such populations contain a substantial proportion of patients whose illnesses would have remitted spontaneously, but it must be remembered that there are a number of non-specific factors which will promote resolution of depressive illnesses among those who put themselves under medical care. The doctor's confidence that he can help the patient – whether based on his own psychotherapeutic powers or his faith in the contents of his pills – promotes hope, and with it an expectancy that improvement will occur. By his offer of return visits he effectively offers to monitor the patient's return to effective social functioning and makes the patient feel that he has a powerful ally, and thus the way becomes clearer for the resolution of both hopelessness and helplessness. The doctor's power to remove social and occupational obligations may allow the patient to rest without a sense of failure; and if sleep can be restored to the patient there is often a considerable improvement in any neurasthenic component to his symptoms. In practice, most patients who have their depressive illnesses detected by their doctors will be given antidepressant drugs, and these provide two further non-pharmacological reasons for improvement. The prediction that 'improvement will occur in 10–14 days' promotes a strong expectancy that improvement will indeed occur, and is in the best traditions of shamans and faith healers. Secondly, the side effects of the drugs provide a constant reminder that the patient is receiving a real drug and not a placebo, and this knowledge is likely to increase greatly the placebo effect since most patients have a strong belief in the power of scientific medicine.

Specific pharmacological treatment

We will not be concerned with an account of the specific effects of antidepressants, and the inter-ested reader is referred to volume 3, especially chapters 25 and 26. It is worth noting that if the decision to prescribe an antidepressant is made, compliance will be very much greater if the doctor anticipates possible side effects, predicts the likely duration of treatment, and explains that the drug will not produce dependence and that cessation of treatment will be an easy matter when the time comes. The clinician is well advised to stick to a few antidepressant drugs so that familiarity is gained with their side effects. If anxiety and insomnia are marked, a sedating antidepressant such as amitriptyline given in a single dose at night is advisable; while if anergia and fatigue are prominent a less sedating antidepressant such as dothiepin may be used in divided doses. There are wide variations between individuals in the extent to which these drugs are absorbed by the gut, and also in ability to tolerate the various side effects. It is therefore a good plan to start with a fairly low dose with an out-patient, and to reassess the patient after a few days and to increase the dose if the drug is well tolerated. In the absence of facilities for measuring levels of drug in the blood, most clinicians will increase the dose if the patient is neither feeling any better nor experiencing side effects.

Specific psychological treatments

It is usual to discover that reactive depression is in an understandable relationship to the patient's life situation or the way in which he handles his interpersonal relationships. It is therefore advisable to take the opportunity of a series of sessions to secure improvements in one or the other of these. It is certainly unhelpful to spend the session endlessly discussing the patient's symptoms, and most prefer to discuss constructive improvements which might be made to the patient's life style, or modifications which should be made in the way in which the patient habitually responds to other people. The research group headed by Klerman and his colleagues (1979) have formalized the way in which such sessions should be conducted, and produced a training manual for clinicians. 'Interpersonal psychotherapy' or 'IPT', consists of approximately 12 weekly sessions for ambulatory depressed patients focused on improving the quality of current interpersonal functioning. The treatment can be carried out by doctors, psychologists, or social workers, and consists of detailed instructions to guide the therapist in his conduct of a session, as well as various techniques for increasing communication, encouraging the expression of affect, use of directive techniques, use of role playing and the setting up of a therapeutic contract. Weissman and her colleagues (1979) have claimed that a combination of an antidepressant and IPT is more effective than either treatment on its own.

In contrast to the more general set of techniques used in IPT Beck's (1976) 'cognitive therapy' for depression is based upon cognitive psychology, and uses behavioural techniques in a frontal assault on some of the self-defeating strategies and unflattering self-concepts typically seen among depressed patients. The negative thoughts the patient holds about himself, his world and his future are held to be a 'cognitive triad', and the therapist and patient work together to identify these negative thoughts and subject them to logical analysis and empirical testing. The cognitive therapist has four tasks: (1) to help the patient appreciate the connections between thoughts, feelings and behaviour; (2) to encourage the patient to monitor his negative thoughts; (3) to examine the evidence for and against these thoughts; and finally (4) to substitute more reality-orientated interpretations for his negative thoughts. The patient is encouraged to keep a diary in which he records activities which are pleasant and those which are associated with a sense of mastery. Rush and colleagues (1977) have claimed that cognitive therapy is equally effective as imipramine in the short-term management of depressed out-patients, and that the improvement is better maintained at six-month follow-up.

Two methods of dealing with grief are reminiscent of Beck's 'cognitive therapy' for depression; the first is the inhibition of painful thoughts by actively avoiding reminders of the deceased, 'selective forgetting', and idealization; while the second is the active evocation of pleasant, or at least neutral, thoughts. In contrast, Lieberman (1978) has described a procedure called 'forced mourning' in which the patient is encouraged to express strong feelings as the therapist explores his relationship with the deceased. Objects which have been avoided, such as photographs or items of jewellery are brought into sessions and discussed. In a final stage the patient reviews both the positive and negative side of his relationship with the deceased, puts aside avoidance behaviour and develops new relationships.

Indications for admission to hospital

If it is thought that the patient is morbidly depressed and there is a risk of suicide with out-patient treatment, the patient should be offered admission to hospital. Most patients accept voluntary admission if time can be spent answering their questions about the hospital, the treatment they are likely to receive, and the probable duration of the stay in hospital. If the patient is reluctant to agree to admission yet there is reason to suspect that he or she intends suicide the situation should be discussed with his or her nearest relative, the risks explained, and another attempt made to secure the patient's agreement to enter hospital. If such agreement cannot be obtained then under English law the relative (or a local authority social worker) should be invited to make application for compulsory admission to hospital under the 1959 Mental Health Act (see chapter 3.5.2).

Prognosis

The concept of a depressive 'reaction' caused by a particular psychic trauma carries with it the implication that after a time homeostasis will occur, and the patient will eventually improve whether or not he has treatment. This is yet another reason for disapproving of the official WHO definition, since minor depressive states are frequently chronic and associated with disadvantageous life situations rather than isolated traumatic events. In such illnesses resolution may not occur spontaneously and indeed they sometimes persist despite the exhibition of psychological, pharmacological, and social treatments. However, the more closely an illness resembles the official definition the more likely it is to resolve spontaneously. We have already seen that depressive reactions following bereavement are very common, but that there is no increase in the rate for referral for psychiatric treatment, and that the majority of the illnesses will have resolved a year after the loss.

Akiskal and colleagues (1978) followed up a group of 100 patients with reactive depression over a period of 3 – 4 years, and showed that those who had recurrent episodes of illness suffered from a wide range of illnesses: 18 had episodes of mania, and over three quarters were not suffering from pure depressive illnesses during the follow-up period. A 'characterological' component was detected at outset in 24 per cent of the patients, and was associated with a poor outcome: 79 per cent of this group have an unfavourable outcome, compared to only 11 per cent of those without such a component. The three suicides in the study all occurred in the 'characterological' group. Patients in this group were described by epithets such as 'pathologically dependent', 'highly manipulative' or 'unstable'; they tended to have hostile depressive outbursts with dramatic behaviour and impulsive suicidal attempts. The authors concluded that patients diagnosed as depressive reactions are a heterogeneous group, and observe that the fact that some patients change from 'neurotic' illness to 'psychotic' illnesses during follow-up challenge the very basis of a simple dichotomy between neurotic and psychotic illnesses.

5.1.4
The impact of depressed parents on their children
SULA WOLFF

Epidemiological findings
Other sections of this volume report on the association between psychiatric disorder in parents and children (Rutter, 1966; Rutter *et al.*, 1970). This association is greatest for pre-school children (Rutter, 1966; Richman, 1977) (see p. 142) and when the mother is the affected parent (Wolff and Acton, 1968; Richman, 1977). Brown and his colleagues (1975) established that working-class women with children under 6 have high rates of depression, often following a stressful event and chronic life difficulties. Four vulnerability factors were found: lack of a confiding relationship with husband or boy friend, having three or more children under 14, not going out to work, and having lost their own mother before the age of 11. The first three may reflect long standing personality difficulties rather than extraneous causes.

Brice Pitt (1975) found that over ten per cent of mothers suffer from puerperal depression after returning home from hospital with their baby. Of these half recovered within a few months while the rest (about four per cent) continued to be irritable, tired, depressed, with loss of sexual and other interests for over a year.

Weissman, Paykel & Klerman (1972) studied the mothering behaviour of 35 acutely depressed women aged 25–60 years. Their scores on a social adjustment scale showed that, in comparison with a matched control group, they lacked emotional involvement with their children, were impaired in their communications, less affectionate and more hostile and resentful. The clinical impression was that their maternal behaviour and the children's responses differed with the age of the children. The depressed mothers of three infants were helpless and either over-concerned or overtly hostile. Mothers of school-age children were irritable, uninvolved, and intolerant of their children's boisterousness. Adolescent children were most overtly disturbed, at times delinquent, in response to their mothers' hostility and emotional withdrawal.

The nature of the association between parental depressive illness and disturbance in the child is complex, variable, and interactional. Maternal depression can itself be precipitated by a child's difficult temperament (Wolkind, 1982). Children in turn react with disturbed behaviour to parental ill health. Moreover, personality disorders predisposing mothers to develop depressive illnesses will contribute also to their children's vulnerability.

General psychiatrists see only a small proportion of depressed patients and it is probable that parental depression and childhood disturbance are often not revealed even to the family doctor. Child and adolescent psychiatrists must be alert to the possibility of depressive illnesses in parents, especially mothers, and general psychiatrists should give consideration to the children of those of their depressed patients who are also parents. Moreover, it is likely that puerperal depression is an important cause for failure of bonding with the painful awareness on the mother's part that her feelings for a particular child are not as they should be.

In a recent study, an excess of psychiatric disorders was found in 3-year-old children whose mothers had been depressed 3 months post-partum, compared with children whose mothers had not been depressed at that time (Wrate *et al.*, 1983).

(i) Depression in association with personality disorder, marital strife and socio-economic privation

Perhaps the commonest circumstances in which child psychiatrists encounter depressed parents, especially mothers, are when a child is referred with a conduct disorder, one or both parents have a history of gross childhood deprivations, there are marital tensions, financial hardship, sometimes excessive drinking, sometimes suicide attempts, and in addition the parents are struggling to bring up a number of closely spaced young children. Unless the depression is severe, general psychiatrists are often more impressed with the parent's personality disturbance or the social pathology of the family and indeed these are the major obstacles to improvement of family functioning. Yet even a mild depressive illness in a young mother can make all the difference between coping and not coping, and its effective treatment can greatly improve the quality of care she can give her children. Most depressed parents are irritable. Some begin drinking excessively. Others take fateful actions they later regret, such as abandoning husband and children or entering into extra-marital relationships. Children will be relieved if they can understand that they have not caused their mother's illness.

The Smith* family were first seen when the mother was 27, the father 31, George 8, Martin 5, and David 3½. The *referral of George* took place during the mother's depressive illness after the spontaneous abortion of a female infant at six months. After David's birth the mother attempted suicide and was in hospital for six months with a serious depression, being treated with medication and then ECT. George was with foster parents, the younger two in a children's home. When the family reunited the mother found George, then 5, disobedient and unhappy. His recurrent stealing then began.

The maternal grandparents had separated in the *mother's* infancy and she was reared in a children's home. At 18 she became pregnant with George and left the home to marry the father. She was later on good terms with her own father who had remarried. She was frigid throughout her marriage. From her children she expected more controls than they could manage. Although attached to them, she could not show her affection openly and she was often irritable. The *father*, a brewery worker, had been in prison for assault. He was violent to his wife when drunk, the children witnessing many fights between the parents. He looked after the children while the mother did an evening job, and only years later she guiltily revealed her knowledge of his apparently playful but quite frightening physical aggression towards the boys.

George, very inhibited, was preoccupied with illness and with his own helpfulness about the house. He said 'when your mum's ill, you have to be very good because noise makes her worse and my wee brothers make a lot of noise. I tell them to stop it. They take their toys out and I put the toys back and do the housework . . . If they have arguments in the living-room, they tell us to wait in the kitchen and one day my mum was crying and I told her not to worry but she was still crying and that . . . When my brothers get lost, I look for them.' George, like his brothers, was afraid of monsters at night. He went on to say 'my mummy had a girl and when she got it, it was dead. That's when she went into the hospital. Because we've all got boys and my dad calls me girls' names for fun. He says he's just playing.'

Unlike George, the younger boys were disinhibited, impulsive, noisy and over-active. David, born after a diffi-

*The name Smith is fictitious.

cult delivery, displayed a lack of concentration and serious specific learning difficulties which persisted into his middle teens and were thought to be constitutional, the result of mild birth injury.

All the boys stole intermittently from inside and outside their home. The violent marriage continued, as did the mother's recurrent depressions and hospitalizations. She was often suicidal and once wandered the streets in a state of clouded consciousness, carrying a knife, thinking she was about to stab someone or herself.

Finally, when George was 12, the parents separated. The younger boys were in one children's home, George in another, the father in lodgings and the mother either in hospital or alone at home. When at home the mother greatly relied on George for help but also upbraided him for minor misdeeds. The father used George as a go-between in attempts to re-establish his marriage. George remained an inhibited, solitary boy, covertly aggressive to his siblings and over-involved with his mother. When she finally remarried she saw him, then 19, engaged and working, as coming between herself and her new husband and 'threw him out' for not helping enough in the house.

The *mother* remarried a patient she had met in hospital and when seen again aged 38, she, now matronly in appearance, and her husband presented as an affectionate and stable couple, both working and providing much more sensitive affection for the younger two boys. These were still in care, Martin with good social and educational adjustment but David still severely retarded educationally and at times dangerously impulsive, frequently playing with matches and once setting a wardrobe alight.

The mother's personality improvement and her recovery from depressive illnesses occurred too late to protect her children from repeated admissions into care and a childhood distorted by violence, threats, and unrealistic demands for early maturity. Whether this mother was able to effect a reconciliation with her oldest boy, which was certainly suggested to her, is not yet known.

(ii) Parental depression and childhood handicap

Many parental depressions are precipitated by their children's handicap, but then in turn affect the handicapped child's behaviour as well as the home atmosphere for the rest of the family.

Mrs Brown, 27, an intelligent and conscientious housewife and mother, had always felt her own needs for mothering had not been met. Her father, reared in an orphanage, was in the Army; her youthful mother led an active social life unaware of the needs of her competent daughter. In late adolescence Mrs Brown left home and married an older Army officer. Despite his supportive understanding, she often wished she had had more time to enjoy freedom in adolescence and had, like her friends, acquired an education. The oldest son, John, developed serious early childhood autism after a squint operation at 14 months. Because of the family's Army postings the maternal grandmother looked after him warmly and conscientiously for four years, during which two further sons were born. The family functioned well until a planned change of educational placement for John, now 8, of which the grandmother disapproved, from special day-to weekly boarding-school became imminent. The father was due for an overseas posting and Mrs Brown became increasingly disappointed at her mother's lack of empathic understanding for herself.

She became depressed and self-accusatory. John, not previously difficult, became noisy and over-active at home, disrupting all conversations. When the children then developed mumps, Mrs Brown began to feel hopeless, unable to enjoy anything, waking in the small hours, and with thoughts of leaving the family and suicide in her mind. What distressed her especially was her loss of enjoyment of, and affection for, the younger children and her quite punitive reactions to them which were out of character. She maintained her usual impeccable appearance and a smiling facade as her self-confidence declined.

Anti-depressants were only slowly effective, she refused a hospital admission for herself, and in the weeks before her recovery, despite much support from her husband, a hospital admission for John, and nursery school placements for both younger children, she engaged in a number of self-destructive acts which perplexed her.

She omitted her contraceptive pills and became pregnant. She left her best handbag containing money and valuables, together with two full shopping bags, at a bus stop as she mounted a bus. Finally, she was caught shop-lifting from a department store. It required psychiatric initiative not only to arrange a termination of pregnancy but also to persuade the Army authorities to defer the father's posting until his wife had recovered, and to certify for the court that the offence had been committed while Mrs Brown's mind was disturbed by illness. In the event the charge was dropped. Mrs Brown did not accept regular psychiatric treatment until her father had a heart attack. She then revealed for the first time ever her father's incestuous approaches to her in childhood and her husband's promiscuity.

(iii) Family catastrophes associated with parental depression

Rare but with more far reaching consequences for the children are the catastrophes occasionally precipitated by parental depression. These disasters are the more tragic because theoretically preventable.

Infanticide is a well known risk of psychotic depression in the puerperium. *Child abuse,* taking the form of *non-accidental injury* or *neglect,* can also, although rarely, occur in the setting of a psychotic depression. Sometimes such mothers present their child spontaneously and repeatedly to the doctor with vague complaints and are very distressed by their feelings that something is wrong with the child and by their awareness of their own lack of affectionate responsiveness or even hatred of their baby. These are the most rewarding cases of non-accidental injury to treat since the mother's personality is often quite adequate and, once recovered, she can provide good child care. It is disturbing that the majority of cases of suspected child injury or neglect are not referred to a psychiatrist (often because they do not have appropriate treatment resources) and are dealt with by paediatricians, social workers, and family doctors, who may fail to make a diagnosis of depression and provide appropriate treatment.

Parental suicide of course has far reaching effects on children but, in child psychiatric practice, more common and more damaging for the children's future self-image, is the *murder of one parent by another*. This very occasionally occurs when the murderous parent is psychotically depressed, and the children may then be objects of attack also. More commonly, murder occurs during episodes of neurotic depression, perhaps with associated alcohol intake, in parents with long-standing personality disorders and in conflict with each other. The child in consequence loses both parents: one dying and the other going to prison. The burdens on grandparents are then often very heavy indeed, especially since they themselves are still struggling with the emotions engendered by a highly traumatic bereavement.

Incestuous behaviour by fathers towards their daughters, which may be totally out of character, also occasionally occurs when the father is clinically depressed. The depression often follows some physical disability and/or unemployment and the incestuous approach is often made under the influence of alcohol.

Suggestions for management

To minimize the harmful effects of parental depression on children, five points must be borne in mind.

(1) *The effect of the illness*, its antecedents, and its consequences on the other parent and on the children need to be considered.

(2) If admission, especially of a sick mother is necessary, the *practical care arrangements* for the children must be reviewed. There should be facilities for the admission of young children to hospital together with their mothers and for all children to visit their parents in hospital under pleasant, child-oriented conditions and with staff available to participate in these encounters. Fathers may need social work help to plan for adequate care arrangements for those children not admitted to hospital with their mother.

(3) *The personality strengths of the healthy parent* need to be assessed and a discussion should take place with him, together with the mother if she is well enough, about the children's reactions to her changed behaviour and to the hospital admission. Parents may need help to understand how young children perceive parental illness and its consequences, to enable the children to voice their anxieties and to provide reassuring explanations.

(4) If neither parent is able to manage this alone, a *joint interview together with all the children* and the parent or parents (provided they are functioning well enough for such a meeting) may be helpful to explore the children's reactions and provide support for them.

(5) Such a meeting may also be very helpful as a basis for *communicating about the special needs of the children during their parents' illness* with other agencies already involved or potentially helpful, such as social services departments, the children's schools or nurseries, and of course the family doctor.

5.2
Anxiety neurosis

5.2.1
Anxiety and phobic disorders, depersonalization, and derealization

M. G. GELDER

Anxiety neurosis

This section is concerned with the syndrome known as anxiety neurosis, anxiety state, or anxiety reaction. It does not deal with the normal emotion of anxiety, nor with the symptom of anxiety which occurs in many kinds of mental disorder; those issues are considered in the section on psychopathology (vol. 1, chaps. 3 and 4). It can be argued that it is rather arbitrary to separate anxiety neurosis from the features of personality which predispose to the development of anxiety symptoms. And it is true that even if the distinction is recognized, it is not easy to define the boundaries of the syndrome clearly – a fact which is reflected in the difficulties in collecting reliable data on the incidence of the syndrome. Despite this, there are good reasons for separating a syndrome of anxiety neurosis: first, many different kinds of personality can predispose to the same group of anxiety symptoms; secondly, treatment is discussed more easily if the distinction is made; and thirdly, the relationship of anxiety and depressive states can be examined more fruitfully.

The syndrome

The idea that anxiety symptoms occur, as the primary feature of mental disorder, often enough to justify the recognition of a separate anxiety syndrome, did not appear until near the end of the nineteenth century. Up to that time, they were encompassed by the syndrome of neurasthenia which had been described by Beard (1880). It was Freud (1895a, b) who suggested the term anxiety neurosis for a subgroup of neurasthenic patients in whom all the clinical features appeared to be related to the central prominent symptom of anxiety. (In fact, the idea, but not the terminology had, as Freud acknowledged, been expressed two years before by Hecker.) Although the clear description which Freud gives in this paper makes it one of the classics of the psychiatric literature, it was some years before the syndrome of anxiety neurosis became widely accepted. Indeed in the First World War, the majority of patients who would now be regarded as presenting with cardiac and respiratory symptoms of anxiety neurosis were diagnosed as suffering from 'irritable heart'. Today the diagnosis of anxiety neurosis is used frequently – so frequently, indeed, that it has lost some of its precision by being applied to patients whose symptoms of anxiety are accompanied by quite prominent obsessions, phobias, or depression. This is not good practice: it is better to restrict the term to cases in which anxiety symptoms make up the whole, or almost the whole, of the clinical picture and to classify these other cases as mixed neurotic disorders.

There is another group of patients, included by Freud in his original description of anxiety neurosis, but who are better considered separately, namely patients with prominent phobic symptoms. Freud later assigned them to his group of anxiety hysterias, and nowadays such cases are classified as phobic anxiety states. They are described on pages 218–23. Recently it has been suggested that another group of anxious patients should be split off from the syndrome of anxiety neurosis. Klein (1964) suggested that anxiety attacks ('panic attacks') should form the central feature of a new grouping. Now to be of value to the clinician a syndrome should help him to decide about treatment or prognosis, and Klein claims that his syndrome is differentially responsive to the tricyclic antidepressant drug imipramine. This claim needs confirmation by other investigators before the established syndrome of anxiety neurosis is broken up in this way, even though the group has been included in the 3rd edition of the American Psychiatric Association's diagnostic manual (DSM III).

Some psychiatrists follow Lewis (1966) in arguing that there is no clear dividing line between anxiety neuroses and depressive disorders, and that pure states of anxiety are much less common than mixed states of anxiety and depression. While this is true of the less severe forms of anxiety and depressive disorders encountered in general practice, it is usually possible to make a distinction when the disorders are more severe. This point of view is supported by a detailed statistical analysis carried out by Roth, Carney, Garside and Kerr (1972). Moreover these authors showed that the prognosis of anxiety neuroses is in general less good than that of depressive disorders (Schapira, Roth, Kerr & Gurney, 1972) which also indicates that the distinction is worth making.

Although anxiety neuroses are encountered frequently, it is not possible to give precise figures about their incidence or prevalence because uniform distinctions have not been made either between anxiety neuroses and anxiety symptoms reported by normal people, or between anxiety neuroses and depressive disorders.

Clinical description

Although the essential concept of the syndrome of anxiety neurosis is clear, there are many variations. The phenomena fall into three groups. The patient complains of feeling anxious, he has other psychological disturbances, and he often has physical symptoms as well. In addition to a sense of fearful anticipation or apprehension, the psychological disturbances include irritability, poor concentration, over-reaction to noise, and a feeling of restlessness. Memory is not impaired but inability to concentrate may lead to complaints of impaired recall. One group of psychological symptoms which has been rather neglected– though Freud mentioned it in 1895 – have been emphasized recently by Beck, Laude, and Bohnert (1974). These symptoms are apprehensive thoughts which relate to, and often appear to be set in train by, the somatic symptoms. For example, a patient who feels his heart beating rapidly whenever he is anxious, may think repeatedly that he is about to have a heart attack; and another anxious patient whose hands tremble may assume that other people are sure to notice this. Such thoughts amplify the original anxiety because they lead to further anxiety which in turn increases the somatic symptoms which set the thoughts in train. Repetitious thoughts of another kind are common in anxiety states, namely ruminations about life problems and about personal inadequacy, and these too can add to the sum of anxiety which the patient experiences.

The somatic symptoms of anxiety neuroses are very variable. Many relate to over-activity of the autonomic nervous system: common complaints include palpitations, dry mouth, nausea, abdominal discomfort, diarrhoea, frequency or urgency of micturition, and sweating. Men often complain of impotence and women of frigidity. Other somatic symptoms relate to the somatic musculature: patients often describe headaches, and these are usually supposed to indicate increased tension in the neck or scalp muscles (though evidence from measurement of muscle potentials suggest that the matter is more complicated than this). Dyspnoea is also common and overbreathing can lead at times to faintness, dizziness, pins and needles in the hands and feet, and occasionally to hyperventilation tetany. A variety of complaints of tension in muscles are encountered, especially related to those of the chest, neck, shoulders and back; undue fatigue is commonly described and so is tremor of the hands. Sleep is frequently disturbed in anxiety neuroses and in a way which is characteristically different from that found in many depressive disorders. Anxious patients describe difficulty in falling asleep, saying that they feel tense, and cannot stop thinking of the events of the day or worrying about the future. Some complain of broken sleep and many report frightening dreams. Any of these symptoms may be the presenting complaint and any one can be the first evidence of organic disorder rather than anxiety. Examination to exclude physical disease is therefore important, but it is the association of the presenting symptom with several other features of the anxiety syndrome which allows the diagnosis to be made on positive grounds.

Many of these symptoms can be studied more objectively by the use of psychophysiological methods. Increased sweat gland activity is reflected in the size of galvanic skin responses: pulse rate, muscle blood flow, and finger pulse volume can also be measured, while electromyographic activity is usually recorded from the forehead or forearm. While these methods are useful for experimental purposes, they are of little value in diagnosis, which depends in the end on careful history taking.

Anxiety neurses can develop in many different personalities. First there are people with anxiety-prone personalities who respond with anxiety to a wide variety of the minor problems of life. Obsessional personalities are also prone to develop anxiety states and so are the schizoid and the dependent. As well as recognizing these personality types, it is important to recognize people who, while not generally vulnerable, nevertheless respond excessively to specific stressors; for example the adult who, because of repeated experiences of rejection in childhood, reacts with anxiety to small indications that others are rejecting him. Such personalities cannot be described in a satisfactory way in any of the existing typologies, but much of the skill of diagnostic interviewing lies in delineating such special sensitivities, and when possible tracing them back to events in childhood which may have caused them.

A clinical description of anxiety neuroses is not complete without some reference to the steps which patients take, knowingly or not, to reduce the unpleasant symptoms of anxiety. Some of these are referred to as mechanisms of defence (see pages 18, 38), others as coping strategies. Neither will be described in detail here, it is sufficient to note that the former, described originally by Freud, arise outside the patient's conscious awareness while the latter, described by Lazarus (1966) amongst others, are arrived at more or less consciously. Finally, the central group of anxiety symptoms is often accompanied by obsessional thoughts, depersonalization, derealization and depressive symptoms. While anxiety neuroses are never completely free from these features, the diagnosis should not be made if they are prominent.

CASE HISTORY: ANXIETY NEUROSIS

The importance of personality can be seen in the following case. A 30-year-old married man sought treatment for recurrent neck and shoulder pains which, on further enquiry, were found to be clearly associated with mental and autonomic symptoms of anxiety. All these symptoms invariably began when he was at work, usually after dealings with his manager whom he disliked. As an adolescent the patient had been hard-working and well-behaved; but he was not obviously prone to anxiety at that time. His relationship with his strict disciplinarian father appeared to have prepared the ground for his subsequent difficulty with authority figures, and his difficulties in expressing anger openly. Moreover he regarded psychological illness as a sign of weakness of character and he was extremely reluctant to admit that his symptoms might have a basis in his emotional life.

While diagnosis depends on thorough history taking, essential information is also obtained from the examination of the patient. At interview he is often restless, fidgeting with his hands or altering the position of his legs, and sitting uneasily on the edge of his chair. His expression is likely to be one of worry or apprehension, with over-activity of the frontalis and masseter muscles. Speech may be rapid and, if concentration is impaired, the history may be given in a rambling or discursive way which can occasionally suggest thought disorder. However, once the interviewer has put the patient more at ease, the logical flow of thinking becomes apparent and there should be no difficulty in distinguishing the thought processes of an anxious patient from schizophrenic thought disorder or the flight of ideas of hypomania. One of the most important tasks in taking the mental state of an anxious patient is to enquire thoroughly about symptoms of depression (for reasons which are discussed in the section on differential diagnosis). It is equally important to assess previous personality from relevant features of the personal history. In patients at or beyond middle age, their cognitive state must also be assessed carefully to exclude an early pre-senile dementia. Physical examination may reveal a fast pulse, moist palms, finger tremor, and brisk tendon reflexes. However the main purpose of physical examination is to exclude organic disease, including, but not exclusively, hyperthyroidism.

Aetiology

It is a convenient generalization to say that anxiety neuroses arise when unusually severe stress is experienced, when the personality is more than usually vulnerable to stress, or when both factors are present. This simple scheme leads first to a consideration of the stressors which may precede anxiety states.

Many different kinds of stress can lead to anxiety neuroses. Most theories distinguish, implicitly or explicitly, between long-term stress which prepares the way for the condition and the stress which occurs immediately before it begins. Most also accept the need to consider not only the objective threat which is inherent in the stressor but also the meaning which this has for the person who experiences it. It is convenient, though again over-simple, to say that much of the psycho-analytic literature on this subject consists essentially of attempts to identify a single central form of psychological experience, which, acting as a long-term stressor, can account for the anxiety state. Such is the diversity of human experience that it is not surprising that none of these attempts has succeeded, although each describes a problem which is important in certain cases. At first, Freud suggested sexual problems as the main causal factors in anxiety neurosis. Whatever the value of this formulation for the patients of his day it cannot now be regarded as a universal feature of patients with anxiety states, and in any case Freud later modified his ideas. Rank emphasized 'birth trauma' or separation

anxiety, Sullivan fear of disapproval by the mother, Adler threat to the individual's image of himself, Masserman and Fromm fears of death and loneliness, and so on. While this cursory account fails to do justice to the complexity and power of the ideas, there is little to suggest that any single psychological factor can explain all anxiety states and much to point to the view that the most striking feature is the diversity of the psychological causes. The reader who wishes to consider this aspect of the problem further is referred to Lief (1967).

An alternative to these ideas which attempt to find unifying features among antecedent psychological problems, is embodied in life-event research. This approach accepts that events of many different kinds can lead to anxiety states and an attempt is made to sum their effects, either by assuming that these are equal and additive, or that each can be given a weighting before they are combined. This approach accords well with everyday clinical experience, particularly in its second form in which events are weighted either according to judgements of their stressfulness to the 'average person' or in relation to their meaning to an individual. The method has been used most effectively by Brown and his colleagues in minor depressive states (Brown & Harris, 1978) and they are now applying it to anxiety states as well. The potential advantages of their methods over those of Holmes and Rahe (1967) are discussed in their monograph.

Reference has already been made to the many different kinds of personality from which anxiety neuroses may develop. In understanding the individual case and in planning the treatment of a particular patient, it is essential to evaluate the personality thoroughly. However, the study of personality has less to teach us about the aetiology of the group of anxiety neuroses as a whole. These can be associated with anxious personalities but also with obsessional, schizoid, and dependent types – indeed, readiness to react with overt anxiety symptoms is a common feature of most personality types except those which are characterized as psychopathic or hysterical.

Genetic studies are hampered by the problem of framing a clear definition of anxiety neuroses which can be used to diagnose the disorder of the proband and the relatives. Evidence from studies of twins and of other families' relationships suggests that anxiety states have a significant genetic component and probably a greater one than that in hysteria (Brown, 1942; Miner, 1973; Slater & Shields, 1969). Genetic predisposition is also reflected in significant hereditability of certain personality types associated with anxiety states, notably neuroticism. The precise nature of the inheritance is uncertain though a polygenic system is usually suggested (Slater & Shields, 1969).

Why do some anxiety states recover quickly while others become chronic? Sometimes the reason is not difficult to find: the stress which provoked the reaction has continued – for example, the patient has continued to live within an unhappy marriage. In other cases, social advantages seem to be perpetuating the symptoms; in one terminology these are secondary gains, in another, similar factors are referred to environmental reinforcers. In many cases, it is the severity of the personality disorder which explains why the anxiety state persists without evidence of any persisting major stress or secondary gain. However, there may be another reason for the persistence of some anxiety states. This is suggested by psychophysiological studies such as those of Lader and Wing (1964) who showed that anxious patients do not habituate to new stimuli at the normal rate. In normal subjects, for example, the response to each member of a series of auditory stimuli is substantially less than that to the preceding one, while anxious subjects' responses decline more slowly. These findings are from short-term experiments using auditory stimuli, but it is tempting to argue that a similar process may take place over a longer period and may involve a wide range of psychological stressors. If that is true, it would have the result that raised levels of anxiety would lead to over-responsiveness to environmental stimuli which in turn would maintain the over-arousal which set the process in train.

A somewhat similar vicious circle is suggested by observations on the cognitive features of anxiety states (Beck, Laude & Bohnert, 1974). We have already seen that apprehensive thoughts about the symptoms of anxiety can serve to make these symptoms worse. In a similar way anxious patients often come to anticipate stress in events which they did not previously view in this way. The idea that such factors prolong the anxiety states is still somewhat speculative, but it accords well with patients' accounts of their experiences and it merits further investigation. In general it can be argued that it is more fruitful at present to study factors such as these, which delay the resolution of anxiety states, than to attempt to discover more about the events which account for their appearance in the first place.

Differential diagnosis

The symptom of anxiety can occur in any psychiatric disorder and patients may complain of this anxiety rather than of the symptoms which are more characteristic of their primary condition. For this reason, the range of differential diagnosis is very wide. In practice, however, certain disorders are particularly likely to be mistaken for anxiety neuroses. The commonest diagnostic problem is between anxiety neuroses and depressive disorders. In practice, the problem can usually be resolved by a thorough search for depressive symptoms in both the present mental state and the recent history, provided that the latter is always taken from a relative or close friend as well as from the patient. Careful enquiry should also be made into the order in which depressive and anxiety symptoms appeared. It is particularly important to distinguish between agitated depressive illness and anxiety state, a problem which is most likely to be encountered in a middle-aged person of anxious or obsessional previous personality: again, a careful history and mental state examination will usually resolve the problem. Schizophrenic patients may also complain of anxiety before they reveal other symptoms, while patients with pre-senile or senile dementia sometimes present with complaints of anxiety as they become aware of failing intellectual powers. Again, the safeguard lies in a thorough examination of the mental state and in an interview with an informant. Patients who are dependent on drugs or alcohol sometimes present with complaints of anxiety. A number of these are anxiety-prone people who began to take alcohol or drugs to relieve these symptoms. Others are giving an account of withdrawal symptoms, a point which should be considered when anxiety is worse on waking. Finally, patients may exaggerate anxiety symptoms to obtain further supplies of barbiturates or other anxiolytic drugs on which they have become dependent.

In a similar way, patients who are experiencing the symptoms caused by physical pathology may present with anxiety rather than the primary physical complaints. This is particularly likely when previous experience has given the symptoms some special significance for that patient. For example, one patient presented with severe anxiety when she began to be constipated; she later revealed that a friend, who experienced similar bowel symptoms, had been reassured by her family doctor only to discover months later that she had a carcinoma of the bowel. A well-known diagnostic problem is between hyperthyroidism and anxiety state. The clinical picture can be very similar, with irritability, restlessness, tremor, moist palms and tachycardia in both. Sometimes physical examination is helpful and especially if there is atrial fibrillation or exophthalmos. Thyroid function tests will usually settle doubtful cases. Phaeochromocytoma and 'spontaneous' hypoglycaemia may occasionally present with an anxiety syndrome, while alcoholism and addiction to barbiturates may also cause diagnostic difficulty when the patient denies these problems.

Prognosis

There is little sound evidence on which to judge the prognosis of anxiety neuroses. General practitioners encounter many short-lived reactions which arise when well-adjusted personalities are subjected to unusual but short-lived stress. Symptoms persist when the stress lasts longer, or when the personality is disordered, and it is from these cases that the psychiatrist's patients are usually drawn. Clinical experience suggests that a useful division can be made at about 3–4 months. Although in Britain few of these short-lived reactions reach the specialist psychiatric services, this is not true in countries which have a less developed system of general practice. For this reason the results of follow-up studies are difficult to evaluate, because they depend on the organization of medical care as well as on the natural course of the condition.

Unfortunately there are other reasons why studies of prognosis are difficult to interpret. Few investigators have studied anxiety states separately from other neuroses and those who have done so have not always made clear their criteria for diagnosis or for assessment at follow-up. With these reservations in mind, it appears that of patients with anxiety neuroses seen in general practice about 75 per cent recover within six to 12 months and that most of those who are unwell at the end of a year still have symptoms two years after that (Kedward, 1969). Of patients referred to psychiatrists and diagnosed as anxiety neurosis, somewhere between a tenth and a quarter recover completely, while marked improvement is noted in about half (Greer, 1969). However, the period of follow-up in reported series is so variable that it is difficult to place much reliance on these figures. Anxiety neuroses referred to hospital have a worse long-term prognosis than depressive disorders (Roth *et al.*, 1972).

Treatment

Rational treatment must be preceded by a thorough assessment of the relative importance of psychological and social stressors and of personality factors. This should make possible a judgement about the chances of spontaneous recovery; a reaction is likely to pass quickly if it is recent, is a response to temporary stress, and occurs in a stable personality. Short-lived reactions are usually dealt with by family doctors. The essential steps with such cases are to reduce anxiety symptoms by simple psychological means – encouraging the expression of emotion about stressful events and giving advice, explanation, and reassurance – aided, if necessary, by an anxiolytic drug. One of the benzodiazepines is usually appropriate, for example diazepam 5 mg three times a day. When peripheral autonomic symptoms are most troublesome, beta-blockers can be used, for example, propranolol 10–20 mg three times a day taking the precautions that are usual with this drug (see British National Formulary, 1981). Night sedation may also be helpful. However, drugs should not be continued unduly and as soon as the patient is calm enough to consider his problems constructively, he should be encouraged to take any practical steps which he can to resolve them and to come to terms with difficulties which he cannot influence.

If symptoms persist for more than a few weeks, if the problems appear from the beginning to be long-term, or if the contribution from the patient's personality is great, other measures must be considered. Nearly all patients can be treated without admission to hospital, though a few days rest and sedation may be an essential first step in treating the most severe cases. In general, long-term medication with anxiolytic drugs should be avoided. Given in small doses, the effects of these drugs diminish with time, while larger amounts carry the risk of psychological, and the possibility of physical, dependence, though the extent of the last problem is not certain. The problem of physical dependence is certainly more serious with the barbiturates which should only be used to produce rapid short-term sedation of the most anxious patients. They should be used rarely if at all, and, when used, prescribed for a few doses only. If anxiolytic treatment is required for a longer period, one of the benzodiazepines can be used but there are two important alternatives. The first is to prescribe one of the antidepressant drugs which has an anxiolytic effect. For this purpose the tricyclic drug amitriptyline is often used in doses of 75–150 mg a day given either in divided amounts or with the larger part at bed time, the latter being especially useful for patients who sleep badly. Some clinicians use one of the monoamine oxidase inhibitors for anxious patients, often phenelzine 15 mg three times a day. The mode of action of monoamine oxidase inhibitors in anxiety states is uncertain but it is possible that the effects are related to the anxiolytic rather than to the anti-depressant effects of the drugs. The same may be true of the tricyclic antidepressants.

An important alternative to drug treatment is provided by relaxation exercises, or the somewhat more elaborate procedures known as anxiety man-agement training. These require more time from trained staff than does the prescription of drugs, at least in the early part of treatment but this can be reduced by treating patients in groups and by the use of tape-recorded instructions. Relaxation exer-cises should certainly be tried for patients who are still taking anxiolytic drugs after three months, although by then it may be difficult to persuade patients to change from one form of treatment to the other. For this reason the plan of treatment should be made clear to patients when treatment begins.

An alternative to simple relaxation exercises is provided by anxiety management training. This treatment has three stages: (a) the patient learns to recognize the symptoms of anxiety and to identify any situations in which they increase ('self-monitoring'); (b) he is told about the ways in which anxiety symptoms can arise, how bodily symptoms are related to the feeling state of anxiety and how fears about the effects of anxiety can create a vicious circle – for example, worry that rapid heart action indicates heart disease leads to more anxiety; (c) he learns to control anxiety symptoms without drugs. Each of these stages needs to be amplified.

Self-monitoring is not only an essential prelim-inary to the other stages of treatment, but probably therapeutic itself because of the increased sense of control over symptoms which it gives. A simple method of recording symptoms is sufficient, for example, a card with columns for a record of time of day at which symptoms occur, their severity, and any events which immediately precede them. The second stage, instruction about the physiology of anxiety and the ways in which fears about symptoms can lead to vicious circles, is a rather complex matter. For this reason, it is useful to provide information for patients to study at home. Various pamphlets are available, but the therapist may prefer to write a sim-ple one of his own.

The methods for controlling anxiety are in three stages. First, the patient learns to evoke anxiety by imagining suitable situations, then he practises ways of arresting this anxiety and finally he practises the same methods with anxiety that arises in his every-day life. It is usual to teach two ways of inhibiting anxiety. The first is to imagine calming situations and then to practise 'switching' from an anxious to a calming image. The second is to relax – the precise form of relaxation training does not seem to matter; various tape-recorded instructions are available commercially, but they can also be made easily by the therapist himself. Although now used quite widely these methods have not been tested rigor-ously in clinical trials with anxiety states. While they work well with mildly anxious people, the main problem about their use in clinical practice is that of motivation: many patients – and clinicians – prefer the effortless use of anxiolytic drugs to the extra effort required for anxiety management.

Psychotherapeutic treatment is important in several ways. At its simplest, in the form of crisis intervention, it helps patients to consider problems which are provoking the anxiety state and the steps which they can take to resolve them. A social worker can help in this way, and also by encouraging the patient to solve the practical problems in his life. If these problems arise in a patient's marriage or in another intimate relationship then conjoint therapy may be appropriate. But psychotherapy is not, of course, limited to the resolution of actual problems, it is concerned also with giving patients insight into the ways in which they habitually attempt to cope with stress and with teaching better ways of coping. It is also concerned in an important way with the patient's perception of himself and with his relation-ships with other people. If these are important, more lengthy psychotherapy may be required either in the form of individual or group treatment. Relevant issues are discussed further in the section on psychother-apy in chapter 3.1.1 of this volume.

Leucotomy has been used in the past for severe and prolonged anxiety states. There is no evidence from controlled investigations that it is effective and if behavioural, psychotherapeutic, and social mea-sures are used with determination it should not be necessary to consider even modified operations for these patients.

Phobic states
Although individual phobic symptoms have been recognized since Hippocrates, the idea of a sep-

arate phobic syndrome began with the description of agoraphobia by Westphal in 1871. Freud (1895a) distinguished 'common phobias', that is, exaggerated fears of things which normal people fear to some degree, and phobias of things which are not part of the fears of ordinary people, for example, agoraphobia. He did not, however, separate either group clearly from the anxiety states. While the recurrent fearful thoughts of phobic patients have led some to consider their relationship to obsessional syndromes, the development of behavioural methods in the last two decades has focused attention on the aspects of situational anxiety and the avoidance of feared situations, and confirmed the practical value of recognizing phobic disorders as a group of distinct syndromes. Although there is still some lack of agreement about the individual syndromes within the group of phobic disorders, three conditions are usually recognized: agoraphobia, social phobias, and other specific phobias. This leaves a group in which fears are part of an obsessional neurosis, for example, the fear of knives expressed by many obsessional patients. The problems of classification have been reviewed by Marks (1969). In the rest of this section these three main groups will be considered separately.

Agoraphobia

Clinical description. This syndrome is the most important of the phobic disorders encountered in clinical practice. Although Westphal (1871) reported the condition in men, at least three quarters of agoraphobic patients seen today are women (Marks, 1969), with the condition usually beginning between the ages of 18 and 35. Anxiety is experienced in situations which share certain common themes: distance from home or from another 'safe' place, crowds and confinement – in public transport, theatre, shops in which the customer must queue before paying, and other situations which are difficult to leave quickly. This anxiety is usually less in the presence of a trusted companion, and sometimes even in the company of a child or a pet. It leads sooner or later to avoidance of the situations which are associated with anxiety. The name agoraphobia is sometimes thought to indicate that fear of open spaces is paramount – and Westphal did draw attention to this fear in his original description – but in fact, it is not the most important feature of the syndrome. In all but the most severe cases, the patient's anxiety subsides quickly once he has left the phobic situation.

In some or all of these situations, typical symptoms of anxiety develop. There is no special feature of the physical components of anxiety, instead it is the accompanying anxious thoughts which are characteristic. The agoraphobic patient typically experiences the recurring thought that she will faint and that if she does she will be the object of ridicule. Fearful expectations of losing control, 'going mad', or sudden death are also reported commonly. As these anxiety symptoms increase, patients begin to avoid the situations in which they arise. Journeys from home are increasingly curtailed until, as the condition progresses, the patient goes out only with a companion and eventually not at all. Social difficulties follow. The mother of young children finds it increasingly difficult to take them to school, while travel by bus or train becomes impossible, and work or social engagements are given up. Some patients say that a car provides a 'safe' form of transport, others that it makes them anxious although they can still travel by cycle or on foot. There are many individual variations around these central themes. Whatever the situations which provoke anxiety, patients almost always say that the symptoms begin when they start to think about what they are about to do. Thus the housewife who is going shopping begins to feel anxious as soon as she thinks about the journey, at first only a few minutes before she goes but eventually many hours in advance of the appointed time. And journeys which are made without warning are, correspondingly, attended by less anxiety.

Agoraphobia, like other neurotic syndromes, frequently includes symptoms which are not directly related to its core symptoms. Depressive symptoms are common, obsessional thoughts are reported quite often, and depersonalization or derealization are not infrequent. Attempts to delineate a separate subgroup of patients with prominent depersonalization (Roth, 1959) have not proved fruitful, nor has Klein's (1964) attempt to split off from the main syndrome a group of panic disorders in which patients experience attacks of severe anxiety in the absence of environmental triggers. That such attacks of 'free floating' anxiety occur in a proportion of patients is beyond dispute, but there is insufficient evidence to create a separate syndrome around this symptom.

The following case history illustrates many typical features.

A 24-year-old married woman sought treatment for typical agoraphobic symptoms. These had begun two years before, when she was shopping in the basement of a large store. She could remember no stressful event on that day, but enquiry revealed that she had been worried for several weeks about the health of her four-year-old son. From that day onward, similar symptoms appeared whenever she was in a large shop, and then, progressively, whenever she travelled by 'bus or car – and most recently when walking alone. She began to ask her husband to accompany her whenever she went out; he was uncertain whether he should agree to her requests or encourage her to manage on her own, but eventually chose the former course. Her previous personality was not obviously anxiety-prone, but further enquiry showed that at school she had been timid and unsure of herself and had worried unduly about her physical health. She had always been rather dependent on her husband who was himself a passive man, uncertain of his abilities at his work and with few friends of his own.

Agoraphobia inevitably affects the life of the patient's family. The husband usually has to accompany his wife when she goes shopping, family holidays may be restricted, there are problems in taking younger children to school and so on. The husband is usually uncertain how far he should protect his wife from anxiety and how far he should insist that she face the situations which she fears. At times this allows an agoraphobic woman to dominate a passive or indecisive husband. Some patients are less active sexually and this may add a further source of friction and misunderstanding. Such problems have led some psychiatrists to emphasize the role of marital disharmony and to regard this as a cause rather than an effect of the agoraphobia. However, a well-conducted survey of marital problems in agoraphobia (Buglass, Clarke, Henderson, Kreitman & Presley, 1977), found them no more often than in controls. However, when marital problems and agoraphobia do coincide, treatment is undoubtedly more difficult. It is presumably these difficult and striking cases which have given rise to the widely held impression that serious marital problems are more common than they really are.

Differential diagnosis. The main differential diagnosis of agoraphobia is from depressive disorders. We have seen that depressive symptoms are common in agoraphobia and it is also true that depressed patients are sometimes reluctant to travel and to enter crowds. It is also important for the clinician to realise that agoraphobic patients often seek treatment at times when they are depressed. When this happens, the depressive symptoms may not be volunteered, and they must be sought in every case, especially by an enquiry about depressive thoughts and by asking a relative or close friend about the patient's behaviour at home. In the occasional case in which the diagno-

sis remains in doubt, a trial of antidepressant drugs may be indicated.

The line which divides agoraphobia from states of generalised anxiety is less clear cut. Nearly all patients with anxiety states describe some situations in which their symptoms increase and at times these have a pattern which is similar to that found in agoraphobia. In separating the two it is usually more useful to pay attention to the circumstances in which the symptoms do *not* appear. In anxiety states, the symptoms are generalized, in agoraphobia the patient will describe some situations in which she is free from anxiety – for example, nearly all are calm in their own homes, although as the condition worsens this may only be true when another person is present. When agoraphobia becomes very severe there may be no situation in which the patient is wholly free from anxiety, but even in these cases a careful history of the earlier stages of the disorder will usually resolve the diagnostic problem.

A less common pitfall, but an important one, is to mistake for agoraphobia the early stages of a paranoid disorder. Such patients may avoid public places because they are unduly sensitive about the opinions of other people or because they have developed definite paranoid delusions. Careful enquiry, in every case, into the content of the patient's thoughts will ensure that this mistake is made rarely, although it is difficult to avoid it altogether because paranoid patients often hide the full extent of their symptoms.

Aetiology. Attempts to explain the origins of agoraphobia are, without exception, unsatisfactory but much is now known about the factors which maintain the disorder once it had begun. Fortunately, treatment appears to depend more on these latter features of the case than on the original causes. Patients' accounts of the onset are characteristic. A single major stressful event is seldom reported; instead the patient is typically out of doors, often waiting for public transport, or in a shop when she experiences sudden feelings of severe anxiety for which she can remember no reason. However, although no immediate stressor is described, these events often take place at a time when the patient is subject to some background of worry, for example, the serious illness of a child, or a marital problem. In a few patients, symptoms begin soon after childbirth, possibly as part of a puerperal depression. In the face of these clinical observations, a simple conditioning theory fails to provide a convincing explanation of the onset of agoraphobia. The most plausible alternative idea is that symptoms are the result of a state of heightened general anxiety, whether due to personal problems or to an affective disorder, which makes it possible for minor additional stress to set off the first sudden attack of anxiety. Accounts of the development of symptoms from that point onwards are more compatible with conditioning mechanisms – for example, the second episode of anxiety very often takes place in the same surroundings as those in which the first was experienced.

Psycho-dynamic theories are, for the most part, founded on the twin concepts of repression and displacement. Much has been written about the possible symbolic significance of the agoraphobic symptoms but, as in the case of anxiety states, it is the diversity rather than the similarity of patients' psychological problems which is striking. Universal explanations whether in terms of fantasies about promiscuity (Miller, 1953) or aggression (Deutsch, 1929) or any other of the many that have been suggested have not proved useful either in understanding the disorder or in developing treatment. These psycho-dynamic hypotheses have relevance to some patients, and because it is impossible to do justice to them in a short space the interested reader is referred to the relevant section in the American Handbook of Psychiatry (Friedman & Goldstein, 1974).

Several attempts have been made to relate the phobic syndrome to attributes of personality which may predispose to it. One approach draws attention to anxiety-prone personalities who have experienced many minor fears before they develop agoraphobia (see for example Ey, Bernard & Brisset, 1974). While this personality can be recognized in some phobic patients, it is not universal. Another approach draws attention to dependency and so-called hysterical traits (for example, a readiness to exploit secondary gain). While these traits can also be observed in a proportion of agoraphobic patients they are not found in every one. They may have more to do with the reasons why some agoraphobic patients find their way to psychiatrists than with the aetiology of the syndrome.

The conditions which maintain a neurotic disorder may have little to do with those which account for its beginnings. Agoraphobia appears to be maintained, invariably, by the patient's habit of avoiding situations which she fears and by fearful anticipation which leads to anxiety long before she encounters them. In many cases family attitudes are also impor-

tant, both in encouraging avoidance and in some, but by no means all cases, through tension engendered by poor relationships and family quarrels. We shall refer to these issues again when treatment is considered.

Prognosis. Although agoraphobic symptoms are less likely to resolve spontaneously than those of anxiety states, there are patients who improve within a few months. Because in Britain many such patients are treated by general practitioners they are under-represented in series reported by psychiatrists. Without treatment, agoraphobia which has been present for a year is unlikely to recover in the next few years, but little is known about the ultimate outcome of these cases. Reported series (Roberts, 1964; Friedman, 1950; Terhune, 1949) vary so much in criteria for improvement, in length of follow-up and in the treatment which patients received, that it is hard to draw firm conclusions. As a rough guide, we can follow Marks's (1969) conclusion that about half the patients whose symptoms have lasted a year are likely to have symptoms causing significant restriction in their lives after five to ten years. Effective treatment speeds up recovery but there is still no evidence that it changes the final outcome.

Treatment. From the beginning, agoraphobic patients should be strongly encouraged to return to the situations in which fear has been experienced and remain there until anxiety subsides. An anxiolytic drug will sometimes be required to make this possible on the first few occasions, but anxiolytics should not be taken regularly. When a drug is needed (diazepam 5–10 mg is appropriate), it should be taken about 30 minutes before entering the feared situation. Drugs should not be used more than a few times for the same situation, and used only to allow new behavioural goals to be reached. Patients who are also depressed may require antidepressant medication. In this case, it is appropriate to use amitriptyline 75–100 mg per day given either in divided doses or, at the smaller dose, taken near bed-time. Claims for the therapeutic effects in agoraphobia of imipramine (Klein, 1964) or monoamine oxidase inhibitors (Mountjoy, Roth, Garside & Leitch, 1977) may reflect their effects on concurrent depression, but they may also reflect the anxiolytic properties of the drugs.

Although in early cases, simple instructions to return to the feared situation may be enough, those which persist will usually require more formal behaviour therapy, which, in one or other of its variants, is the treatment of choice for agoraphobia. The evidence now points to the value of simple exposure methods (see page 84) carried out in a way which encourages patients to take as much responsibility as possible for their own treatment. Desensitization given alone is less effective, but some use it as a preliminary to exposure methods. However there is no evidence that this adds to the effect of exposure, although it is sometimes a convenient way of dealing with situations which the patient can enter only occasionally. Flooding (page 84) is no more effective than the less distressing forms of exposure treatment and there is no reason to use it. Most patients are also helped by learning a way of reducing anxiety. For many, simple relaxation training is enough, but others seem to be helped more by anxiety management (see pages 217–18). Few agoraphobic patients can succeed in a programme of exposure treatment without help. However, if the therapist does too much, dependency develops and improvement ends as soon as the therapist stops seeing the patient. An alternative, which avoids this problem to some extent, is to encourage the spouse or a close friend to help. This can only be done if the helper is instructed thoroughly in his role and if he attends with the patient each time she sees the therapist. If the spouse is the helper there is the added advantage that the couple are given constructive goals which they can share. Provided that marital difficulties are not severe, these shared activities often help to improve the relationship of the couple as well as bringing about improvement in the phobias. If severe marital problems preclude such collaboration, conjoint therapy should be tried before behaviour therapy is attempted. In a similar way, individual or group psychotherapy used as the sole treatment has little effect on agoraphobic symptoms, though such treatment may be indicated when there are prominent difficulties in personal relationships. If the relationship problems are severe, the psychotherapy may need to come first, otherwise it is convenient to start with behaviour therapy and review progress after a few weeks.

Social phobias

Clinical picture. This syndrome encompasses patients who are anxious in circumscribed social situations. Unlike the anxieties of patients with self-insecure personalities, these fears have not been present since early years; instead most have begun in the patient's late teens or early twenties. Social phobics are not anxious in the whole range of situations which affect agoraphobic patients, although most of the latter describe some degree of social phobia. This point is often misunderstood, with the result that some agoraphobic patients are misclassified as social phobics. The condition is about equally common in men and women.

The situations which provoke anxiety include busy restaurants or other places in which the patient has the idea that others may watch him as he eats or drinks; public transport in which he has to sit facing other passengers; and any other place in which aspects of his social performance are open to public scrutiny, for example, at the hairdressers, in a seminar, or at a board meeting. In such circumstances, patients may experience any of the usual physical symptoms of anxiety, although complaints of blushing, trembling of the hands, difficulty in swallowing, and nausea are particularly common. Some patients fear that they will vomit, while others have the fear that they may see another person vomiting. Patients are usually preoccupied with the idea that others will notice these signs of anxiety and will therefore form unfavourable opinions. Such ideas increase further the patient's anxiety and the associated blushing, trembling, or other symptoms, and as in agoraphobia, the ideas often precede the patient's entry into the feared situations. When severe, these symptoms lead to avoidance of social intercourse which can seriously restrict the patient's life. Accompanying symptoms of depression, obsessions and depersonalisation are encountered less frequently than in agoraphobia. Many patients use, and some abuse, alcohol to control their symptoms.

Aetiology. The origins of social phobias are uncertain. The cause of the first episode of anxiety is difficult to explain in the majority of individual cases, and no general explanation is convincing. However, as with agoraphobia, the development and spread of symptoms takes place in a way that is consistent with conditioning mechanisms.

Prognosis. The prognosis of social phobias has not been investigated thoroughly and there is little which can be said with confidence. Clinical experience suggests that a substantial proportion of patients whose symptoms have persisted for a year are likely to have symptoms up to four years after that. However the majority appear eventually to improve.

Treatment. Treatment is broadly similar to that of agoraphobia. In cases of recent onset, patients should be encouraged to face the situations which they fear. For this some will need the prescription of a benzodiazepine or other anxiolytic drug given in a moderate dose and for a limited period. Beta-blockers are more useful here than with agoraphobia for they control the peripheral autonomic symptoms which are prominent in so many patients. Anxiolytic drugs should not be taken regularly nor should they be continued routinely for more than about three months. Patients who are taking alcohol to reduce symptoms should be advised strongly to stop doing this and particular care should be taken in prescribing anxiolytics for such patients. If longer-term anxiety reduction is required, a sedative antidepressant may be tried but it is usually preferable to teach relaxation exercises.

Apart from simple instruction in relaxation, behaviour therapy is of value although there is no general agreement about the best methods. No differences have been found between the outcome of patients treated with desensitization, flooding, and social skills training (Shaw, 1979). It is possible that simple exposure methods (pages 84–5) are as effective as any of these more complicated methods. Anxiety management training (page 218) is also found helpful by many patients. Social skills training has also been advocated but it is time-consuming and does not appear particularly well suited to the disorder because patients do not usually lack social skills, instead they are too anxious to express skills which they possess. Group psychotherapy is also used for patients with social phobias, but it is less suitable for them than it is for people with insecure personalities whose difficulties lie in a wider range of social interactions.

Specific phobias
Patients with isolated but severe phobic symptoms occasionally ask for psychiatric treatment. The objects of these fears are innumerable and no useful purpose is served by attaching names to the different phobias. Instead they can be divided broadly into fears of animate objects, for example, spiders, snakes, birds, dogs; fears of natural phenomena, for example, darkness, thunder, rainstorms; and a miscellaneous group including fears of heights and confined spaces, admission to hospital, dental treatment, injections, or obstetric procedures. However, even this grouping is of little value since it relates neither to prognosis nor to treatment.

Aetiology. The aetiology of persistent specific phobias is obscure. Nearly all start in early childhood, at a time when such fears are common. Thus the important question is why some of these fears persist into adult life, rather than why they begin. Neither the severity of the original childhood fears nor the response of the parents towards the child have been proved to explain why some persist, though presumably these factors are of some importance. Psychodynamic theories suppose that the fears are related to the manifest objects in only a superficial and unimportant way and that they are really displacements of other sources of anxiety. Starting with Freud's analysis of 'Little Hans', great ingenuity has been shown in suggesting the symbolic meaning of specific phobias. It is impossible to test these ideas at all rigorously, but the response of the majority of specific phobias to deconditioning suggests that simpler mechanisms are at work. A fuller account of the clinical picture and aetiology is found in Marks (1969).

There is no systematic information about *prognosis* but clinical experience indicates that severe specific phobias encountered in adults last for many years, if no treatment is given.

Treatment. This is by the 'exposure' form of behaviour therapy (see chapter 3.1.2). However before embarking on this, it is important to look for evidence of a depressive disorder. Patients who have tolerated the anxiety and inconvenience of specific phobias for many years sometimes seek treatment not because the fears are more severe, but because depressive mood change has caused the patient to feel less able to cope with them. When this happens, successful treatment of the depression will often bring the patient to say that he no longer feels that the phobias require treatment. Some of these phobias are little more than a nuisance, but those related to dental treatment, operations, and childbirth may require urgent and determined treatment.

Anxiety and phobias in childhood: the childhood origins of phobias
Anxiety and fear is as much a part of the normal life of children as it is of the life of adults. Discussion of anxiety as a normal emotion can be found in the volume on psychopathology (vol. 1, chap 4). This section is concerned with abnormal states of anxiety in childhood and with phobic states. However, the important special case of school phobias is

not considered here because it appears in chapter 4.2.1 of the present volume. In adults the division between normal anxiety responses to stress and the pathological reactions which make up anxiety states and phobic disorders is difficult to define and rather arbitrary. In children the distinction is even less easy to make because there are other sources of variation. These are the parents' response to the child's complaints and behaviour, and the severity of the disorder which prompts them to seek help. In other words, the child has to complain to the doctor through one of the parents – usually the mother – and there are times when the complaint is related more to the parent's own anxiety than to that of the child. It is particularly important to bear in mind that a depressed mother may bring her child for help for problems with which she would cope herself if she were well.

Anxiety states
Clinical description. Although the specific syndromes of anxiety neurosis, obsessional neurosis and hysteria can all occur in children, mixed neurotic disorders are more common. These mixed disorders are sometimes labelled 'anxiety states', with the result that terminology is used less precisely than it is with adult patients. In this account a narrow definition of anxiety states is used for the same reasons that a narrow view of anxiety states was preferred in the discussion of adult patients.

Older children can often give clear descriptions of the psychological and physical symptoms which are familiar in adult patients with anxiety states. However, with younger children the clinician must often rely on observations of behaviour: apprehensiveness, irritability, timidity, restless sleep sometimes broken by nightmares or 'night terrors', trembling, sweating, and rapid pulse. Instead of complaining of anxiety the child may describe physical symptoms, including nausea, abdominal discomfort, giddiness, paraesthesiae, vague complaints of ill-health, and excessive fears, for example, fears of the dark. These complaints may be sustained as a chronic anxiety reaction or appear as acute episodes. The latter may occur at night, when the child wakes from sleep confused, sweating, and apparently terrified. He may describe vivid and frightening dreams or appear to be experiencing visual hallucinations. Some children walk in their sleep at these times.

Aetiology. Anxiety states develop in children who have been emotionally stable in the past but are now

experiencing severe stress; or in children who for years have shown signs that they are unusually prone to react to stress. These latter may also be unduly sensitive to noise, and they often appear to worry unduly when faced with new experiences. It has been suggested that these temperamental patterns are directly related to certain features observed in young infants: the tendency to startle easily, to react adversely to minor change in routine and to cry readily.

Many different stresses can provoke abnormal states of anxiety in small children. Of these, separation from the mother has received much attention and it is clear that it is not only the fact of separation which is important, but also the reasons. When separation is the result of another event which is itself stressful, then anxiety is even more likely. Obvious examples include admission to hospital, and separation from the mother because she is unwell – whether with a physical or mental illness. In other children, anxiety is a reflection of the parent's own anxiety, which acts in two ways: as a source of stress to which the child reacts, and as a model which encourages anxiety responses in situations in which another parent would act in a reassuring way. Eisenberg (1958) has pointed out these mechanisms in school phobias, but it is likely that they apply more widely although Rutter's (1966) study indicated that the relationship between mental disorder in patients and children cannot be explained on either hereditary or environmental factors alone – both are important.

The extent to which, in children, anxiety arises from intrapsychic conflict, rather than obvious psychological and social stress, is more difficult to determine. Psycho-analytic theories have sought to explain both the immediate anxiety reactions and the state of excessive readiness to react. Explanations have ranged from the condition of birth itself ('birth trauma') to disturbances of the relationship between the child and one or other of his parents (for example, 'Oedipal situation'). Some of these ideas, especially those related to events at the time of birth, are difficult to reconcile with current knowledge about the state of cognitive development in young infants, while others, such as the Oedipal complex, are better regarded as allegorical rather than explanatory. They are set out at length in psycho-analytic writings and will not be considered further here.

These psycho-dynamic explanations do, however, contain two important ideas which are now being pursued more objectively. First, that readiness for anxiety develops in a cumulative way in which the effects of later experiences are determined by those which have gone before. Secondly, that the events of the first few weeks of life are important in shaping the secure relationship which the child needs with his mother.

Prognosis. The prognosis of anxiety states in children not only depends on the severity of the disorder, how long it has been present, and on the child's temperament, but also on the reaction of the parents. An over-protective attitude on their part reinforces the child's anxieties and delays recovery, while lack of understanding of his feelings deprives him of the security which he needs if he is to overcome his fears.

Follow-up studies show that, in general, emotional disorders of childhood do not persist into adult life, and this probably applies also to anxiety states. The few which do persist develop into neuroses in the adult but these may be depressive as well as anxiety states (Hersov, 1976).

Treatment. Treatment must take into account the reactions and problems of the rest of the family and not just those of the child who is presented as the patient. Drug treatment has little part to play except as an occasional short-term measure when symptoms are severe. When this is needed one of the benzodiazepines is appropriate. Psychotherapy with the child is better directed to his or her expressed anxieties than to interpretation. As much time should be spent with the parents as with the child, giving advice about the way in which they should respond to him, and discussing their own anxieties. This will often require a review of the whole family and some therapists prefer to see them together (Bentovim, 1979). Older children may be able to learn relaxation exercises, otherwise a behavioural approach is often most usefully directed to examining how the reactions of the parents may be prolonging the disorder in the child.

Phobic anxiety states

We have seen that this section excludes school phobia which is considered in chapter 4.2.1. When this condition is set aside, most phobias in childhood are specific fears – often of animals, insects, and the dark. These phobias merge into milder fears which are so common among children that they are best considered as a normal part of psychological development. Thus Cummings (1944, 1946) found that 33 per cent of children under four showed specific

fears, 22 per cent of those under six and 13 per cent of those aged six to eight. Nearly all were short-lived. At each age, fears were observed more frequently in girls than in boys. Fears which are abnormally intense or which persist beyond the age at which they are commonly encountered in other children with similar backgrounds are the phobic disorders of childhood. Phobias of situations (which include fears of school) are as commonly reported in boys as in girls and are quite common at about the age of ten (Rutter, Tizard & Whitmore, 1970). Specific phobias of animals are much more common in girls and about half as frequent as situation phobias (Rutter *et al.*, 1970). The syndromes of agoraphobia and social phobia are not observed in childhood, although the retrospective accounts of adult phobic patients suggest that the former may perhaps have some relation to some of the complaints of car-sickness among children.

Just as the normal fears of early childhood resolve spontaneously, so do most phobias respond to sensible reassurances from the parents (Rutter *et al.*, 1970). In treatment, therefore, as much attention should be paid to the parents' reactions to the child and to their own emotional problems, as to the direct treatment of the patient. Once a calm and reassuring atmosphere has been established in the home, the phobias often resolve and if they do not, simple behavioural measures are usually effective. In these the child encounters a carefully graduated series of the situations or things which make him anxious. Modelling calm behaviour in the presence of the phobic objects is important in treatment in children – more important than it is with adult phobic patients. Most children with phobic symptoms have other emotional problems so that each case should be investigated thoroughly and treatment should not be focused too narrowly on behavioural measures for the fears.

Although child psychotherapists often find that phobic children are 'a pleasure to treat in that, like Hans, they are generally alert, inquisitive and resourceful in the therapeutic situations and make full use of all the symbolic equations in play' (Anthony, 1967), there is no evidence that analytic treatment yields results which are better than those of the kind which we have just outlined.

Childhood origins of adult phobias

Finally, what is the relationship between childhood phobias and phobic disorders of adult life? The uncommon specific phobias of adult life begin, almost invariably, in childhood. The few which persist into adult life are therefore the remains of a much larger number which disappear by about the age of ten. Why a few specific phobias persist into adult life when the majority resolve, is not known, but the relationship between childhood symptoms and those in the adult is a direct one.

The same cannot be said of social phobias, for although shyness is common in childhood, social phobias are not. Indeed they usually begin in the teenage years. Most shy children overcome their fears and those who do not are more likely to grow into an adult with a personality disorder than a person with a social phobic state. In other words, general shyness in childhood does not narrow down to the specific areas which characterize the adult with social phobias.

Agoraphobia also begins in early adult life rather than childhood. Although a proportion of agoraphobic patients say that they were shy children, and others say that they had specific phobias, the condition can seldom be traced back to a similar syndrome in childhood. Some agoraphobic patients report that they experienced school phobia as children, but they are a minority: 10 per cent according to Tyrer & Tyrer (1974); 22 per cent according to Berg and co-workers (1974). Moreover the proportion of agoraphobic patients who report school phobia is not significantly greater than the proportion of depressed patients who do so (Berg *et al.*, 1974). Some agoraphobic patients also report that as children they experienced car-sickness on long journeys or that they fainted in assembly at school and it is possible that such symptoms reflected anxiety about travelling or about crowded places. This association and that with school phobia probably reflects a general neurotic predisposition rather than any specific causal link with agoraphobia. We must conclude that from the uncommon specific phobias, there is no regular continuity between phobic disorders in childhood and adult life.

Depersonalization and derealization syndromes

The symptoms of depersonalization and derealization, are encountered in many psychiatric conditions and occasionally in healthy people at times when they are tired. The individual symptoms are considered in the volume on phenomenology (vol. 1, chap. 3); in this section we are concerned with the question of whether there is a distinct depersonalization *syndrome* and with the measures which can be used when the symptom appears as a prominent part of another neurotic syndrome.

Clinical picture The clinical features were well described by Shorvon, Hill, Burkitt & Halstead (1946). Of their 66 cases, two-thirds were women and in about half the condition began before the age of 30. The onset, which is usually sudden, is often related in time to the appearance of symptoms of anxiety, so that it may be difficult to decide which symptom came first. Shorvon and co-workers obtained descriptions in which depersonalization was followed by anxiety – which they regarded as a response to the alarming feelings of lack of reality – but the reverse sequence can also be observed. Indeed it has been suggested that depersonalization appears when anxiety reaches a critical level as a kind of shut-down of sensory input. Derealization may or may not accompany depersonalization, but it does not commonly appear on its own. Patients usually find it difficult to describe their experiences; they express in one form or other the idea that they feel strange, that perceptions no longer have the familiar quality of reality, that emotions are dulled and that actions feel mechanical. They no longer feel love or hate in a normal way and cannot feel intense pleasure. Paradoxically patients often complain that this dulling of feeling is extremely distressing. It is important to note that all this is expressed in terms of 'as if'; there is no loss of insight. Depersonalization and derealization are distressing symptoms and they are accompanied by varying degrees of anxiety and depression. Other features which accompany depersonalization include changes in the experience of time and *déjà vu* experiences. Some patients experience the changed quality of sensory experience not in the whole body but in a single part, often the head or limbs. Patients may complain that the whole head, or some part of it such as the nose, feels as if made of cotton wool, seems to be without proper sensation, or is distorted in size. Once established, the disorder may last for years, often with periods of remission, though it usually subsides eventually.

A 20-year-old single woman described intense feelings of depersonalization which began nearly a year before, during an argument with her boy-friend. She complained that she could no longer feel any emotion in a normal way, and that at the same time her surroundings had taken on an unreal quality. This lack of feeling was described as being intensely distressing and she said that she had at times felt so desperate that she had thought of taking her life. Her previous personality was the kind often called schizoid: she had never succeeded in forming close relationships and to her family seemed often detached and unfeeling. In her relationship with men she had avoided real intimacy. Her evident distress was not accompanied by any clear evidence of a depressive disorder or anxiety state.

Aetiology The aetiological problems centre round the question whether there is a primary depersonalization syndrome or whether the clinical picture which has been described is always secondary to another condition. Shorvon and co-workers (1946) claimed to have identified a distinct syndrome but their evidence is based on clinical observations made at a single time, and they presented no follow-up information to show whether the cases remain distinct from anxiety state, depressive disorder, schizophrenia, and organic states.

Ackner (1954), in a comprehensive study, allocated all his patients with prominent depersonalization to organic, schizoid, depressive, tension, and hysterical syndromes. Of these it is the last which is the most difficult to assess because of the well known vagueness of the concept of hysteria. It can be argued that these cases could equally well have been assigned to a primary depersonalization syndrome, for Ackner classed them as hysterical largely on the grounds of secondary gain, the absence of affective or organic features, and lack of evidence of a schizoid personality. To argue this is not to deny that depersonalization can occur in patients who are demonstrative and demanding and that when this happens, the management of the condition is more difficult. However, whatever the nature of these cases, the patients are probably a minority of those who present with severe depersonalization – in Ackner's series only ten of 54 patients were categorized as hysterical depersonalization syndrome.

Ackner also regarded depersonalization as a secondary phenomenon when it appeared in schizoid personalities (five in his series of 54). As Mayer-Gross, Slater, and Roth (1960) observe, such cases have attracted an interest out of proportion to their numerical importance, probably because these patients often give particularly interesting descriptions of their experiences. Since depersonalization usually starts abruptly in these as in other cases, it does not appear logical to regard the condition as a personality disorder which implies a condition

stretching back into early years. Mayer-Gross and colleagues (1960) regard this group, arising in schizoid personalities, as the primary depersonalization syndrome, and suggest that it includes the cases described in adolescents by Meyer (1961).

Differential diagnosis. The differential diagnosis has been referred to already. Depersonalization and derealization can be the presenting symptoms of organic states, schizophrenia, depression including bereavement reactions, hysteria, obsessional neurosis, anxiety states, including – and according to Mayer-Gross and colleagues (1960) especially – phobic states, and in schizoid personalities. It can also occur in organic states such as temporal lobe epilepsy. In connection with the obsessional states we can note that anxious self-scrutiny, which is a feature of the obsessional, was stressed by Schilder (1935) as an important element in all cases. Finally it can occur as a transient experience in normal people (Sedman, 1966) especially when they are tired. The diagnostic problem is usually settled by a careful examination of the mental state seeking for symptoms of the primary disorder. Occasionally, however, depersonalization is the sole symptom for many months and a firm diagnosis has to be delayed. In each of the conditions we have listed, depersonalization occurs in only a minority of patients and it is not known why these few develop the symptom while the majority are spared.

The mechanisms by which symptoms begin is also obscure. At times, symptoms begin during heightened anxiety and it has been suggested by Lader (1969) that they represent a form of restriction of sensory input which serves to reduce anxiety at the time and which fails to return to normal afterwards. However, this attractive idea does not explain why, in other cases, the symptoms begin at a time when the sensory input has already fallen and the patient is relaxing after a period of stress (Shorvon *et al.*, 1946), or why some patients report that the established symptoms are made worse by relaxation. Other explanations, couched in terms of the integration of the body schema (Schilder, 1935) cannot be tested rigorously.

Treatment. The treatment is that of the primary disorder if such can be identified. In the rare cases which appear to represent a primary depersonalization neurosis, it is unusual for any treatment to be effective. This has not prevented psychiatrists from applying the whole range of treatment including sedative drugs, abreaction, narcosis and ECT. None has proved to be effective and ECT may make the condition worse (Shorvon *et al.*, 1946). However, a trial of benzodiazepines or antidepressant medication is often appropriate. The patient's evident distress, espcially when coupled with an immature and demanding personality, not infrequently lead to overtreatment. When a primary condition is found – as it will be eventually in most cases – appropriate treatment should be given. Otherwise, the doctor needs to do what he can to relieve his patient's distress by reassurance and supportive psychotherapy, but should not heap one ineffective measure on another.

5.2.2
The impact of anxious parents on their children
SULA WOLFF

Anxiety states

Anxiety states are not commonly encountered among parents of psychiatrically disturbed children and their effects on children are not especially harmful. Perhaps this is because the illness tends to be time limited and not life threatening. Its symptoms, often understandable as expressions of mental discomfort, rarely involve the child.

Bruce was almost 12 on referral to a child psychiatrist because of obsessional rituals present for two and a half years. He had a habit of flicking his right hand, breathing oddly, and having to hop several times as he walked. The symptoms were most marked on the football field, always just as he was about to score a goal. In addition he had repeatedly to check his homework.

He was on poor terms with his older brother, James, resenting the fact that this boy could do a lot of things still out of reach for Bruce. Throughout his life he had had mild asthma and his appearance was delicate like his father's. He was his father's favourite to the extent that the mother felt impelled systematically to support James, each parent resenting the other's apparent rejection of their favourite son and thereby contributing to the bitterness between the boys.

The *father*, 36, had recently set up on his own as a plumber. He worried about the business. Following the death of a man whose house he had replumbed, he developed attacks of panic with tachycardia and sweating, sleeplessness, loss of libido, and a recurrent thought that he could not swallow. These symptoms resembled those he had had at 18 after his father's death from cancer. His father had always favoured an older brother and our patient's father had resented his own position as the black sheep of the family. His mother did not make up for his father's lack of affection. On the contrary, it was she who urged him to become a plumber, rather than follow his own wish to join the Army.

While his illness, precipitated by a constellation of circumstances which revived for him his childhood conflicts, did not in itself contribute to Bruce's obsessional state, it increased the marital tensions and precipitated the subsequent break-up of the family.

Bruce's symptoms responded well to clomipramine hydrochloride. But the father's psychoneurosis did not improve with psychiatric treatment until he decided to give up his business and become a wage-earner once more. A series of family interviews failed to improve family relationships. The mother, more intelligent than her husband but with her own personality difficulties (she often presented herself like a provocative teenager) stemming from a grossly abnormal and violent childhood, felt rejected by her husband but also taunted him for his timidity. Finally she entered an extra-marital relationship. The father then left the family to live with his mother. Bruce and James became more harmonious but Bruce, still resentful and now disapproving also of his mother, engaged in some minor delinquency with another boy.

Phobic illnesses

Phobic states especially in mothers are more likely to affect the life of a family and to involve the children.

Mr Jones, an ambitious businessman, a weekend golfer, initially described a happy childhood wishing that he could give as much time to his children as his father had given to him. Yet he resented his wife's appeals that he should be at home and talk to her more, finding himself irritated and constricted by her dependency. When she was pregnant with her second son, his mother died of cancer and it was at this time that *the older boy*, then 2½, developed serious night terrors. These persisted for some years.

Finally the father changed his work to be at home more but felt increasingly resentful and became irritable with his sons, especially the older, less able boy. At this stage he had an accident at work sustaining a serious burn. *The mother*, herself the product of a quarrelsome marriage, now developed a depressive illness with much irritability. The couple ceased intercourse and were very unhappy.

When the older boy was referred to a psychiatrist because of school refusal, the father revealed that when he was 12 his mother had developed a street phobia. Because his father was unsympathetic to her, *he* became her 'right hand man', accompanying her everywhere. He never once resented her dependency on him, which lasted until he left school and deprived him of all social activities with his peers.

He himself had made no connection at all between this experience and his resentment of his wife's dependency on him, which he had labelled as such and which he knew was more legitimate.

In the second interview he reported that he and his wife had had things out with his dependent and inactive business partner. Both felt and were communicating better. He now revealed his academic ambitions for his not very able son, recognizing these as a great burden on the boy.

Both these case histories illustrate the inner continuities between childhood and adult experiences of anxiety in the individual parent. They show in particular how abnormal reactions to stress in adult life (whether in the form of psychoneurotic symptoms or maladaptive behaviour) can be associated with a perceived recapitulation of painful, childhood circumstances, personal and unique, which are often still interpreted by the individual with the pre-rational, animistic logic of his childhood self.

If we shift from the experiential to the objective viewpoint, we find that parental psychiatric symptoms are most harmful to children when they involve the child or when both parents are psychiatrically disturbed. Parental personality disorder is most strongly associated with childhood psychiatric disturbance (Rutter, 1966) and of course many parents with phobic and anxiety states have associated personality disorders.

Berg and co-workers (1974) found no difference between the rates and types of maternal psychiatric illness in school phobic and other youngsters in an adolescent in-patient unit.

There is however some evidence for continuity of psychoneurotic symptoms from childhood into adult life. Patients who had attended both child and adult psychiatric clinics at the same hospital usually had the same type of disorder on each occasion (Pritchard & Graham, 1966). Tyrer and Tyrer (1974) found significantly more adult psychiatric patients with phobias, anxiety states, and depression to have had a period of school refusal than orthopaedic and dental patients. The incidence of truancy in childhood was the same for both groups. Both childhood symptoms were reported more often by women than men. But, while a history of school phobia is elicited in 16–22 per cent of psychoneurotic adults, agoraphobics are no more likely to have had this childhood disorder than other psychoneurotic patients (Berg, 1982).

6
Hysteria

6.1
Childhood origins of hysterical personality disorder and of hysterical conversion syndromes: Hysterical conversion symptoms in childhood

SULA WOLFF

Childhood origins of hysterical personality disorder

Child and adolescent psychiatrists have excellent opportunities to witness the processes of personality development. They have access to the recollected childhood experiences of young parents and can trace connections between these recollections and the parents' current aspirations, emotional responses, and behaviour in relation to each other and their children.

Child psychiatrists also see many youngsters with enduring characteristics of behaviour usually thought of as constituting hysterical personality. Only systematic follow-up studies can show how permanent such characteristics will turn out to be and how many affected children will in adult life display personality disorder as opposed to hysterical personality traits without functional impairment.

The features of hysterical personality clinically apparent even in childhood are: over-eagerness to be liked and accepted, with great investment in personal appearance and accoutrements (earrings, bracelets, handbags, hairstyle, and other fashion equipment); escessive sensitivity to criticism or perceived slights with fear of rejection; excessive curiosity combined with prudishness in relation to sex, often with undue concern about destructive and hurtful aspects of intercourse and procreation; a tendency to find frankness in human relationships difficult, with excessive inhibition of anger and assertiveness. Parental behaviour clearly contributes to such patterns. Relationships with peers are often impaired by the child's mistrustful lack of openness. Denial is a common defence mechanism. These traits are, as in adults, more often seen in girls than boys, perhaps because of different parental expectations. A common family constellation is a mother not unconditionally accepting of the child, who instead turns to the father (see also Chodoff, 1974). In some cases the mother is rejecting of male sexuality and the father either absent or seductive towards the child.

The crucial life experiences which help to explain this mode of being usually take place between 2½ and 6 years, when the individual is beginning to be aware of life and death matters, of family relationships and sexuality, but is not yet able to comprehend the environment in rational terms.

Michele, a seven-year-old, whose parents separated after many violent quarrels when she was four, had a sudden onset of crying, fear of the dark, and regular nightmares after her father requested access and her mother's solicitor asked her whether she wanted to see him again. For over a year the mother had complained of the child's bad temper, fearing she might become 'psychopathic' like her father, reacting punitively to the temper outbursts and with irritation to the nocturnal disturbances.

Michele, a large, attractive, bright-eyed child, with carefully varnished nails, was over-eager to please. She sat herself down and opened the first interview with 'I'd like to tell you all about my father. In my bed one night he told me to turn the hall light off and I was only two years old.' When she was three he had once locked her and her mother into their house. Once he had thrown an ashtray and cut the diningroom chairs with a knife, had fallen downstairs and had to go to hospital. She has recurrent dreams 'about my father throwing the ashtray and my mum doesn't want to go over it again. My mum didn't want a wee girl, but my dad made me watch TV films and a girl with a tarantula and a thing on her tummy, and I started screaming. One night my mum went to a dance . . . and he forced me to eat mince and stabbed me with a fork in the arm and I couldn't bear it.' She told her grandfather and the police were called. Once her father tried to stab her with a knife. 'It still happens in my mind. I'm frightened to leave my mum.' When she grows up she wants to be an army nurse 'helping all the men and old ladies'.

The mother described her appalling marriage at length and also her own frigidity and her wish to remain single. Referring to a previous child, she whispered 'there's another one like her in the world'.

Childhood origins of hysterical conversion syndromes

In contrast to parents, especially mothers, with hysterical personality disorders, adults with hysterical conversion symptoms do not often cross the child

psychiatrist's path, perhaps because the conditions are usually time limited. The exceptions are chronic complaints of body pains, globus hystericus, and dissociative states mimicking epilepsy.

Two sisters, both referred in early childhood with enuresis and separation anxiety, in one associated with soiling and educational retardation and in the other followed in middle childhood by panic attacks and screaming whenever her mother had visitors, were being brought up by a single mother. This woman, the oldest of two sisters, developed grand mal epilepsy at 19 and felt 'my whole nature changed'. She was classed as 'disabled', warned by her father to avoid heights and machinery, and stopped working. She married a man younger than herself and became fat and frigid. When her husband left her for another woman she refused divorce and developed very frequent 'blackouts', many of which were not epileptic. She also now engaged in obsessional checking each night that no man was under her bed.

She became totally dependent on her mother and social security, raged frequently at the children and felt neglected by the many professionals intent to help her. In later years she had a succession of young boy friends, her house was always full of people and she talked mainly about failed sexual and family relationships.

Both girls did much housework, never had their mother to themselves, worried constantly about her health and often complained to their psychiatrist about their mother's anger and lack of appreciation of their own efforts to help.

The childhood origins of adult hysterical psychoneurosis can only be inferred. Children themselves tend to recover from hysterical conversion symptoms (Caplan, 1970); and the opportunity for childhood observation of subjects destined to develop these in adult life must be quite rare.

Hysterical conversion symptoms in childhood

It seems to be agreed that, as in adults, hysterical conversion symptoms in childhood have become uncommon. Mildred Creak (1969) believed this to be because we now respond more sensitively to children's anxieties when they are ill. A further reason may be that crippling illness and early death have become rare, and invalidism is no longer seen as a possible way of life.

Accounts of hysterical psychoneurosis in childhood stress the aetiological importance of physical illness in the child or others (Caplan, 1970; Creak, 1969; Dubowitz & Hersov, 1976). In Caplan's (1970) series, even among the fifteen pre-pubescent children who had no organic basis for their conversion symptoms, the psychoneurosis was precipitated by a personal experience of accident, physical illness, or medical intervention in six, and by the death or illness or another person in four.

Children often express anxiety in terms of the physical symptoms of others by the process of identification. Episodic attacks of mass hysteria in schools (Sirois, 1974) which cease during the holidays bear witness to this.

A girl of six with an hysterical limp had a father with a congenitally short leg. A boy with body pains and panic attacks after drinking what he thought was coca cola (but was really coke and rum), feared he would become alcoholic like his father. His physical and anxiety symptoms were exactly those which had led the father to seek psychiatric help.

Conversion hysteria in referred children is commoner in girls (1.6:1, as reported by Robins and O'Neal, 1953); is more often associated with a diagnosis of hysteria but less often with other psychiatric disorders in close relatives than other emotional disorders (Caplan, 1970); is very often accompanied or followed by a diagnosis of organic illness related to the symptoms (in 13 or 28 pre-pubescent children, Caplan (1970)); and is very rarely accompanied by conduct disorders (Caplan, 1970) but, in contrast with adults, always by symptoms or signs of anxiety (Robins & O'Neal, 1953). In Caplan's out-patient series, recovery was the rule in the absence of organic illness, although the outcome was less good in Robins and O'Neal's in-patient series (1953). The diagnosis of hysterical amblyopia must be made with great caution since a number of cases were subsequently found to have progressive organic blindness.

Management involves an active, behavioural treatment approach to the symptom itself in addition to psychotherapy for the child and her family. Organic pathology masked by, or masquerading as, hysteria should never be overlooked. But Dubowtiz and Hersov (1976) caution paediatricians against the iatrogenic effects of too many physical investigations, bed rest, and immobilization when they really know the child has a psychological disorder. Paediatricians, child psychiatrists, physiotherapists, psychologists, and social workers can effectively collaborate in the management of this condition.

6.2
Hysteria
R. E. KENDELL

Physicians have recognized since the time of Sydenham that many of the patients who consulted them with symptoms which purported to be those of bodily disease were not in fact suffering from the diseases whose symptoms they displayed. Sometimes they assumed that such patients were simply pretending or imagining that they were disabled or in pain. More often, either because the patient's distress and suffering seemed so real, or perhaps because the opportunity to prescribe and charge a fee was irresistible, the assumption was made that the patient's complaints were the result of a nervous affliction. Explanations of how a nervous disorder could generate so wide a variety of insistent complaints were inevitably rather vague, but by the middle of the eighteenth century the two ancient concepts of hysteria and hypochondriasis were regularly invoked to account for this state of affairs, and in 1765 the Scottish physician Robert Whytt was driven to observe that physicians 'have bestowed the character of nervous on all those disorders whose nature and causes they were ignorant of'. More recently several new concepts have been added to the list. As well as hysteria and hypochondriasis we now have neurasthenia, psychophysiological, psychosomatic, and somatization reactions, organ neuroses, the 'functional overlay' of the general physician, and plain malingering. All these terms, except perhaps the last, are inadequately defined and overlap with one another. Thomas Dover's sardonic remark that 'what we call hypochondriacal in men we call hysterical in women' is almost as true now as it was when he made it in 1733.

Of all these muddy concepts hysteria is the most ancient and the most ambiguous. The term is derived from the Greek word *hystera* for womb. Egyptian physicians in the second millennium BC and their Greek descendants believed that the phenomena of the disease were caused by the uterus wandering away from its proper station and sought to entice it back by the local application of fragrant potions, or alternatively to drive it back by administering nauseous draughts by mouth. Thus arose the tenacious concept of hysteria as a disease of women and the theme of reproductive pathology. Less than a hundred years ago Freud's teachers in Vienna ridiculed the idea that hysteria could occur in men and even Kraepelin regarded a convulsion precipitated by pressure on the ovary as one of the hallmarks of the condition.

During the last twenty years the confusion surrounding the concept of hysteria has been as remarkable as at any time in the past three thousand years. The term is applied to several different syndromes, most with ill-defined boundaries, and related only tenuously to one another. Indeed it is sometimes applied to phenomena like trance states in which there is little evidence that the subject is ill, or even wishes to be regarded as such. Very varied assumptions are also made about the aetiology of the condition. In the words of Paul Chodoff, one of the most perceptive of recent writers on the subject, 'Entities that are clinically quite different are being held together artificially by little more than the authority of an ancient name . . . it is a fossil encrusted with and obscured by successive layers of meaning' (Chodoff, 1974). Indeed, it would probably be all to the good if the term hysteria were to be abandoned. It has in fact been omitted by the American Psychiatric Association from the current version of its official nomenclature (DSM–III), along with hypochondriasis and neurasthenia, but the term has already survived a series of scathing attacks going back at least to the beginning of this century and, as Lewis (1975) dryly observed, it is a tough old word which tends to outlive its obituarists.

In this situation the most sensible course for the author of a textbook account of 'hysteria' is probably to describe the various syndromes which are traditionally subsumed under that rubric, if only because they will not be described elsewhere, and then, having done so, suggest what alternative concepts might provide a more appropriate framework for considering the phenomena in question.

Conversion hysteria

The uterine concept of hysteria, which survived almost unchallenged from before the time of Hippocrates until the latter half of the nineteenth century, was based explicitly on somatic pathology. It was a disease of the body, not of the mind. The same was true of Charcot's hysteria. Despite his preoccupation with hypnosis and his demonstration that all the symptoms of the condition could be produced or removed at will under hypnosis he remained convinced that hysteria was a degenerative and hereditary disorder of the nervous system. So did Janet (1907), despite his greater understanding of the role of psychological influences on the behaviour of hysterics, and his conviction that all the symptoms of the condition were due to a 'dissociation' of consciousness. The idea that hysteria was a purely psychological disorder was introduced by Breuer and Freud in their famous *Studies on Hysteria* (1896), and the opposition to their views owed almost as much to the abandonment of neurological pathology as it did to the introduction of novel and disturbing ideas about infantile sexuality.

According to Freudian theory, hysteria is a specific clinical entity arising from sexual conflicts originating in the oedipal stage of psychosexual development. Failure to relinquish the incestuous tie to the opposite sexed parent that develops during infancy leads to sexual conflicts in adult life because the sexual drive, or libido, retains its forbidden incestuous quality. The drive is therefore subjected to the defensive psychological manoeuvre of repression and its energy is *converted* into a hysterical symptom, which not only protects the patient from conscious awareness of the drive, and hence from the anxiety that would otherwise result, but simultaneously provides a symbolic expression of it.

At the time it was first proposed the concept of 'psychic energy' and its conversion into a physical symptom was not as far fetched as it sounds today. In the 1890s Cajal had only recently convinced the leading scientists of the German-speaking world that the brain was composed of distinct neurones and was not a reticulum as Golgi had believed. The mechanism of neural conduction was quite unknown; the neuronal resting potential was not discovered until 1910. In this climate Freud's assumption that energy was transmitted from one neurone to another like water down a pipe, and that the only way a nerve impulse could be prevented from arriving in one site was by displacing it to another, did not appear unreasonable to the neurophysiologists of the day. His assumption that the structure of the mind reflected that of the brain, and that psychic energy was transmitted in analogous ways to physical energy, was equally plausible. It is much harder, however, to understand how these ideas persisted for so long after neural conduction had been shown to depend not on transfers of energy but on the propagation of impulses, excitatory and inhibitory, by small changes in membrane potentials. The explanation is to be found partly in the isolation of most psychiatrists from developments in neurophysiology and neuropsychology, and partly in the general immunity of psycho-analytic theory to refutation by observation or experiment. It may also be significant that, as the first-born child of psycho-analytic theory, the concept of conversion hysteria was invested with a historical and emotional significance which prevented it from being quietly abandoned as it might otherwise have been. But although we are no longer prepared to give credence to Freud's explanatory theory, and regret the fact that it has been enshrined in the term 'conversion symptom', the observable phenomena still present the practitioners of many different branches of medicine with an unresolved clinical and theoretical challenge.

The term conversion symptom is applied to disturbances of motor or sensory function arising in the absence of any demonstrable lesion of the relevant neurological pathways. The patient complains of a failure of sensation (blindness, deafness, or loss of cutaneous sensation), or of muscular weakness or paralysis, despite the fact that no abnormal neurological signs can be elicited or any abnormal neurophysiological responses demonstrated either peripherally (for example, nerve conduction times or electromyography) or centrally (for example, cortical evoked potentials). By convention the term is restricted to disturbances referable to somatic afferent or efferent pathways though, largely for historical reasons, convulsions are also included.

The presentation of conversion hysteria varies considerably from generation to generation and culture to culture. The commonest motor symptoms are usually weakness or paralysis of one or more limbs – monoplegia, hemiplegia, or paraplegia. Sometimes the patient is unable to walk or stand, or does so only with a bizarre staggering gait. In chronic cases contractures and muscle wasting may develop but oth-

erwise there are no neurological signs and often it is apparent that the patient is using affected muscle groups, for sitting up or turning over in bed, for example, which he or she does not use on formal examination. Some patients present with abnormal tic-like movements or tremors rather than weakness and sometimes the weakness is restricted to the laryngeal muscles (hysterical aphonia). Characteristically, the disability corresponds to lay concepts of paralysis rather than with the distribution of peripheral nerves or spinal segments. In hysterical aphonia, for example, although the patient is quite unable to talk in a normal voice he can often enunciate perfectly in a whisper and coughing is unimpaired. Sensory symptoms are analogous. Disturbances of cutaneous sensation may affect pain sensation only or all modalities and are usually restricted to one or more limbs or the whole of one side of the body. Blindness is much commoner than deafness and often peripheral vision is grossly restricted while central vision remains relatively unimpaired (tunnel vision). As with motor disturbances, the anaesthesia corresponds to lay ideas rather than to neurological reality: hemianaesthesia stops abruptly at the midline, limb anaesthesia has a 'glove and stocking' distribution, and vibration sense is lost on one side of the head and preserved on the other. Hysterical seizures likewise reflect lay concepts of epilepsy. Generally they consist of a fall to the ground followed by a few minutes of uncoordinated thrashing of all four limbs with eyes shut. There is no sequence of tonic and clonic movements, it is rare for the patient to void or injure herself, and the EEG does not change even after a series of fits. They also tend to occur in public rather than when the patient is alone or asleep. It has often been observed that unilateral hysterical (and also hypochondriacal) symptoms are commoner on the left side of the body than on the right. This intriguing finding may be a reflection of functional differences between the two cerebral hemispheres or, alternatively, of the different and deeply rooted connotations of right and left (*dexter* and *sinister* in Latin).

Patients with hysterical symptoms often show a striking lack of concern about their disability – the 'belle indifférence' of nineteenth-century French physicians – although they show normal anxiety about other matters. A girl of 16 who has suddenly become paralysed from the waist down may seem quite unconcerned at the prospect of a life of invalidism with hopes for career and marriage blighted, and equally unconcerned to know why she has lost the use of her legs. This is, of course, readily comprehensible in terms of the psycho-analytic theory of conversion but other equally plausible explanations are available and when autonomic indices of arousal, like pulse rate and psychogalvanic skin response, are measured hysterics tend to be over-, rather than under-aroused.

The ease with which hysteria can be distinguished from neurological disease varies considerably with the nature of the symptom and the setting. Often the incompatibility between the patient's complaint and his other behaviour makes it possible to establish the diagnosis without hesitation. The blind man crosses and recrosses the room without ever falling or bumping into the furniture and the paraplegic's hamstrings contract whenever he is asked to lift his paralysed legs off the bed. But dystonic movements are commonly misdiagnosed as hysterical and sometimes hysterical fits can be realistic enough to deceive the most experienced and sceptical of observers. It is when neurological disease is already present and the question at issue is whether all or only part of the patient's disabilities are organic that the difficulties become formidable. The most important general rule is to preserve an open mind as long as possible. Mistaken decisions either way have usually been taken too quickly.

Little is known of the epidemiology of conversion symptoms, largely because they are so varied in nature. It is generally believed that they are commoner in children than in adults, commoner in women than in men, commoner in the naive and unintelligent than in the sophisticated, and less common in this century than in the nineteenth. None of these statements can be made with confidence, however, because all are based simply on clinical impressions. No one has ever measured the incidence or prevalence of conversion symptoms in a random sample of a population. Such symptoms characteristically develop in response to stress and tend to be contagious. This is seen most dramatically in time of war because the stress is obvious and affects many people simultaneously. In the First World War in particular hysterical tremors, gait disturbances and convulsions were commonplace, particularly in infantry units which had been in the trenches for months on end and suffered heavy casualties.

Psychophysiological reactions

Although as originally conceived the symptom into which psychic energy was converted in Freud's conversion hysteria was invariably 'neurological' in character later generations of psycho-analysts became convinced that other symptoms like pain, nausea, vomiting and dizziness could also be produced by the same mechanisms of repression and conversion. Some writers, however, continued to maintain that symptoms of this kind – referrable to the viscera and mediated by the autonomic nervous system – were 'psychophysiological reactions' rather than conversion reactions; they were simply the physiological correlates of unconscious affects and lacked the symbolic quality of true conversion reactions. It is doubtful, of course, whether there could ever be a sharp demarcation between the two, because symptoms like abdominal pain and vomiting involve both autonomic and somatic pathways. More important is the expansion of the concept of psychogenesis to include pain and visceral symptoms as well as neurological deficits. Willingness to regard pain as a hysterical symptom is particularly important, for pain which is not accompanied by unequivocal evidence of organic disease is commonplace and it is not nearly so easy as it is in the case of paralyses and anaesthesias to be confident that no relevant organic disturbance is present. One is reminded again of Robert Whytt's remark about physicians bestowing 'the character of nervous on all those disorders whose nature and causes they were ignorant of.'

Dissociative reactions

The concept of dissociation of consciousness was introduced by Pierre Janet in the closing years of the nineteenth century at the same time as Breuer and Freud were formulating their concept of conversion. To Janet, dissociation was the fundamental disturbance underlying hypnosis and all hysterical phenomena, and although he himself paid little attention to the infant school of psycho-analysis in Vienna the two concepts – conversion and dissociation – were eventually incorporated side by side in an uneasy synthesis which has somehow survived for most of this century.

What Janet meant by dissociation or 'disaggregation' of consciousness was essentially a failure of integration of different elements of consciousness, producing either a disturbed or restricted sense of personal identity or a restriction of conscious awareness to certain themes of immediate emotional importance in a setting in which memories of past personal events were often inaccessible (Janet, 1907). Retrospective amnesia for events during the period of dissociation was a further characteristic feature. Although this dissociation was nearly always temporary, and did not affect either intellectual ability or a wide range of acquired skills, it was assumed, at least by Janet himself, to be due to a hereditary 'degeneracy' of the nervous system. Its most dramatic manifestation was the rare phenomenon of multiple personality but equally clear examples were to be found in fugues, amnesic episodes and trance states, either arising spontaneously or induced by hypnosis.

Multiple personality

This is a rare phenomenon, though as multiple personalities always arouse great interest when they come to medical attention there are over 200 case reports in the literature, and several examples in fiction (for example, Robert Louis Stevenson's Dr Jekyll and Mr Hyde). Usually there are only two personalities, the second arising at a time of emotional crisis and replacing the first for anything from a few hours to several years. The two personalities are always quite unalike and unaware of one another, and each has amnesia for the period when the other is in control. Typically, the original personality is timid and inhibited and the alter ego strikingly more adventurous and assertive. Occasionally three or more quite distinct personalities emerge in sequence. When this occurs each of these subsidiary personalities may be aware of, and make disparaging remarks about, the original timid, conforming personality but they still remain unaware of one another and the original personality remains unaware of them. Sometimes the emergence of the alter ego is ushered in by a fugue and the new personality builds up an entirely new life, acquiring a new job and a new circle of friends in a different community, but more commonly the two alternate in the same setting. As with other hysterical phenomena, it thrives on the fascination it engenders.

Hysterical amnesia

Hysterical amnesia usually develops as a direct response to severe, and sometimes overwhelming, stress. It may extend over a few hours or days and serve to blot out a particularly frightening or painful incident, it may extend over several years, so taking the subject back to a happier stage in their life, or it may go right back to early childhood so that the subject temporarily loses all sense of personal identity and may then present at a hospital or police station complaining that they don't know who they are or where they come from. Short-lived amnesia is particularly common in time of war. A soldier who has been

trapped inside a burning tank, for example, and who perhaps has fought with his surviving companion to escape through the hatch, has no memory of the incident when restored to his unit, but continues to have nightmares until he relives it under hypnosis or sedation. People who present with complete loss of memory are likewise usually escaping from stressful situations – marital conflicts, money troubles, the exposure of sexual or financial misdemeanours, and so on. Sometimes, however, the escape is from an intolerable mood – usually deep depression – rather than a life situation. In many of these patients presentation with amnesia is preceded by a fugue, emphasizing the close links between the two phenomena. Some also have organic brain disease – epilepsy, recent concussion, or early dementia. Indeed, there is considerable overlap between hysterical and organic amnesias and any patient presenting with loss of memory requires careful neurological assessment, whether or not there is presumptive evidence of psychogenesis.

Sometimes the psycho-dynamics of the amnesia are more complicated than merely the relief of anxiety or the avoidance of stress:

A woman of 40 who was drinking heavily and whose marriage was disintegrating lapsed into a drunken sleep after a bitter row with her husband. On waking in the small hours of the morning she couldn't understand why the street lights were on and ran round the house drawing all the curtains and talking of the black-out. She failed to recognize her husband when he appeared and addressed her 18-year-old son, of whom she had always been inordinately fond, as 'darling' and sought protection in his arms from the presumptuous stranger in their house. Throughout that day she behaved as if it were 1944 rather than 1964, except for one brief moment when she suddenly noticed her son ironing his own shirt in desperation and said spontaneously 'You mustn't iron that, it's nylon'. The next morning, after being sedated and sleeping for ten hours, she had recovered.

With or without treatment hysterical amnesias do not usually last longer than a few days and occasionally, if the subject is bluntly told that he or she is pretending to have lost their memory, they will confess that this is so. During the amnesic period the subject may appear somewhat dazed but usually retains memories which are not explicitly personal, and also skills like driving a car and playing cards acquired during the 'forgotten' part of their life.

Fugues

A fugue is a journey, or period of aimless wandering, undertaken in a state of dissociated or restricted consciousness. It usually lasts a few hours or days, but occasionally for much longer. Sometimes the subject wanders aimlessly, sleeping rough and eating little; sometimes behaviour is much more purposive and organized, involving long, complicated journeys and even periods of gainful employment. Occasionally the subject behaves during the fugue in ways that are strikingly uncharacteristic and it is tempting to see in this a *forme fruste* of the related phenomenon of multiple personality. As with uncomplicated hysterical amnesias the onset is usually directly related to stresses of readily understandable kinds. The subject is confronted with an immediate threat which he cannot either evade or combat. He becomes depressed and his thought content becomes increasingly restricted to the insoluble dilemma confronting him. In this setting dissociation occurs and the fugue begins. Sometimes the motive is simply to escape but it may be more complicated. The soldier who deserts his unit may enrol in another regiment in the course of his fugue, or travel to a distant place associated with happier memories, like the town where a kindly grandparent used to live. As with amnesias and trance states, the subject often appears rather dazed and is usually left with an absent or incomplete memory of the journey afterwards. Those who embark on fugues are often described as having hysterical or psychopathic personalities and often come from broken homes and have a previous history of epilepsy, head injury, alcoholism, or pathological lying. It is uncertain which of these relationships is of aetiological importance, and whether the significance of epilepsy, head injury, and alcoholism is that they have produced enduring changes in brain function, or simply that they have provided an earlier model of amnesia, and the possible advantages thereof.

It is not uncommon, of course, for people who feel themselves surrounded by insoluble problems or realize that they are in danger of ignominious exposure, to desert their homes and families, temporarily or permanently. A fugue should only be diagnosed, therefore, when it is fairly certain, either from the subject's mental state at the time or on the grounds of subsequent amnesia, that consciousness was impaired during the flight. As with amnesic states, however, there is no clear border between what is conscious and what is unconscious, or between the hysterical and the organic. In particular, what may start as a fugue may develop into a conscious decision not to return home, a sequence of events which may well underlie some of the fugues which appear to last for weeks or months and involve what to the observer may appear to be a series of decisions and behaviours shrewdly calculated to evade retribution.

Trance states

A trance is a state of dissociation in which responsiveness to environmental stimulation is greatly reduced and for which, like other dissociative states, the subject has no memory afterwards. It may arise, or be induced, in a variety of different ways. A somnambulistic trance has its onset during sleep, the subject rising from his bed night after night and behaving in a stereotyped way which usually portrays some important emotional conflict, like Lady Macbeth tormented by her guilt at Duncan's murder. The subject is oblivious of any watchers, cannot be roused by ordinary means, and has no memory for the event afterwards. Trance states may also be induced simply by the exclusion of environmental stimuli. The Eastern mystic sitting silently in a posture which promotes immobility and concentrating on a single thought does so deliberately. The lorry driver or airline pilot driving silently through the night with nothing to look at but his instruments and the unchanging vista ahead does so involuntarily, sometimes with disastrous results. Paradoxically, the same effect can be induced by a combination of powerful emotional arousal and massive rhythmical sensory stimulation, as in a variety of religious ceremonies in which the participants dance and chant together for hours on end. Hypnotic trances are essentially similar and are usually induced either by monotonous rhythmical stimulation or by concentration on a single unchanging stimulus, aided by powerful suggestion.

Mass (epidemic) hysteria

Although the most dramatic and famous examples of mass hysteria were the 'dancing manias' of the fourteenth century, over ninety similar outbreaks have been reported in the medical literature of the last hundred years, including several in the last decade. Most of these involved girls or young women and took place at a time of stress in a tightly knit community – a school, a convent, or a nurses' home. A typical and well-documented outbreak occurred in a girls' secondary school in Lancashire in 1965 (Moss & McEvedy, 1966). A mood of apprehension was created by an outbreak of poliomyelitis in the neighbourhood and newspaper reports of lorry drivers refusing to enter the town. In this emotionally charged setting several girls fainted while standing waiting for a church service and shortly afterwards, over the course of a few hours, dozens of girls collapsed complaining of dizziness, headaches, weakness, shivering, and paraesthesiae. When sent home they quickly recovered, but there was a second outbreak when the school was re-assembled a few days later, and a third later still. As in other similar epidemics the onset of symptoms was in a public setting rather than at home, and no viral or bacterial pathogen could be incriminated. The essential elements are suggestibility and shared apprehension and the key figures in the outbreak frequently have personalities of so-called hysterical type.

Briquet's syndrome (St Louis hysteria)

Although it was first described by the French physician Briquet in 1859, and again by the English physician Savill in 1909, this syndrome owes its contemporary recognition to the St. Louis school of psychiatry in the United States (Purtell, 1951). As described it occurs almost exclusively in women. The patient presents in early adult life with a series of symptoms referrable to different bodily systems for which no adequate organic cause can be found. Complaints of headaches, abdominal pains, dizziness, backache, palpitations, generalized weakness, and so on, are made, singly or together, over several years and often to several different doctors. Characteristically, though not invariably, the symptoms are dramatized. The headaches are 'agonizing', the abdominal pains 'like red hot knives' and the weakness so extreme the patient 'can hardly stand'. She nearly always has menstrual symptoms and sexual problems (frigidity or dyspareunia) as well and is typically either unmarried or divorced. Sometimes hysterical personality traits are prominent and sometimes classical conversion symptoms develop but neither is an integral part of the syndrome. As described by the St Louis school these women have often exhibited delinquent behaviour in adolescence and family studies reveal a high incidence of Briquet's syndrome in other female relatives and of alcoholism and antisocial personality disorder in male relatives.

The behaviour of these women is very persistent. Most continue to present with an endless series of somatic symptoms at least until late middle age. They accumulate thick files, have multiple operations which rarely relieve their symptoms for very long, and often become addicted to drugs unwisely prescribed to relieve their pains. Psychiatric treatment is rarely successful, largely because of their refusal to accept that their symptoms may not be due to organic disease, and their habit of changing doctors whenever their complaints are not accepted at face value. It is, nevertheless, important to recognize the syndrome in order to minimize the number of unnecessary investigations and operations that are performed, and prevent the prescribing of potentially addictive drugs.

Other related syndromes
Factitious disorders

Most physicians have experience of occasional patients who present with symptoms which appear initially to be manifestations of serious organic disease but which eventually prove to be the result of deliberate deception. Recurrent skin lesions are produced by self-imposed trauma, a pyrexia is feigned by manipulating the thermometer, a tourniquet is used to produce recurrent swelling of a limb, diarrhoea is produced by the secret ingestion of purgatives, or palpitations and weight loss by ingestion of thyroxine. The patient is usually a young woman and usually unmarried. She is hardly ever dishonest or antisocial in other respects; indeed she is often a conscientious and effective worker of above average intelligence, though often lonely, emotionally immature, and from a disturbed family background. Several authors have commented on the high proportion of these patients who are nurses or members of other paramedical professions. Doubtless this is partly attributable to their familiarity with medical procedures and their access to drugs like thyroxine, but other factors are also involved. Many of these unhappy young women have become nurses in an attempt to conquer their own deeply rooted dependency needs but find, particularly at times of stress, that they cannot sustain the role. Although their self-image is that of the provider of love, care, sympathy, and attention for others their underlying need to receive rather than to give makes the 'invalid role' very tempting, and under stress they assume by deceit that which their innate good health denies them. Successful management calls for great psychotherapeutic skill, for the patient cannot admit to herself, still less to anyone else, that her symptoms are bogus and accusations or exposure usually lead only to tears and stubborn denial. Only after the subject's trust and confidence have been slowly and painfully won can the delicate question of the nature and function of the original symptoms be broached, and even then a wise physician is content with an implicit rather than an explicit confession.

Munchausen's syndrome

This term was coined by Richard Asher (1951) to describe an ill-defined group of people who repeatedly present in hospital emergency departments with dramatic symptoms simulating an acute medical or surgical emergency like renal colic, a perforated ulcer, or a heart attack. Often they move from hospital to hospital using a series of assumed names but presenting with much the same symptoms each time. Their motivation is obscure. Their behaviour often results in their being repeatedly subjected to painful investigations and operations, and although they may obtain opiates or make fools of unsuspecting doctors neither of these consequences seems of central importance to them. Attempts to stop this behaviour by psychotherapeutic or other means are usually ineffectual.

Malingering

This term is best reserved for situations in which disease or disability is feigned for obvious and straightforward reasons, and in which there is no doubt that the subject is fully aware of what he is doing and why. It is probably commoner in military than in civilian life. Certainly the word is used more often by military doctors, and more often by surgeons than by psychiatrists, though it is likely that some of the patients whom psychiatrists assume to be suffering from hysteria or 'compensation neurosis' are well aware that they are acting, and why they are doing so. (Many psychiatrists are curiously reluctant even to consider the possibility that their patients' disabilities might be deliberately assumed.) Some of the best-documented and most ingenious examples of malingering have been prisoners of war seeking repatriation on medical grounds, largely because this is the one situation in which malingering meets with social approval.

Compensation neurosis

People who have sustained injuries or become ill in the course of their duty, or as a result of the particular hazards of their occupation or the folly or incompetence of others, are often eligible for financial compensation for the harm they have suffered. No one disputes the appropriateness of this and the general principle of financial compensation for injury is widely and increasingly implemented. Doctors involved in assessing the disabilities of people seeking such compensation, however, or trying to treat them before the legal issues have been resolved, have long been convinced that the possibility of financial gain often makes symptoms which would otherwise have been mild or short-lived much more extensive and intractable. The term 'compensation neurosis' was coined to describe this situation and implies that the individual concerned is not simply pretending to be more severely disabled than he really is, but is in the grip of a mental illness of some kind.

The basic facts are best documented in the case of head injuries, largely because they are common and often the subject of compensation claims. As Henry Miller has shown, men seeking compensation often have far more extensive and long-lasting complaints than those whose original injury was more serious but who are not seeking, or eligible for, financial redress (Miller, 1961). The cumbersome legal process with its attendant medical assessments often drags on for two years or more, and throughout this time their symptoms fail to respond to treatment or even to wane with the passage of time. Moreover, those who seek compensation after apparently minor injuries tend to have a number of striking features in common; they are unskilled or semi-skilled, employed by large impersonal corporations rather than by small firms or farms, and usually middle-aged. And although they insist that they are incapable of working until their symptoms have cleared they rarely seek treatment spontaneously. Once their claim is settled, whether they win or lose, their complaints generally fade away within a few months, unless they are paid a pension whose existence or size is dependent on continuing disability. Physicians are often convinced that the unhappy invalids they are asked to assess, or to try unavailingly to treat, would have been better off and far happier had the possibility of financial compensation never existed, or if they had been given a small sum quickly after the event, but the legal process once set in motion is not easily influenced by considerations of this kind.

The most effective treatment is generally to try to convince the patient's lawyer to settle the claim as quickly as possible and to embark on energetic reha-bilitation as soon as this has been done.

Writer's cramp and other occupational neuroses

Many different 'occupational neuroses' have been described. Writer's cramp is the best known but telegraphist's, goldbeater's, piano player's and vio-linist's cramps are all essentially similar. In each case the subject's livelihood depends on the occupation, which involves finely co-ordinated hand movements maintained for several hours a day. The onset of symptoms is gradual and usually starts when the subject is tired, or short of time. In the case of writ-er's cramp the muscles of the hand and forearm become increasingly painful and writing becomes slow, laboured, and jerky. The pen may be held so tightly that it is driven into the paper and in advanced cases writing is made impossible either by tremor or spasm of the muscles of the hand and sometimes the whole arm. There is no evidence of neurological or muscular disease and other related activities like painting are characteristically unaffected. The sub-ject is usually an anxious person and often it is evi-dent that they were finding their job increasingly tedious and burdensome before the onset of these symptoms. Perhaps for this reason the natural course of the condition is usually unfavourable and pro-longed rest is usually ineffective even when it is fea-sible. Attempts to overcome the disability by learn-ing to type, or to write with the other hand, are more often successful, though it is not unknown for these new skills to be affected also. Behavioural treatments are usually more effective. Sylvester and Liversedge (1960) employed negative conditioning procedures, using an apparatus designed to give the patient an electric shock if he gripped his pen too tightly or deviated from the track on a writing board, and obtained lasting improvement in the majority of cases. Other workers have found that negative con-ditioning is ineffective in very anxious subjects, and that relaxation exercises may give better results.

The relative contribution of neurological and psychological factors in the genesis of these cramps is still uncertain. The fact that all the occupations that give rise to cramps involve finely co-ordinated hand movements for hours on end suggests a common neurological basis, but the frequent observation that the subject was fed up with his job before the onset of the symptoms suggests that psychological factors are also involved.

Ganser syndrome

In 1897 the German psychiatrist Ganser described three men who had developed auditory hallucinations and other symptoms suggestive of a florid psychotic illness while in prison awaiting trial or execution. Largely because this state was short-lived and followed by retrospective amnesia he was convinced it was a hysterical phenomenon rather than a conscious attempt to subvert the course of justice. The term Ganser syndrome has subsequently been used by some authors for any behaviour simulating madness or dementia which is thought to have a hysterical basis, though others restrict the term to cases which occur in a forensic setting. The latter are rare and most cases in the English literature were already psychotic or brain damaged before the onset of the Ganser symptoms, for example, a man with a psychotic depression who was convinced, quite wrongly, that he was responsible for his wife's death and about to face trial. Ganser's name is also associ-ated with the phenomenon of *Vorbeireden*, that is, giving absurd answers to questions which neverthe-less make it clear that the question has been under-stood, like saying five when asked how many legs a horse possesses. Although *Vorbeireden* was displayed by Ganser's original three patients it is an inconstant feature of simulated psychoses. As with other hys-terical phenomena the speech and behaviour of a patient simulating madness or dementia vary con-siderably with their sophistication and cultural back-ground. *Vorbeireden* may also be the product of aphasia or acalculia. The most florid example I have ever encountered was in a young woman with exten-sive brain damage from carbon monoxide poisoning who was not simulating insanity either consciously or unconsciously.

The need for a new conceptual framework

The various syndromes described above are a rather motley collection with very little in common with one another. Dissociative reactions in particular have little in common with the others. Their inclu-sion is largely a matter of history. Charcot was con-vinced, quite incorrectly, that only hysterics could be hypnotized and Janet believed that dissociation of consciousness was the fundamental disturbance underlying both hypnosis and all the 'major symp-toms' of hysteria, within which he included fugues and trance states as well as what are now called con-version symptoms (Janet, 1907). If we put dissociative states on one side, however, the remaining syndromes have one thing in common: the patient is presenting with symptoms which purport to be those of bodily disease (or madness, in the case of Ganser's syndrome) but no evidence of disease is to be found.

Medicine has never had an adequate understanding, or classification, of patients of this type and at the present time in this confused area six or seven different terms are used more or less interchangeably at the whim of individual clinicians. The multiple meanings and archaic conceptual basis of hysteria itself have already been discussed. The concept of hypochondriasis (see chap. 8.8, and vol. 1, chap. 2.6) is almost equally muddled and in addition to these we have neurasthenia, the 'functional overlay' of the general physician, psychophysiological and psychosomatic reactions and organ neuroses, all overlapping with one another and all inadequately defined. Part of the problem is that doctors are conditioned by what social scientists call their 'medical model' to assume that every bona fide patient must have an illness of some kind. If the patient's complaints can be related to a physical lesion no problem arises. But if they can't most doctors tend to oscillate uneasily between two alternative attitudes – either there is nothing wrong with him, or he is psychiatrically ill. The former may be true in organic disease model terms but does not explain why the patient is behaving in this way, nor does it relieve his suffering. The latter immediately invites the questions – what is the psychiatric illness? And what is its cause? Until recently we were not much nearer to answering these questions than we were 200 years ago.

The 'sick role'

The concepts of the 'sick role' and 'invalid behaviour' developed by sociologists like Talcott Parsons and David Mechanic provide the basis of a better understanding of the problem. Such writers have emphasized that the 'sick role' in our society carries with it many valuable privileges. Invalids are exempted from normal social obligations; children don't have to go to school and adults don't have to go to work, and may even continue to be paid for months on end despite not doing so. They are also exempted from responsibility for their behaviour, and so can't simply be told to pull themselves together. Indeed, other people are under an obligation to be kind and sympathetic to them, and often to take over their responsibilities as well. (The patient's wife takes

over the business as well as the housekeeping, the neighbours cut his lawn for him, and the hire purchase company waits for its money with uncharacteristic patience.) The only obligation on the patient, on the other hand, is to seek and accept appropriate treatment so that he utilizes the privileges of the sick role for as short a time as possible.

One of the most basic principles of learning theory is that patterns of behaviour which are rewarded tend to increase in frequency at the expense of those which are not, and the rewards of the sick role are so substantial, and are experienced by most of us so frequently in childhood, that it is hardly surprising that not all those who consult doctors with bodily symptoms have objective evidence of disease. This has, of course, been recognized for a very long time. But in the past it has generally been attributed by doctors unused to thinking in behavioural terms either to malingering, or more commonly to ill-defined mental or nervous disorders. It is probably more accurate, and certainly more straightforward, to regard it primarily as a matter of training. People who behave as if they were ill when the demands of everyday life become too heavy for them may well be doing so for the same reason they feel hungry three times a day and look both ways when stepping off the pavement – because, without realizing it, they have been trained to do so in the past.

Figure 6.2.1 provides a tentative classification of illness behaviour in the form of a Venn diagram. Reality is undoubtedly considerably more complex than this, but the relationships between the three overlapping populations shown here illustrate some important principles. Most illness behaviour is generated by recognized disease (including well-defined psychiatric syndromes like schizophrenia and melancholia). But substantial parts of the whole are generated either by fear of disease, or by the 'positive reinforcement' provided by the advantages of the invalid role. There are large and important overlaps between these three populations, and the main recognized disease population is surrounded by a penumbra of unrecognized but genuine disease (mainly people with accepted but as yet undiagnosed illnesses, like occult neoplasms, but perhaps also including subpopulations with as yet unrecognized syndromes, like people with narcolepsy in Janet's day). The management of individual patients depends on which of the eleven populations formed by the intersections of these four circles they come from, rather than on which of a few mutually exclusive diagnostic categories they belong to. In very broad terms illness behaviour generated by fear of disease corresponds to hypochondriasis and illness behaviour motivated by the advantages of the invalid role to what we call hysteria (though fear also plays an important part in some hysterical phenomena, especially mass hysteria).

Put in its simplest form, the sick role is attractive, and so liable to be adopted, whenever the balance of its advantages and disadvantages outweighs those of health. To some people the normal demands of life are so onerous – either because they lack the ability or the energy to cope successfully, or because only when ill do they receive sufficient love, sympathy or attention from other people – that the sick role is preferable most of the time. To many more the sick role becomes attractive only in situations in which their responsibilities are abnormally great (for example, soldiers in battle), or when they are in trouble (impending exams, debt, the fear of prosecution, and so on), or when the possibility of financial gain increases the attractions of illness further still (compensation neurosis). The very high incidence of hysterical phenomena in time of war suggests that everyone is potentially capable of developing hysterical symptoms, just as everyone is capable of devel-

Fig. 6.2.1. A tentative classification of illness behaviour.

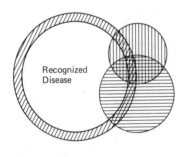

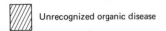

Illness behaviour motivated primarily by fear of disease or death

Illness behaviour rewarded by the advantages of the invalid role

Unrecognized organic disease

oping epilepsy, but that people vary in their liability to do so. This variation presumably depends partly on constitutional variables like suggestibility and capacity to dissociate, but the subject's current social role and past experience are probably equally important.

This view of hysteria provides a plausible explanation of what we know of the epidemiology of hysterical symptoms. The reason why these are seen mainly in the young and the immature is probably that the role of child and the role of invalid have much in common, and because the adoption of a role which involves being dependent on others and cared for by them comes most readily to those who have only recently been required to forgo the privileges of childhood and are least experienced at coping with the demands of the adult world. The predominance of conversion symptoms in women probably has a similar explanation. Until recently women were expected to be dependent on their husbands or fathers and to turn to them for help in times of trouble. This dependent role was, of course, much more clear-cut in the nineteenth century than even a generation ago, which may explain why Charcot and many of his contemporaries were convinced that hysteria occurred only in women, whereas most of the descriptions of conversion symptoms published in the last thirty years show a female predominance of no more than 2:1. The frequent coexistence of hysteria and organic disease is also readily explained, for those who are genuinely ill or handicapped are the very people who are likely to have most difficulty coping with the demands of everyday life, and also the most vivid and recent awareness of the potential advantages of invalidism.

Recovery is likewise dictated primarily by the balance of advantages and disadvantages involved. Indeed, recovery from most illness is greatly affected by the social setting in which it occurs. If the situation which precipitated the symptom resolves itself recovery will quickly follow, particularly if the patient is provided with a setting in which this can take place in response to treatment. If the situation persists, or if the enduring inadequacies of the subject herself are paramount, the advantages and disadvantages of the chosen symptom become important as well as those of the invalid role itself. This is why disabling symptoms like blindness and inability to stand or walk have a comparatively good prognosis, whereas those which can be switched on or off as occasion demands, like fits and vomiting, or cause little disability, like tremors, are more intractable. According to psycho-analytic theory the choice of symptom is determined by its symbolic meaning for the patient. The woman who develops hysterical convulsions, for example, does so because she is expressing in the rhythmical movements of the fit her fears or phantasies of coitus. Doubtless this is sometimes so. More often, however, the choice of symptom is determined by the subject's past experience, or by his experience of illness in others. The nurse who develops hysterical blindness had severe conjunctivitis as a child, and the young man who loses the use of his legs had a grandfather who was bedridden for years after a stroke. In mass hysteria, of course, the choice of symptom is determined entirely by example, except in the instigators.

Diagnosis and clinical management
The clinical diagnosis of hysteria

The first task is obviously to exclude the possibility that the patient's symptoms are due to organic disease and the ease and confidence with which this can be done vary considerably with the presenting complaint and general setting. For some neurological symptoms it can be done with confidence on clinical examination alone. In other cases, particularly where the patient's complaint is simply of pain, the problem is much harder. Not infrequently all that can be said, even after very thorough investigations have failed to reveal any evidence of relevant pathology, is simply that no evidence of organic disease can be found, and by itself this is a wholly inadequate basis for a diagnosis of hysteria. Some physicians and surgeons regard a histrionic manner as good evidence that symptoms are hysterical but this is usually unwise and it is important to remember two things. First, no one other than the patient can possibly know how severe the pain really is. More important still, people with organic disease which physicians have failed to detect are not infrequently driven to dramatize their symptoms in an attempt to persuade their doctors to treat them seriously. People with porphyria, for example, are commonly labelled as hysterics on the strength of their supposedly histrionic manner before the correct diagnosis is finally made.

Variability is another feature of some diagnostic significance. It is obviously significant if a patient who can barely stand on one occasion is observed to walk the length of the ward on another, and it is sometimes possible by playing on the patient's suggestibility to induce either improvement or deterioration in his or her symptoms almost at will. It is important not to rely on this too much, though. The symptoms of organic disease, particularly pain and sensory losses, can also fluctuate in response to suggestion, and the disabilities produced by conditions as diverse as osteo-arthritis, myasthenia, and multiple sclerosis may vary considerably from day to day. The same applies to the lack of concern, or *belle indifférence*, which characteristically accompanies hysterical symptoms. It may be very striking and a valuable diagnostic clue, but not everyone reacts to adversity with obvious alarm and it is dangerously easy for a physician who believes his patient's symptoms to be hysterical to convince himself that her emotional reactions are inappropriate.

Unless the bizarre nature of the patient's complaints, or the disparity between the complaint and the lack of disability observed outside the consulting room, are virtually incompatible with organic disease a diagnosis of hysteria can never be made with certainty. The probability is high, however, if, as well as an absence of evidence of bodily disease, there is good evidence from the social context in which the symptoms have developed of advantages for the patient in being regarded by others as ill. The diagnosis is strengthened further if the patient has a previous history of conversion symptoms, or of multiple somatic complaints for which no adequate cause could be found. Most people who develop hysterical symptoms start to do so in childhood or early adult life. For this reason one should be cautious about making the diagnosis for the first time in middle age unless the patient has been under intolerable stress. Most cases of hysteria developing *de novo* in middle life or beyond are secondary either to a depressive illness or to brain disease, and the latter may not be apparent initially (Slater, 1965).

Management and treatment

The treatment of hysterical symptoms depends in essence on eliminating or counteracting the situation which evoked them in the first place. This is done by manipulating the patient's environment in such a way as to maximize the advantages to the patient of regaining their health and to minimize those of remaining an invalid. Before this can even be attempted a detailed history must be obtained, not only from the patient herself but from friends and relatives as well, because it is necessary to understand not just the stresses affecting the patient at the time the symptoms developed but also the ways in which other people's attitudes and behaviour towards her changed when she became ill, and how they reacted on similar occasions in the past. Often the stress which precipitated the illness behaviour is self-limiting. For this reason the first question that has to be asked is whether it is wise to treat the patient at all. Hysteria fascinates doctors and it is all too easy to make the problem worse by admitting the patient to hospital or focusing attention on her symptoms by repeated examinations. For obvious reasons medical attention easily serves to confirm the patient in the invalid role. Sometimes, however, the instigation of some innocuous but plausible treatment, with or without admission to hospital, serves the invaluable function of enabling the patient to discard without loss of face a symptom which she no longer needs.

Unfortunately, hospital admission is often unavoidable because a period of observation and extensive investigations are needed to establish the diagnosis and exclude the possibility of organic disease. It may also be necessary, in order to gain sufficient control over the patient's environment, to eliminate the rewards which invalid behaviour is receiving from solicitous friends and anxious relatives in the outside world. Within the confines of a hospital ward, particularly if the staff are familiar with the general principles of behavioural treatments, it is usually possible to provide sufficient incentives for recovery and sufficiently widespread and sustained disincentives for remaining ill to induce the patient to recover. If these incentives cannot be maintained outside hospital, however, the symptoms will almost inevitably recur when the patient returns home. For this reason successful treatment of chronic or recurrent hysterical symptoms nearly always has to involve other members of the patient's family. They have to be helped to see how their own behaviour and attitudes are sustaining the problem, and helped to behave differently without becoming either angry or guilty. Florid and long-standing examples of invalid behaviour usually prove to be sustained by some key figure, usually a parent or spouse, who is consistently rewarding invalidism and in subtle ways discouraging normal behaviour because of his or her own neurotic need for a child or invalid to care for. In such cases, because the neurotic needs of the two participants match each other so well, it may well be impossible to alter the situation, and sometimes wise not even to try. Indeed, there are some situations in which the patient's invalid behaviour produces such widespread benefits, for themselves and others, that

it is positively meddlesome to attempt to restore them to health:

A woman of 54 with a mild but lifelong fear of travelling and of being alone tripped and fell headlong down an escalator on a rare visit to London. On admission to hospital she was found to be paralysed from the waist down. At first she was thought to have broken her back but, although as time went by an increasingly confident diagnosis of hysteria was made, she failed to regain any useful power in her legs. When first seen by a psychiatrist four months after the accident she was in a wheelchair in a rehabilitation unit but in good spirits and surrounded by the flowers brought by her many visitors. Her husband, a recently retired civil servant, had been encouraged to take her home at weekends and she had found that, provided he was always there to help her, she could cook and run her household without leaving her wheelchair. He, for his part, seemed glad to have a new role in his retirement and perfectly happy to help her hang out the washing and push her invalid chair round the supermarket.

When last seen a year later she was still in a wheelchair. She was able to walk a few steps around the house by herself but she never went out without her husband, or he without her in case she fell in his absence.

In the past hypnosis has often been used in the treatment of hysterical symptoms, and with dramatic success in the short run. The suggestibility of many hysterical subjects makes them readily susceptible to hypnotic suggestion, and to other less dramatic means of suggestion also. In the long run, however, little is gained by removing symptoms in this way. What matters are the relative advantages and disadvantages of health and illness. If the patient no longer has good reasons for remaining ill the symptoms will soon fade away and any plausible treatment will suffice. But if the original reasons persist or recur the symptoms will almost certainly return in one form or another, and receiving an exciting and mysterious treatment like hypnosis may increase the attractions of invalidism still further.

It has already been pointed out that some symptoms are much harder to diagnose confidently as hysterical than others, and that some involve greater disadvantages than others and are therefore less likely to become chronic. This is usually the only significance of the symptoms themselves. What matters is not whether the patient has paralysed legs or abdominal pain but the fact that he has adopted the invalid role and one of the cardinal principles of management is to pay as little attention as possible to the symptoms themselves. Initially, while the patient is being investigated to exclude organic disease, attention is inevitable, but thereafter it should be studiously avoided except to confirm that recovery is taking place.

As soon as the possibility of serious organic disease has been reduced to the point at which it can safely be ignored the patient should be reassured that he is not seriously ill and that recovery will not be long delayed. If possible, explanations and diagnostic labels are best avoided. Patients are always sensitive to insinuations that their symptoms are not genuine, particularly when they have doubts, or worse, on that score themselves. All too frequently discussions about the cause of their symptoms end in disaster with a hurt and angry patient convinced she has been told that her pain is imaginary, or that her disabilities are bogus or exaggerated. If an explanation is unavoidable the best approach is generally to explain that the symptoms are emotional in origin and probably developed when they did because of the stress the subject was under at the time. If pressed further and asked, for example, how stress can possibly cause paralysis of an arm or abdominal pain it is probably sensible to take refuge in a frank confession of ignorance, but at the same time to emphasize that, although we do not fully understand the mechanisms involved, the situation is a thoroughly familiar one and that recovery is almost invariable. While awaiting recovery, and trying to manipulate the patient's environment in order to expedite this, it is important not to lose one's nerve and continue to re-examine the paralysed limbs and order further investigations in order to reassure oneself and the relatives that the patient does not have disseminated sclerosis or a cerebral tumour after all. It is pointless telling the patient that you are sure she doesn't have anything serious the matter with her if your behaviour makes it clear that you are not.

An important advantage of this behavioural approach to the management of hysteria is that it is unnecessary to decide, or even to ask oneself, whether the patient is aware that his or her symptoms are assumed. One of the major disadvantages of the psycho-analytic concept of hysteria is that it requires a distinction between conscious motivation (which is malingering, and so subject to strong disapproval) and unconscious motivation (which is an illness – hysteria – and so worthy of sympathy and concern) in spite of the fact that it is frequently impossible to distinguish the two. Indeed, the degree of awareness the patient has often varies from time to time, so that what is initially unconscious becomes conscious, and vice versa. The old aphorism that a hysteric is an actress who has become so convinced by her own performance that she has joined her audience illustrates this very well. In the last resort the only way one can tell for certain that fits or amnesia are feigned rather than hysterical is if the patient decides to confess. Faced with the need to decide whether motivation is conscious or unconscious, but lacking any means of distinguishing the two, most psychiatrists simply assume that their patients' motives are unconscious. Others are less gullible but no better equipped to make the distinction. As a result their opinions about their patients' motivation are usually determined by how sympathetic they feel rather than by any insight into the psychological mechanisms involved. If they can empathize with the patient they accept the motivation as unconscious, and if they cannot they are reluctant to do so.

Prognosis

It is as difficult to make firm statements about the prognosis of conversion symptoms as it is about their epidemiology because they are ways of behaving under stress rather than the symptoms of an illness, and therefore subject to all the cultural influences and contingencies that affect behaviour in general. Ljungberg (1957) studied 380 patients with conversion symptoms in Stockholm and found that 80 per cent, and almost all those with basically normal personalities, recovered within twelve months. Most of those who did not recover within a year retained their symptoms indefinitely, however, though two-thirds of these chronic cases were still capable of working. Barham Carter (1949) found a better prognosis in 90 patients whom he had seen in London in the early 1940s and treated with nothing more elaborate than skilful suggestion, but this was probably because most of his patients were basically normal people reacting to the abnormal stresses of war. Both authors found that tremors, fits, and vomiting were more likely to persist or recur than more incapacitating symptoms like blindness or inability to walk or stand.

Usually a more accurate indication of the likely prognosis in an individual patient is provided by his own past history and a detailed assessment of the relative advantages and disadvantages for him of health and illness than by the literature. It is important to bear in mind, however, that conversion symptoms rarely arise for the first time in middle age or later except in response to overwhelming stress, and that that stress may be some form of organic brain disease which is not yet producing obvious physical signs.

The prognosis of Briquet's syndrome has been discussed already and is much worse than that of conversion symptoms. Most of the women who fulfil the criteria for the diagnosis of this syndrome continue to behave in the same way at least until late middle age, whether or not psychiatric treatment is attempted.

Concluding remarks

The behavioural approach to the puzzling and multifaceted phenomena of hysteria advocated here falls some way short of providing a comprehensive understanding of the problem. It sheds no light on the phenomenon of dissociation and merely ignores the patient's fears, phantasies, and degree of insight. It does not adequately explain why some people develop conversion symptoms under stress while others develop headaches, others become anxious, and some rise to the occasion and cope unaided. Nor does it provide either an explanation of or an effective treatment for the intractable somatic complaints of many patients in whom repeated investigations have failed to reveal any evidence of organic disease. Its advantages are that it focuses attention on the crucial significance of the 'invalid role', avoids untested and untestable assumptions about intrapsychic mechanisms, leads directly to a comprehensible and relatively effective strategy for management, and allows scope for the incorporation of concepts and therapies derived from other fields – pharmacological, physiological, or psychological.

6.3
The hysterical (histrionic) personality
R. E. KENDELL

The concept of the hysterical personality arose out of the clinical observation that the women who developed conversion symptoms tended to have certain personality characteristics in common. Janet listed a desire for attention, a tendency to lie extravagantly, emotional shallowness and a need for praise and attention among the 'common stigmata' of neuropathy and in his textbook in 1924 Bleuler associated these characteristics specifically with hysteria. Since that time a fairly consistent behavioural description has evolved.

The subject's behaviour is histrionic and exhibitionistic. She dresses in a striking and sometimes outlandish manner, casual acquaintances are warmly embraced, everything is dramatized and exaggerated. At times exaggeration is taken to the point of overt falsehood so that the subject's account of her own past life becomes a saga of tragic deaths, wicked stepmothers, exotic settings, and attempted rape, and in a medical context her symptoms are often equally dramatic. Inconvenient facts, those aspects of the subject's own past behaviour and current circumstances which are incompatible with this romanticized self-image, are simply ignored and denied. Her emotions are as labile and exaggerated as her behaviour. Infectious gaiety is transformed by minor frustrations or disappointments into sobbing grief or angry tantrums, yet despite their intensity these displays of emotion strike other people as shallow and unconvincing, like bad acting. Relationships with other people are unsatisfactory and often shortlived.

Though the subject is often superficially charming and vivacious and quick to form friendships, she is too demanding and egocentric and shows too little consideration for the wishes and feelings of others for these to endure for long. She is also prone to behave in a dependent, helpless manner, forcing friends and relations to care for her and solve her problems for her whether they want to or not. Finally, and perhaps most characteristically of all, she is flirtatious in her dealings with men and prone to flights of romantic fancy. However, she is rarely a satisfactory or even a willing sexual partner, because basically it is attention, admiration, and parental affection she seeks, not sexual gratification, and despite the coquetry she is commonly frigid and sexually naive. Although women with hysterical personalities usually marry – a consequence of their good looks and flirtatious behaviour – their marriages often break down. They frequently remain childless and when they do have children they are often poor mothers. They are too egocentric and unstable, and although they lavish affection on their children intermittently they are unable to respond consistently to their emotional needs, or to cope for long with the never ending cycle of chores which motherhood involves.

The strong feminine (and anti-feminine) emphasis in this description is not accidental, for the concept of the hysterical personality arose at a time when hysteria was still regarded as a predominantly, if not exclusively, female disorder. As a result the personality traits associated with it, as Slater and others have pointed out, constitute a kind of caricature of femininity. Although there is a wide measure of agreement amongst psychiatrists on the characteristics of the hysterical personality the objective evidence that the traits in question cluster together in reality, occur almost exclusively in women and carry with them an increased liability to develop conversion symptoms, is fairly slender. The relationship between hysterical personality traits and hysterical symptoms is probably similar to that between the obsessional personality and obsessional symptoms. There is no doubt, in other words, that the majority of those with these traits never develop either conversion symptoms or dissociative states, and that many of those who develop these symptoms do not have noticeably hysterical personalities; but nevertheless the relationship is a real one in the sense that hysterical personality traits are commoner in those who develop hysterical symptoms than in the population at large.

Despite the consistency of textbook descriptions of the hysterical personality the practical application of the term is extremely lax, and almost invariably derogatory. Chodoff (1974) has justly described it as 'one of the most loosely used phrases in the lexicon of a profession not famous for the scientific rigour of its concepts'. He also comments on the tendency of young male doctors to use the term to describe any attractive woman with whom they come into therapeutic contact. In similar vein, others have commented that the epithet 'hysteric', and 'gross hysteric' even more so, often signifies only that a male doctor has become irritated with a female patient, either because he thinks she is exaggerating her symptoms, or determined to cling to them, or because she is manipulating him. Lay use of the term hysterical to describe any display of emotion which incurs the commentator's disapproval devalues the term even further. Indeed, it would be far better if the term hysterical personality were to be abandoned, as it has been in the nomenclature of the American Psychiatric Association (1980), and replaced by the more prosaic and less emotionally charged term histrionic personality.

In view of its pejorative overtones and past misuse a diagnosis of hysterical (or preferably histrionic) personality should only be made if clearly stipulated criteria have been met. The American Psychiatric Association's DSM–III lists three characteristics, all of which must be present:

(1) Behaviour which is attention seeking and histrionic
(2) Demanding interpersonal behaviour
(3) An affect which is overly reactive and intense in its expression.

Although this choice is somewhat arbitrary the need for explicit criteria of some kind is clear enough. It is also important that the behaviour should be characteristic and manifest in a wide range of situations, and not restricted to episodes of depression or relationships with male doctors.

Despite its title and historical origins the main importance of this personality type for psychiatry is not as the soil from which conversion symptoms arise. It breeds other more frequent and more troublesome offspring. Three of the most fundamental features of the so-called hysterical personality are the subject's need for affection and attention, her dependency, and her tendency to manipulate other people. The first two of these traits bring the subject into frequent contact with doctors and the third makes these contacts mutually frustrating. The reasons why the 'invalid role' is attractive to people with strong dependency needs, and why they frequently present to doctors with somatic symptoms for which no organic cause can be found, have been discussed in the previous chapter. Others present directly to psychiatrists complaining of depression or anxiety, or in the aftermath of an impulsive overdose. Their relationships with physicians in general, and inexperienced psychotherapists in particular, tend to pursue the same course as their other relationships. Things start very well because the subject is glad to be accepted as a patient, and often flatters her doctor and seems anxious to please, but before long she begins to make increasingly unreasonable demands, often in situations in which, although the doctor does not want to comply and is irritated to have to do so, he feels that under the circumstances he has little choice.

Manipulation

The patient often starts by telling her physician that no one has ever understood her so well before, or that she has been able to tell him things she has never been able to confide in anyone else. After preparing the ground in this way she asks for a prescription for a sedative drug, or for permission to ring him at home if she becomes too panicky before her next appointment. The initial requests often seem harmless enough and the doctor accedes to them. However, as time goes on they become less and less reasonable and sooner or later, perhaps after being visited at his home, or woken by a telephone call at 2 a.m., he refuses, or tells the patient indignantly that her behaviour is unacceptable. There are then tears and recriminations, accusations that the doctor 'doesn't really care' and hints of suicide. At this point an inexperienced therapist finds himself in a quandary. If he lets the patient have her way he feels he is either losing control of her treatment or exposing himself to intrusions on his private life or other inconveniences; but if he denies her he will be increasing her distress, running the risk that she will terminate treatment and perhaps the further risk of her attempting suicide. If two physicians are involved the situation is even worse, because almost invariably the patient succeeds in splitting them, so that the one who is minded to take a firm line has to contend with his colleague's pleas not to be obstinate or foolhardy as well as with the patient herself. As Murphy and Guze (1960) have emphasized in an invaluable discussion of the management of manipulative patients, it is essential to set limits and, having done

so, essential not to allow these to be transgressed. If the therapist does not set limits, or loses his nerve and retreats, he does not avoid a painful confrontation with his patient by doing so; he merely postpones it and makes his eventual task that much harder. Nor in the long run is the risk of the patient attempting suicide, or indulging in other destructive behaviour out of despair or pique, reduced by giving in. Most important of all, the doctor is powerless to treat his patient effectively until he has established that he will make the decisions and not be cajoled or frightened into letting her do so instead. Undoubtedly there are situations in which it takes some courage to stand firm, but if the situation is handled skilfully the risks are much less than they usually appear to the inexperienced. If the therapist calmly insists that, although he is not going to accede to the patient's demands, that does not mean that he does not understand how she feels or that he is not trying to help her; and if when threatened with suicide he can convince her that he recognizes that she may kill herself, and her right to do so, but hopes that she will not and will return to see him next week instead, then usually the battle is won. And generally this only has to be done once. If the therapist is genuinely concerned about the patient his concern is usually apparent to her and reduces the risk of her angry threats being carried out. Conversely, if the patient does make a serious suicidal attempt, or behaves in other dangerously destructive ways, it is often because she has in reality been rejected by an angry doctor.

Manipulation, of course, is not peculiar to relationships between patients and their doctors. It is a characteristic of most unequal relationships. Fundamentally, it is a strategy for achieving power in a setting in which power is not normally available. This is why patients manipulate their doctors, children manipulate their parents, and Victorian wives manipulated their husbands, rather than the other way about. Those who are in a position to issue orders, or even to negotiate on even terms, have no need to manipulate. The preceding discussion of the management of manipulative patients was based on the assumption that the doctor was male and the patient female. In reality either doctor or patient can be male or female, but in practice manipulation is usually only a prominent feature of relationships between male doctors and female patients because historically, as a result of the culturally enforced dependence of women on their menfolk, it has been an integral part of relationships between men and women generally. Successful manipulation requires some degree of willing acquiescence by the person being manipulated and to some extent men tolerate, and even encourage, manipulation by women, particularly if they find them attractive. (Adults of either sex do the same with children.) It is no accident that so many of the women with histrionic personalities are strikingly attractive, or were when younger. They behave as they do because in a very real sense they were trained to behave in this way by the rewards which previous manipulative behaviour brought with it, and had they not been attractive, or had unusually indulgent parents, these rewards would not have been forthcoming. We may find, therefore, that as the social role of women becomes more nearly equal to that of men the need for manipulative behaviour will wane and with it the more florid manifestations of the histrionic personality, so that such patients may seem as strange to our successors as Charcot's hysterics do to us.

Depression

People with histrionic personalities, male or female, often come to medical attention complaining of recurrent bouts of depression. This depression is nearly always 'neurotic' or 'reactive' in type, and usually relatively mild. Part of this apparent liability to depression is simply a consequence of the tendency of histrionic personalities to consult doctors with symptoms which other people endure, but this is probably not the whole explanation. Certainly the inability of these people to form stable relationships with others often makes their lives very stressful, and these depressive episodes are usually related to disappointments or frustrations.

Like phobic and obsessional symptoms, histrionic personality traits often become much more obvious and troublesome when the subject is depressed. Moreover, it is not uncommon in psychiatric practice to encounter a depressed patient behaving in a floridly histrionic manner, and make a confident diagnosis of hysterical personality disorder on that basis, only to discover that the histrionic behaviour fades away as the depression lifts and that when the patient is her old self again hysterical traits of any kind are hardly in evidence at all.

Alcohol and drug abuse

This is also a common complication of histrionic personality disorders. Drinking starts as social drinking but is often excessive and if the subject's

relationships with other people are seriously disturbed, and her life becomes progressively more unsatisfying as her physical charms fade, she often starts drinking regularly and becomes addicted in middle age. Abuse of other drugs follows a similar sequence. The subject's dependency needs bring her into frequent contact with doctors and all too often her manipulative skills ensure that she is provided with a supply of hypnotics to take at night, anxiolytics to take by day and analgesics for her numerous bodily pains as well. This motley collection of drugs is then taken in overdoses at times of emotional stress. It is also not uncommon for histrionic personalities to become addicted to barbiturates or morphine-like analgesics if physicians are unwise enough to prescribe them. It is important to keep all prescribing to a minimum when treating patients of this kind, despite their incessant pleas.

Parasuicide

Several references have already been made to the liability of histrionic personalities to threaten suicide, or take overdoses of tablets. Many of the people who take overdoses, perhaps as many as a third, do not have personality disorders and are not psychiatrically ill. They are essentially normal people under severe stress who have temporarily reached the end of their tether. But of those who make repeated attempts the majority have personality disorders and, at least in women, histrionic personalities predominate. There are many reasons for this. Most acts of parasuicide arise out of disturbed relationships between close relatives or sexual partners, and because of their demanding, egocentric behaviour and their dependency the interpersonal relationships of people with personalities of this type are characteristically stormy and fragile. They are also prone to fluctuations in mood in response to stress and, as we have just seen, are often well supplied with psychotropic drugs. But most important of all, parasuicide is *par excellence* a manipulative act. This is not to doubt that some suicidal attempts by histrionic personalities take place in a mood, albeit short-lived, of genuine despair, but usually it is clear from the circumstances in which the overdose was taken that its main purpose, and effect, was to coerce someone else into behaving in a way more to the patient's liking. The teenager swallows a handful of tablets when her errant boy-friend goes out with someone else. The middle-aged woman does so when her long-suffering daughter announces that she is moving into a flat of her own, or simply after a row with her husband.

Although these recurrent overdoses characteristically pose little threat to life it is not uncommon for histrionic personalities to die by suicide in the end. Sometimes this is simply a misjudgement, but not always. Like most other personality disorders histrionic personalities tend to mature slowly and lose their more conspicuous abnormalities as they reach middle age. Certainly the diagnosis is not often made after this stage of life. Even so, the problems some histrionic personalities create for themselves get steadily worse. As their physical charms fade so does their ability to obtain attention and affection from men and to manipulate them. They become increasingly more lonely, prone to increasingly severe bouts of depression, and sometimes addicted to alcohol as well, and the final fatal overdose is taken in this setting.

Self-mutilation

It is not uncommon for young women with personality disorders to cut themselves repeatedly, usually with razor blades or bits of broken glass, or sometimes to burn themselves deliberately with cigarette ends. The commonest site is the wrist but the cuts may extend up the anterior surface of the arm to the antecubital fossa or be restricted to other sites – face, thighs, or abdomen. Sometimes this is indistinguishable from other forms of parasuicide: the subject behaves as if she were trying to kill herself and intends other people to believe that she is. But more often she makes no such claim. She insists that suicide was not on her mind, and usually the cutting or slashing takes place in private.

The young women who do this usually come from severely disturbed family backgrounds and cut themselves at a time when circumstances suggest that they are disappointed or angry. Usually, however, they do not themselves describe feeling either depressed or angry. Instead they describe either a steadily mounting tension or else an unpleasant depersonalization in which they feel 'numb' or 'empty'. Either way this intolerable mood is effectively terminated by cutting themselves. Usually they are not aware of feeling pain and it seems to be the sight of blood, or the gaping wound, which brings relief. Sometimes there is pain and this itself seems to be the crucial experience. Either way there is a cathartic quality to the whole episode and when it is over the subject will quietly submit to having her wounds dressed and sutured. Usually there are multiple parallel cuts, the damage is fairly superficial and nerves and arteries are not severed, but repeated episodes often produce disfiguring scarring of arms or face.

Self-mutilation of this kind is relatively common in psychiatric hospitals and is often precipitated by an unhappy encounter with a doctor or nurse, which the subject interprets as rejection. There is also a strong imitative element so that it tends to occur in epidemics. For both these reasons one should always hesitate before admitting anyone with a history of self-mutilation to a psychiatric ward.

The management of histrionic personality disorders

Many of the principles of management have already been discussed under other headings but it is perhaps worth summarizing them here. The difference between an experienced and an inexperienced therapist, or between a really good psychiatrist and the rest of us, is nowhere more evident than in his or her management of patients of this kind. Part of the reason is that they provoke strong feelings in doctors which, if not recognized and allowed for, easily lead to inappropriate courses of action. A doctor whose parental feelings are aroused may easily allow the patient to become too dependent and manipulative, one who is annoyed may dismiss someone who is genuinely in need of help, one who is sexually attracted may prolong a professional relationship that ought to end, or terminate one that needed to continue.

Because of the risk of dependence and overdoses, drugs of all kinds should be prescribed as infrequently as possible. This applies particularly to hypnotics, sedatives, and analgesics which, of course, are usually those the patient most wishes to receive. Admission to hospital may be necessary during severe bouts of depression, in the immediate aftermath of an overdose and during crises to forestall dangerously impulsive behaviour, but all admissions are best kept brief. If the patient is allowed to remain in hospital for weeks or months on end in pursuit of elusive psychotherapeutic objectives the result may easily be a patient who has added a number of new techniques to an already formidable repertoire of manipulative behaviours, and also learnt to regard a lengthy sojourn in hospital as her right when life in the outside world gets too difficult, but is not noticeably different in other ways. Some people with personalities of this kind can benefit considerably from interpretive psychotherapy but they have to be carefully chosen, and not only because of their capacity for 'acting out'. Although they may appear perceptive and sensitive this may prove to be a temporary phase adopted to win the interest and esteem of the therapist, and their capacity for denial may prevent them ever acknowledging the realities of their inner feelings and behaviour. For most such people a supportive relationship is more appropriate, in which the doctor establishes early on that although he or she is not prepared to be manipulated he does recognize the patient's distress and is willing, within prescribed limits, to do all he can to help for as long as may be necessary. The 'prokaletic' techniques used so effectively by Kräupl Taylor (1969) may also, in skilled hands, be a very potent means of controlling undesirable behaviour.

6.4
The impact of parents with hysterical personalities on their children
SULA WOLFF

In a comparative study of primary school children referred to a psychiatric department and children in the community it was found that, in addition to sociopathy of mother or father, the type of parental psychiatric disturbance which distinguished the referred group most highly was hysterical personality disorder of the mother (23 out of 100 mothers of clinic attenders were given this diagnosis, compared with 5 out of 100 in the control group). An independent rater reading the parental life histories written by the interviewer in this study agreed quite well with the interviewer's diagnostic categorization of the parent's personality disturbances (Wolff & Acton, 1968). Hysterical personality disorder without sociopathic features (addiction, sexual deviation, violence, or criminality) occurred much more often in the mothers than the fathers of the disturbed children.

There is no one to one correspondence between the type of personality disorder of a parent and the occurrence and form of psychiatric disturbance in a child. Many people with hysterical personality traits are not disturbed in any way. Their personality patterns do not interfere with their marital, parental, other inter-personal, social, or work activities. Even among parents with hysterical personality disorders, that is with some constriction of life adjustment, the degrees of this will vary and we do not at all know how often it contributes to psychiatric disturbance in the children. Other life events and circumstances affecting parents and children introduce so much diversity that only a few generalizations are warranted on the basis of clinical experience, none as yet supported by objective research.

In the study referred to (Wolff & Acton, 1968) mothers of clinic attenders reported poor relationships with their own mothers in childhood very significantly more often than mothers of controls, and the pattern of poor relationships with their mother and exceptional closeness to their father was also significantly more common in mothers of the disturbed children. It was not however established whether these patterns were found particularly among the mothers with hysterical personality disorders, although clinical experience suggests this might be so.

Many mothers with hysterical personality disorders encountered in child psychiatric practice reveal experiences of inadequate mothering in their own childhood with a continuing sense of distance from, and unfulfilled longings for closeness with, their mothers. Often they turned to their fathers for protective care. This relationship is then likely to have been coloured by sexual guilt. Incestuous behaviour had sometimes occurred; more often a more light hearted 'daddy's girl' experience is reported. The subsequent marital choice seems frequently to have been predetermined in such a way that the children's father turns out to be unsatisfactory, not matching in any way the mother's picture of her own idealized father and proving to her that her own mother's disapproval of her choice had after all been justified.

In child psychiatric practice many mothers with hysterical personality disorders have parted from their children's father and have not subsequently made adequate second marriages. In other cases, although the marriage is stable, the sexual relationship between the parents is disturbed by the mother's frigidity.

Such mothers may find it as difficult to be unconditionally accepting of their children as of themselves. For some such mothers their appearance, that is their presentation of themselves to public gaze, and what other people think of them is of crucial importance and they display their children impeccably dressed and equipped, insisting at the same time on excessive politeness and good manners. Their intolerance of normal childish oppositional behaviour, of messiness and aggression, can interfere with their emotional closeness to their children and induce these children to attempt excessive inhibition of aggressive and sexual impulses, with

consequent emotional or conduct disorders. Some mothers with hysterical personality disorders have persistent vague fears that something is wrong with their child, presenting the child repeatedly to doctors with physical complaints for which there is no organic basis. These complaints resemble hypochondriacal symptoms. The mother is preoccupied with her small daughter's possible sexual precocity, repeatedly warning the child about 'men' or 'strangers', perhaps also over-concerned about masturbation, or seeking repeated investigations of the child for a vaginal 'discharge'.

A mother with a hysterical personality disorder may be excessively flirtatious with and intrusive towards her son or, alternatively, may identify him with his unsatisfactory father and distance herself from him in expectation that he will follow in his father's footsteps.

Some boys who present with a homosexual orientation and also some delinquent boys have been reared by such mothers.

Mrs Jackson, 48 and very obese, was first seen because her daughter, Mandy, then 7, and under long-term paediatric surveillance for recurrent urinary infections, was bedwetting, overweight and complaining of frequent abdominal pain.

Mrs Jackson, a competent cook/housekeeper, had been brought up together with an older brother in a family where the maternal grandmother was constantly fostering children. About this Mrs Jackson did not complain. Her relationship with her mother had, however, always been distant and this still hurt her greatly. She had turned to her father for affection but he was the less powerful of her parents. She wept as she recalled his death ten years previously.

She married at 18 and was unhappy from the start. In fact she had 'a breakdown' two weeks after the marriage. She never enjoyed sex. Her husband drank, was promiscuous, and did not work. The couple were allowed to adopt a girl, who was later taken over against Mrs Jackson's wishes by the maternal grandmother at a time of marital discord.

A boy was born after six years of marriage.

Mrs Jackson recalled with vivid horror once witnessing her husband have intercourse with a young relative of his employer in the cowshed. She had been rooted to the spot and then suffered from recurrent 'blackouts'. Finally she left her husband, taking her son with her. During the year following her father's death she was raped by the village taxi-driver who, drunk, had gained entry into her home. She concealed the resulting pregnancy and continued in her job. Finally, two weeks before Mandy's birth she 'collapsed' at work, was rushed into hospital and remained there until her confinement. When she refused to give up the baby for adoption, her mother and brother 'disowned' her.

When Mandy was 2, Mrs Jackson married a widower with five children, all grown-up, except the youngest, Jean, then 4 and in foster care. Mrs Jackson reclaimed Jean but, although Mandy and Jean were very close, she herself was always critical and distrustful of this child.

To the discomfort of both girls, Mandy was over-protected and Jean rejected. Mrs Jackson later revealed that these attitudes were based on a misunderstanding. She had *thought* (but never attempted to verify) that Mandy was being followed up for possible cancer of the bladder, because urine was repeatedly tested and she overheard the doctor's comment once that there was no 'growth' this time.

The relationship with Jean never improved; over the years the step-father was perceived as unaffectionate and much less competent than Mrs Jackson (a realistic assessment); and when Jean was pubescent, her oppositional attitudes and incipient sexual interests evoked so much hostility from both parents that she was placed in a children's home and then joined her oldest married sister. Mandy remained obese (as was her mother) and inhibited, although her enuresis and abdominal pain disappeared. Jean, after great initial misery, became more outgoing once she had left her father and stepmother and evoked much affection from others.

Throughout our contact with each other, Mrs Jackson flourished when her own needs, past disappointments, and present troubles were understood and she was given credit and respect for her practical competence. She was however totally unable to appreciate Mandy's needs for independence or to tolerate expressions of oppositional views or negative feelings from either Mandy or Jean. While at first reluctant to part from Jean and then guilty about her own negative feelings towards her, she made no subsequent attempts to effect a reconciliation and was insensitive to Jean's feelings about her broken relationship with the parents.

This mother displayed the common association of features of oral-dependency as well as hysterical personality traits (Tyrer & Alexander, 1979). Under stress she episodically developed symptoms of depression and dissociative states. She often acted impulsively, dissolving into tears if her feelings were hurt and voicing angry threats (that she would leave or become ill, or that they would have to pack their bags) towards her children and her husband, if her own wishes were thwarted. Twice she had taken in other people's children (the adopted girl and Jean) in attempts to create a happy family and become their mother. On each occasion the child was eventually rejected. Yet she denied totally any resentment about her own mother's repeated fostering of other children at a time when she herself was still in need of total care.

7
Obsessional disorders

7.1
Childhood origins of obsessional disorders, stereotyped behaviour, tics & Tourette's syndrome, and stuttering

JOHN CORBETT

Childhood origins of obsessional disorders

Obsessional ideas, minor rituals, and other forms of repetitive, apparently purposeless behaviour (stereotypies) are relatively common in childhood. Although they may be prominent symptoms of a number of psychiatric disorders, they infrequently present as single disorders, with sufficient pathological intensity to require treatment in their own right.

Several different types of clinical phenomena need to be distinguished:

(1) *Obsessional or ritualistic behaviour as part of normal child development*

Many young children go through phases when they must only jump on, or between joints of paving stones or touch every other tree or say some special jingle on occasions. Old superstitions may be resuscitated and persist in this form in the games and folklore of children in most countries (Opie & Opie 1969). In a more private context excessive orderliness, ritualistic behaviour, and bedtime ceremonials are seen in many young children. These phenomena have been associated by psycho-analytic writers with the 'anal phase' of development, diminishing when 'the relevant drive and ego positions have been outgrown'.

Preoccupation with favourite toys or objects such as pieces of a favourite blanket with a particular smell, so called 'transitional objects', whose temporary loss may cause considerable distress, also occurs at this time and such attachments may persist into later childhood. It is very doubtful whether this form of behaviour can be considered obsessional or ritualistic. Boniface and Graham (1979) in a total population survey of three-year-old children found that 16.4 per cent were currently using such an attachment object and concluded that whether a child uses an attachment object may well be determined by a more general tendency to use oral modes of comfort in situations of stress and distress and is, in itself, of no pathological significance.

There are marked individual differences in the appearance and persistence of ritualistic behaviour. Longitudinal studies of temperamental development in children suggest that less fastidious children with marked irregularity in sleeping, eating, and bowel habits are more prone to develop psychiatric disorder in later childhood and it seems most likely that these rituals serve to reduce anxiety by introducing an element of sameness, security, and comfort into a changing and uncertain world. These developmental phenomena are most prominent between the ages of three and five years and, like other habits such as food fads and thumb sucking, they tend to decline gradually after this time.

(2) *Obsessional symptoms as part of a neurotic disorder in children*

Although there are many accounts of neurotic illness in adult life in which obsessional symptoms can be traced back to childhood, it is uncommon for children to present for treatment before the onset of puberty. Judd (1965) suggests that the onset is insidious and symptoms have usually been present for several years before the child presents for treatment. He makes the distinction between this and compulsive behaviour appearing during normal play, which is not experienced by the child as alien or incongruous: children report no internal need to combat or resist the compulsion in a way which is characteristic of true obsessional neurosis, although this distinction has been queried by other authors. Also this type of ritualized behaviour is abandoned under mild external pressure and perceived by the child as pleasant and enjoyable.

On the other hand, true obsessional neurosis interferes with the child's functioning and may present as school non-attendance in the child who is so consumed with obsessional rituals that she is unable to get out of the house.

Beryl, aged 13, had always been considered by her parents as a very fastidious but model child. Following a change of schools at the age of 11 years she became increasingly withdrawn and preoccupied with a fear of dirt and germs. She would, for example, only eat off a special plate or go into a room if the door handle had been wiped. Initially her parents acquiesced in these rituals but later as they became more disruptive of family life any attempt to limit them would result in angry outbursts from Beryl. She involved her mother in prolonged rituals of handwashing and combing her hair which eventually prevented her getting to school and precipitated her referral. Admission to hospital with a combination of behavioural and family therapy resulted in slow improvement and enabled the family to set limits on her obsessional behaviour, but she remained intermittently preoccupied with her ritualistic behaviour.

Although obsessional symptoms are seen in children with various psychiatric disorders, the frequency of obsessive compulsive neurosis of childhood in the general population is unknown. Clinical studies suggest that it accounts for around 1 per cent of referrals (Judd, 1965; Adams, 1973). It differs in two main ways from the same disorders seen later in life, in that the child involves others, particularly his parents, in the rituals, and initially, it may be more difficult to elicit any subjective feeling of resistance on the child's part.

Families often acquiesce in the child's ritualistic or compulsive behaviour to a remarkable degree, so reinforcing the symptoms. This causes marked family disruption and when the rituals are interfered with, considerable anger is elicited, often with aggressive behaviour and temper tantrums.

Treatment. It follows that treatment should always involve the family to some degree. It is customary to use a combination of psychotherapeutic techniques aimed at reducing anxiety and minimizing the disruption and impairment of family relationships, resulting from the child's illness, with more specific behavioural techniques to eliminate or reduce the time spent in ritualistic behaviour (Weiner, 1967). Rarely, more severely afflicted children may require admission to hospital to focus on their behaviour and reduce the family tensions which increase the frequency and severity of symptoms.

The prognosis of severely affected children is poor, with substantial improvement in less than one-third of cases (Warren, 1965), although the outlook is better in cases with single episodes of minor obsessional symptoms (Adams, 1973). Children and adolescents with long-standing symptoms tend to become increasingly withdrawn and depressed, while obsessional symptoms may be secondary features of depressive illness. In a recent follow-up study, seven of ten children who had suffered from severe obsessional neurosis in childhood reported serious problems with social life and peer relationships, which persisted into later life (Hollingsworth *et al.*, 1980). Although obsessional symptoms may be a presenting feature of schizophrenia, there is no indication that this is more common in childhood than in adult life.

(3) *Ritual and routines in childhood autism*

Quite distinct from the occasional presentation of schizophrenia with obsessional symptoms is the occurrence of rituals, routines, and abnormal attachment to material objects which are an integral part of childhood autism. These symptoms were related by Kanner (1943) to the child's 'intense desire for the preservation of sameness' which appears to derive from the autistic child's inability to make sense of the world and his excellent memory for things as they were first experienced (Wing, 1976).

They differ from the rituals and routines of normal childhood in their persistence, the degree of distress which results when they are interfered with, and their bizarre and unusual nature. Thus, the child may hoard objects whose function is irrelevant to the attachment (Marchant *et al.*, 1974), such as pieces of metal or stone which do not so clearly have the comforting function of normal transitional objects. Sometimes these routines interfere to a major extent with the child or his family's life, requiring the use of behaviour shaping procedures to modify them (Marchant *et al.*, 1974).

Repetitive speech patterns, in particular delayed echolalia, in which the child repeats phrases he has heard previously, are also seen in this condition, and in more able, autistic children with Asperger's syndrome (autistic psychopathy), the child may be preoccupied with quite elaborate bizarre and repetitive ideas, for example, collecting railway timetables (Asperger, 1944).

This needs to be distinguished from obsessive compulsive disorders, and as with other forms of repetitive behaviour in childhood autism, there is no obvious resistance to carrying out these activities.

(4) *Stereotyped motor behaviour*

Although some forms of stereotyped behaviour, such as rocking or hand flapping, may occur as transient phenomena in normal child development,

they are rarely persistent, except in psychotic or severely retarded children. Such stereotyped behaviour is increased in barren, unstimulating environments where there is limited opportunity for personal interaction and play activities (Baumeister & Forehand, 1973). Hand flapping and other forms of manneristic behaviour may occur in similar situations and they may also increase with anxiety in autistic children.

Such stereotyped behaviour is seen in up to 40 per cent of severely retarded children but does not usually require specific treatment unless it is associated with severe repetitive self injury (Corbett, 1975).

(5) *Tics and Tourette's syndrome*

Tics or habit spasms are sudden brisk involuntary contractions of individual muscle groups, usually around the eyes or lower part of the face, and may spread to cause jerking of the neck, trunk, or limbs. They are repetitive, non-purposeful, and resemble the normal motor accompaniments of the startle response, for example, to a sudden loud noise.

The typical age of onset is between 5 and 10 years and they are usually transient, lasting for a few weeks or months. By the age of 7 years, 5 per cent of children have been noticed to have tics at some time of other (Kellmer Pringle *et al.*, 1967). Children whose tics are sufficiently severe to be referred to a paediatrician or a child psychiatrist usually show other symptoms of emotional disturbance, and often considerable tension is found in the family (Corbett *et al.*, 1969). Anxiety increases the movements, concentration often decreases them, and they cease during sleep. They are more frequent in boys and are not related to intellectual ability. Encephalitis is the only organic condition clearly associated with tics, although some authors have suggested an association with minimal signs of neurological dysfunction (Shapiro *et al.*, 1978), and it is occasionally possible to identify a clear-cut emotional precipitant to the tics.

Tics may be associated with developmental disorders such as speech impairment and, conversely, emotional symptoms, such as tempers and aggression, are less frequent. Thus, they may have a developmental basis, but it has also been suggested that they represent an alternative form of emotional expression or a learnt form of behaviour. Tics may be a cause of anxiety, but independently of this it has been found that there is an increased rate of affective illness in the mothers of children referred for treatment (Corbett *et al.*, 1969).

Very occasionally, around the time of adolescence, tics may worsen and become associated with vocalizations which may develop into compulsive swearing (coprolalia) or obscene gestures (copropraxia). This combination of symptoms is known as Gilles de la Tourette's syndrome and tends to be associated with more severe emotional disturbance.

Peter, aged 15, first developed eye blinking and lower facial tics at the age of six. This was said by his parents to have followed seeing his pet dog run over by a car. The tics subsided after a few weeks but recurred at the age of eleven after his mother had been taken ill with a severe depressive illness. On this occasion he had generalized body tics associated with grunting and monosyllabic swear words. He became very withdrawn and depressed. He was admitted to hospital where treatment for his depression and symptomatic treatment with pimozide for the tics resulted in improvement. He required intermittent treatment throughout adolescence but lost his tics completely in early adult life.

Treatment. Most simple tics respond to explanation of the mechanism to the family, to the appropriate management of any associated emotional disturbance, and to the parents obeying instructions to ignore the tics. Where they persist, fuller psychiatric treatment is required and major stresses such as educational problems should be dealt with before symptomatic treatment is attempted.

Psychotherapy alone is of little value but combined with behaviour therapy based on mass practice, may be effective in the case of simple facial tics (Jones, 1960). In more severe cases with multiple tics, treatment with haloperidol is indicated and there are now a large number of reports of its efficacy (Corbett, 1977). Although with simple tics a dose of 0.5 mg t.d.s. may suffice, in more severe cases, daily doses of up to 20 mg have been used with effect (Craven, 1969). It seems possible that this drug has a more specific effect than can be accounted for by mere reduction in anxiety, and it has been suggested that it is effective through its dopamine blocking effect. There is, as yet, no definite proof of this theory, but for this reason pimozide has also been used and it has recently been reported that clonidine is effective in doses of 0.05–0.15 mg daily in children unresponsive to haloperidol (Cohen *et al.*, 1979).

Only 10 per cent of patients with troublesome tics continue with their symptoms unchanged or worsening into adult life, but not infrequently one tic is replaced by another during the course of the condition. It is rare for tics to appear for the first time in adult life and in this case in anxious subjects the prognosis tends to be worse.

(6) *Stuttering*

Stuttering comprises interruptions to the free flow of speech, which interfere with communication, without mechanical impairment of the organs of speech. Stuttering (or stammering) refers to speech interruptions beyond normal levels at each age, and differs from the hesitancies and repetitions of the young child, in that physical or emotional tension makes the stuttering worse as the stutterer tries to overcome his handicap. Eventually social situations, which are associated with difficulty in speaking, are avoided and this further increases the social handicap.

Aetiology. The age of onset is usually less than eight years and seldom over the age of thirteen years (Morley, 1957). About 3 per cent of children develop a stutter at some time but only about 1 per cent become persistent stutterers (Andrews & Harris, 1964).

Normal infantile stuttering may persist as a result of anxiety or parental interference, but more severe stuttering lacks a satisfactory explanation. Delayed auditory feedback of speech can produce a speech abnormality similar to stuttering, which has been attributed to a defect in the perception of auditory feedback from the sound of the speaker's own voice (Cherry & Sayers, 1956). It is, however, unrelated to organic factors such as brain damage or convulsive disorders, neither is it related to handedness (West, 1958).

Particular situations or words arouse anxiety in stutterers and may thus interfere with fluency. It has been argued that when speech stutters to a halt, anxiety may decrease, so that the stuttering is reinforced. Furthermore, parents' anxieties about the child's speech, and attempts to make him speak more clearly, often make the stuttering worse. Personality tests have shown no consistent differences between stutterers and controls, except that stutterers show more non-specific anxiety.

Treatment. The contribution of emotional disturbance to the maintainence of the symptom must be assessed and the patient helped to cope with environmental stresses and to deal with anxiety in alternative ways. The parents must stop exhorting the child to 'speak more clearly and distinctly' or 'take a big breath before speaking'.

Regular intensive speech therapy will help the child to develop more fluent speech. Drugs do not affect the stuttering but can reduce tension and anxiety, and improvement has been reported with haloperidol (Wells & Malcolm, 1971).

Contemporary speech therapy techniques for the management of stuttering include a variety of rhythmical procedures which attempt to increase the predictability of vocalization. Syllable timed speech (Andrews & Harris, 1964), the electronic metronome (Wohl, 1968), and regulated breathing (Azrin & Nunn, 1974) can be included in this category. Operant procedures for the treatment of stuttering have been developed by Ryan (1971) into a systematic programme which can be implemented at home by trained parents.

In recent years Fransella (1975) has advocated the use of Personal Construct Theory as a means of understanding the difficulties of the stutterer.

Increasingly there is a shift towards intensive group therapy for adolescent stutterers, which may include a variety of treatment techniques ranging from specific training in speech control to social skills training. These two-week programmes offer the opportunity to tackle both the specific symptoms of stuttering and address the social and/or emotional difficulties of the individual (Rustin, 1978).

7.2
Obsessional illness and personality

J. E. COOPER

Introduction

The specific psychiatric use of the word 'obsessional' is closely related to the lay meaning, which is usually given in dictionaries as being harassed, preoccupied or haunted by a thought or topic. Qualities of repetition, unpleasantness, and something not wanted are present in these definitions, and it should be noted that these are all qualities of style rather than details of content. A group of psychiatric patients with these themes pre-eminent in their complaints have been recognized for the last hundred years or so. Those with the more severe conditions have stimulated many psychiatrists to add to the definition, as the essentially morbid criterion, an unpleasant and complicated experience of feeling compelled to think or act while at the same time knowing that the thoughts or acts are senseless and should be resisted.

A problem at present unresolved, largely due to lack of epidemiological information, is whether obsessional conditions can be regarded as distributed in the general population according to a normal distribution model, or whether their distribution is uneven. If the latter, then obsessional personality types, obsessional personality disorders, and obsessional illness should be regarded as separate although related conditions rather than as a continuum. In psychiatric clinical practice they often appear to be comparatively discrete, but this could well be due to the many selection processes through which patients pass before coming to a psychiatrist. In spite of this uncertainty, obsessional conditions will be subdivided in this chapter in the above fashion for convenience of discussion. In addition, the view is taken here that there is no essential difference between obsessions (as thoughts) and compulsions (as the acts derived from or countering against obsessional thoughts): obsessions and compulsions are very closely connected and very few patients do not have them both, at one time or another.

Is an obsessional illness a neurosis or a psychosis? This question cannot be answered in any simple way, because of the problems of definition of these two traditional terms. Ever since their recognition it has been conventional to regard obsessional symptoms and illnesses as neurotic, presumably because in most patients, insight is retained, anxiety is prominent, and a surprising degree of social functioning may be preserved. But in the more severe varieties of obsessional illness, insight may be very limited and incapacity may be complete; the label of neurosis sometimes seems very strange indeed.

The thought processes of patients with obsessional symptoms have some similarities to the 'magical thinking' commonly found in myths and legends, and in pre-scientific, religious, and intuitive ways of viewing the world. Freud and a number of his pupils drew attention to this, and clinicians using more general and descriptive frameworks have continued to emphasize this resemblance: for instance 'The half-beliefs of obsessional patients are similarly steeped in assumptions that their thoughts, words and deeds may be magic charms and spells magically right or wrong, the magic instruments of finding salvation or suffering damnation' (Taylor, 1979). However, the morbid obsessional thoughts of the patient are usually private and often shameful, in contrast to the magical or religious rituals which are usually public, shared, and often praiseworthy. In addition, the ritual actions derived from the morbid obsessional thoughts are time-consuming, intrusive, and comparatively inefficient in warding off harmful influences, instead of being limited to specific occasions and places,

Obsessional symptoms

The following more detailed description of obsessional disorders starts with the definition of obsessional symptoms, since they provide the themes and contents of both obsessional illnesses and of obsessional personality disorders. The next section deals with obsessional personality types and obsessional personality disorders. The final section describes obsessional illness, the term illness implying those states in which the predominant symptoms are obsessional. The distinction between symptoms and illness is necessary because obsessional symptoms can occur as a subsidiary or additional feature during the course of illnesses of other types, notably depressive and schizophrenic.

Westphal (1878), Janet (1903), Schneider (1925) and Lewis (1936) have all contributed in their turn to the list of criteria which follows:

Obsessional symptoms are based upon contents of consciousness, variously labelled ideas, thoughts, impulses and experiences, which:

(1) come repeatedly into the patient's consciousness against his will,
(2) are usually unpleasant and often abhorrent and frightening,
(3) are always recognized by the patient as his own thoughts in spite of these first two qualities already described,
(4) cannot be accepted by the patient as inevitable and harmless. The patient therefore tries constantly to push the thoughts out of his mind, and tries to resist the implications of their content.

The result is an internal mental struggle almost always accompanied by tension and anxiety, which may be obvious but which may sometimes be concealed by the patient to an extraordinary degree.

To counteract the unpleasant or dangerous nature of the obsessional thoughts, secondary rituals may be developed which seem to the patient to diminish the likelihood of the thought becoming an act, or of harm resulting from an apparently innocent act already carried out by him. Secondary rituals may again be thoughts (counting, checking, or the repetition of special words or phrases) or may be physical acts (touching, cleaning, or the placing of objects in special positions).

It should be noted that the content of the thoughts or acts does not enter into these criteria. The obsessional symptom as defined here is a unique style or type of experience, with many different types of content. Nevertheless, within a wide variety of content of symptoms, there are several common and related themes such as cleanliness, tidiness, contamination, checking, repeating and blasphemy, upon which each patient produces his own personal variations. There is some limited evidence that the first three of these themes are useful ways of classifying both personality traits and symptoms (Cooper & Kelleher, 1973; Stern & Cobb, 1978; Murray, Cooper & Smith, 1979).

Lewis, Taylor, and a number of other authors have also recognized another feature of obsessional symptoms which serves to avoid confusing these patients with other and different groups sometimes labelled as 'impulse disorders' or 'self-indulgent manias'. Gamblers, alcoholics, 'kleptomaniacs', and persons with some sexual disorders may often complain that they are subject to powerful impulses they do not want and cannot control. Their problem is that they do carry out the act consequent upon the impulse, and the act in itself is pleasurable (often intensely so), giving immediate and often profound relief from the impulse and any associated tension. This is in contrast to obsessional thoughts as defined above, which hardly ever give rise directly to acts (except to the rituals designed to ward off the harm). Furthermore, the performance of ritual acts is not itself pleasurable; at most, the patient experiences a partial and temporary lessening of the internal struggle and tension.

Related concepts

In Janet's classical descriptions of his syndrome of 'psychoasthenia', emphasis was given to a process of weakening of the will, by which the endless vacillations and thought trains of the morbid state were facilitated. The concept of will-power has gone out of fashion, and so the formulations of Janet and his contemporaries are now difficult to convert into modern ideas. But it is clear that Janet was well aware of commonly associated features in his patients that would now be classed as traits or symptoms of hypochondriasis and depersonalization; *'folie de doute'* and *'sentiment d'incomplétude'* were additional key phrases in Janet's clinical descriptions. These are closely related and refer respectively to the inability of the patient to convince himself that he has actually done or not done the act or thought that has to be repeated, and the feeling of incompleteness and dissatisfaction that accompanies the whole process.

Obsessional as described and defined here overlaps a great deal with 'anankastic' (from the Greek *anankasmos,* necessity of fate, compulsion) a term much used in German psychiatry. Anankastic is now preferred to obsessional in the psychiatric section of the latest (ninth) revision of the International Classification of Diseases, (WHO, 1978) and this term usually carries with it additional emphasis on marked traits of sensitivity and insecurity.

The condition that Kretschmer delineated as the 'sensitive delusion of reference' (*sensitiver Beziehungswahn*) has some elements in common with both obsessional personality disorder and with obsessional illness as discussed here. But the overall resemblance is not very close, because of the complicated set of additional concepts used by Kretschmer in constructing a framework of related ideas of which the clinical state of 'sensitive delusion of reference' is only one part (Kretschmer, 1927, 1974).

Erwin Straus (1966), a proponent of phenomenological and existential views, has suggested that feelings of disgust, acting 'as a defence against invasion by decay' is the central theme or mechanism of obsessional disorders, but this approach does not appear to have proved popular, and has had no practical consequences in terms of methods of treatment.

Obsessional personality traits, types, and obsessional personality disorders

Minor variants of the morbid obsessional symptoms can be recognized fairly frequently in persons who are not regarded as ill or in need of treatment by themselves or by others. The mildest grade of severity commonly recognized is that of obsessional personality traits, such as over-conscientiousness, tidiness, regularity, and other attitudes and behaviours expressing a strong tendency towards rigidity and inflexibility. Someone possessing a number of such traits to a striking but not troublesome degree can be conveniently called an obsessional personality type. 'Perfectionist personality' and 'houseproud housewife' are often used to express some of these qualities. When such traits are so marked that they override and dominate other aspects of the personality to a troublesome degree, it becomes legitimate to speak of obsessional personality disorder.

Obsessional traits: distribution in the general population

The frequency of persons with different combinations of obsessional personality traits in the general population is not known. Measurements of obsessional traits by means of special inventories given to selected groups of non-patients has provided some indication that the same trait clusters and patterns exist as can be found in obsessional patients, but numbers studied are up to now inadequate for generalization. (Cooper & Kelleher, 1973). Cultural differences may exist, although they may not be of any great magnitude; one study found that Irish subjects had significantly higher obsessionality scores and trait patterns than English subjects (Kelleher, 1972).

The possession of marked obsessional traits, and even minor degrees of obsessional illness, can be consistent with great ability and achievements and indeed the presence of such traits and symptoms may be seen to contribute to the personal drive and application that are needed. Lewis (1957) uses the writings of Martin Luther, Amiel, John Bunyan, and Dr Johnson to provide vivid examples of this.

The pre-morbid personality of patients with obsessional illness

Janet (1903) was the best known of a number of French psychiatrists around the beginning of this century who provided vivid descriptions of the pre-morbid personalities of obsessional patients. Between one-third and one-half of patients with obsessional illness have a strikingly obsessional personality, often at the level of personality disorder, so it is understandable that this subject has remained a favourite topic for clinicians. But systematic and comparable information is meagre, and there remains the puzzle posed by the other two groups of patients who demonstrate no such link: those who develop obsessional illness but whose pre-morbid personality has no obsessional traits, and those with very marked obsessional personalities whose traits do not develop into troublesome obsessional symptoms even when they are subject to severe stress.

Lewis (1957) extended the descriptions of pre-morbid personality of obsessional patients by suggesting that two separate types could be identified. Vacillation, doubting, and uncertainty are the hallmarks of one type, and such a person would also be slow and indecisive. A morose, gloomy, and pessimistic outlook is said to be the main feature of the second type, coupled with traits of meanness and irritability. Both types are said to share a general rigidity of attitudes and marked stubborness once decisions have been made.

Obsessional personality traits and types are not differentiated from obsessional symptoms and illness in Freud's approach to the subject, which is centred around the concept of anal-erotic personality. Papers on this theme have always formed an important part of psycho-analytic literature in spite

of the therapeutic disappointments (Freud, 1895, 1908, 1913; Jones, 1918; Abraham, 1921; Stekel, 1949).

Obsessional personality disorders

Patients with obsessional personality traits sufficiently obtrusive to be troublesome to both the patient and to others, but yet without the symptomatic features of repetitiveness, senselessness, and resistance, are sometimes encountered in clinical work. There is a strong clinical tradition that such persons are particularly prone to develop depressive illnesses (of the 'endogenous' and agitated type), and it is the depressive change that brings them forward, not the personality pattern in itself.

There is no epidemiological information available to allow estimates of the frequency in the community of persons with obsessional personality disorders. They are encountered in clinical work only occasionally in their own right, since a lack of insight into the viewpoint of others and a marked distaste for psychiatrists and psychological enquiry of any sort are often found to be among their outstanding characteristics. When such individuals present clinically with either depression or an obsessional illness, it sometimes seems that they have been precipitated into their morbid state by changes in status at work, particularly if these involve increased responsibility; for instance, promotion into a post carrying more occasions for making important decisions or maintaining an open mind and a flexible approach would be understandably stressful for someone with an obsessional personality disorder.

When assessing the family relationships and stresses of teenage or young adult patients with other disorders, it is not uncommon to find that the source of much of the stress lies in the rigid attitudes and intrusive, dominant behaviour of a parent with a strikingly obsessional personality.

Management. It is notoriously difficult to influence the behaviour and personal interaction of persons with obsessional personalities, even in the minority who accept that they themselves should try to change. In those in whom some understandable life change seems to be implicated, discussion and guidance about the nature of changes and how they can be circumvented and coped with may be helpful, but in practice it usually turns out that the patient chooses avoidance or retreat rather than attempts at constructive change.

In families in whom an obsessional parent is

found to be a major source of stress for others, the problems are often seen to be resolved only when the younger member leaves home to be more independent. A good deal of help can be given, often through casework from a psychiatric social worker (at both strategic and tactical levels), to ease the various family members through the processes of parting and separation. Several unsuccessful attempts to live independently may be made by the children of obsessional parents before they finally succeed, and during the whole turbulent process it is often the parent that needs the professional support just as much as the child.

Obsessional illness: clinical, epidemiological and aetiological aspects

Some patients are able to hide their symptoms from even their relatives and close friends for years. Patients who do not have extensive behavioural rituals of cleaning, repeating, or checking often appear to be able to function reasonably well at work and at home, even though their minds are full of complicated trains of thoughts and counter-thoughts. Their motivation for hiding their symptoms as much as possible may sometimes come from the obscene or horrific nature of their thoughts, but fear of being ridiculed as silly and weak-willed for being unable to push such senseless thoughts out of their mind is often a large part of the explanation.

Consequently, obsessional patients sometimes present to psychiatric attention many years after the onset of their symptoms. During such periods of hidden suffering, close relatives often report that the patient changed in non-specific ways, appearing to be quieter and more withdrawn. An increase in vague physical aches and pains, irritability, and even frank hypochondriacal worries about serious physical illness are quite often reported by the patient and observed by relatives, and a general change of this type also often accompanies the onset of obsessional symptoms that are declared from the start.

The very common ritual behaviour seen occasionally in most healthy children, in which they count and check, sometimes carrying rituals from traditional games over into other activities, is not a predictor of later obsessional symptoms.

The age of onset is often quoted as having an average value in the early twenties, but there is a fairly steady incidence rate by age between the ages of about 15 and 35 years, judged by hospital-based series (Black, 1974). By the age of 30, about three-quarters of cases have declared themselves, and only a few cases arise afresh after the age of 50.

Minor episodes of obsessional symptoms, lasting a few weeks or months only and not severe enough to compel the patient to seek help, are quite commonly reported by patients when they finally come forward with their main illness. This, together with the already noted tendency to hide symptoms, means that generalizations about typical modes of onset are of limited value. However, a very acute onset, in terms of a few days, is very rare, and most patients report the gradual appearance of a few symptoms, followed by a gradual worsening of associated preoccupation and disability.

Many other aspects of both the onset and the aetiology of obsessional illness have been examined in detail by Skoog (1959, 1965)

Types and severity of obsessional symptoms

Some main themes of contamination, obscenity, blasphemy, and checking have already been mentioned. Each patient produces his own individual variation of these common themes, often with unique additions. Contamination may be feared from urine, faeces, sweat, or menstrual blood, or it may be from 'germs', viruses, or other ill-defined agents presumed to be present by the patient. Obscene sexual thoughts may be simple words and phrases, or may be complicated trains of swear words; complete scenes and actions involving several persons in sexual acts may be visualized. Similarly, thoughts of violence or harm coming to close relatives may be experienced as either thoughts or visual imagery. Trains of thought in which the patient stabs, slashes, or dismembers close relatives and friends may be sparked off by random encounters with kitchen knives, hammers, or axes. One well-recognized subgroup of obsessional patients consists of mothers with infants, who are very distressed by experiencing thoughts and images in which they throw their baby out of the window or into a fire, or harm it by any one of a variety of methods.

Sexual and religious thoughts may be combined to such an extent that the patient is too shocked and embarrassed to express them even when it is clear that he trusts and accepts the therapist in every other way.

Incapacity is usually connected with the development of behavioural rituals, in addition to the thoughts and images. The checking and repeating of virtually any activity, not only cleaning, may occupy hours. In the more extreme cases, hands may be washed fifty or more times a day (producing troublesome dermatitis) and clothes may be changed, washed, and ironed several times daily. Admission to hospital as an emergency is occasionally necessary because patients reached the stage of spending many hours a day at home naked, washing and bathing themselves and cleaning the house in a vain attempt to get rid of feelings of contamination.

A feeling that harm may come to others if some thought or act is not performed or if the dreaded contamination is not contained, is sometimes a central and particularly distressing part of the patient's experience. In the patient's mind, the consequences of his not performing the rituals may become extraordinarily enlarged and widespread, putting his whole family or neighbourhood at hazard. Similarly all-pervading is the rare feeling that something harmful but unnamed has been left behind when leaving a room or a house.

Where harm to others and self is a prominent feature of the symptoms, the patient may discover certain counter-thoughts or actions which, if carried out exactly and repeatedly, have the effect of reducing or even cancelling out (at least for a short while) the possibility of harmful consequences. The countermeasures may take the form of repeating numbers of phrases a certain number of times, or may be ritual actions performed in a certain order or frequency. After a few months, a once successful countermeasure may lose its effectiveness, but another one may be developed in its place.

Numbers, symbols, and formulae are another subject for obsessional trains of thought. Repeating set sequences of numbers, or always doing or thinking something a set number of times are common examples. Motor-car number plates often catch the patient's attention, and may need to be added up, squared, and worked out in various ways before the patient can pass on to anything else.

Most obsessional patients have one or two symptoms at the forefront of their attention at any given time, but systematic enquiry will almost always show that they also have many more in the background. Patients suffering from long illnesses often change the focus of their attention from one obsessional theme to another as the years go by. It is in the chronic illnesses that the feelings of resistance tend to fade away, becoming far less troublesome than in the first few years. However, there is always some feeling of resistance experienced in relation to whatever happens to be currently the most prominent theme. Patients who have struggled for years with their thoughts and rituals will often express their experience more in terms of recognizing their senselessness than in active feelings of resistance, but a detailed discussion with them will make it clear that the one experience is really a less acute form of the other, and that nothing has changed fundamentally.

Obsessional patients tend to be of high intelligence, whether this is measured by educational and professional attainment or by more specific tests. Ingram (1961) gave special attention to this point in his study, but as always, generalizations are hampered by unknown selection processes. But this finding, and a long-standing clinical impression, does seem likely to have substance, although no particular explanations have ever been put forward. The obvious associations between high educational attainment and social class may explain the less firmly established suggestion that obsessional patients also tend to be more frequently classified as of upper or middle class than expected.

Most obsessional patients have some sort of sexual problem, but no common theme emerges as typical of the whole group. The most that can be said is that a turbulent and often excessive sexual drive is common, with a tendency to complain of a poor level of satisfaction. This sexual dissatisfaction is probably one contributing cause to the unusually low marriage rate in patients with obsessional illness. Several studies report only about half of their patients to be married (Kringler, 1965; Blacker & Gore, 1955; Ingram, 1961), which is well below the rates both for other neurotic categories of psychiatric patients and the general population.

There is no overall evidence to suggest that men and women differ in their susceptibility to obsessional illness, although findings in different studies vary markedly.

Incidence and prevalence

Information about the incidence and prevalence of obsessional illness in populations is very scanty. Estimates of its prevalence in German and North American populations give a figure of 0.05 per cent (Rüdin, 1953; Woodruff & Pitts, 1964) and a similar figure was also estimated for Hong Kong Chinese (Lo, 1967). Anecdotal evidence from clinicians working in many cultures suggests that obsessional patients are easily recognized in very diverse cultural settings, but one of the few systematic community surveys done on a large sample of subjects from a non-Western culture (aboriginal Taiwanese) found, surprisingly, no obsessional patients (Rin & Lin, 1962)

Hospital statistics can show only that obsessional illness is comparatively rare compared to conditions such as depression, anxiety neurosis, and the major psychoses. Problems of definition and selection are presumably responsible for the wide differences in figures quoted, for instance, for the proportion of in-patients with this diagnosis; Pollitt (1957) found four per cent, but five other authors (amongst them another British study of Ingram (1961) found less than one per cent. There is more agreement about the relative preponderance of obsessional patients amongst all those mental hospital in-patients labelled as neurotic, and around three or four per cent seems to be the case for the UK.

The aetiology of obsessional illness

Genetic, familial, social, and organic influences have all been identified as contributing towards the development of obsessional illness, but in assessing their relative importance it must be remembered that most surveys of patients with the condition also demonstrate that the aetiology is unknown in the majority of cases. Necessary or sufficient causes of obsessional illness cannot be identified in any simple sense.

Genetic and familial influences. Since obsessional illness is so rare, very few twins with it are available for study. Almost all published reports of twin studies are also bedevilled by poor standards of information for both diagnostic criteria and for zygosis; this is particularly so in those studies finding the highest rates of concordance in monozygotic twins (Tiernari, 1963; Ihda, 1965; Inouye, 1965). The information of good quality is on too small a scale to allow generalizations, but is best exemplified by a report from the Medical Research Council Genetic Unit. In six pairs of monozygotic twins, three were concordant and three discordant for obsessional illness (Shields, quoted by Marks *et al.*, 1969).

Because obsessional symptoms are so often expressed in domestically disruptive behaviour, an obvious and intrusive model of behaviour is present for developing children. An interaction of genetic and environmental influences therefore might be expected, producing a familial increase of obsessional personality traits or illness. In addition to such a specific link, the presence of an obsessional patient in a family can be regarded as a general stress, encouraging the development in other family members of other psychiatric illnesses. Both the general and the specific effects have been found in surveys of such families, but again the lack of uniform diagnostic criteria and varying quality of information prevent any firm conclusions. Studies by Brown (1942) and Greer and Cawley (1966) produced some evidence in favour of the more general correlation, but the evidence becomes less convincing the more it is examined in detail. The widespread clinical impression that the relatives (particularly parents) of obsessional patients often have marked obsessional traits if not frank illness, is supported by the study of Lewis (1936) and to a lesser extent by the studies of Brown (1942), Rüdin (1953) and Rosenberg (1967). But to separate out the genetic, familial, and environmental components of this association is impossible on present knowledge.

Social influences as precipitants. In spite of differing ideas about what constitutes a reasonable period of time between the onset of illness and an event that can be considered to be a precipitant, there is a common finding from a number of studies that about half of the patients studied have had some fairly obvious recent stress or life change, in the areas of sex, domestic and marital relationships or responsibilities, or work. Illness or death of a close relative, and pregnancy and the puerperium have been specifically linked with this onset of obsessional illness in some studies (Pollitt, 1957) but have not been identified in others (Ingram, 1961). Even the highest estimates of the frequency of precipitating events suggest that they are present in only about half the patients studied, so our knowledge of the precipitating mechanisms of obsessional illness is still very incomplete.

The identification of precipitating causes is made even more uncertain by the onset of obsessional illness being particularly difficult to time in many patients. It is often found, for instance, that the patient comes to psychiatric notice after a long period of gradual worsening of pre-morbid personality traits. In addition, the late presentation of many patients means that the details of the start of the illness are obscured simply by the passage of time.

Brain damage as a contributing cause. Schilder (1938), Lewis (1946), and more recently Grimshaw (1964) have all drawn attention to the presence of neurological disease or previous brain trauma in as many as one-third of some series of obsessional patients seen in psychiatric clinics and hospitals. Schilder in particular emphasized the importance of basal fractures of the skull and various ill-defined forms of encephalitis; epilepsy has also been incriminated. Damage to the basal ganglia is the common factor in the great majority of reports, so there is probably a general but not very strong relationship between the appearance of obsessional symptoms and damage to this part of the brain.

A more specific link, but still with the same anatomical basis, probably exists between obsessional symptoms and encephalitis lethargica. The above-mentioned authors noted this link, which takes the form of the appearance of obsessional symptoms of any type occurring alongside the Parkinsonian syndrome which may develop as a late sequel to the acute encephalitis. As might be expected, a number of publications in the late 1920s recorded this mixed syndrome, some years after the period when encephalitis lethargica was particularly frequent.

Obsessional symptoms may come and go during the development of pre-senile and senile dementias, but as with other forms of brain damage, the organic condition usually overshadows the obsessional symptoms in importance; the question of treatment of the obsessional symptoms in their own right usually does not arise.

Differential diagnosis

The differentiation of obsessional symptoms from other types of symptom

If the above criteria are used, then it is unusual to find much difficulty in deciding whether a particular thought or action should be called obsessional. In only the occasional patient may there be difficulty in differentiating obsessional symptoms from delusions, schizophrenic thought intrusion, or depressive ruminations.

The differentiation from a delusional belief is occasionally difficult because some obsessional patients fluctuate in their degree of insight and in their resistance to their ideas, particularly about contamination. In the more intense phases of their illness, some patients will appear to be quite convinced at times that, for instance, they are dangerously contaminated, but a few hours later or the next day they will express the usual recognition of the senselessness of the idea, together with some resistance to it. Such fluctuations in insight about one or two symptoms should not be allowed to have much diagnostic weight. The overall diagnosis should rest on the summary impression gained from a consid-

eration of all the symptoms, and such patients will usually have a variety of other symptoms typical of one condition or the other which clarify the diagnosis.

Schizophrenic patients with the experience of thoughts being put into their minds from elsewhere occasionally protest about it, and say that they wish the thoughts were not there. This gives them a superficial resemblance to obsessional patients describing how they are trying to push the unwanted thoughts out of their mind, but the attribution to self or to others is usually clear, and is the overriding point.

Depressive ruminations are often unpleasant for the patient to bear, particularly if suicide is being considered, and so at first sight the patient appears to be resisting the thoughts. However, the clue to the basically depressive nature of such thoughts is that the patient will admit that even though the act of suicide itself would be frightening, it would also be justified or deserved.

Obsessional doubting, one of the rare obsessional symptoms, is sometimes present alone, with none of the more familiar themes or rituals. In patients who are not skilled at expressing their inner thoughts and feelings, this symptom is easily missed, but it may explain quite disabling degrees of slowness, indecision, inefficiency, and social withdrawal. The patient's mind is filled with questions and doubts about almost any action and decision. In some patients, the focus is on everyday trivial decisions about what to wear, what to eat, and what to do next, and in others, the doubts and questions may be about philosophical issues such as the purpose of life, the meaning of existence and the creation of the universe. Thoughts of this last variety produce no specific behavioural component.

The choice of an overall diagnosis for patients with a mixture of symptoms

Patients sometimes present with a mixture of obsessional and other type of symptom. Mixtures of obsessional, depressive, and schizophrenic symptoms are the most familiar clinical examples, and of these the mixture with depressive symptoms is the most common.

Two separate clinical issues need to be distinguished. First, there may be some difficulty in deciding which is the primary or major condition when several symptoms of each type may be present. Secondly, the question may not be one of 'either' – 'or' but more simply one of assessing the significance of the presence of one set of symptoms as a minor component of a major illness of another type. The first issue is one of differential diagnosis and is considered here. The second issue is dealt with in a later section on the appearance of obsessional symptoms in other conditions.

In patients with both depressive and obsessional symptoms, there is often considerable difficulty in deciding which type is the most important, since a number of symptoms of both types may be present (and both may fluctuate for no obvious reasons). In spite of these difficulties, the decision as to which is the major component is worth some effort because of important treatment implications. If the illness is basically depressive, there is no point in treating obsessional thoughts or rituals that will probably disappear in any case when the underlying depressive illness is treated. If the illness is basically obsessional, the mistaken use of electroconvulsive therapy may well make the patient feel worse; this is because the usually prominent tension and anxiety are often associated with a poor outcome of electroconvulsive therapy (which has no effect upon the obsessional symptoms).

Severely affected obsessional patients are usually distressed, resentful, and unhappy because of their symptoms, but these emotions have to be differentiated from the morbid characteristics that denote the depressive illness process. The diagnosis of a primary depressive illness should not be made only because of the presence of depressive affect. It should depend upon the clear presence of some of the symptoms known to be closely associated with depressive affect, (such as poor concentration, loss of interests and enjoyment, unjustified hopelessness and guilt, and the so-called 'biological' symptoms of early morning waking, loss of libido, loss of appetite and weight, and motor retardation).

Patients with both obsessional and schizophrenic symptoms present a very different problem, largely because of the traditional diagnostic precedence given to schizophrenia over other functional psychiatric disorders and particularly over the neuroses. The presence of even one delusional idea or 'first rank' symptom of Schneider will indicate that the illness is basically schizophrenic.

Obsessional symptoms and depressive illness
Obsessional symptoms are fairly common in severe depressive illnesses, and obsessional illness without obvious depressive symptoms sometimes resembles manic-depressive illness in that it may occur periodically without any clear precipitating influences. These connections have led to assumptions that there is a special relationship between obsessional and depressive illnesses; Henry Maudsley, for instance, asserted that obsessional illness was no more than an atypical variant of manic-depressive psychosis. Possible genetic and familial links between the two conditions have been studied by examining the frequency of manic-depressive psychosis and other forms of depression in obsessional patients and their relatives, and comparing this with the frequency of depressive conditions in the general population, and in other non-obsessional illnesses. (Brown, 1942; Rüdin, 1953; Rosenberg, 1968). These studies all find very weak or no evidence for a specific relationship between the two types of illness.

In contrast, there is no doubt that some obsessional symptoms are common during the course of about a third of severe depressive illness; in about one patient in six the obsessional symptoms may precede the more obvious and severe depressive symptoms (Gittleson, 1966). The presence of obsessional symptoms is associated with a lowered risk of suicide attempts. In most of these patients, the obsessional symptoms clear up with treatment of the depression, but in a few patients the obsessional symptoms disappear spontaneously before this. In a few others the obsessions persist after the depression has gone, and whereas this is in part understandable if the patient had an obsessional personality before he became ill, it is quite puzzling in the few patients who showed no hint of this before their depressive illness.

Obsessional symptoms and schizophrenia
As with manic-depressive psychosis, there is no evidence of any special relationship between schizophrenia and obsessional illness, but there are many reports, confirmed by ordinary clinical experience, of patients presenting with a few obsessional symptoms who then develop a clearly schizophrenic illness.

As Lewis (1936) observed, it is perhaps surprising that obsessional illnesses do not change into schizophrenia quite frequently, simply by the patient giving up the struggle and losing insight into the origin of the intrusive thoughts. In fact this happens rarely, and there is no evidence to suggest that schizophrenia develops more often in patients with established obsessional illness than it does in patients with other psychiatric illnesses.

The presence of obsessional symptoms in a schizophrenic patient is important nevertheless, because a better than usual prognosis is usually implied (Stengel, 1945; Rosen, 1957). These patients also often have prominent affective symptoms, and their illness follows the general rule for schizophrenia that the prognosis is better, the more unusual features are present. The protective effect of obsessional symptoms may have a psycho-dynamic explanation (Stengel, 1948), and it can also be regarded as due to the presence of the pronounced affective symptoms (anxiety, tension, and variable depression) that almost always accompany the obsessional symptoms.

Forensic aspects

Both doctors and patients are sometimes concerned lest the startling obsessional thoughts should lead to dangerous actions. There is no systematic information on this problem, but the absence of specific reports and the rarity of finding obsessional patients charged with any sort of crime are convincing indications that the feared actions do not occur. Clinical experience suggests that only those patients whose obsessional symptoms are complicated by other conditions, such as schizophrenia, brain damage, or psychopathic personalities, are at even a slight risk of giving way to their impulses. In Courts of Law, mention is sometimes made of 'irresistible impulses' but this concept is not usually brought into the arguments by psychiatrists.

The treatment of obsessional illness

Specific treatments for obsessional symptoms have only begun to emerge in the last few years, and the non-specific therapies such as anxiolytic and antidepressive drugs and supportive psychotherapy that have been used with obsessional patients have been unpredictably and often only marginally effective. The more recently devised behavioural methods are still mainly experimental and also are often unpredictable, but have opened up a new approach that deserves enthusiastic development and exploration. Most obsessional patients require a mixture of several types of treatment, but for simplicity the different approaches available will be described separately under the headings of psychotherapy, chemotherapy, brain surgery, and behavioural treatment.

Psychotherapy

In this discussion, psychotherapy will be classified as suggested by Cawley (1971, 1974) into:

(1) *extensive,* as ordinary doctor–patient interaction focused upon personal and psychological aspects of illness, as found in any clinical discipline, not implying any special psychiatric training,

(2) *informal,* as the various forms of psychotherapy practised by most general psychiatrists,

(3) *formal,* as the more highly developed psychological techniques, based upon a theoretical framework and practised by specialized psychotherapists who have usually had a personal analysis of some sort.

Formal psychotherapy is ineffective in helping obsessional patients, in spite of early hopes and persistent efforts. Freud studied a number of obsessional patients in great detail, and clearly became fascinated by the symbolism and the psychological processes that are so readily available for interpretation (Freud, 1895, 1908, 1913). But clinical experience appears to have produced a fairly uniform practice among specialized psychotherapists, in that it is unusual for patients with obsessional illness to be accepted for treatment by units or departments of psychotherapy. Fenichel (1945) wrote extensively on the problems encountered in the analysis of obsessional patients. He pointed out that, in analytic terms, the symptoms represent a very intellectualized, isolated, and all too conscious form of the conflicts and drives of the patient, far removed from their origins and basic emotional cathexis. In more ordinary terms, obsessional patients are usually found to be argumentative and stubborn, and are quite unable to respond constructively to the interpretation of their symptoms.

In spite of the continued interest of psychoanalysts in this field (Sandler & Joffe, 1965; Anna Freud, 1966) there is still no evidence to justify the use of formal psychotherapy in the treatment of obsessional patients. A similar conclusion was reached by Cawley (1974).

Informal and extensive psychotherapy. Most obsessional patients feel supported and obtain temporary relief from some of their anxiety by talking about their thoughts and rituals with someone whom they can trust not to ridicule them. Regular, supportive, and non-interpretive interviews during which other forms of treatment such as drugs or behavioural regimes are discussed and planned are almost inevitable at some stage of the management of obsessional patients, but it is when the other more active measures come to an end that the fondness of the patient for the simple supportive contact often becomes clear. Patients often wish to continue to have such support, but whether it is justified is an individual matter between the therapist and the patient, depending upon the patient's distress and disability and the availability of the therapist. If such interviews are continued at, say, monthly intervals for several years, the psychiatrist will see a new and longitudinal view of the patient. He will probably witness the waxing and waning of different groups of symptoms within one patient, together with mood swings (mainly depressive) of several months duration. These are resistant to antidepressants, and while they are present the patient is gloomy and pessimistic. The patient's complaints, questions, and demands for reassurance usually become repetitive and stereotyped, and it is often clear that the interview and the psychiatrist's responses have become part of the patient's system of ritual activities.

Long-term support of this type is an activity familiar to most psychiatrists, but can equally well be given by a general practitioner who has developed an interest and skills in supporting patients who are not likely to change.

Chemotherapy

Almost all the available psychotropic drugs have been recommended for the treatment of obsessional illness over the last decade or so, which is a good indication that no specific drug action exists.

Complaints of tension, feeling 'on edge' and an inability to relax are common in obsessional patients, so anxiolytic drugs such as chlordiazepoxide or diazepam are often given. Only a temporary and minor reduction of complaints is usual, and there is rarely any effect at all upon the obsessional symptoms themselves. Phenothiazines and related drugs are similarly ineffective, but most obsessional patients are in any case markedly intolerant of the subjective side-effects of this group of compounds, and stop taking them after a few days.

Tricyclic antidepressants, particularly clomipramine, pose some important but yet unanswered problems in the treatment of obsessional illness. Over the last ten years or so, clomipramine has been marketed as a specific treatment for obsessional and phobic conditions, and a number of preliminary but enthusiastic reports have appeared describing its use. Unfortunately the promised long-term follow-up studies with adequate comparison groups have not appeared, and the evidence available for any specific action on obsessional symptoms is still anecdotal.

Three of the major clinical points that make it particularly difficult to demonstrate a specific antiobsessional effect for clomipramine or any other tricyclic antidepressant are:

(1) the frequent coexistence of depressive and obsessional symptoms (already noted),
(2) that all antidepressant drugs (including monoamine oxidase inhibitors and tetracyclics) also have a marked anxiolytic effect in most patients,
(3) that illnesses which are eventually regarded as basically depressive in nature quite often present in the first instance with anxiety, obsessional, or other symptoms.

None of the published studies deals thoroughly with these complicating possibilities, and none of them has the status of more than preliminary reports. In particular, the claims for the effectiveness of intravenous infusion of clomipramine have not been properly substantiated. There remains, however, a tantalizing series of individual case-reports and anecdotes which justify further investigation of the actions of clomipramine and other related drugs in both obsessional and phobic symptoms.

Behavioural treatments

The various forms of behavioural treatment that have been developed over the last two decades are described elsewhere (see chapter 3.1.2), so the details of how each technique is carried out with the patient will not be repeated here. This discussion will be limited to comments on the place of the different techniques, and of the whole 'behavioural approach' to treatment, in relation to obsessional symptoms.

Most obsessional patients present with obvious behavioural symptoms, so they were naturally included in the first trials of various forms of behavioural therapy. Results were at first disappointing (Wolpe, 1958; Cooper, Gelder & Marks, 1965) and it has subsequently become clear that the various forms of desensitization and relaxation first developed for the treatment of phobic symptoms, have little or no effect upon obsessional symptoms. More recently, however, some significant progress has been made, and the newer behavioural techniques may be divided into those used for rituals, for thoughts and for slowness.

Behavioural treatment of rituals. The development of various forms of 'response prevention' (apotrepic) treatment by Meyer and others (Meyer, 1966; Hodgson, Rachman & Marks, 1972) has resulted in a specific and often effective method of reducing the time spent by patients on their rituals. The presence of a therapist who gives instruction, support, and encouragement, while also providing a model of behaviour for the patient, creates a complicated situation, which can be interpreted in several ways. Depending upon the type and frequency of the rituals, an additional element of 'flooding' can be introduced by increasing exposure to the particular stressful stimulus during sessions (sometimes also called 'confrontation'). The earlier forms of response prevention techniques relied upon close individual supervision by a therapist, often a trained nurse, during virtually all of the patient's waking hours, but further experience has shown that total supervision is not necessary. However, many hours a week of skilled work from nursing, psychological, and psychiatric staff need to be available for this form of treatment, particularly in the early stages. It is usually necessary to start treatment as an in-patient but since some rituals are specific to a domestic setting treatment sessions may need to be arranged in the patient's home.

There are now many published reports which demonstrate that response prevention can be effective. In some individual patients the effect is dramatic and long-lasting, even when the symptoms have been disabling for many years. Unfortunately, some patients respond little or not at all, usually because they are only partially co-operative in carrying out the details of the behavioural programme. These patients are often found to have a variety of other interpersonal, sexual, and family problems, and it may become clear that a simple improvement in their symptoms would not necessarily bring any major benefit.

Behavioural treatment of obsessional thoughts. Thought stopping is a behavioural technique for patients with troublesome obsessional thoughts not associated with ritual behaviour, and was one of the many treatments tried by Wolpe in his pioneering efforts (Wolpe, 1958). Although individual case reports show that this can be effective in some patients, more systematic studies have failed to show any very specific effect (Stern, Lipsedge & Marks, 1973). This cannot

yet be regarded as a technique of established effectiveness, and further trials are needed.

Thought satiation (variously called saturation, paradoxical intention and prolonged exposure in the imagination) may turn out to be more useful than thought stopping, but more detailed studies are needed before it can be recommended with confidence (Emmelkamp & Kwee, 1977).

Behavioural treatment of obsessional slowness. The marked slowness of obsessional patients has been put forward as a major feature in its own right, and some experimental techniques of 'pacing' have been reported (Rachman, 1974; Marks, Hodgson & Rachman, 1975). Again, more systematic studies are needed but this could be a promising area for development.

Practical issues in the behavioural treatment of obsessional patients. Although each treatment technique can be conceptualized and assessed as if it were separate from the others, an analysis of what is actually experienced by the patient usually shows that the techniques overlap a good deal of practice. It also becomes clear that the intense and repeated interaction between the patient and therapists leads to close and crucial relationships that inevitably have either a good or a bad effect upon the patient's motivation to co-operate. In other words, a behavioural treatment programme usually turns out to be much more complicated than just the carrying out of a series of prescribed techniques.

The initial decision whether to plan a behavioural approach should rest with the pyschiatrist in charge of patient, although he may well choose to give a great deal of responsibility for this to a clinical psychologist with whom he is accustomed to work closely. The detailed assessment and analysis of symptoms and the design of the programme of sessions can be carried out by either a psychiatrist or a clinical psychologist, so long as the individual concerned has a special interest and training in behavioural approaches. The same therapist should initiate the treatment sessions, but it is often useful to involve a co-therapist, together with one or more of the nursing staff who will inevitably become involved in observing and interacting with the patient. Recent experience has shown that a proportion of trained psychiatric nurses are well able to develop the additional skills needed to play a central part in the treatment programme (Marks *et al.*, 1977). In practical terms, these various considerations imply that specially experienced and trained therapists who have comparatively generous amounts of time available are needed before this type of treatment can be planned with any confidence of success.

The detailed and systematic analysis and description of the patient's symptoms and behaviour that form the basis for planning the treatment programme usually involve counting or timing of behaviour; that is, a degree of quantification. This lends itself readily to the preparation of charts, diagrams, or graphs upon which the patient's symptoms are recorded (hourly, daily, or sessionally as appropriate) as treatment proceeds, thus giving an objective and permanent record of response to treatment. All the therapists directly interacting with the patient should be encouraged to contribute to these records of treatment and response, since to do so increases the feelings of contribution and commitment that may be needed to sustain the therapeutic team during a trying task.

Obsessional patients usually have other problems in addition to their current symptoms. Close relatives may need to be brought directly into the treatment programme so that, for instance, response prevention programmes can continue at home. Such a development immediately tests out the quality of relationships, and considerable contact with and instruction of wives, husbands, or parents may be needed before a satisfactory programme can go forward. It may be necessary to spend as much time and effort on various forms of individual and joint psychotherapy or family casework, directed at these other problems, as on the behavioural programme itself.

Brain surgery

If all other treatments have been tried and have failed to relieve the patient's distress and disability, there is then a choice between some form of leucotomy or simply waiting in the hope of a natural remission. The common therapeutic effect in the various forms of leucotomy is usually regarded as relief of psychic tension and preoccupation with symptoms, so it is not surprising that some patients who are very disabled and distressed by obsessional symptoms obtain marked relief from leucotomy. Sykes and Tredgold (1964) confirmed the findings of previous, less selective, studies, but also found that only about half of their obsessional patients maintained their initial improvement. The comparatively non-specific effects of leucotomy are confirmed by the lists of points associated with good or bad outcome of the operation – they are virtually the same as the points associated with comparatively good or bad outcome of any other sort of treatment (or presumably none at all). Stable personality and domestic circumstances, strong motivation to recover and return to work, and an illness of acute and recent onset in a patient under forty years of age are the principal points associated with a good result. After surgery, even in patients with only moderate degrees of symptomatic improvement, there may be a surprising lessening of the resulting disability; such patients often comment that although they still have just the same thoughts and impulses, they are less troubled by them. As with leucotomy for any other condition, it seems likely that the outcome is largely dependent upon favourable post-operative management facilities and long-term social circumstances. Brain surgery also has a small but definite mortality and post-operative complication rate, not possessed by other forms of treatment; in Sykes and Tredgold's series, mortality was 1.4 per cent and there was a temporary post-operative epilepsy rate of 16 per cent.

The most recent British series (Mitchell-Heggs, Kelly & Richardson, 1976) used the technique of stereotactic limbic leucotomy, which appears to be superior in both effectiveness and safety to earlier methods. Twenty-seven of their patients were severe obsessionals, twenty-four of whom were reported to show considerable symptomatic improvement sixteen months after the operation. In their total series of one hundred patients with various conditions, there were no fatalities and remarkably few adverse neurological or psychological effects: this certainly seems now to be the surgical technique of choice. These workers also took great care to make thorough and objective symptom measures before and after the operation, and are clearly aware of the importance of post-operative support and follow-up. Their figures probably represent what can now be achieved with high-level facilities plus considerable expertise and enthusiasm.

Course, prognosis and outcome

All varieties of course can be found, but the pessimistic prognosis often given for obsessional illness arises because just over half the patients have a more or less permanent and unremitting illness (Ingram, 1961; Black, 1974). The remainder have phasic or fluctuating courses, according to the main studies that have been reported.

Some of the follow-up studies of obsessional patients already quoted have been used to identify indicators of good and bad outcome, but there are many inconsistencies and contradictions between the studies. In addition, those points which have been identified with a good prognosis are the usual ones which are found in the study of almost all psychiatric illnesses; that is, a good previous personality, known precipitating factors, a short illness before presentation, an episodic course, and atypical mixtures of symptoms. Some measure of agreement emerges on the poor prognostic significance of definite obsessional symptoms since childhood and a very severe degree of illness on admission to hospital, but these are probably no more than an expression of a general factor of severity.

Most clinicians tend to be pessimistic about the long-term prospects of obsessional patients, but the sudden recovery of severely ill patients is also a well-known clinical observation. The tendency of feelings of resistance to fade as the years go by has already been noted. It is surprising how few obsessionals become long-stay patients; somehow or other the great majority of those admitted leave hospital whatever their disabilities, and stay out. With the recent advent of behavioural treatments, and the likelihood of ever more varieties of tricyclic and related 'antidepressant' drugs, the treatment prospects of obsessional illness may be improving.

7.3
The impact of obsessional parents on their children
SULA WOLFF

Obsessional disorders are rarely encountered among parents of child psychiatric clinic attenders. When a father has to engage in ritualistic checking behaviour or is obsessionally preoccupied with food hygiene, the effect on a son from middle childhood onwards can be like that of other incomprehensible psychiatric symptoms: to undermine his respect for and pride in his father and induce feelings of inferiority in relation to other boys.

Obsessional personality traits are more common among mothers and fathers of referred children. Such parents tend to be coercive and to expect excessively early impulse control.

E. J. Anthony's neat hypothesis (1957), that children with discontinuous encopresis, that is, children once toilet-trained who relapse in response to stress, are excessively anxious and fastidious and had coercive mothers with inordinate aspirations for early sphincter control, whereas children who never attained bowel control are non-anxious but insufficiently trained, is not borne out in practice (Olatawura, 1973). Coercive toilet training and obsessional maternal attitudes are not identified in most discontinuous soilers, and most soilers of whatever type are anxious. Yet obsessional personality traits are found in some mothers of encopretic children and are then of great significance both in understanding the multifarious aetiology of the symptom and in its management. And there are, of course, children with other types of behaviour problems who have obsessional mothers or fathers, but this is only one among many aetiological factors.

James, aged 6, presented with continuous soiling, mild constipation, and a number of minor physical complaints. He was an intelligent, left-handed boy, physically healthy and well adjusted socially and at school, where he was generally continent.

Toilet training was started at eighteen months (that is, *not* early), he disliked his pot and his mother had to coerce him to use it. These interactions, while by no means violent, were unpleasant for mother and child. At this time both began hospital visits to James' cousin, Mary, three months younger than himself. She was the child of the mother's favourite brother and had cystic fibrosis.

When James was 3½, Mary's father fell through a plate glass window in a block of flats and died. James' mother could not cry about the loss of her favourite brother, became irritable to her husband, emotionally preoccupied, and withdrawn. Her placid husband was a great support to her. Three months later James's brother was born. James asked about procreation and his mother knew he did not fully understand her explanations. At 6 he still believed babies were born through the umbilicus. When James was 4, Mary died and when he was 4½ his mother conceived for the third time, was at first distressed but then looked forward to a girl. A third boy arrived.

She was a most capable mother, affectionate, orderly and an excellent time keeper. She found herself disgusted by James' dirty pants, and irritated by his obsinate 'go slow' manoeuvres when she tried to get him up and off to school each morning. He in turn was very tidy (even in the playroom he meticulously brushed away grains of sand) and good at helping her about the house.

While continuing to pressure him about his toilet habits she also identified with his public shame. She remembered being teased about a squint she had in childhood and she then recalled a further source of insecurity. At the time of her marriage she discovered a fact her parents had not known how to convey to her earlier: that she was her mother's illegitimate child and that her father was not her real father.

Our patient, James, with perhaps a mild maturational delay in acquiring sphincter control, had experienced a series of anxiety-inducing events (the major one being Mary's illness and death) during his oedipal stage when he would be attempting to understand with pre-rational logic the biological facts of family life and to cope with rivalry feelings. His mother at that time, still trying to toilet-train him, was depressed, irritable, and over-burdened with young children. Her obsessionality, so clearly present, was the least of his troubles, merely contributing perhaps to raise his anxiety about his symptoms. Like many soilers he wished he never had to pass 'jobbies' at all and lived his life attempting to deny this fact.

8
Patients presenting with bodily complaints and disturbances

8.1
Psychosomatic medicine and liaison psychiatry

HENRY WALTON

Historical review of the concept of psychosomatic disorder

Psychosomatic medicine, a term some would consider misleading or even obsolete (Grinker, 1973), deals with an area of physical illness in which psychiatry has a large part to play. Psychiatrists working in general hospitals have been closely implicated in this sector of illness which has been intensively studied in the context of general hospital psychiatry. The term 'liaison psychiatry' refers to the work of the psychiatrist in the general hospital.

The course of development of psychosomatic medicine has been absorbing and eventful, with extreme shifts of direction which are exceptionally informative to follow, these transitions reflecting the changing relationship between psychiatry and its parent discipline of medicine.

Concepts linking body and mind

The notion (mistaken as we now realize) that it is possible to split nature into two separate parts, mind on the one hand and matter on the other is associated with the seventeenth-century French philosopher, Descartes, and hence is known as Cartesian *dualism*. The body, and the brain in particular, is the material aspect of the person, in this view; Descartes postulated a separate self in addition: the mind. The human being was to be seen as a machine (the body) with a ghost in it (the mind). Many doctors, wittingly or not, adopt this position.

The other popular position about the mind–

body problem is *materialism*. The American behaviourist Skinner holds that the entire concept of mind should be discarded as a mere superstition, an 'epiphenomenon'. There is a third possible approach, propounded by Spinoza in the seventeenth century, Schopenhauer in the nineteenth, and now by O'Shaughnessy: *dual aspectism* (1980). The material aspect of the person, his body, is undoubtedly a physical object, part of the external world, but it is that part of the material world which is incorporated within the self: no person regards his body as 'outside' himself. Body and mind are twin partners. No aspect of a person's behaviour can be reduced to either physical or psychological aspects. Aspects of mind are connected with each other, but always and indissolubly with the body as well. A person is endowed with two general orientations about his body: one, from the outside (through the senses), perceives it as material, a physical entity – the other, from the inside, experiences the body mentally. As Wittgenstein wrote: 'One *knows* the position of the limbs and their movements . . . just as one knows the place of a sensation (pain) in the body.' The enduring body-image that a person has is of a different order from the awareness he obtains about his body through the sense perceptions.

Psychosomatic medicine

The earlier preoccupation with taking all possible steps to exclude physical illness before making a psychiatric referral of a patient (still followed by some physicians) is misplaced and should be obsolete. A patient can suffer simultaneously from both physical and psychiatric illness. In fact, disorders of both psychiatric and somatic types cluster in a section of the population (Hinkle & Wolff, 1957). This recognition had led increasingly to greater provision of psychiatric liaison services (see below) in general hospitals. As psychiatrists have worked more often and regularly in association with physicians, interest has grown in the relationship of physical illness with emotional disorder. By common agreement among clinicians, there came to be certain physical illnesses in which emotional states of the patient were seen to play a large part; these 'psychosomatic' illnesses were viewed as due to a chronic exaggeration of physiological accompaniments of emotion. The visceral effects of prolonged, intense emotion were held eventually to lead to tissue changes and damage.

W. B. Cannon early in the century proposed that in emergency conditions of 'fight' or 'flight'

autonomic and vegetative systems become activated (1920). If the anger can be expressed as aggression, or the fear relieved by flight, these visceral reactions are dissipated. However, Cannon postulated, if such outlet or action is not possible, the visceral changes are likely to persist, and give rise to organ pathology. The concept of organ specificity was explored: Deutsch (1939) considered that childhood emotional experiences were responsible for determining which body part would later become the target for stress-induced physical disease ('organ neuroses').

Helen Flanders Dunbar, of the Columbia University Medical Centre, supported a personality profile theory (1935). She proposed in the 1930s that certain 'psychosomatic diseases' were associated with particular personality types, for example, coronary thrombosis was held to occur in ambitious, confident, forceful men. Her theory that a specific personality type would emerge for each of the psychosomatic disorders (she wrote about the 'hypertensive character', and 'ulcer personality', and so on) has not been supported. The concept, however, has been revived recently in the field of research into myocardial infarction. Friedman and Rosenman in 1960 described the Type A behaviour pattern in which the person has pronounced traits of aggressiveness, ambitiousness, and competitiveness: this type of person is not only exaggeratedly work-oriented, but often works with a great sense of urgency. Other traits such people exhibit are hostility and continual impatience. The converse Type B individual, free of these pronounced personality traits, generally feels no pressing conflict over time or competition with other people, and does not constantly experience a sense of urgency. The description of these two types depicts a style of overt behaviour which is the habitual way that these individuals confront, interpret and respond to their life circumstances. In a return to the 'personality profile' approach, these authors hold that the Type A person is at greater risk of coronary artery and other myocardial disease.

Characteristic personality types have been associated with other 'psychosomatic disorders' as well. Engel (1958) described the rigid attitudes he found in patients with ulcerative colitis, pointing out their conscientiousness, neatness, orderliness and punctuality.

Franz Alexander, a psycho-analyst in Chicago singled out a group of illnesses: coronary disease, hypertension, bronchial asthma, peptic ulcer, thyrotoxicosis, rheumatoid arthritis, and ulcerative colitis as 'psychosomatic'. He advanced a different causal proposal, that the psychological disorder in the psychosomatic illnesses should be sought not in the personality type, but in the reaction pattern of patients (1950). This was the 'conflict specificity' approach: by it, unconscious emotional conflicts were held to activate autonomic nervous system reactions; the latter was proposed as the mechanism producing organ disease. A person with a peptic ulcer, for example, was postulated to suffer from unexpressed dependency needs (such as unmet wishes to receive love); anxiety results as an expression of the unresolved conflict; the anxiety is discharged through the parasympathetic nervous system, with increased gastric secretion and ulceration as consequences. Alexander associated asthma with an unconscious persisting terror of loss of closeness to the mother. His theories sought to link repressed emotional conflicts with autonomic imbalance and visceral lesions, thus attempting to relate defined psychological processes (a characteristic unconscious emotional conflict) with organ pathology through the autonomic nervous system. At this stage of historical development in the search for the aetiology of the different disorders, the expectation was that characteristic patterns of emotional response would prove to be associated with each of the specific physical disorders. A distinct and fairly unitary psychological causation for each of the different conditions was still being pursued, but now at the level of varying emotional states and their physiological accompaniments (rather than at the level of any specific personality profile).

This approach, aiming to establish a specificity theory, has not been sustained either. For example, the theory that the activation of a peptic ulcer is directly related to psychologically-mediated increase in the secretion of gastric acid has not been confirmed: the patient with peptic ulcer has a high secretion of gastric acid whether his ulcer is active or not; thus a psychogenic increase in acid secretion cannot be the factor responsible for a peptic ulcer becoming active.

Harold Wolff and Stewart Wolf at the Cornell Medical College adopted a non-specific approach to the study of organ or tissue damage occurring with emotional maladaption (1943). They did not set out to link personality profiles or characteristic psychological conflicts with organic illness. Instead, they did experiments to study the physical changes in various bodily organs in response to psychological stimuli. They investigated the effects of emotional stress on the nasal mucosa, the stomach, and the colon. They postulated that tissue swelling, increased blood flow, and increased motility were the basis for the pathological changes seen in psychosomatic diseases. They concluded that psychosomatic disease results in a person as a result of organ responses under threatening life circumstances. Rather naive symbolic implications were suggested for the physical changes they observed: for example, nasal obstruction from increased blood flow was viewed as representing a tendency by the person to shut himself off from stressful life events.

The investigation of emotion-linked somatic illness in humans was augmented by ingenious experiments inducing conflicts in animals. Pavlov in pioneering research had produced experimental neuroses in dogs. Gantt (1944) induced psychosomatic disturbances such as respiratory disorders in dogs and farm animals. Brady and his colleagues in 1958 reported duodenal ulcers and other gastrointestinal disturbances in experimental animals ('executive monkeys') required to maintain constant alertness during a conditioning procedure, in which electric shocks could be avoided by lever-pressing (1958).

Still concentrating on the seven-or-so 'psychosomatic diseases' which Alexander has especially emphasized, the social circumstances of these patients began to be more carefully studied. Evidence began to accumulate about the relation between the onset of certain physical illness and significant life crises, such as the death of a spouse, or the loss of one's job (Holmes & Rahe, 1967; Kasl & Cobb, 1970). As awareness of the relation between life crises and illness grew, clinicians more systematically enquired whether patients had experienced misfortune, and how they coped with and adapted to it. The loss of security, diminished status, and lowered self-esteem of physically-ill patients who had experienced social misfortune came to be accorded clinical relevance, more so than hypothetical linkages between mind and body.

The current view
The present approach is no longer based on the preconception that certain diseases are 'psychosomatic'. Instead, any physically-ill patient may require to be studied clinically to determine whether psychological disorder or social problems are also present. The degree of the emotional component in patients with 'psychosomatic disorder' varies greatly

with different patients, and cannot be considered the only causative factor. However, it must be said that in many of these patients emotional antecedents, particularly related to fear of estrangement from a loved person or to the control of hostility, are often prominent in the precipitation or the exacerbation of the physical illness.

Classification of psychosomatic disorders

In the Ninth Revision of the International Classification of Diseases (World Health Organization, 1978) two diagnostic categories refer to psychosomatic disorders. Section 306 is labelled 'Physiological malfunction arising from mental factors'. It includes physical disorders usually regarded as related to emotional conflict (but not the illnesses with actual tissue damage). Section 306 thus includes psychogenic torticollis, hyperventilation, psychogenic pruritis, cyclical vomiting, and psychogenic dysmenorrhoea. Section 316 of ICD–9 includes physical conditions, usually involving tissue damage, in the aetiology of which mental disturbance or psychic factors are thought to play a part. The glossary indicates that the mental disturbance implicated is usually mild and non-specific and psychic factors (worry, fear, conflict, and so on) may be present without any overt psychiatric disorder. That is to say, the psychological accompaniments become evident if the clinician actively explores the less overt aspects of the patient's self-experience and his interpersonal relationships. Asthma, eczema, gastric ulcer, ulcerative colitis, and urticaria are among the conditions included in this section.

The American Psychiatric Association, in turn, has produced a new Third Edition of its Diagnostic and Statistical Manual of Mental Disorders, DSM–III, (American Psychiatric Association, 1980). This widely-used system of classification includes a category 'Psychological factors affecting physical disorder' and proposes that this rather unwieldy circumlocation be used to describe disorders which in the past have been referred to as either 'psychosomatic' or 'psychophysiological'. The category includes obesity, migraine, neurodermatitis, acne, rheumatoid arthritis, asthma, gastric ulcer, duodenal ulcer, ulcerative colitis, and hyperthyroidism.

The clinical approach

The psychiatrist's responsibility, therefore, to physically-ill patients referred to him is to detect any psychological disorder or social difficulties which may accompany the somatic illness. The psychiatrist explores the psychological and the social sectors using his proper investigative method, the psychiatric interview.

In the case of physical illness, it opens by an exploration with the patient of his symptoms. The patient may often be puzzled, confused, or resentful over talking with a psychiatrist at all, and convey still more bewilderment or distress as the clinical enquiry moves from the physical symptoms into discussion about the patient's main current personal relationships and life circumstances, his problems at work or in his personal life, and his private preoccupations about which he may speak only with hesitation, reserve, or great difficulty.

As the psychiatric enquiry proceeds to explore the emotional and social sectors of the patient's experiences, significant and highly relevant aspects of the case history begin to emerge, which the patient may not have thought to mention to his physicians, nor they have sought to discover.

A man aged 48 years was referred by a cardiologist following a myocardial infarction. He should have recovered satisfactorily, on all physical counts, but instead he was inactive at home, excessively worried over trifles, his efforts to return to his work did not succeed (the patient repeatedly returned home early and dreaded going to work in the morning), and his formerly close and warm relationship with his wife had deteriorated to irritability and querulousness. The cardiologist considered the patient incapacitated, not obviously because of his physical state, which was one of recovery.

Psychiatric enquiry showed that before the myocardial infarction the patient had been told that his work might be terminated by redundancy, 'a statement which has never been retracted': he was inwardly furious that his long service had been regarded as of little account when his former trusted senior colleague was succeeded by a younger, more critical superior. The patient, particularly following his heart attack, could not bring himself to challenge his employers about his insecurity of employment. Formerly 'aggressively confident', he found himself not thinking clearly, and anxious and diffident when giving orders.

Both at home and at work, he felt that the 'low status' consequent on his invalidism 'disqualified' him socially: he would sit only a few minutes with visitors, and no longer initiated encounters with other people.

He was both more dependent on his wife, a former nurse, and also demanding and reproachful when she seemed insufficiently protective, as the following incident illustrates. It was a weekend. His wife took him into the kitchen, to remove some hairs off a black tee-shirt he was wearing. He turned on her furiously because the back door happened to be open, and he considered that she exposed him 'to a howling gale'. Neither spoke to the other during the rest of the weekend. 'You know how it goes! Who's to blame . . . I'm sorry, but not sorry enough to apologize. I can tell my wife had a dreadful time during my illness, and now she feels she is in need of some sympathy and consideration for herself.'

Turning to exploration of his early life, it emerged that the patient had ambitions which his father had disregarded. He had wanted to become a doctor. Instead, although the family was not poor, he was required to go into commercial work after leaving school. The psychiatrist suggested that he had probably been very disappointed that his father minimized his hopes for his life, and failed to encourage him in his ambitions. Bitterly the patient said that he was the one who cared most now that the father was old; his brothers and sisters occasionally 'gave him biscuits', and that was all.

As the psychiatric interviews continued (the patient's wife had separate discussions with the social worker), he expressed extreme indignation that the psychiatrist was suggesting that his father had been negligent of the patient's welfare in youth. He claimed that his interpretation had been wrong and distasteful. 'In my opinion, my father is this good guy – my mother was the poor one.' The patient could then discuss how emotionally deprived his relationship with his mother had been. He could consciously recognize his hostile responses towards her. But about his father he could feel only apparent regard. It then became evident (supporting a hypothesis of repressed hostility) that he was pathologically guilty about his father, whom he could never visit at the Aged Home without an inner struggle to bring his demented parent away with him. He castigated himself for not doing enough for his father.

The disorder in the psychological sector thus became increasingly evident: this man had never resolved his regressed anger towards his father, his overt disappointment at being unloved by his mother, and his resentment that his siblings failed to take on part of the reparative, misplaced dutifulness which he felt was owing to his father. In this psychic condition the patient, with the support deriving from his dependent attachment to his competent, maternal wife, had succeeded at work until there was a threat of dismissal through redundancy, followed by the devastating impairment of his reliance on his physical integrity when the cardiac catastrophe occurred.

The opportunities for discussing his previously unacknowledged psychological conflicts, the progressively frank and assertive steps he took at his work about his employment status and his working relationships, and the greater frankness fostered between him and his wife by occasional joint interviews, resulted in very satisfactory return to his former physical and social vigour. He actively resumed the treasureship of his local brass band as a leisure activity; his cup was full when he was in the Albert Hall and the band was judged the twelfth best.

Clinical management: liaison psychiatry
The role of the psychiatrist

Feinstein (1970), in a famous paper, has given emphasis to the absence in medicine generally of a science of clinical management: almost no attention is paid to steps necessary for reducing observer variability, developing a taxonomy of managerial decisions, or establishing criteria for clinical judgements, therapy, or prognosis in direct clinical work with patients. The absence of a systematic specification of the necessary concepts and methods is equally prominent in the practice of liaison psychiatry. Only a few of the crucial technical procedures will be mentioned.

The psychiatrist called to investigate a physically-ill patient is not the primary physician. Besides being perceived at times by the patient as an intruder (sometimes an unwelcome one), the referring physician, surgeon, obstetrician, and so on, has the right to hear from the psychiatrist what his findings are and what further psychiatric investigation or management is proposed. The psychiatrist, therefore, establishes clinical communication not only with the patient, but also with the referring physician. Many potential advantages follow, but hazards also. The psychiatric consultation is therefore complexly interactive.

It is thus on request of the referring physician that the psychiatrist interviews the patient (Macleod & Walton, 1969). The effectiveness of the consultation, inevitably, is dependent on the communication between the psychiatrist and the consultant making the referral, and the mutual confidence which obtains (Crisp, 1968). It is not to be expected that the referring clinician will necessarily be aware of the nature of the patient's psychological disorder. The liaison psychiatrist need not adhere to the letter of a referral made to him; nor would the referring clinician expect him to respond narrowly to the immediate medical perception of the clinical problem. Non-psychiatrist colleagues cannot be expected to define all psychiatric problems which may be present; they expect that the psychiatrist will identify the specific psychological information relevant in the case only after he has brought his own investigative skills to bear. The liaison psychiatrist is therefore called upon to interpret the referral, and to see it in context as an initial communication. As his knowledge of the case progresses, he will frequently engage in a dialogue with the referring clinician, and he may convey a series of reports about the interventions he comes to perceive as necessary, as his acquaintance with the patient's problems extends. To communicate effectively with non-psychiatrists the liaison psychiatrist needs to rephrase psychiatric concepts in terms which are generally intelligible and acceptable. Failure to recognize these requirements is one of the main obstacles to effective clinical collaboration.

The psychiatrist in the general hospital errs at times by expecting that he can contribute satisfactorily to the care of the patient merely by deploying skills appropriate for psychiatric hospital work. The liaison psychiatrist who expects to deal with generally-known psychiatric syndromes will overlook much emotional and social disorder which his hospital colleagues expect him to recognize and respond to clinically (Lipowski, 1967). All psychiatrists, who increasingly will be expected to do part of their work in general hospitals, should receive training in a liaison psychiatry setting. In the first place, general hospital patients frequently do not present with identifiable psychiatric syndromes; instead, they often disclose interpersonal problems, subjective distress, or agitating preoccupations to the psychiatrist: these then become the focus of clinical attention.

The occupational hazard to which many psychiatrists succumb is the adoption of one or other ideology, the most notorious being the undue espousal of either the 'medical model' or a psychodynamic approach. Such simplistic views can be a crippling limitation in general hospital work. Many referred patients in general wards have difficulties in their relations with people close to them as their main psychiatric impediment. Such interpersonal failures will go undetected by the type of psychiatrist only alert to defined psychiatric disease entities. In turn, the psychiatrist who insists on a narrowly descriptive psychiatric approach (Havens, 1973) can be altogether unhelpful to his medical and surgical colleagues. To assist patients referred to him, and be useful to the staff making the referral, the psychiatrist does well to adopt the perspective that whatever the terms of a referral, his task is to explore all appropriate approaches including those not immediately explicit, by which his specialist skills can contribute to the clinical management of the case, and augment the capability of the other clinicians to achieve their investigative, therapeutic, or management goals.

The theory of *intentionality* holds that an emotion is always directed at an object, a specific person. An angry individual feels hostile towards somebody. Therefore, the exploratory interviews should properly discover which people the patient is most closely concerned about, and reveal to which individuals his strongest feelings are directed. Any of the patients in the categories indicated on p. 279 may be found to be emotionally disturbed, and enquiry will disclose the individuals in their lives who are implicated. Psychiatric investigation does more than discover that such patients are trapped in life situations engendering desperation, intense frustration, rage, or resentment: the persons significantly associated with the patient in these situations become identified. The

extreme frustration and anger any employee experiences may be directed at a colleague with authority over him at his work, by whom he is regularly humiliated and dominated. A patient found to be depressed may have been left recently by his wife. A woman with depersonalization may disclose that her father, with whom she lived following her mother's death, is contemplating marrying again and detaching his affections from her.

The necessary approach in liaison psychiatry is to investigate impairment in any of the three sectors: the somatic, the social and the psychological. The psychiatrist is of course not unconcerned with the somatic sector; certain psychiatric disorders are organic in type. However, the psychiatrist's knowledge and his clinical skills equip him to contribute understanding about the patient's social and psychological state which may be critically important for a full appraisal of the physical illness. What he discovers is frequently a problem in living, the more difficult to arrive at when the patient himself does not have any clear appreciation of his conflicts prior to the psychiatric consultation.

Much of this information will be qualitatively different from that elicited by a somatic approach. It will refer to the patient's personal life, his 'lived experience', and depends on the facts emerging about the more intimate aspects of the patient's associations with those close to him. Unless seen in such a biographical context, when the meaning is discovered which the patient attaches to particular aspects of his existence, only a partial and often a misleading grasp of his mental life results. In this sense, psychiatry is a hermeneutic (i.e. subjectively interpretative) as well as a biological science: it contributes a clinical method whereby the patient can reflect on his own experience and enable the psychiatrist to clarify whether the patient is failing to acknowledge an aspect of his own life. An obvious example is a bereaved person who fails to identify and respond to the emotional effects of his loss.

Of equal importance is the fact that such extension in understanding which is achieved by the psychiatrist is intersubjective, that is, it is clinically important that the patient also grasps that he has been understood. The fact-finding of the psychiatric examination is accompanied by shared understanding between the patient and psychiatrist, and the assignment of meaning to the patient's experience. A clinical relationship is established which is based, to a greater or less extent, on mutual understanding. The patient possesses the biographically relevant facts: imparting (or withholding) them often determines how accurate and effective the psychiatrist becomes in clarifying the psychological disturbance and social difficulties applicable to the individual patient.

The psychiatrist, therefore, both investigates and begins to treat the patient as he investigates the social and psychological circumstances accompanying the onset and progression of the physical illness. His interviews, which frequently elicit life-experiences that the patient has not thought to disclose previously to other clinicians, permits the patient to experience feelings which had been wholly internalized. With such communication of emotion considerable relief can result.

Patients referred

Patients with physical illness are frequently found to be psychiatrically disordered as well, when enabled to talk about their personal circumstances in a psychiatric interview. Only a small proportion of such patients are identified by physicians and referred to see a psychiatrist (Shepherd *et al.*, 1960; Maguire *et al.*, 1974).

A large range of conditions occur in general hospitals calling for collaboration between psychiatrists and the specialists primarily responsible for the care of the patient. Liaison psychiatric services can assist with the following types of patient, to indicate only some:

(1) patients who present to physicians with physical symptoms for which insufficient organic cause is detected,

(2) patients with combined physical and psychiatric diagnoses,

(3) patients with primary psychiatric disorders or symptoms for whom referral to psychiatric hospital is unacceptable,

(4) patients with organic illness who have emotional difficulties in complying with the necessary treatment,

(5) patients with physical disease secondary to emotional or mental disorder, for example the consequences of suicidal attempts, alcoholism, and so on,

(6) patients for whom the illness or its treatment causes such profound changes in their lives that a considerable emotional readjustment is necessary; for example, patients undergoing renal dialysis or patients with crippling neurological disorders.

AN ILLUSTRATIVE CASE HISTORY

A 32-year-old married man, a senior hospital technician, had complained of abdominal symptoms for over a year. At times he was convinced that he had carcinoma of the head of the pancreas. He described a constant 'crushing' and 'rawness' in the upper abdomen, with occasional vomiting at times of 'high stress'. Continuing to quote the patient's own phrases, the referring physician reported that the patient described himself as 'emotionally drained'. His symptoms were extremely distressing, amounting at times to panic. Repeated examinations by the general physician and extensive laboratory and radiological investigations had failed to elicit any definite abnormality.

The patient told the psychiatrist that he had a feeling of irritation, which he thought was inflammation in the right upper abdomen. He had been investigated for gall bladder disease. He had bypassed his general practitioner to get the physician with whom he worked to do further tests. Once the general practitioner had said disparagingly that his real problem was 'working in the health profession', but the patient considered that the physician was properly concerned about possible serious physical illness. 'I have this constant burning'. The patient insisted that his symptoms were certainly organic. He explained that he had been neglected professionally before. A year after he began to work in the hospital he developed a 'renal carbuncle'. He was treated as an in-patient, but when his symptoms persisted he was told to stop working in hospital where 'there are always infection problems'.

The patient's family and personal history were highly relevant. He described his father as a hairdresser who had 'one or two health problems of late – he thinks he's got a serious heart complaint, but I don't think there's an indication of that'. The patient had started his secondary schooling late – because of illness. He explained that at eight and a half years of age Perthe's disease of the hip was diagnosed belatedly. Since the age of five he had suffered from pain in his knee, presumably referred from the diseased hip. It was his father who insisted on the patient being referred to hospital, where a surgeon correctly diagnosed his condition. 'I wasn't the only one who was unhappy for the time it took for referral.'

Having communicated the childhood counterpart of the current dilemma, akin because in both experiences of sickness the patient dreaded serious physical disease that his doctors appeared to ignore, the whole atmosphere of the interview altered (a shift the clinician awaits in every first interview with a physically-ill patient primarily under the care of another physician). Instead of being defensive and waiting for questions to be put to him, he gave information with a confidence absent from the opening phase of the consultation. He explained that he was a reticent person, used to working matters out for himself – 'but the physical thing had become such a nightmare . . . I suppose it relates to living with a high level of pain for such a long time as a child, before the Perthe's disease was discovered. I was an active child, but I had to pay with the pain afterwards. Then I had to spend two years in hospital, until I was eleven'. He proceeded to amplify his account of his renal illness nine years previously. 'I was unhappy for the time it took for referral. I had complained of being unwell for a very long time before losing my left kidney. Whenever I got myself referred to the Out-patients, I was told there was nothing wrong. I got to the stage that I wasn't allowed back to my own laboratory in the hospital to do my job. I was advised to give it up and never resume working in a hospital. After all that I was admitted as an emergency, and the surgeon confided that when they operated they did not know what was wrong. I have no desire to take issue with the profession, but I felt bitter because I thought there was little or no support. After the nephrectomy I was never booked properly into clinics, never followed up properly.'

The mental state. Further examination showed that the patient had been depressed in mood, 'difficult to be at peace with myself', inactive whereas he had been a person 'always on the go', tense, his sleep poor, and incapacitated by hypochondriacal ruminations that his abdominal discomfort betokened fatal internal disease, in fact, cancer. His wife, when interviewed, confirmed his loss of zest, and gloom and anxiety over his state of health.

The diagnosis was that of a depressive illness arising largely as a result of earlier illness experiences. The patient's medical neglect in childhood was being re-enacted in his own mind. Moreover, he had not readjusted occupationally following surgical removal of a kidney nine years previously. He had come to consider his general practitioner as neglectful and offhand, while the physician who made the referral was spared such censure. 'I am quite satisfied with the way he is handling the problem.'

His polarization of his doctors, one execrated and the other idealized, had psychological reference to the patient's father. When a sick child he overtly revered his father as the agent vainly seeking remedy from neglectful doctors until the effective paediatric surgeon emerged. The patient entered and succeeded in a health profession. The recent psychiatric illness followed a repetition of clinical mismanagement and muddle, in the patient's view. Meanwhile, his father had declined, also to a hypochondriacal state, to which the patient reacted with tolerant scepticism.

Action taken. Aware that he could be viewed either as dismissive or as an ally, the psychiatrist insisted that his contribution was not to adjudicate whether or not physical illness was present, but to explore and help with the patient's psychological state.

Antidepressant medication was prescribed. At subsequent out-patient interviews at fortnightly intervals, psychotherapy aimed to review and clarify how the content of the patient's illness related to the disabling physical disease in childhood, reactivated first by the experience of the kidney operation and subsequently by his work difficulties and his father's hypochondriasis.

Outcome. After three months the patient reported that 'everything was improved'. He slept better and had gained a stone in weight. He was now content and able to relax. He reported himself as 'aware of my problems in one sense, but I did not know where the problems lay'. He continued to have some abdominal discomfort, which he now attributed to being tense, but was no longer so concerned about it. He was trying to make himself relax more. He was now able to confide in his wife, with improvement in their marital relationship.

8.2
Chronic pain: the role of the psychiatrist

ISSY PILOWSKY

Introduction

The role to be played by a psychiatrist in the management of chronic pain is influenced by two important factors. The first, rather obvious one, is the patient's overall health status, and the second is the context in which the clinical encounter occurs. Although these two factors are usually interrelated, this is not always the case, and while the relevance of the patient's physical and psychological status to treatment decisions is self-evident, the crucial contribution of the setting in which the clinical encounter occurs, is not always recognized. For example, a patient seeing a psychiatrist who is only one of a group of consultants attached to a multidisciplinary pain clinic reviewing the problem, will come with quite different attitudes and expectations from those of the patient who has been sent to the psychiatrist by a physician who has 'not been able to find anything wrong' and has therefore concluded that the problem must be a 'psychiatric' one.

It is a truism that the approach to pain management is relatively uncomplicated if the complaint is clearly associated with either a physical disorder or a psychiatric disorder. In other words, if a circumscribed somatic pathological pattern, or a psychopathological pattern can be recognized, subsequent steps in the clinical decision-making process may be straightforward. However, the presence of a prominent pain complaint often distracts clinicians from considering or recognizing psychiatric illness, because of the powerful association in people's minds of pain and physical illness.

In practice, therefore, it is most helpful to focus on the patient's 'pain experience' and to consider all those influences which may be determining its characteristics and the patient's associated behaviours.

Definitions

Two definitions of pain have been formulated which are of particular utility to the clinician. The first is that of Sternbach (1968) who defines pain as 'an abstract concept which refers to (1) a personal, private sensation of hurt; (2) a harmful stimulus which signals current or impending tissue damage; (3) a pattern of responses which operates to protect the organism from harm. These responses can be described in terms which reflect certain concepts, i.e. in neurological, physiological, behavioural and affective languages'. The second definition is due to Merskey (Merskey & Spear, 1967) who regards pain as 'an unpleasant experience which we primarily associate with tissue damage or describe in terms of tissue damage, or both'. More recently, Pilowsky (1978a) and Wall (1979) have also emphasized the essential inseparability of pain and 'illness behaviour'. In Wall's (1979) words, 'just as hunger is associated with the search for food and eating . . . pain is associated with the search for treatment and optimal conditions for recovery'. By 'chronic pain', is usually meant pain which does not respond to standard conventional therapies and is usually present for at least four weeks.

In the light of these definitions, it can readily be appreciated that the diagnostic process in relation to chronic pain complaints requires a multidimensional approach, with an appraisal of the somatic, intrapersonal, interpersonal, and social factors contributing to and determining the characteristics of an individual's pain experience and illness behaviour.

It is worth emphasizing that attempts to decide whether a patient's pain is 'organic' or 'psychogenic' are not worthwhile, and may be positively antithetic to the achievement of appropriate diagnosis and management. Indeed, the situation is further complicated by the fact that the relative contributions made by somatic and psychological processes to a patient's pain, can vary from one phase of an illness cycle to another, so that the clinician needs to be prepared to review from time to time what may have appeared to be the situation at the time of the initial appraisal.

Psychiatrists are generally consulted for pains whose descriptions do not conform to known somatic pathologies; or when the patient behaves in relation to a pain, in ways which the clinician regards as inappropriate. For example, a patient may continue to complain of pain despite the provision of what is believed to be adequate treatment, or may appear unable or unwilling to co-operate in a rehabilitation programme aimed at reducing impaired functioning.

Pain problems presenting to the psychiatrist can, therefore, be grouped in terms of a few broad clinical presentations, which reflect the fact that such patients are generally referred by colleagues who find themselves unable to deal adequately with the pain.

Pain associated with psychiatric syndromes

Pain is not an uncommon feature of all psychiatric syndromes. When it is prominent it may render the syndrome less typical and, as a consequence, it may not be readily diagnosed. It needs to be added, however, that in some instances, there may be a reluctance on both the patient's and the clinician's part to acknowledge the presence of a psychiatric illness and a preference to focus on somatic complaints as a more socially acceptable basis for gaining access to the sick role.

From a survey carried out by Spear (Merskey & Spear, 1967) in a Sheffield psychiatric clinic we can obtain some idea of the prevalence of pain amongst such populations. It was found that 53 per cent of new admissions had pain as one of their symptoms, and that depression was the commonest associated diagnosis. However, 'anxiety/hysteria' was also prominent. Amongst psychiatric in-patients and day-patients, he found that pain was experienced at some stage of their stay by 65.6 per cent of the population surveyed.

It would not be appropriate to discuss in great detail the somatic component of the pains complained of by patients suffering psychiatric illness. The commonest sites for these pains are the head and back, but any part of the body can be involved. In some cases, the pain seems clearly related to musculo-skeletal disorders, such as muscle tension and arthritic changes associated with ageing. Syndromes such as 'spastic colon', dyspepsia, and aerophagy may also play a part. Indeed, such 'psychophysiological' entities, which are often overlooked, may require attention at the somatic level.

The proper management of pains associated with psychiatric illness depends on the diagnosis and treatment of the psychopathological state. Since these syndromes are fully described elsewhere, comments will be restricted to the special features associated with the presence of pain.

At this point, it is worth mentioning a particular type of patient who, while relatively amenable to a psychological approach to the understanding of his pain, will emphasize that stress never produces the pain. In these instances, careful history-taking often reveals that these individuals are using the word 'stress' to refer to situations of high activity and task involvement. For example, a patient who worked as a maintenance engineer illustrated the fact that stress was unrelated to his headaches by describing a day at work, during which innumerable machines had broken down, with danger to personnel safety, requiring him to rush from one part of the factory to another to avert 'catastrophes'. Despite all this, he had not experienced a headache until he was 'relaxed' at home. It soon became clear, however, that such 'stress' situations represented occasions when he felt more competent, in control, and adequate, and that they did not represent 'stresses' at all. This realization led to the possibility of understanding the nature of situations which were more truly stressful for him.

In other cases, the pain complaint may be part of a psychotic illness but, none the less, not integrated with the predominant psychopathology. Thus, patients with a psychotic depression or schizophrenic illness may complain of headaches or other pains, but not be deluded about their significance. Here, again, the pain complaints may recede into the background once the diagnosis is made and treatment begun.

The complaint of pain as a depressive equivalent has been described (Bradley, 1963). Certainly, this may occur, but it is important to make the diagnosis of a depressive syndrome, especially of the endogenous type, on positive grounds before antidepressants are prescribed. It must be acknowledged, however, that in the presence of pain, it may not be possible to elucidate all the usual criteria for the diagnosis of endogenous depression. Often a prevailing mood of despondency and irritability is the main clue to the diagnosis, and should not be simply attributed to the pain.

Patients with schizophrenia may complain of pain in various locations, particularly in the early stages of the illness. Some authors have suggested that pain complaints may protect against personality disintegration and withdrawal by providing a rela-

tively acceptable complaint for the purposes of interpersonal contact (Cowden & Brown, 1956). Clearly, a complaint of pain is a better basis for ordinary social conversation than the reporting of hallucinations or paranoid delusions.

The concept of 'abnormal illness behaviour'

Abnormal illness behaviour (AIB) may be defined as: 'the persistence of an inappropriate or maladaptive mode of perceiving, evaluating and acting in relation to one's own state of health, despite the fact that a doctor (or other appropriate social agent) has offered a reasonably lucid explanation of the nature of the patient's health status and the appropriate course of management to be followed, based on a thorough examination and assessment of all parameters of functioning (including the use of special investigations where necessary) and taking into account the individual's age, educational and socio-cultural background' (Pilowsky, 1978b).

Patients are commonly referred for a psychiatric opinion when a presumptive diagnosis of 'abnormal illness behaviour' has been made by a clinician, even though, of course, this term may not be used. It is indeed more common for such patients to be described as 'hysterics', 'hypochondriacs', or in even more overtly pejorative terms. Certainly, these patients, more than most others, have a capacity for evoking hostility from the medical profession, and it is a crucial prerequisite of any management programme that the determinants of this doctor–patient conflict be clearly understood.

Essentially, this strain on the doctor–patient relationship may be seen as arising out of the patient's maladaptive need to cling to the sick role and the doctor's need to respond to complaints with efforts to alleviate them. However, since the patient is utilizing illness behaviour (albeit maladaptively) to achieve some degree of psychological equilibrium, in much the same way as another patient may use abdominal guarding and rigidity to control the pain of peritonitis, it is not surprising that he recoils from the doctor's attempt to divest him of his primary strategy for survival, even though, at one level of awareness, he may realize that it is an attempt to help him.

It can be seen, therefore, that the management of pain depends to a considerable degree on the early clarification of the presence or absence of abnormal illness behaviour.

In a certain percentage of patients AIB can soon

be excluded since there is a ready acceptance of a reformulation of the illness in psychiatric terms. Indeed, patients may indicate that they have for some time suspected that their pain should be approached in this way, but were reluctant to offer this option to their doctor. For example, some will make the observation that their pain is worse when they are upset, for some reason or another, and they deduce, therefore, that psychological factors are significant.

Abnormal illness behaviour syndromes

These syndromes may be grouped into psychotic and neurotic forms.

Psychotic AIB. The best recognized forms of psychotic AIB are those associated with psychotic depression and schizophrenia. In the case of the former, the patient may manifest hypochondriacal delusions such as the belief in the presence of cancer, blocked bowels, and other abnormalities. In the case of schizophrenia, the complaint of pain may point to the presence of somatic delusions such as the belief that a part of the body is being influenced and damaged by malign forces outside the patient. Generally, these pain complaints will subside, as part of the patient's overall response to treatment, although they may persist in an attenuated form over prolonged periods after the acute illness has resolved.

Neurotic AIB. The commonest forms of somatically focused neurotic abnormal illness behaviour are the hypochondriacal and conversion reactions.

Hypochondriacal reactions present as two patterns: phobic hypochondriasis and somatic hypochondriasis. In both cases, the patient reports being preoccupied with thoughts of illness. In the phobic type there are fears about the possibility of falling victim to specific illness, such as 'heart attacks', 'strokes', and cancer. There is also anxious concern over the significance of physical symptoms, but usually some degree of insight into the irrational nature of these fears is present. In certain patients there may be a reluctance to communicate these concerns for fear of having them confirmed.

Patients with somatic hypochondriasis show a preoccupation and concern with symptoms. They usually deny anxiety and depression. They may also deny concern over any specific illness, although if pressed, they may acknowledge that the possibility of a particular disease has occurred to them. In some ways, this group is equivalent to those diagnosed as

having 'primary hypochondriasis' (Pilowsky, 1970), and the phenomenology of their mental state suggests an overvalued idea or, perhaps more accurately, a morbid preoccupation. This ideation may be difficult to distinguish from a hypochondriacal delusion, especially where this represents a monosymptomatic hypochondriasis.

Conversion reactions may be distinguished phenomenologically from hypochondriacal reactions in that the patient denies any concern over, or preoccupation with, disease. The focus tends to be on the pain as such and the disability it causes. Anxiety and depression may be totally denied, or if acknowledged, attributed to the pain. The serene attitude described as *'la belle indifférence'* is not invariably present, but when it is, it can be seen to be a somewhat fragile and brittle state with other affects, such as anger and depression, not far beneath the surface. It can be appreciated, therefore, that pain can be presented to the clinician in much the same manner as a classical conversion symptom such as limb paralysis.

In some patients, while it is possible to diagnose 'abnormal illness behaviour' of the neurotic type, it may be extremely difficult to decide whether it is a conversion or a hypochondriacal reaction because there are features of both syndromes and, indeed, 'abnormal illness behaviour' may be a reasonable interim diagnosis, corresponding to Engel's 'pain-prone' patient (Engel, 1959).

Management

A prerequisite to the success of any clinical management goals, is the achievement of a treatment alliance between doctor and patient. This process involves arriving at reasonable agreement as to the nature of the illness, its origins and its proper management.

In the case of chronic pain, the psychiatrist is presented with a particularly difficult task from the outset, since the patient almost invariably regards his referral as evidence that his pain is not accepted as 'real' and that it is the psychiatrist's task to demonstrate that it is a figment of his imagination.

This attitude on the patient's part must be dealt with from the very outset and this can be done in two ways. The first is direct, and the second, indirect. The direct approach is to encourage the patient to ventilate his feelings over being referred to a psychiatrist by pointing out that many patients take this to mean that their reports of pain are not believed. It should be made clear that the patient's pain is accepted as a real experience, and that the psychiatrist's task is to try to understand the effect which the patient's life situation is having on his pain and his capacity to cope with it and, also, to elucidate the effect which the pain is having on his life. It should be emphasized to the patient that any situation which influences his capacity to cope with the pain must be delineated in the hope of possibly modifying it. It should also be made clear that complete removal of the pain is unlikely to be a realistic objective. Patients usually react to such a statement by emphasizing their wish to cope even in the presence of some degree of pain which they do indeed believe they will be able to tolerate.

The less direct approach to reassuring the patient that his pain is being taken seriously is to make efforts to ensure his physical comfort during the interview. In the case of back pain, for example, the patient should be asked if the chair offered is satisfactory and another obtained if possible. The patient should also be told not to hesitate to stand and move around if he needs to at any stage of the interview. While all these measures may seem obvious, it is an unfortunate fact that clinicians often make no reference to them, even when the patient is making very 'loud' non-verbal signals of physical distress.

Apart from these strategies relating to the interview itself, it is important to consider the context most likely to facilitate the effectiveness of the psychiatric contribution. In the case of chronic pain where neurotic abnormal illness behaviour is prominent, the psychiatrist will function best in the context of a multidisciplinary pain clinic (Pilowsky, 1976). Bonica (1974) has provided excellent descriptions of the working of such clinical facilities, and the importance of their role in the treatment of chronic pain cannot be overemphasized, since they are in a position to arrive at a comprehensive assessment of the pain, and to present the patient with a definitive statement.

Most patients with chronic pain can be managed as out-patients. The treatment programme will depend on the pathologies demonstrated, and may often be a mixture of ingredients, such as individual brief psychotherapy, conjoint marital therapy, antidepressants, biofeedback relaxation training, and physiotherapy. In the case of biofeedback-assisted relaxation the patient is helped to learn how to relax by providing him with information as to the degree of tension (activity) present in selected muscles. This data is obtained by electromyograph and can be presented to the patient through earphones in the form of a tone which changes in intensity according to the degree of muscle tension present. (Of course the information can also be presented visually.)

In-patients are admitted when invalidity is marked and analgesic intake is excessive. On the ward, the approach tends to be a combination of psychotherapy and behaviour modification (Fordyce, 1976). Pain charts are kept using visual analogue scales and exercise gradually increased to 'quota' and not to 'tolerance'. Thus the maximal physical effort possible is first established ('tolerance' level) and the patient is then required to achieve about half this amount of exertion ('quota'). The quota is then gradually increased. (The approach shares much with the technique of systematic desensitization.) Analgesics are given on a fixed time-contingent basis and gradually reduced. In most instances, this approach results in a rapid improvement in activity levels and a reduction of analgesic intake over a three-week period.

Prognosis

It is obviously difficult to make general statements about prognosis in such a heterogeneous collection of problems. Clinical impressions suggest that of the order of one-third of patients referred to a pain clinic report some degree of improvement (Hallet & Pilowsky, 1982). It is important to stress that in evaluating progress and the necessity for further treatment, the patient's capacity to cope and function in the broad sense must be appraised, in addition to the nature of the pain experience. Failure to do so may result in the continued application of therapeutic measures long after the patient has decided that the amount of pain is tolerable and the quality of life is acceptable.

Illustrative of the type of patient who may be seen for the treatment of chronic pain is the 48-year-old woman who was referred to the pain clinic with the complaint of pain in the back and neck which had been present for 5 years. Although it fluctuated in intensity, the pain was always present to some degree and she took analgesics irregularly to obtain relief, with little success. The pain had worsened in the past year.

The patient described an unsettled and unhappy childhood. Her parents divorced when she was 4 years old and she had always felt unwanted. At the age of 3 years she spent 8 months in hospital because of 'rheumatic fever'.

She was married, with 3 children. The older two had left home and the youngest daughter was planning to do so. In recent months the pain had been increasingly disabling, and she was no longer able to maintain the high standards of cleanliness and tidiness which she had always demanded of herself. Her husband was extremely supportive.

She was found to have no marked somatic abnormalities apart from degenerative vertebral changes consistent with her age. She was admitted to the psychiatric ward for observation and treatment. Her stay was short and she soon established a psychotherapeutic relationship in which she was able to ventilate her feelings of grief at the impending departure of her daughter. She was also treated with physiotherapy and graduated exercises to improve her mobility and muscle tone.

Three months later she reported that her pain was only slightly improved but she felt far better able to cope with it. She was more active and used fewer analgesics. She was discharged from the pain clinic to the care of her general practitioner on the understanding that she would contact the clinic if she felt she needed help in the future.

The management of this patient demonstrates the importance of a 'mixed' approach with the use of both somatic and psychotherapeutic modalities (Pilowsky & Bassett, 1982), as well as the usefulness of having the background support of a multidisciplinary pain clinic. Indeed, the possibility of success in the treatment of chronic pain is limited unless those involved have accumulated considerable experience and maintain a close working relationship with each other. At the very least, this approach should have the effect of sparing the patient any further operations or investigations which may not be strictly necessary.

Finally, the role of the family should not be overlooked. A range of interventions involving the family may be appropriate, and these should be considered in every instance. They may include conjoint marital therapy, advice on the response to illness behaviour, family therapy, or simply the provision of clear information as to the nature of the patient's illness and prognosis. (The reader is referred also to volume 2, chapter 7.)

8.3
Anorexia nervosa and bulimia nervosa
GERALD F. M. RUSSELL

Anorexia nervosa is one of the few psychiatric disorders which can readily be defined by clear-cut diagnostic criteria. In its classical form it develops most frequently in adolescent girls after puberty, when it is characterized by a severe and self-induced loss of weight, a cessation of menstruation and a specific psychological disturbance. Although the occurrence of the illness in boys is rarer, its general features in the male are very similar to those in the female. Bulimia nervosa is an eating disorder closely related to anorexia nervosa of which it is often a late and chronic form. In common with anorexia nervosa the bulimic patients are fearful of becoming fat. The other characteristic feature of bulimia nervosa is periodic overeating which the patient seeks to counteract with devices such as vomiting or purging. This account will be divided into two main sections – classical anorexia nervosa, including a note on the illness in the male, and bulimia nervosa.

Historical note
Morton is credited with the first convincing account in 1694 of self-induced starvation attributable to 'an ill and morbid state of the spirits'. It was William Gull, however, who in 1874 named the disorder 'anorexia nervosa', and concluded that 'the want of appetite is due to a morbid mental state' and that 'young women at the ages named are specially obnoxious to mental perversity'. Gull provided sound advice on treatment: 'the patients should be fed at

regular intervals, and surrounded by persons who would have more control over them, relations and friends being generally the worst attendants'. Lasègue in 1873 also drew attention to the disturbed family relationships of the patients afflicted with *'l'anorexie hystérique'*. Loudon (1980) has put forward the interesting idea that anorexia nervosa and chlorosis are two closely related conditions, each representing a psychological reaction to the turbulence of puberty and adolescence. He has suggested that the disappearance of chlorosis during the early years of this century has coincided with the emergence of anorexia nervosa.

Classical anorexia nervosa
Causes

The fundamental causes of anorexia nervosa are unknown, but there is growing evidence that a multiplicity of factors, interacting with each other in a complex manner, contribute to the genesis and perpetuation of the disorder. Many of the theories advanced are speculative, but will nevertheless be mentioned if they contain the seeds of useful ideas. These putative causes will be grouped under the headings of psychosocial and biological factors, but it would be a crude over-simplification to consider them as mutually exclusive.

Psychosocial factors. The incidence of anorexia nervosa in Britain is estimated as 0.6 to 1.6 per 100 000 of the whole population per year (Kendell *et al.*, 1973). This represents a rising incidence during recent years and confirms the earlier finding by Theander (1970) of a five-fold increase in Malmö, Sweden, from the 1930s to the 1950s. The illness may manifest itself with a much higher frequency in certain groups at special risk: 1 in 250 of schoolgirls in England aged 16 and over, rising to 1 per cent of girls in independent or boarding schools (Crisp *et al.*, 1976); 3.5 per cent of fashion students and 7.6 per cent of professional ballet students in Canada (Garner & Garfinkel, 1980). The highest incidence was found among groups of girls who felt under considerable pressure to achieve a slim body shape and succeed professionally. These observations support the view that culturally determined attitudes contribute to the origin of anorexia nervosa. The increased incidence of the illness may also reflect an aesthetic preference for thinness in western cultures. Anorexia nervosa is commoner among upper social classes, but the social class bias may be modest (Kendell *et al.*, 1973).

The role of social factors in influencing the incidence and distribution of anorexia nervosa provides strong evidence in support of psychological determinants. Clinical observations also permit the identification of precipitants of the illness, varying from one patient to another but having in common an experience of stress of particular significance for the individual. They include bereavements, broken families, physical illnesses, and demands for academic achievement. A more fundamental basis for the psychogenesis of anorexia nervosa has been postulated by a number of writers. One of the oldest psycho-dynamically-based theories is that anorexia nervosa is a defence against unconscious fears of pregnancy (Waller *et al.*, 1940). This view had been virtually discarded, but similar conflicts can sometimes be elicited in married patients with anorexia nervosa (see case history 2). Bruch (1974) has stressed features of individual psychopathology: a disturbance of body image and a faulty interpretation of bodily stimuli such as the signs of nutritional need. She has also described in patients a 'paralyzing sense of ineffectiveness' which she attributes to the parents' failure to encourage self-expression. The patient's lack of autonomy, and her feeling that she will never come up to her parents' high expectations, have led Bruch (1978) to describe her as 'the sparrow in the golden cage . . . who wants to fly around and take off on its own'. Minuchin and his colleagues (1975) have postulated that certain kinds of family situations are conducive to the development and maintenance of the eating disorder. The family members are locked in patterns of interaction in which the daughter's symptoms play a major part in avoiding conflict and maintaining family homeostasis. These theories have become the basis of various psychotherapeutic methods, but still require firmer supportive evidence. They are consistent with clinical observations of a lack of self-reliance in the patient or disturbed relationships within families, but it is often difficult to know whether these precede or follow the onset of the illness. Another theory bridging psychological and biological determinants of anorexia nervosa has been put forward by Crisp (1980). He proposes that the avoidance of carbohydrate foods and the resulting weight loss lead to an interference with the central nervous regulation of menstruation and hence to a form of regression into a simpler existence, avoiding the conflicts of growth, sexuality and personal independence. Thus, the avoidance of food is reinforced and perpetuated. This explanation cannot readily be applied to the very young girls in whom the illness commences before puberty.

Biological determinants. The most relevant are the genetic and neuroendocrine mechanisms.

Genetic aspects: Information on this subject is limited. There is a higher incidence of anorexia nervosa (6.6 per cent) among the sisters of patients (Theander, 1970). Concordance for the illness in identical twins is more frequent than discordance, but the number of twin pairs is still too small to permit reliable conclusions.

The hypothalamic disorder: It has long been recognized that neural regulatory mechanisms control eating behaviour, the onset of puberty, oestrus and menstrual function. The evidence is derived from experimental lesions in the hypothalamic centres of animals (Anand & Brobeck, 1951), and from chemical interference with neural pathways, especially those concerned with the release of the neuro-transmitter dopamine (Marshall, 1976). The approximate equivalence between the deficits in these experimental animals and the symptoms of anorexia nervosa has led to the hypothesis that the illness is in part due to a disorder of hypothalamic function (Russell, 1965, 1972). There is strong evidence for a hypothalamic disorder in anorexia nervosa, especially one involving the hypothalamic-anterior-pituitary-gonadal axis (see below). The point at issue, however, is whether this disturbance of endocrine function which underlies the amenorrhoea of anorexia nervosa is entirely secondary to the weight loss, or whether other factors, including psychological determinants, interact with the nutritional disorder in a manner not fully understood. It is unlikely that anorexia nervosa is generally caused by gross hypothalamic lesions although in one autopsy report of a patient who died from the illness a small astrocytoma was found on the inferior surface of the hypothalamus (Lewin *et al.*, 1972).

Psychogenesis and pathogenesis

There is often convincing evidence for the psychological origin of anorexia nervosa. The patients readily disclose that they do not eat normally because they fear becoming fat or losing control over eating, or they feel guilty after having eaten. Their worst fears appear to be confirmed by a misperception of the size of their body, whereby they do not see themselves as emaciated and may even consider themselves fat. Experimental observations have confirmed that

wasted patients, when asked to estimate their body size, see themselves as wider and fatter than they actually are (Slade & Russell, 1973; Crisp & Kalucy, 1974; Goldberg *et al.*, 1977). Yet this perceptual disturbance becomes diminished if the patient gains weight as a result of treatment. Food intake in anorexia nervosa is unduly dependent on the patient's awareness of her body size (Russell *et al.*, 1975). But this awareness is a distorted one with the patient seeing herself as unduly large so that it becomes understandable why she should seek to attain, by starvation, proportions which are more acceptable to her. In turn the starvation and weight loss worsen the patient's distorted awareness of herself. Here therefore is a self-perpetuating mechanism which explains at least the persistence of the illness.

The nutritional disorder is clearly secondary to the avoidance of food and may be aggravated by the metabolic sequelae of vomiting and purging. Nevertheless, the malnutrition itself causes tiredness, depression, and other psychological symptoms, and so contributes to the self-perpetuation of the illness.

Evidence of a disorder of hypothalamic function comes from clinical and experimental observations. Amenorrhoea is an early symptom at the onset of anorexia nervosa and in a minority of patients may even precede loss of weight (Kay & Leigh, 1954). That the cessation of menses is due to a specific disorder of the hypothalamic-pituitary-gonadal axis has been shown by studies conducted during treatment which leads to a correction of the malnutrition. At the stage when the patient is still undernourished, the urinary and blood levels of gonadotrophins and oestrogens are invariably found to be low or undetectable (Bell *et al.*, 1966; Crisp *et al.*, 1973). Even at this stage, however, it is possible to show that the anterior pituitary remains reponsive to the administration of synthetic gonadotrophin-releasing hormone (LHRH), which is followed by rises in the serum levels of luteinizing hormone (LH) and follicle-stimulating hormone (FSH), confirming that the site of the disorder is in the hypothalamus and not in the pituitary (Mortimer *et al.*, 1973). The loss of weight is certainly an important cause of the endocrine disorder, as shown by a gradual return of normal activity in a definite sequence after a return to normal weight. First there is a rise in serum levels of LH, FSH, and oestrogens. There follows a return of the capacity of the hypothalamus to respond to the negative-feedback effects of oestrogen. The final step is the return of the hypothalamic response to the positive-feedback effects of oestrogen which results in a peak surge of LH and a later resumption of cyclical menstruation and ovulation (Wakeling *et al.*, 1977). This final evidence of endocrine recovery may be delayed for several months, with amenorrhoea persisting in spite of weight gain. This evidence, together with the early onset of amenorrhoea occasionally antedating the loss of weight, indicates that non-nutritional factors contribute to the hypothalamic disorder. Their nature is uncertain but a more fundamental disorder of hypothalamic function or, more probably, the effects of the psychological disturbance itself should be considered (Russell, 1977).

The complex interactions between the psychological disorder, the endocrine disturbance and the malnutrition in anorexia nervosa are shown in figure 8.3.1. The thickness of the lines reflects the solidity of the evidence for each interaction. Best established is the fact that the mental disorder causes the reduced food intake and weight loss (a) which in turn interfere with the hypothalamic-pituitary-gonadal axis and cause amenorrhoea (b). It is also likely that malnutrition worsens the mental disorder (c). The adverse effects of the abnormal mental state on endocrine and menstrual function is shown by pathway (d). The original postulate that the food refusal of anorexia nervosa might in part reflect disordered hypothalamic control of food intake is represented by the dotted line (e). The weakest link in the chain (f) is that postulating that the patient's mental state may be influenced by a neuro-hypothalamic disorder so as to give rise to her abnormal attitudes to eating and body size. The diagram, although simplistic, serves to illustrate the important role of self-perpetuating disturbances in anorexia nervosa.

Clinical features

Anorexia nervosa usually occurs in girls within a few years of the menarche so that the commonest age of onset is between 14 and 17. Occasionally the onset is a later age in a woman who may have married and have children. Very occasionally the illness begins in late childhood before the menarche. The patient's previous personality may have been trouble-free. In some instances, however, there is a preceding history of food fads or evidence of maladjustment (for example, excessive tidiness, an inability to make friends).

The onset is insidious. The patient reduces her intake of foods such as bread, potatoes, pastries, and sugar. She takes more exercise and walks instead of using public transport. At first these changes of habit may be mistaken for healthy pursuits, as the girl explains persuasively that she is aiming to improve the appearance of her figure. She may add that someone at school has teased her about being fat even though her initial weight would probably be normal (50 to 60 kg). At this early stage the parents may notice nothing amiss, but within a few months their daughter's weight will have fallen to 45 kg and her menses have ceased. In a few patients, amenorrhoea may be the first symptom, preceding the loss of weight.

It is commonly noted that parents and other close relatives seldom react until weight loss has been considerable, and may wait as long as three to six months or until the weight is as low as 35 kg. They will then report a newly acquired restlessness, irritability, and preoccupation with schoolwork. The patient may still appear not to understand the concern of others. If she has a boy-friend she drifts away

Fig. 8.3.1. Interactions between the psychological disorder, the endocrine disturbances and the malnutrition of anorexia nervosa.

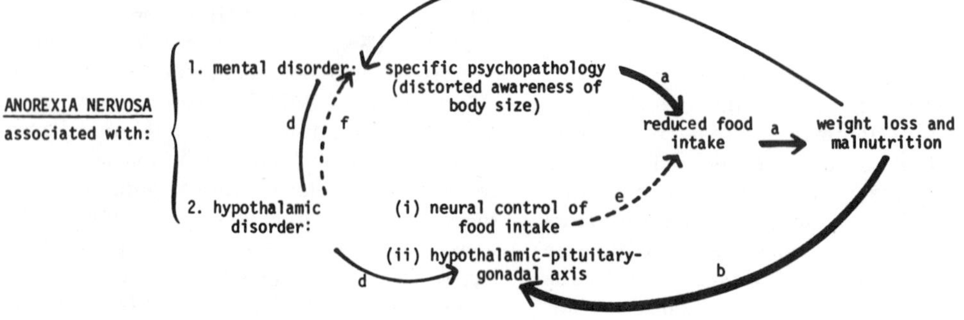

from him and withdraws from other social contacts. In a more advanced stage of undernutrition she will admit to symptoms of depression, insomnia, failure of concentration, and sensitivity to cold. It may only be at a late stage that she will reluctantly allow her parents to seek medical advice. A dietary history will reveal that she is subsisting on a diet of vegetables, fruit, and cheese. On some days she may ingest only black coffee. It is often necessary to ask searching questions to elicit that the onset of 'dieting' followed an emotional upset such as the stress of examinations, or an increase in tensions within the home threatening the stability of the family.

CASE HISTORY 1 (age 17: Figure 8.3.2)

When aged 14 the patient weighed 56 kg (8 stone 12 lb) and decided to diet because the other girls at school said they were concerned about their weight, and in any case the school dinners were 'awful'. Within six months her weight had dropped to 44 kg (6 stone 13 lb) and she had missed two menstrual periods. Her mother eventually took her to her general practitioner who for a while succeeded in persuading her to regain some weight, which she then kept at 48 kg. At the age of 17, however, while on holiday and before entering her final A level year at school, she lost weight again and her menses ceased. She applied for a university place but confined her enquiries to nearby colleges as she resolved not to leave home. In spite of out-patient supportive treatment she rapidly lost weight and in the course of a few weeks weighed only 36 kg, and was admitted to the Maudsley Hospital. She disclosed that she had begun 'dieting' at a time when there had been arguments between her parents and she had feared that they would separate. She was also worried about her mother's health.

When encouraged to accept treatment she declared that her desired weight was 41 kg (6½ stone) and that she would never return to her former weight of 56 kg. She feared that she might lose control over eating. She expressed concern about having no periods, but at the same time was worried lest they return.

The treatment resulted in a gain in weight from 36 to 52 kg in 50 days. After discharge from hospital she returned to school and later entered a teachers' training college accessible from her home. She continued with outpatient treatment but her weight slowly fell to 43.75 kg. Thereafter she gradually improved and recovered fully within two years.

In a patient who is older and married, sexual conflicts may be evident, or there may be an undeclared dread of pregnancy which is not communicated to the husband.

CASE HISTORY 2 (age 31)

This lady married at the age of 24. In the course of three years she twice became pregnant but had both pregnancies terminated on the grounds of financial difficulties. Soon after the second termination the marriage deteriorated and the couple separated for six months. The patient then returned to her husband and there followed what appeared to be a mutual agreement to begin a family– she stopped using contraceptives. Her weight had been stable at around 51 kg (8 stone), it increased to 54 kg (8½ stone) and she decided to follow a diet. This marked the onset of the anorexia nervosa at the age of 28. Within a few months her weight had fallen to 46 kg and her menses stopped. At first she thought she was pregnant. She sought medical advice, was told she was not pregnant, and there followed one year's treatment for her 'infertility', including a course of clomiphene. She subsequently attended out-patient psychotherapy sessions but lost more weight and defaulted from treatment. When referred to the Maudsley Hospital she weighed 37.5 kg. She and her husband at first denied marital problems, but they later confided sexual difficulties and indicated that the future of their marriage was uncertain. She was admitted for treatment, which resulted in a gain in weight to 50.4 kg. When it was suggested that perhaps she was not fully reconciled to the idea of pregnancy and motherhood, she reacted with apparent consternation, but in subsequent interviews she spontaneously returned to this theme. Her husband said he had been keen to have children but had not imposed his wishes on his wife. It was concluded that the onset of the illness was related to the marital conflicts, and the patient's rejection of pregnancy combined with her need to conceal her feelings from her husband and indeed herself.

Mental state. The most characteristic and diagnostic feature of the anorexic patient's mental state is her dread of becoming fat. Her concern may be expressed in terms of a sensitivity about a particular part of her body such as her stomach, thighs, hips, legs, breasts, or face. In addition, she will often look upon fatness in herself as a condition to be ashamed of, equating it with the expression of self-indulgence, a sign of social failure, or a state which merits condemnation by others. There is often an associated fear of losing control over eating, so that the pursuit of thinness may be a means of securing a 'margin of safety' against the risk of fatness. Not only does the avoidance of fatness become an overvalued idea, but the patient defines it in extremely harsh and precise terms. The interviewer will be able to elicit the weight which she considers 'right' for her. Inevitably, this idealized weight will be several kilos below any reasonable standard: even more significantly, it will be far below her own premorbid weight. The patient may deny that she looks thin and may even assert that her wasted body and limbs look fat to her. These clinical observations are paralleled with the misperception of body size already described on page 287.

It is also common for the patient to be anxious about her sense of individuality. This is shown by great indecision when faced with the inevitable steps marking gradual separation from the parental home. Thus, acquiring a boy-friend, taking a job, or leaving home are viewed as events of momentous importance over which she hesitates. Allied with this reluctance to leave home is an increase of emotional ties and dependence on a particular member of the family, usually the mother.

In spite of the patient's evident ill-health, she is likely to minimize her problems, deny her illness, and question the need for treatment. This resistance may diminish when she begins to suffer from bodily fatigue, insomnia or other distressing complaints. Among these, depressive symptoms are most frequent and severe. Obsessional thoughts and rituals may also occur and often centre around the food eaten and its preparation, when she keeps an exact count of the calories ingested.

Physical state and special investigations Body weight will be markedly low. Wasting is likely to be severe, resulting in gaunt facial features, stick-like limbs, a hollow belly, flat breasts, and buttocks. The hands and feet are blue and cold to the touch, and the patient may suffer from chilblains in winter. The skin is dry, and in older patients minor knocks to the extremities or limbs may result in patches of bruising resembling 'senile' purpura. There is an excess of downy hair (lanugo) over the cheeks, the nape of the neck, the forearms, and legs. The heart beats slowly (50 to 60 per minute) and the blood pressure is low (for

Fig. 8.3.2.(*a*) shows the 17-year-old patient described in the first case history before treatment and weighing 36 kg; (*b*) shows this patient weighing 52 kg after 50 days' treatment in hospital.

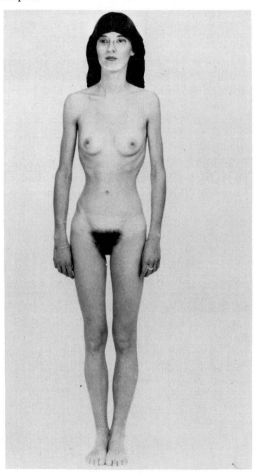
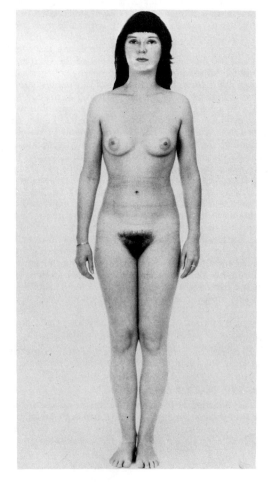

example, 90/60 mm Hg). There are no other signs of significant endocrine disorder although a slight reduction in thyroid activity, or an elevation in plasma growth hormone or cortisol may be found, probably the result of the deficient food intake or malnutrition. The initial haemoglobin level is likely to be normal. Serum electrolytes are normal unless the patient has repeatedly induced vomiting or purging when the potassium level may be low and the bicarbonate elevated.

Anorexia nervosa in the male

Although precise estimates of the incidence of the illness are not available, it is probably 10 or even 20 times less common in the male than in the female. There is a close similarity in the main features of the disorder between the sexes (Beumont *et al.*, 1972). The commonest time of onset in the male is soon after puberty. The young boy's morbid preoccupations with fatness are strikingly similar and he will also avoid carbohydrate-rich foods so as to lose weight. Even the endocrine disorder in the male parallels that in the female. The disturbance of the hypothalamic-pituitary-gonadal axis causes a decline and then a disappearance of the recently acquired sexual interest and potency. This is reflected by low blood and urinary levels of gonadotrophins and testosterone.

Diagnostic criteria of classical anorexia nervosa

The following three sets of clinical disturbances constitute essential diagnostic criteria of anorexia nervosa.

(1) *A considerable loss of weight which is self-induced.* The commonest method is the extreme avoidance of foods considered "fattening" (i.e. rich in carbohydrates), but weight loss may be aggravated by self-induced vomiting or purging, or by excessive exercise.

(2) *A specific psychopathology.* The patient holds the overvalued idea that fatness is a dreadful state. Her definition of fatness is extremely harsh and she will not let her weight rise above a very low threshold.

(3) *A specific endocrine disorder.* This varies according to sex. In the female: amenorrhoea occurs at an early stage of the illness. In the male: sexual interest and potency are lost.

The occasional departures from these clinical features are readily explained. In the very young

patient the endocrine disorder expresses itself as a delay in puberty: primary amenorrhoea and failure to develop breasts in the female; arrest of secondary sex characteristics in the male. In the more mature female patient on a contraceptive pill, menstruation may continue, due to the replacement of deficient oestrogen and progesterone by the hormones contained in the contraceptive.

Treatment

The treatment of anorexia nervosa is of necessity empirical. It consists of a regime of general management divided into three overlapping stages, each with its principal therapeutic aim:

(1) to gain the patient's co-operation
(2) to induce a return to a normal weight
(3) to reduce the likelihood of relapses and a chronic course.

(1) *Securing the patient's co-operation.* Patients are often reluctant to seek medical help and are brought to their doctors by distraught relatives. They may not consider themselves ill and are most fearful that they will be made to gain weight by abandoning their 'diet' or entering hospital. They may resist psychiatric treatment from an exaggerated concern with the stigma of mental illness. Yet this is usually the most appropriate treatment and an admission to a psychiatric unit is often indicated. It is advisable to proceed one step at a time and first establish a relationship of trust with the patient. This may require two or three interviews devoted to an exploration of the most distressing antecedents and consequences of her illness. Sympathy should be expressed over her painful preoccupations with food and body weight, but without condoning her wish to remain thin at the cost of her health. She should gradually be persuaded that treatment will relieve symptoms of depression and insomnia, increase her chances of success with her studies or work, and improve her social relationships. It is also important to anticipate the emotional pressures that a young patient may exert on her parents, whereby she seeks to avoid treatment. She may, for example, threaten that she would never forgive them if they agreed to a hospital admission. Preliminary discussions with the patient should thus be followed with a joint interview including the parents. This combined approach usually leads to a consent to come into hospital.

Wasted patients sometimes present as emergencies when it may be tempting to abandon the usual methods of persuasion and opt for a compulsory admission. So long as body weight is not below 35 kg (in the case of females), it is best to persist with attempts to secure a voluntary admission. It may, however, be appropriate to resort to Section 26 of the Mental Health Act when life is endangered by the risks of suicide, severe inanition, or the metabolic complications of induced vomiting.

(2) *Restoration of a normal weight.* This will be discussed under the appropriate out-patient and in-patient settings.

Out-patient treatment: The first few out-patient interviews are occasionally so successful that the patient can be persuaded to increase her weight. Such satisfactory progress may be due to the patient dreading an admission to hospital even more than a gain in weight. She should then be set definite goals, and advised that an admission can only be avoided if she succeeds in returning to a normal weight. The clinician may adopt an expression of moderate pessimism and say that he does not expect his patient to overcome her resistance to weight gain. He adds that he is willing to wait two or three weeks in order to convince her that in spite of her good resolutions she will inevitably require treatment in hospital. In milder cases, this kind of challenge may succeed. In this event it is best to continue out-patient treatment and adopt the psychotherapeutic methods discussed on page 294.

In-patient treatment: This is discussed under four headings below.

(a) *Nursing care.* The sheet anchor of successful treatment is a well-trained nursing staff working as a team. The medical staff's role is subsidiary and consists of setting a high level of expectation in terms of restoring the patient's weight to a normal (or healthy) level. At the same time it is necessary to give the nursing staff full moral support and help them develop their confidence and skills. There is no profound theoretical basis for the nursing treatment. Groen and Feldman-Toledano (1966) have described a similar therapeutic approach as 'educational' and have postulated that success depends on the physician and nurse acting as 'substitute parents' to the patients whose family life may have been deprived of love. Other workers stress the virtues of applying the principles of behaviour therapy with a system of rewards and removal of privileges (Agras & Werne, 1977; Pertschuk, 1977). The treatment described in this account relies mainly on practical psychotherapeutic measures, with the nursing team establishing

a relationship of trust with the patient. The nurses need to become conversant with the clinical features and psychopathology of anorexia nervosa. The senior nurses are given details of the patient's case history so that they can understand her individual problems and needs. They express concern for her distress and sympathize with her preoccupation over the size and appearance of her body. They should be aware that the anorexic patient may resort to subterfuges to avoid food or exercise to excess. It is better, however, to stress the positive supportive aspects of the nurse's relationship with her patient rather than the undoubted need for careful supervision. If the management is structured to render it difficult for the patient to dispose of food, she will soon give up any attempt to do so with resulting feelings of relief.

A recommended way for the nurse to establish the required relationship and express concern for the patient's dread of fatness is to say that she will become responsible for judging how much food should be eaten: 'Leave these decisions to me. I shall choose the amount of food you require and I shall make sure you do not become fat.' The patient is encouraged to accept this arrangement on trust and not stipulate a limit to the optimum weight gain. If the patient insists on discussing her weight the nurse expresses regret that she should be worried about precise weights and interpret this as a sign of persisting illness. Care is taken not to bargain with the patient over any weight level which she may regard as desirable or 'ideal'. With weight gain she is likely to express distress at what she considers to be a big stomach, fat legs, or large breasts. Once again the nurse offers the most appropriate reassurance such as 'the weight does tend to go first to the stomach, but in time it will become generally distributed'. There is indeed some substance to this kind of reassurance, for abdominal distension diminishes in time. Moreover, one can be absolutely truthful in complimenting the patient on regaining her good looks once her gaunt emaciation has been corrected. She is encouraged to take a pride in her new appearance by the use of cosmetics and a visit to the hairdresser. When weight has returned to normal the nurse should anticipate another source of concern – the discovery that she can no longer get into her former clothes. The parents' help is obtained to enable the patient to spend generously on new clothes fitting her more shapely figure, and her older clothes are donated to Oxfam (a charity) as a symbolic gesture of the need to maintain a normal weight.

It has already been said that the degree of supervision necessary to discourage recourse to subterfuges need not be oppressive. It should be in keeping with a friendly and relaxed relationship between the nurse and her patients. This is best achieved by an early understanding that the patient will remain in the ward and will forgo outings and home visits for the whole period of weight gain. All meals are taken in the ward in the presence of one or more nurses, seated at table: they will distract the patient in a friendly way from anxieties that may reappear when she is confronted with large helpings of food. From the beginning of the treatment the patient learns that she is expected to consume all the food placed before her, and to return to her occupational therapy or leisure activities only after this has been achieved. On rare occasions the patient may be suspected of hiding food or purgatives, for example when her weight remains static or she unexpectedly develops diarrhoea. It may then be appropriate to search her locker and belongings, but there must be no hint of punitiveness. The nurse may say 'I know that you are basically an honest girl but your illness and your anxiety about your weight may lead you to deceptions which are not in your nature'. Following this explanation, the nurse carries out her search in the patient's presence. In the event of food or purgatives being uncovered the nurse remains sympathetic and proposes further discussions aimed at alleviating anxieties. In other ways there should be as few restrictions as possible. Full facilities for occupational therapy or study should be made available on the ward. Visiting is generally encouraged unless the patient's restlessness is such that visits by her parents rekindle her anxiety and ambivalence, and lead to appeals for her to be discharged from hospital. In these circumstances the parents may require reassurance that their daughter's resistance to gaining weight is likely to last only for a few days and that visits may be resumed thereafter.

(b) *Dietary treatment:* the patient's food requirements to restore her weight to normal are often underestimated. Metabolic studies have shown that for each kilo weight gain a surplus calorie balance of 7500 calories is needed (Russell & Mezey, 1962). It is prudent to provide a moderate calorie intake (1500 to 2000 calories daily) during the first seven to ten days in order to avoid the rare but dangerous complication of gastric dilation. Thereafter the patient is encouraged to consume about twice the food intake of an average adult (3000 to 5000 calories daily). No special diets are needed and care must be taken to include carbohydrate-containing foods. Concentrated foods may be used to achieve the high caloric

intake (for example, Complan, Metrecal, or Carnation breakfast food), adding them to water or preferably milk. There is no virtue in prescribing additional vitamins. The positive energy balance at this stage should amount to 1500 to 3000 calories daily, leading to a daily weight gain of 200 to 400 g.

(c) *Drug and other physical treatments:* There is usually little to be gained from the administration of drugs. An earlier practice of giving large doses of chlorpromazine to reduce the patient's resistance to eating can be dangerous in malnourished patients and should be abandoned. Smaller divided doses of chlorpromazine (not more than 300 mg daily) may sometimes facilitate the nursing treatment if the patient is very agitated. Anti-depressants are seldom beneficial: a relief of depressive symptoms usually occurs spontaneously within a few days or weeks of weight gain. Endocrine therapy has a limited place in the treatment of persistent amenorrhoea after the restoration of normal weight and will be discussed on page 295. There is no place for tube feeding. It is also doubtful whether even modified forms of leucotomy are ever justified, and the risk of suicide is greater after such procedures (Dally *et al.*, 1979).

(d) *Assessment of progress:* The most useful way to check the patient's progress is to weigh her daily. Weighing should be a set procedure before breakfast, after emptying the bladder and in standard clothing. Figure 8.3.3 shows a typical weight chart with the optimum weight gain of 200 to 400 g daily and a total weight gain of 16 kg in seven weeks. The photographs of this patient (described in case history 1) show her before and after treatment (Figure 8.3.2, p. 290). In most patients psychiatric symptoms diminish or disappear, eating becomes unconstrained and the preoccupation with body size and shape becomes reduced by the time they leave hospital. This paradoxical psychological improvement is partly due to the correction of malnutrition, and partly the result of encouraging the patient to accept a higher body weight – a form of 'exposure treatment' to her former body size and shape. The aim is to restore body weight to normal within six to eight weeks and to provide a further two weeks in hospital to allow the patient to test her own ability to maintain her weight on leave-days at home. During the last weeks of the in-patient stay psychotherapeutic support should be initiated, and this will become the mainstay of treatment after leaving hospital.

(3) *Prevention of relapses and chronicity.* Whereas the results of in-patient treatment are impressive in terms

of weight gain and psychological improvement, the subsequent course of the illness in an individual patient is almost unpredictable. It must be conceded that the efficacy of *long-term treatments* has not so far been established. Nevertheless the clinician will do his utmost to mobilize whatever resources are available in an attempt to improve the subsequent prognosis. In the event of relapses and the patient's weight again sinking to a precarious level, he will readmit her to hospital and repeat the previous course of treatment. Among the measures calculated to prevent relapses and chronicity, individual supportive psychotherapy and family therapy are the best tried.

(a) *Individual supportive psychotherapy:* The patient is treated as an out-patient, once every two weeks or more frequently. At its most basic level the

Fig. 8.3.3. Weight chart of patient 1 (shown in Figs. 8.3.2(a) and (b). This satisfactory weight gain was obtained during the course of in-patient treatment.

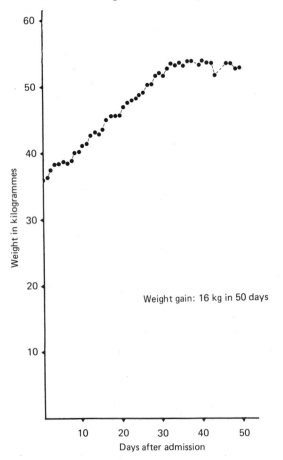

supportive treatment is directed at maintaining regular eating habits in a normal social context, and ensuring that weight remains at a normal level. Weight is recorded on every visit and the clinician warmly compliments the patient if she maintains a healthy weight or succeeds in improving a low weight. Loss of weight, on the other hand, elicits from him the expression of extreme concern for his patient's welfare. She is warned that further losses will lead to readmission to hospital, although it is better to keep up the struggle until body weight drops once again to a low level, rather than precipitate an admission in the hope of halting the downward trend. She is reminded that healthy nutrition promotes physical stamina and prevents unpleasant psychological symptoms. She is reassured that she looks attractive and feminine when heavier, but is chided for her skinniness when she loses weight.

The psychotherapy should be directed into spheres of the patient's life most likely to engender conflicts. In the case of younger patients these will include the problems of growing up, relationships within the family, and ambivalent attitudes towards achieving independence, themes well discussed by Bruch (1978). These conflicts are particularly evident in patients of obsessional temperament who become painfully indecisive about the future and the various options between a professional career on the one hand and marriage and domesticity on the other. Married patients may drift into intractable marital problems. A reluctance to embark on a pregnancy may lead to the perpetuation of the illness and its associated infertility, a device usually concealed from the husband and denied by the patient herself. In all these patients psychotherapeutic support has to be delicately balanced avoiding a threatening approach which might lead to the abandonment of treatment.

(b) *Family therapy:* It has already been shown that the clinican should take the patient's parents into his confidence when negotiating her admission to hospital. Further explanations and reassurance are needed throughout the treatment, especially at times when the patient shows distress and pleads with her parents to have the treatment interrupted. It is essential that all the staff involved in the patient's management should remain attuned to the distress experienced by the parents of an adolescent who is starving herself for reasons which are obscure to them. Their ordeal is often associated with feelings of guilt and anguish.

Whereas the behaviour of the parents can be

viewed to a large degree as an understandable reaction to their daughter's illness, there are occasions when their attitudes are much more complex. They may appear to collude with their daughter's desire to achieve a low weight and an idealized figure. They may resist medical advice on the grounds that psychiatric treatment would carry too great a stigma. In rare instances the parents may even allow their daughter to reach a state of inanition close to death before seeking help. There is evidence that neurotic symptoms in parents may increase as their anorexic daughter begins to respond to treatment (Crisp *et al.*, 1974). It is important to recognize these more abnormal reactions of parents and take them into account when planning the programme of management.

A more theoretical approach to family therapy has been advocated, based on an 'open systems' model which assumes that certain kinds of family situation are closely related to the development of symptoms (Liebman *et al.*, 1974; Minuchin *et al.*, 1975). The family are treated as a unit with the aim of promoting healthier patterns of interaction between its members, and reducing the patient's need to solve the family's problems by starving herself. One of the first sessions may consist of a 'family lunch' in which the therapist participates, thereby witnessing how the family members try to deal with the patient's most salient symptoms and intractable behaviour. Many family therapists apply their method throughout the course of treatment and claim good results in terms of weight gain as well as more fundamental changes of attitude. It would appear more appropriate, however, to reserve family therapy as a long-term treatment for the purpose of improving the outcome of the illness, once the weight loss has been corrected by the more predictable methods outlined on pages 292–293.

(c) *Treatment of persistent amenorrhoea:* Although endocrine therapy seldom has any effect on the course of anorexia nervosa, it has a useful role when amenorrhoea persists in spite of weight gain. Most patients who have succeeded in maintaining their weight will welcome the return of normal menstruation. In general, it is best to wait up to six months for a spontaneous resumption of the cycles. With longer delays, one or two courses of clomiphene (50 to 100 mg daily for 7 days) may be effective. An intravenous infusion of LHRH (synthetic hypothalamic gonadotrophin-releasing-hormone) is more reliable in inducing menstruation and ovulation, and can even be effective in underweight patients if high doses are given (Nillius & Wide, 1977). Patients of low weight fail to benefit generally from the induction of menstruation, so that in them this treatment is not indicated.

Prognosis

The course of anorexia nervosa is variable. Even when the eventual outcome is favourable, the illness lasts two or three years, during which much distress is experienced by the patient and her relatives. During the more acute stages cause for concern may arise that the malnutrition might cause death directly or through complications such as hypothermia, irreversible hypoglycaemia, or secondary infection. With modern treatment, however, such deaths are rare during the acute stage.

Long-term prognostic studies show that up to one-half of patients recover completely with a return to cyclical menstruation and normal fertility, and about one-quarter improve sufficiently to have only minor residual eating problems or menstrual irregularities (Morgan & Russell, 1975; Hsu *et al.*, 1979). In the remaining quarter or so of patients, however, the illness runs a chronic course with serious weight loss, amenorrhoea, and disabling psychological and social handicaps. An unknown proportion of patients who do not recover develop bulimia nervosa. In any of these patients running a chronic course, suicide is the main cause of death, and this may indeed also occur during the acute phase. The mortality rate has been estimated to be around 5 per cent in the longer follow-up studies. It is extremely difficult to forecast the outcome in any individual patient, although it has been shown that poor prognostic signs are a later age of onset (early twenties as opposed to early teens), an illness lasting longer than five years, the advent of bulimia, and a markedly disturbed pre-morbid personality. A very low weight during the course of the illness may also signify a worse prognosis. Even after a prolonged illness, surprisingly good results can still be obtained from careful and thorough treatment.

Bulimia nervosa

Bulimia nervosa is a syndrome which occurs in a minority of patients with anorexia nervosa who enter a chronic phase of the illness. Its main features are recurrent bouts of gross overeating, and a persistence or even an accentuation of the psychopathology characteristic of anorexia nervosa (Russell, 1979). A similar disorder occasionally arises in patients who have not previously experienced an episode of anorexia nervosa. Thus the bulimic syndrome may have a number of different origins. Its incidence is unknown but according to clinical impression it may have become commoner in recent years.

Psychopathology and pathogenesis

It is unknown why some patients with anorexia nervosa fail to recover fully and become bulimic when food avoidance is partly replaced by overeating. It may be postulated that when a suboptimal weight has been maintained for long by the patient, there occurs a physiological response which drives her to overeat. If the dread of fatness and the overvaluation of thinness persist, she will seek to avoid the fattening effects of the food ingested by inducing vomiting, purging, or resorting to some other device. This may be partly successful from her point of view, inasmuch as weight gain may be relatively small. The weight of bulimic patients will range from a very low level (overlapping with that of anorexic patients) to relatively normal or even elevated levels. Serious complications are likely to arise, however, from the loss of body fluids during vomiting or purging, causing a depletion of potassium and an alkalosis. They in turn may lead to urinary infections, impairment of renal function, epileptic seizures, and tetany.

Clinical features

Many patients who develop a bulimic disorder do so within one year of the onset of the original anorexic symptoms. In others the interval may be longer, up to several years. The patient reports that she is almost constantly preoccupied with distressing thoughts of food. For much of the time she succeeds in avoiding 'fattening' foods, but then succumbs to bouts of overeating. The quantities of food consumed at one sitting are enormous whether estimated by weight (for example, 7 lb), caloric content (15 000–20 000) or cost (for example, many pounds worth of cheap food). The foods eaten are usually those she endeavours to avoid at other times (for example, bread, biscuits, chocolate, pastries, or icecream). The eating bouts vary from once weekly to several times daily, and are usually terminated by the patient's chosen method of avoiding the fattening effects of the food. The commonest method is self-induced vomiting, achieved by deep insertion of the fingers inside the mouth and throat, or by use of an instrument such as a toothbrush. With repeated practice some patients no longer need to stimulate the pharynx mechanically and simply induce vomiting by bending forwards and exerting pressure on the abdomen. Purgative abuse is the second preferred method of preventing the absorption of food. This would appear less effective but patients may regard purging as 'turning food into water'. Senokot and Exlax are favourite laxatives, with 12 to 20 or even more tablets ingested daily. Other patients purge themselves once weekly with a single dose of 100 tablets which begins to take its devastating effect within three hours of ingestion. Most patients combine self-induced vomiting and purging. One unfortunate young woman, who acquired her eating disorder after already suffering from diabetes mellitus, discovered that she could avoid gaining weight after bulimic episodes simply by neglecting the required administration of insulin. Finally, a few bulimic patients may abuse diuretics or thyroid-containing preparations.

The bouts of overeating followed by vomiting and purging take place in secret, and may be so frequent as to fill much of the patient's day. Her personal and social relationships suffer and she becomes depressed. When the switch occurs from anorexia nervosa to bulimia nervosa there is some gain in weight, but the patient endeavours to keep her weight below a self-imposed threshold which is usually several kilos below her 'healthy weight', that is, the weight prevailing before the onset of her illness. Nevertheless if weight gain is sufficient, there may be a resumption of regular menstrual cycles. The patient may achieve a satisfactory sexual relationship. Fertility may also return.

CASE HISTORY 3 (age 20)

At the age of 14 this girl became self-conscious about her weight (57 kg; 9 stone) and 'went off' her food. Her weight fell to 44 kg and her menstruation ceased for the next two years. When aged 15 she began overeating: 'I suddenly went out of control. I felt that if I continued to eat I would explode.' Her weight climbed to 70 kg within a year and she resumed an even stricter diet (for example, one peach a day). At 17 she began to induce vomiting with a toothbrush pushed into the throat, and abused purgatives (3 to 4 Senokot daily). On one occasion she felt she could not bear making herself sick after having overeaten and took a mixture of 15 tablets of Valium and Paracetamol instead. She received psychiatric treatment and there followed an improvement when she completed a secretarial course, found work, and left home to live with her boyfriend. Leaving home had in some ways been a positive step because of tense relationships between the parents, and between the patient and her three sisters. The family history was complicated by the occurrence of depressive illnesses and anorexia nervosa in several of its members: the youngest sister also had anorexia nervosa. Within a year the patient relapsed. She would buy and eat sweets and cakes after work and make herself sick, choosing to do this at her parents' home rather than her flat, and repeating the sequence up to three times in an evening. She tended to overestimate her weight and declared that she had to keep it under 47 kg or she would feel unattractive and depressed. Treatment in hospital was aimed at getting her to accept a moderate weight gain with equanimity. Her weight rose to 52.5 kg and she remained symptom-free for three months after discharge from hospital. At Easter, her boy-friend gave her a chocolate egg, which precipitated a relapse of overeating, vomiting, and depression, with a return to her pre-treatment state.

Mental state. The bulimic patient's preoccupations closely resemble those of the anorexic patient, but they are likely to be even more intractable. She will declare that she thinks almost constantly about food. She denies that the overeating is a result of hunger but attributes it rather to a habit she cannot break. Her behaviour causes her great distress and shame. Depressive symptoms are commonly severe and include sadness, irritability, impaired concentration, and suicidal ideas. The bulimic patient sets herself a sharply defined weight threshold which she fears exceeding. The dread of fatness is an overvalued idea and she equates it with ugliness, greed and lack of femininity.

Physical state and special investigations. The patient's weight may not be very low but is often several kilos below its premorbid level. Occasionally there is bilateral swelling of the parotids and other salivary glands. Signs of latent tetany may be detected. Ulcers and calluses of the skin may appear over the fingers or the dorsum of the hand as a result of repeated friction against the upper incisors while inducing vomiting. Serum potassium may be low and serum bicarbonate elevated. Creatinine clearance may be reduced, indicating an impairment of renal function which is nevertheless reversible. The electroencephalogram may show small sharp waves or epileptiform discharges.

Diagnostic criteria of bulimia nervosa

(1) *Preoccupations with food, irresistible cravings for food and repeated episodes of overeating.*

(2) *Devices aimed at counteracting the "fattening" effects of food.* Among these the commonest are self-induced vomiting and purging, often combined. The patient may alternately starve herself and overeat. Abuse of diuretics and thyroid preparations are more indirect means of lowering weight.

(3) *A psychopathology resembling that of classical anorexia nervosa,* but even more entrenched. The patient has the overvalued idea that fatness is dreadful and she strives constantly to regulate her weight below a self-imposed threshold.

(4) *A previous overt or cryptic episode of anorexia nervosa.*

Treatment and prognosis

The treatment of bulimia nervosa presents many difficulties, especially when viewed in the context of the uncertain natural course of the illness. Follow-up studies have not been undertaken but there is an impression that the prognosis tends to be unfavourable with a relatively high risk of suicide. In contrast with anorexia nervosa it is rare for an impressive response to follow any of the available methods of treatment. This may reflect the fact that when bulimia nervosa occurs it is a late phase of the anorexic illness.

Treatment falls into three stages, each with a principal aim:
  (1) to enhance the patient's co-operation
  (2) to arrest habitual bulimia and vomiting or purging
  (3) to maintain improvement and encourage eventual recovery.

(1) *Securing the patient's co-operation.* The bulimic patient usually appears ready to seek treatment but this is often only on her own terms. She tends to reject sound advice to let her weight rise and may be reluctant to accept admission to hospital if this is necessary. She may even default from out-patient treatment. It is therefore essential to gain the patient's confidence during the first few interviews before tackling the basic problems.

(2) *Control of bulimia and self-induced vomiting/purging.* When overeating and vomiting (or purging) are frequent and habitual, and especially when physical complications arise, it is advisable to admit the patient to hospital. The best results are obtained in a psychiatric unit where nursing staff are trained to provide a supportive and supervised regime, based on a therapeutic relationship with the patient. Because overeating is the primary abnormal behaviour, treatment is directed at this symptom rather than the vomiting. Thus the patient is confined to the ward without access to food apart from the regular meals. She thus avoids the temptations of the hospital shop.

Visitors are requested not to bring any food. She is encouraged to take regular and full meals in company of other patients and vomiting is rapidly brought under control. If the serum potassium level is initially low, it rapidly returns to normal so that potassium supplements are unnecessary.

(3) *Attempts to induce more fundamental changes.* The bulimic patient is likely to resume her disordered eating habits soon after being discharged from hospital. One method of trying to prevent relapses is based on the theoretical view that overeating is a physiological response to the patient's prolonged maintenance of a sub-optimal weight. Most bulimic patients attempt to keep to a 'desired' weight, several kilos below their original or 'healthy' weight. By encouraging the patient to let her weight rise, it is postulated that the excessive drive to eat may be subdued. The nurse endeavours to persuade the patient that she should accept a higher weight, using the argument that her cravings for food are the result of her deprived body rebelling and demanding to be fed. With reassurance from the nurse she is gradually 'desensitized' to her dread of gaining a few pounds. When successful, this treatment may result in a diminished preoccupation with food and weight, and a loss of depressive symptoms, which may last for several months.

Other methods of preventing rapid relapses are psychotherapeutic and aim at inducing fundamental changes in the patient's life. Individual supportive psychotherapy or family therapy should be attempted, and the same principles apply here as in the treatment of anorexia nervosa.

A variety of behavioural methods of treatment are currently being investigated. They include increasing control over eating, the structured regulation of meals, exposure to foods otherwise avoided, and improving attitudes to body weight and shape (Fairburn, 1981). Antidepressants are indicated in patients with persistent depressive symptoms of at least moderate severity. These symptoms may be relieved but the eating disorder itself is seldom improved by simple drug treatment.

8.4
Obesity
GERALD F. M. RUSSELL

Definition

The definition of obesity is no simple matter, as even an attempt to describe physical adiposity must distinguish between normal and abnormal obesity. Garrow's (1974) definition of obesity, 'a condition caused by an excessive amount of adipose tissue' must be qualified by criteria for the adjective 'excessive'. For practical purposes it is useful to decide whether or not the patient's health would benefit from a reduction in weight and, in cases of cardiac or respiratory disease, an increase of only 10 per cent above the desirable weight might be unhealthy. In healthier subjects obesity would only be considered if there was an increase in body weight of at least 20 per cent, although the problem is complicated by the unreliability of weight as an index of obesity, even if allowance is made for height and body frame. Skinfold thickness measurements are sometimes used as an alternative. The commonest measure is that of 'relative weight' which is the observed weight expressed as a percentage of 'desirable weight' derived from tables such as those compiled by the Metropolitan Life Insurance Company. This method overestimates adiposity in muscular individuals and underestimates it in women over 60 years old (Garrow, 1974). The tables are based on actuarial findings that at all ages excessive weight increases mortality rates in proportion to the degree of obesity (Donald, 1973). The more severe degrees of obesity are easily recognizable, and Kekwick and Pawan (1956) define obese persons as those about whom no lay observer would have any doubt!

It is even more difficult to define the aspects of obesity relevant to psychiatry, and opinion ranges widely about psychological factors as causative. At one extreme, Kaplan and Kaplan (1957) state that

the overwhelming majority of causes of obesity are simply the result of overeating, which is caused largely by emotional disturbances that abnormally increase the intake of food.

At the other extreme, Silverstone (1973) concludes

psychiatric factors are unlikely to be of primary aetiological significance . . . although they may well play a secondary part.

There is greater agreement on the association of neurotic symptoms with obesity, the resistance to treatment of obese patients, and the psychological effects of weight loss in these patients, and it is clearly important to distinguish between these interactions. But obesity is not a homogeneous disorder and, in contrast with anorexia nervosa, need not invariably be accompanied by psychiatric disorder. Each obese patient must be studied individually to ascertain whether psychopathological features are present and, if so, whether their role is primary or secondary.

Incidence of obesity

The most precise studies have been carried out in the United States by the Metropolitan Life Insurance Company (1959). They found that about 30 per cent of men in their twenties and 63 per cent in their fifties weigh at least ten per cent more than the 'best' weight for their height. For women in their twenties, the corresponding figure is 23 per cent, rising to over 67 per cent, for women in their fifties. With a more stringent criterion for obesity (20 per cent or more above the 'best' weight) the incidence is one in twenty for males aged 20 or over and one in nine for females in the same age distribution.

Causes and classification of obesity

The control of energy balance

Obese subjects do not defy the law of conservation of energy: changes in the amount of adipose tissue in the body are the consequence of imbalances between total energy intake and output, and an excess intake over output will inevitably lead to increased adiposity. Garrow (1974) explains the control of energy balance as follows. Energy expenditure in an individual depends partly on innate metabolic activity and partly on the habitual level of physical activity. In early life, the food intake pattern is determined by the amount needed to satisfy hunger and allow for growth, but in adults the intake tends to follow this previously established pattern with short-term modifications caused by sensations of hunger and satiety. Garrow postulates a *non-physiological control* of long-term energy balance: 'when energy imbalance occurs during adult life it is corrected by more or less conscious effort at a stage when the change in body weight is no longer acceptable'.

A different view is expressed by Shapiro (1973) that each individual conserves a certain mass of adipose tissue but the form that the regulation of this process takes is unknown and has been questioned, because the 'set point' is hard to establish and shifts with time (Garrow, 1974). In favour of the 'set point' hypothesis are the findings of Miller and co-workers (1972), who showed that fat babies tend to become fat adults.

Classifications of obesity

The causes of obesity are diverse and will vary in importance according to which of the several types is being considered.

Bierman's (1979) simple classification recognizes two forms: lifelong, with onset in childhood, further increases during puberty and pregnancies, a failure to maintain any loss of weight, and a tendency to gross obesity; and adult-onset obesity, which reflects the much commoner weight gain associated with a more sedentary way of life and resultant reduction of energy expenditure in middle age.

The classification of Van Itallie and Campbell (1972) includes these as well as rarer forms: *'metabolic obesity'* includes endocrine disorders such as hypothyroidism, hypogonadism, and hyperadrenocorticism, and some forms of lipodystrophy. *'Constitutional obesity'* corresponds to lifelong obesity and allows for genetic mechanims or the role of fat cell hyperplasia postulated by Hirsch and Knittle (1970). *'Regulatory obesity'* rarely follows hypothalamic lesions in sites which Hetherington and Ranson (1940) demonstrated as controlling food intake in animals, but also includes the much commoner obesity of sedentary middle age. Under this heading should also be considered psychological and social influences leading to increased food intake. A specific cause can be identified in less than 1 per cent of obese subjects.

Genetic causes

Genetic factors may contribute to all forms of obesity, and Mayer (1965) has said that genetic factors are of paramount importance whatever the contribution of environmental influences. Reviewing several studies, Foch and McClearn (1980) found that one or both parents of obese patients were overweight in around two-thirds of cases. Withers (1964) found a closer correlation between the weights of adopted children with their natural parents than with the adoptive parents, and concluded that genetic factors were of more importance. This finding was supported by twin studies which show the weights of monozygotic twins to be closer than those of dizygotic twins, even when the twins had been brought up apart, although there were some exceptions (Newman et al., 1937; Shields, 1962). In any case, it should be recognized that the data from twin studies support an hereditary determination of weight but not necessarily of obesity.

Social factors

An association has been shown between socio-economic class and obesity, with, in western affluent society, lower class status being associated with a higher prevalence of obesity. For example, in the Midtown Manhattan study (Srole et al., 1962), the percentage of overweight women was 30 per cent in lower, 16 per cent in middle, and 5 per cent in higher social classes, whether determined by the subjects' socio-economic status or that of their parents. This suggests that the relationship is causal, not merely the result of obese subjects dropping down the social scale. Among men the same relationship holds, but to a lesser degree. Similarly, Silverstone and co-workers (1969) found twice the prevalence of obesity in London women of lower (IV and V), compared with higher (I and II), social class.

However, in less affluent or underdeveloped countries, as would be expected, higher weights result from the higher standard of living, as shown by studies of Indian and Latin American adults and among Navajo Indian children in the United States (Garb et al., 1975). Thus, the prevalence of obesity according to socio-economic status is represented by an inverted U-shaped curve, with a peak frequency among the poorer members of western urban society. The prevalence of obesity decreases from this peak because of diminished availability of food in underdeveloped countries. But in affluent societies obesity is controlled by the influence of fads and fashion (Stunkard, 1975). In an article 'Fat is a dirty word', Allon (1975) states the view of fatness as a sinful deviation by middle-class women in the United

States, and its contention by the National Association to Aid Fat Americans, Inc. which aims 'to challenge and change thin norms which discriminate against "fats" in clothing, in schools, and in jobs'.

Psychological disturbances associated with obesity

Personality development. Attempts have been made to ascertain the development and structure of the personality that may lead to obesity. Bruch and Touraine (1940) looked at the effect of the family, stressing parental disharmony. The mothers were generally domineering and rejecting and attempted to compensate for emotional insecurity by overprotection and excessive feeding. Food acquired exaggerated importance and stood for love, security, and satisfaction, and to withhold it might upset the precarious balance in relationships. This early study of family influences requires to be replicated using a more stringent methodology than clinical impressions. Nevertheless there is evidence that the effects of overfeeding in early life can be serious. Obesity persists into adult life in 80 per cent of obese children, and it is during the first year of life that overfeeding is most deleterious while adipose tissue can react by multiplication of adipose cells (Brook et al., 1972). It is this mechanism which Hirsch and Knittle (1970) suggested as leading to the perpetuation of obesity into adulthood.

Psychophysiological function. A peculiarity of psychophysiological function was investigated by Stunkard and Koch (1964), who observed an inability of obese women to associate reports of hunger with changes of gastric motility. They suggested that obese subjects are less responsive to the normal visceral signals of hunger, while Schachter, Goldman, and Gordon (1968) proposed in addition a heightened susceptibility to perceived cues such as the sight or smell of food, or the approach of mealtimes. They found that a speeded-up clock could deceive obese students into eating much more than normal students, and noted that overweight students were more likely to miss eating breakfast and occasional meals at times relatively devoid of food-related cues such as weekends. Related findings in obese subjects are their lack of distress after missing meals (Goldman et al., 1968) and resistance to the temptation of available food kept out of sight (Nisbett, 1968). The latter behaviour is similar to that in rats rendered obese by hypothalamic lesions: the rats appear unmotivated to overcome minor obstacles in the way of their food (Miller, 1955). On the other hand obese subjects are more likely to leave clean plates when supplied with large helpings of food. This suggests that there is a relative insensibility to cues of both food deprivation and satiety, which contributes to the inability to equate food intake with energy needs (Nisbett, 1968).

Obesity as a reaction to distressing events. Obese subjects may be unduly vulnerable to distressing events, such as the death of a close relative, accidents, or operations which may be followed by 'reactive obesity'. Weight gain may result from a married woman worrying over her straying husband, a mother awaiting the return home of her adolescent daughter, or a father adjusting to the birth of his child (Bruch, 1974). These reactive weight gains are more likely where there is a predisposition to obesity, as was shown in a group of women attempting to lose weight after major events in their lives: it seems that over-eating provides comfort when it is not possible to solve the problem (Lipinski, 1975). In seeking a connection between obesity and neurotic problems, the simplest hypothesis proposes that eating provides comfort in anxiety, depression, or loneliness. A more complex view is that the obese existence protects from demanding responsibilities and difficult relationships. In fact, surveys usually fail to show any difference in neurotic symptoms between obese and normal subjects, perhaps because the surveys conducted in hospital clinics or general practice include only a few markedly obese patients (for example, 45 per cent overweight or more) (McCance, 1961; Shipman & Plesset, 1963; Silverstone, 1973). In one London general practice survey (Crisp & McGuinness, 1976) low levels of anxiety were found in obese men and women and low levels of depression in obese men. In 'massive' obesity, profound psychiatric disturbances may be present, but are revealed only after weight loss, defence or denial mechanisms having previously concealed the disorder (Crisp & Stonehill, 1970).

Obesity as a cause of psychological disturbance. Psychological disturbances may be the consequence of obesity itself or its treatment. Disturbances are more common in patients whose obesity dates from childhood or adolescence, and often consist of impaired interpersonal relationships and heterosexual adjustment, often accompanied by what has been called a disturbance of body-image. This is a harsh disgust with one's appearance and a resulting lack of confidence in relationships (Mendelson, 1966). The actual appraisal of body-size is distorted, with obese persons usually exaggerating the degree to which they exceed normal size (Glucksman & Hirsch, 1973).

Especially if the decision to lose weight follows the breaking up of an important relationship, dieting may be followed by severe disturbances of mood, a period of elation being followed by anxiety and 'dieting depression' (Stunkard, 1957), and suicide may be a rare complication (Crisp & Stonehill, 1970). Psychiatrists see only a selected group of patients with relatively severe symptoms, and general surveys suggest that these are rare but that minor symptoms such as anxiety, restlessness, weakness, and irritability are much commoner (Stunkard, 1957).

In conclusion there is strong evidence that psychological disturbance forms an important part of the clinical picture in many obese patients, sometimes as a cause and sometimes as a consequence of the obesity.

Clinical features

It is not possible to generalize on the significance of psychological disturbances in obese patients: one patient may experience neurotic symptoms whereas another may be entirely free from them. It is therefore necessary in every obese patient to determine whether psychological disturbances are present and whether they play a primary or secondary role in the obesity. They are most likely to be detected in patients whose obesity first became manifest in childhood or early adolescence, and has reached considerable proportions

Pattern of eating

A stereotyped pattern of eating in an obese patient may indicate a neurotic disturbance. Food may be consumed at a specific time of day or night. At these times enormous quantities of high-calorie foods may be eaten, especially pies, biscuits, bread, cakes, chocolate, and ice cream. The episode of overeating is similar to that described in patients with bulimia nervosa (see page 296) but there is unlikely to be vomiting or purging. There may be a clear association with emotional upsets, especially domestic rows and interpersonal difficulties, or with loneliness and isolation. The patient will probably be ashamed of what he perceives to be a weakness, and may make food purchases from several different shops to avoid the embarrassment of the accumulation of food being noticed.

Sensitivity and self-criticism

The obese person's attitude to his large body is the aspect most likely to be disturbed in a specific way, especially if the obesity was of early onset and hence present during adolescence, a period of maximum vulnerability to the butts and sallies of others. The patient may be self-critical, see himself as monstrous or elephantine, disgusting to others, shunned by the opposite sex, and particularly ashamed of his reflection in the mirror. That there is some truth in these sentiments adds to the difficulties in relationships. Self-criticism may encompass other aspects such as a voracious appetite: a middle-aged woman compared herself to a garbage can – 'I eat everything in sight. It all goes down the hatch'. Some obese patients, however, especially if the disorder is of late onset, show little concern about their obvious size. Indeed, the indifference may be abnormal, suggesting that denial mechanisms are at play.

Disturbances of mood

Less specific and even more variable are minor affective symptoms. They may contribute directly to the obesity, causing the anxious or depressed patient to seek solace from eating. Or the affective symptoms may arise from a disordered personality which renders the patient prone to both neurotic symptoms and overeating. Or the symptoms may be a reaction to the patient's excessive size and his struggle to control overeating, or later in life may be a reaction to the physical complications of obesity. He may react adversely to criticism or ostracism, or to difficulties in personal relationships.

The affective symptoms may appear only after commencing a diet, begun in a phase of mild elation and at first resulting in a profound sense of achievement as weight is lost. The patient may proudly proclaim success at meetings of Weight Watchers, or in the media. However, the early elation may give way to feelings of depression or weakness or, more rarely, to severe depression and suicidal feelings, although it is commoner for the early resolve to be lost and replaced by despondency and a sense of failure. Patients who succeed in losing a considerable proportion of their excessive weight may appear to undergo a change of character, with irritability and dissatisfaction appearing for the first time. The newly expressed difficulties often concern personal, and especially marital, relationships.

The complexity of some of the abnormal psychological mechanisms is illustrated by the following patient.

CLINICAL EXAMPLE: (age 40)

The patient's obesity began at the age of 10 when she would regularly obtain three breakfasts by visiting relatives on her way to school. Her father was obese himself and tolerated this behaviour but her mother warned her that she would not find a husband if she became too fat. When she did marry at the age of 20, she escaped her mother's dietary checks and gained weight rapidly. 'I was an animal let loose.' She preferred bread, chocolates, biscuits, Swiss rolls, and ice cream, and would eagerly devour chunks of bread torn from the loaf and covered with butter. Overeating occurred in particular during the late afternoons before the family returned home. Periodically she would wake up during three or four successive nights with a craving for sweet foods in which she indulged. She was on good terms with her husband and two sons, but her increasing obesity earned the strong disapproval of her father-in-law who had, for several years, refused to speak to her. At 37 she sought surgical treatment for varicosities in the legs but to her distress this was refused on the grounds of her obesity. She sought treatment to help her lose weight and at first obtained behavioural treatment which involved keeping a diary and recording her daily weight and food intake. At first she lost weight, but recalled how later 'I got very crafty – I cheated with the bathroom scales – the doctor never weighed me – I felt too ashamed to tell him'. The psychiatrist then interrupted the treatment. She attended Weight Watchers with more success and lost 24 kg but this was soon regained. At 40 she again sought psychiatric treatment, now weighing 125 kg and worried about her arthritic knees and breathlessness. She was moderately depressed and mentioned how she avoided seeing her reflection which made her think 'My God, is that me?'. She accepted admission to hospital, where she became so enthusiastic as to refuse part of her meagre 400 kcal daily diet. In two months she lost 20 kg, thereafter attending first as a day-patient and later as a weekly out-patient. She continued to lose weight until she reached 75 kg (Fig. 8.4.1,), some four months later, but described herself as becoming more selfish – 'I answer back my husband and no longer pamper my 10-year-old son'. Despite out-patient care her weight increased to 85 kg during the next year and she then ceased attending. Two years later she consulted a physician, 'I live in hope that my fatness is from thyroid trouble', but subsequently sought another psychiatric consultation. She was sensitive about her weight which she estimated as 119 kg, refused to be weighed, and complained that a nurse had called her obese. She declined the offer of in-patient treatment, making the excuse that her family could not cope without her.

This patient illustrates how emotional factors become intertwined with the course of obesity which may have been largely constitutional in origin, in view of the childhood onset and positive family history. A psychiatric assessment must include the early history, family relationships, weight gain following important life-events and milestones, and any situation or mood state which favours excessive eating. Nevertheless, the emotional difficulties may remain hidden until a major reduction in weight brings them to light (Crisp & Stonehill, 1970).

The management of obesity

Assessment

As treatment is so difficult and the results so unpredictable, it is necessary to assess soberly the importance and possible benefits of weight reduction. In the presence of diabetes mellitus or congestive cardiac failure, this will reduce symptoms and incapacity, and in otherwise healthy obese subjects may prevent physical disease and increase longevity.

Insurance companies recognize the higher mortality rates in overweight subjects (Donald, 1973), and in the 18-year prospective Framingham Massachusetts Heart Disease and Epidemiology Study (Kannel & Gordon, 1975) obesity was associated with most of the major cardiovascular diseases and a doubled incidence of brain infarction and congestive failure. Several atherogenic metabolic changes were thought to be implicated, including impaired glucose tolerance, hyperlipidaemia, hypertension, and hyperuricaemia. As obesity is also thought to predispose to diabetes mellitus, gout, arthritis, and gall-bladder disease, its treatment assumes an important prophylactic value.

Fig. 8.4.1. Weight chart of a 40-year-old woman, showing a reduction of body weight from 120 to 75 kg in response to treatment.

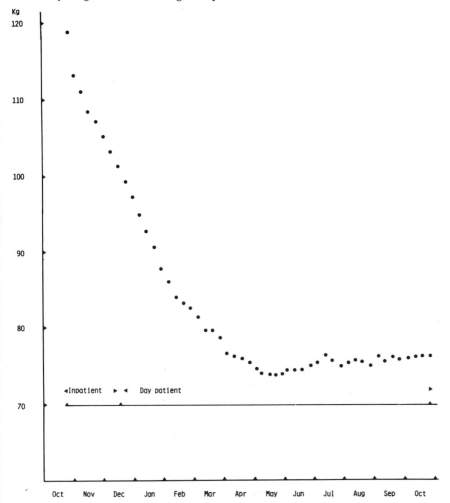

The patient's own attitudes to weight loss must be carefully considered. He may resist a dietary regime, rationalizing his obesity as 'glandular' or finding excuses for being unable to comply with advice. The patient described on p. 302 sabotaged her treatment. On the other hand a patient suffering bitterly from the social and sexual restrictions imposed by his obesity may have unrealistic hopes that all his problems, however personal, will be resolved by weight loss alone, and may press for drastic surgical procedures to achieve this. Thus a realistic assessment must include an estimation of the patient's strengths and weaknesses, of episodes of depression or neurotic symptoms following previous attempts at weight reduction, and of long-standing personality problems. Shipman and Plesset (1963) considered that the presence of such factors militated against therapeutic success, whereas Stunkard and McLaren-Hume (1959) found no relationship between anxiety and induced weight loss. Unfortunately it is in those patients with massive obesity and early onset that there is least doubt about the desirability of treatment, but also the greatest resistance to therapeutic measures.

In-patient and dietary treatment

The two basic principles in the treatment of obesity are to reduce weight to a level optimal for health, and to re-educate eating habits in order to stabilize weight at this new level. Weight loss is achieved by establishing a negative energy balance, for instance by increasing energy expenditure by an additional daily walk of 30 minutes, although it usually also requires a drastic reduction in food intake. Most severely obese patients, given this advice, fail to achieve a satisfactory weight loss, usally through a failure to adhere to the diet. Garrow (1974) observes that no patient is resistant to weight loss if complete control of the diet can be established, and predicts an average weight loss of 9.5 kg over 40 days on a daily diet of 550 kcal. This degree of control usually necessitates hospital admission, particularly for the severely obese housewife constantly tempted by available food in her kitchen. By removing her from this environment and with moderate nursing supervision, a predictable degree of weight loss can be achieved and the patient surprised by the absence of craving for food, but in addition psychotherapeutic support and an occupational therapy programme designed to strengthen resolve should be provided. The dietary restrictions should be strict and consis-

tent – daily intake of 400 to 600 kcal achieving the optimal reduction in weight. Harsher regimes or starvation should be avoided because of the risk of cardiac or renal failure in predisposed patients. The composition of the diet does not affect successful weight reduction (Russell, 1962), although it is customary to have a low carbohydrate content, which facilitates the inclusion of essential nutrients and is reported by patients as more satisfying. Such a regime is most commonly provided on medical units, but the extended duration of treatment may discourage physicians from using 'acute' beds and result in inadequate treatment. Although the necessary therapeutic and occupational skills are available, the patient may fear the stigma of admission to a psychiatric ward, despite the advantage of following such an admission by a period of day care.

Psychological treatments

Psychological support and encouragement are an integral part of the inpatient regime described above, and assume even greater importance if inpatient treatment is impossible; but the results of even a systematic application of alternative psychological treatments without admission have proved disappointing.

Psychotherapy. Psychotherapy with a psycho-dynamic orientation is often used as a 'non-specific' treatment for obesity in the United States (Stunkard, 1977), while in Britain the aim is less ambitious and consists of supporting and educating the obese patient. Obese patients tend to deny emotional problems, and it may only be after a substantial weight loss that the patient, discovering that an improved adjustment to life is not immediately achieved, becomes amenable to a more exploratory psychotherapy (Crisp & Stonehill, 1970). Advice and reassurance about the return of sexual feelings may be necessary. Hilde Bruch (1974) describes a more intensive psychotherapy of obese patients and stresses the effect of family relationships, particularly in children or adolescents, in perpetuating the disorder.

Behavioural treatment. The usual method is of behaviour modification by operant conditioning techniques: a detailed and precise record of eating patterns and associated mood states is compiled (Levitz & Stunkard, 1974), and several manoeuvres may then be employed to change the pattern: planning meals in advance or eating only at a specific time and place, removing superfluous food, altering the rate of eating itself or routinely leaving untouched food, instituting a reward system, and finding alternative ways to combat boredom, fatigue, or distress. Although such techniques may be effective in the short term, the benefits tend to be of limited duration (Stunkard, 1977), and they are not as predictably effective as in-patient treatment.

Self-help treatment: Weight Watchers. Numerous organizations exist in Britain and the United States which utilize group factors such as mutual encouragement to aid weight loss (Weight Watchers, TOPS – Take Off Pounds Sensibly). The programme usually includes weighing, the announcement of weight losses (or gains), approbation or criticism, and discussion of nutritional or weight-related subjects. There is a regular fee, and may be a fine for weight gains. The effectiveness of such groups is limited – defaulting is common and the average weight loss small (Stunkard, 1977).

Drug treatments

The clinical value of appetite suppressants is low, with generally only a disappointing induced loss of weight, and considerable dangers in their use. Munro (1979) counsels against their use where there is a previous history of psychiatric disorder or drug abuse. There are two types of drug:

(1) *Amphetamine and amphetamine-like drugs.* These cause a general stimulation of the central nervous system as well as acting on hypothalamic feeding centres, by stimulating amine receptors directly or by releasing catecholamines from nerve endings. Diethylpropion (Tenuate, Apisate) (given as a 25 mg tablet three times daily one hour before meals or as 75 mg once daily in a sustained release form) and phentermine (Duromine) cause less central nervous stimulation and lessen the high risk of addiction with amphetamine itself, a risk which can be further reduced by the equally effective intermittent use of diethylpropion (4 weeks on, 4 weeks off).

(2) *Fenfluramine (Ponderax).* This (in a dose of 40 to 120 mg daily) causes no central stimulation and probably acts by releasing 5-hydroxytryptamine and blocking its uptake, but may cause nausea, diarrhoea, drowsiness, and depression; abrupt withdrawal increases the risk of depression and it cannot be used intermittently.

Surgical measures

Splinting the teeth so as to restrict the patient to a fluid diet is a drastic measure which does nothing to re-educate the patient's eating habits; removal of the splints is likely to be followed by further weight gain and the method is not recommended.

Of the intestinal bypass operations which have become more popular recently, the jejuno-ileal bypass has been most extensively performed, the first 14 or 15 inches of the jejunum being connected to the terminal ileum, 4 or 5 inches from the ileocaecal valve. This decreases caloric intake by reducing drastically the available absorptive surface of the small bowel. A marked and sustained loss of weight usually occurs, partly because of malabsorption but also because food intake is generally reduced, particularly in the early post-operative months (Mills & Stunkard, 1976; Pilkington *et al.*, 1976; Robinson *et al.*, 1979). It is surprising that few of these patients, most of whom are massively obese and show neurotic disability, show psychosocial problems after the procedure (Crisp *et al.*, 1977). The operation carries a significant mortality, however, and a minority of patients continue to be at serious risk from late physical complications including liver failure, while many experience persistent diarrhoea. It is too early to reach a judgment about the surgical treatment of obesity, but caution is essential with emotionally disturbed or isolated patients, who may seek eagerly for an easy solution to their difficulties. Before any heroic operation, the patient should be persuaded to try at least one admission to hospital for a prolonged period of determined conservative treatment.

Prognosis

It is all too easy to confirm the obese patient's conviction of hopelessness and to abandon the therapeutic struggle by adopting a gloomy outlook. The much quoted review of Stunkard and McLaren-Hume (1959) indicated poor short-term responses to treatment and even poorer long-term prospects of maintaining weight loss, but the patients received comparatively perfunctory treatment, attending a 'nutrition clinic', being offered a diet sheet and asked to return at intervals of 2 to 6 weeks. Garrow (1974) has questioned the pessimistic outlook and data of these authors. Moreover, an individual prognosis is hard to determine in a disorder of such varying severity and intractability, and the reported studies fail to allow for complex factors of selection and bias in the sample studied. There is agreement that massive obesity of early onset usually carries a worse prognosis, but the advent of physical complications such as arthritis or heart failure may finally motivate such patients to reduce weight. An important if obvious lesson which emerges is that an attentive approach to patient care, including treatment in an authoritarian setting, is likely to succeed where previous casual attempts have failed.

Acknowledgement. I am grateful to Dr David Hirst for considerable help with the text.

8.5
Premenstrual syndrome
ANTHONY CLARE

Definition and prevalence

Ever since the first systematic description of cyclically occurring physical and psychological symptoms and changes in behaviour during the week or so preceding the onset of the menstrual period (Frank, 1931), the reported prevalence of the condition has shown remarkable variation. (Table 8.5.1). A major explanation for such variation is the lack of agreement concerning the precise definition of the premenstrual syndrome. Virtually any symptom which appears after ovulation, worsens right up to menstruation and is relieved or disappears with the onset of the menstrual period, may qualify as a premenstrual symptom. However, not every symptom eases or disappears with menstruation. Indeed, some persist over several menstrual days with the result that the term 'paramenstrual' has been coined to describe symptoms which occur during the days immediately preceding the period *and* during the period itself (Dalton, 1969). A further problem is posed by those women who do have symptoms at other times during the menstrual cycle but who experience an exacerbation of these same symptoms during the premenstrual phase. However, a useful and common definition of the premenstrual syndrome is the recurrence of symptoms on or after ovulation, increasing during the premenstruum and subsiding during menstruation, with complete absence of such symptoms from the end of menstruation to ovulation.

While a bewildering array of symptoms and behaviours have been associated with the premenstruum (Moos, 1969), there are a number of classical symptoms which commonly occur around this time. Common *physical* symptoms include painful or tender breasts, subjective feelings of swelling or bloatedness (which may be accompanied by weight gain), backache, headache, skin eruptions, and premenstrual stomach cramps. Common *psychological* symptoms include tension, irritability, depression, tiredness, sleep disturbance, mood swings, forgetfulness, and feelings of loneliness. A significant relationship between the premenstrual phase of the cycle and a variety of specific and defined behaviours has been reported in a number of studies. Correlations have been demonstrated between the menstrual or premenstrual phase and aggression (MacKinnon & MacKinnon, 1956; Ellis & Austin, 1971), the commission of violent crimes (d'Orbán & Dalton, 1980; Dalton, 1961, 1980), suicide and attempted suicide (MacKinnon *et al.*, 1959; Tonks *et al.*, 1968), the illness behaviour of mothers with young children (Dalton, 1966, 1970; Tuch, 1975), road and industrial accidents (Dalton, 1960; ROSPA, 1977) impairment of sporting performance (Williams & Sperryn, 1976; Zaharieva, 1965; Wearing *et al.*, 1972), alterations in sexual interest and behaviour (Udry & Morris, 1968; Kopell *et al.*, 1969), and impaired performance on psychological tests and scholastic examinations (Dalton, 1968). However, few of the studies in this area are without serious flaws and a number of critics have cautioned against too ready an acceptance of such links and premature assumption of causal connections. (Birtchnell & Floyd, 1974; Parlee, 1973).

Psychiatric ill-health and the premenstrual syndrome

Given that several of the symptoms commonly associated with the premenstrual phase are psychological in nature, it is understandable that an association has been claimed claimed between psychiatric ill-health and premenstrual complaint. There is an array of studies supporting the view that in many women recurrent mental conditions of a psychotic nature, whether affective, cognitive or mixed, flare up premenstrually more often than would be expected if time of recurrence were a chance phenomenon. (Smith, 1975). Individual case studies and groups of such patients have been described (Gregory, 1957; Sletton & Gershon, 1966; Altschule & Brem, 1963; Linghaerde & Bredland, 1954; Janowsky *et al.*, 1967). Dalton (1959) studied 276 mental hospital admissions and found distinct peaks at the premenstrual, menstrual, and ovulatory phases, while an analysis of 435 admissions to a Danish mental hospital (Kramp, 1968) found that 183 (42 per cent were immediately premenstrual. A connection between manic-depressive illness and premenstrual complaint has been suggested, the existence of bipolar symptoms in a number of patients with premenstrual mood change having been noted (McClure *et al.*, 1971). However, a careful study, comparing women with previously diagnosed affective illness with a healthy control group, found no difference with regard to somatic symptoms reported around menstruation, while so-called 'dysphoric' symptoms showed only a slight trend towards increased reporting by the affective group (Diamond *et al.*, 1976). There was a tendency for women to be hospitalized for depression during

Table 8.5.1. *Prevalence of premenstrual syndrome*

Authors	Nation	% with PMS	Study sample
Bickers & Woods (1951)	US	36	Factory workers
Rees (1953)	GB	20	'Normal' women
Lamb *et al.* (1953)	GB	73	Student nurses
Pennington (1957)	US	95	'Normal' women
Appleby (1960)	GB	29	General practice attenders
Kessel & Coppen (1963)	GB	80	Community survey
van Keep & Haspels (1979)	Holland	47	National probability sample
van Keep & Lehert (1981)	France	77	Community survey
Clare (1981)	GB	77	General practice attenders

the late premenstrual phase of the cycle. The authors of this study suggested that women predisposed to affective disorders, but not suffering from a current episode, experience menstruation in much the same way as healthy women. On the other hand, patients in the middle of an affective episode may experience a premenstrual exacerbation of their current symptoms so that hospital admission is often precipitated at that time. To date, this does appear to be the most acceptable explanation concerning the association between psychosis, particularly affective psychosis, and premenstrual symptomatology.

A number of studies (Coppen, 1965; Rees, 1953) suggested that premenstrual symptoms occur more frequently in neurotic than in healthy women but such studies were not random, employed variable definitions of premenstrual tension, and relied on questionnaire response, tests of personality, and/or daily self-report ratings, rather than on standardized diagnoses arrived at by experienced psychiatrists. However, a recent study of the psychological and social status of women attending general practitioners and the identification of premenstrual symptoms did involve the participation of a clinical psychiatrist using a standardized, semi-structured psychiatric inventory together with a modified version of the Moos Menstrual Distress Questionnaire, the best known schedule used in the identification of premenstrual complainers (Clare, 1977; Moos et al., 1969). This study did find a statistically significant and positive association between premenstrual complaint and psychiatric morbidity. The direction of the association merits comment in that whereas psychiatrically healthy women had an even chance of complaining of at least one of the 34 symptoms and behaviours on the modified Moos Menstrual Distress Questionnaire, nearly 90 per cent of the psychiatrically-ill women complained of one or more such symptoms (Clare, 1981).

Several explanations have been advanced for the relationship between psychiatric ill-health and premenstrual complaint. The simplest suggests that the premenstrual disturbance causes the psychiatric ill-health. However, Clare's general practice study found little convincing evidence to support such a view in other than a small proportion of psychiatrically ill complainers. Alternatively, psychiatric ill-health may serve to 'sensitize' women to premenstrual fluctuations which might otherwise be tolerated or even ignored. In support of such a suggestion is the finding in a number of studies to the effect that the great majority of women do notice some alterations in physical and psychological functioning premenstrually (Clare, 1981; van Keep & Lehert, 1981), together with the clinical impression that many women under psychological stress for other reasons regard these ubiquitous alterations as 'the last straw'. Then again, psychiatric ill-health and social stress may actually aggravate and exacerbate normal premenstrual variations in mood and behaviour. To date, unequivocal evidence in favour of any one of these explanations is lacking but greater attention to distinguishing between psychiatrically ill women and those complaining of relatively 'pure' premenstrual complaint (Steiner et al., 1980) may help clarify the picture.

Aetiology and treatment

One of the earliest causal theories postulated an imbalance in the premenstrual phase between the ovarian steroids, oestrogen, and progesterone. Dalton has been the most consistent and vigorous of those who argue that the underlying factor in the syndrome is a relative deficiency of progesterone (Dalton, 1977). Several studies have reported low levels of progesterone in the premenstrual phase (Backstrom & Carstensen, 1974; Munday, 1977) but the findings are not consistent. Nevertheless, the administration of progesterone to premenstrual sufferers is enthusiastically endorsed (Dalton, 1977; Lever et al., 1979). Because it is reportedly inactive if administered by mouth, progesterone is usually given in the form of rectal or vaginal suppositories, 200 mg in strength, and on a daily basis of 1–2 suppositories during the 7–14 days of the premenstrual phase. Dalton also administers progesterone by injection in doses ranging between 50 and 100 mg daily and claims that 90 per cent of her patients improve (Dalton, 1981).

However, many women dislike taking medicine by suppository or pessary and find the prospect of daily injections of a hormone daunting. A number of synthetic progestogens are available which can be taken by mouth and which are reported to be quite effective. The most notable of such progestogens is *dydrogesterone*. The symptoms which are reported to show particular benefit are those which also appear responsive to progesterone and include feelings of swelling and bloatedness, depression, tension, and irritability. Dydrogesterone is normally given in a daily dose of 10–20 mg during the premenstrual phase.

A third hormonal approach to the problem involves the administration of an oral contraceptive and a considerable literature now exists testifying to the efficacy of such a therapeutic approach (Grant & Mears, 1967; Goldzieher *et al.*, 1971; Herzberg & Coppen, 1970). A number of studies (Kutner & Brown, 1972; RCGP, 1974) have shown that women taking oral contraceptives report fewer premenstrual symptoms than do non-takers. However, surveys of users and non-users of the pill may reveal a misleadingly favourable picture of therapeutic efficacy as a consequence of the tendency of patients who tolerate oral contraceptives badly or whose premenstrual symptoms are exacerbated by it to discontinue its use and turn to other methods of contraception. Nevertheless, the administration of an oral contraceptive to a patient with premenstrual symptoms is worth trying with one of the following results to be expected: (a) relief of symptoms; (b) continuation of symptoms but limited to one or two days premenstrually; (3) intolerance of the oral contraceptive (for example, depressive side-effects); (d) no change. Suitable oral contraceptives include low-dose combination preparations such as Microgynon–30, Minilyn or Loestrin 20 or a progestogen-only compound such as Micronor or Noriday.

More recently it has been suggested that raised prolactin levels could account for some premenstrual complaints (Horrobin, 1973; Carroll & Steiner, 1978) and the prolactin-suppressant drug, bromocriptine, 2.5 mg once or twice daily, has been recommended (Benedek-Jaszmann & Hearn-Sturtevant, 1976). However, apart from relieving disabling premenstrual breast tenderness, bromocriptine has not been found particularly helpful and its use is somewhat limited by the unpleasant side-effects associated with higher dosage.

Energetic research efforts have failed to reveal a consistent relationship between fluid retention and premenstrual complaints (Bruce & Russell, 1962; Golub *et al.*, 1965; Reeves *et al.*, 1971). Yet, diuretics are still commonly used to relieve symptoms and a number of uncontrolled studies support the use of ammonium nitrate and chlorothiazide (Stieglitz & Kimble, 1949; Appleby, 1960). However, double-blind trials of potassium chloride (Reeves *et al.*, 1971) and chlorthalidone (Mattsson & von Schoultz, 1974) failed to demonstrate their superiority over placebo. More recently, a causal role in the appearance of premenstrual symptoms has been suggested for aldosterone, and the aldosterone antagonist, spironolac-

tone, has been reported to be a significantly better than placebo in relieving symptoms associated with premenstrual weight gain and psychological symptoms (O'Brien *et al.*, 1979).

High levels of plasma monoamine oxidase (MAO) activity have been demonstrated in some premenstrual women (Klaiber *et al.*, 1971). It has also been noted that oral contraceptives with high progestogen content induce major elevations in endometrial activity of MAO, whereas the more oestrogenic preparations do not (Grant & Pryse-Davies, 1968). This has led to speculation that progestogenic stimulation causes generalized changes in MAO activity which could be a factor in the occurrence of depression and loss of libido in susceptible women. To date, however, no adequate studies of the use of psychoactive drugs, such as monoamine oxidase inhibitors, tranquillizers, and antidepressants, in the treatment of premenstrual symptoms have been reported. Good therapeutic results have been claimed with lithium (Sletton & Gershon, 1966) but two controlled trials (Singer *et al.*, 1974; Mattsson & von Schoultz, 1974) and one uncontrolled one (Steiner *et al.*, 1980) have failed to sustain this claim.

It has been suggested that the depressed affect which has been reported to accompany some oral contraceptive use might be related to a functional deficiency of pyridoxine and that a similar problem could be the basis for premenstrual dysphoria. Preliminary reports of the use of the vitamin in doses ranging from 50 mg to 150 mg daily suggest that it may be helpful in the treatment not merely of psychological symptoms but also of headache, swelling, and weight gain (Winston, 1973; Kerr, 1977; Day, 1979).

More recently, a reaction against what some see as a premature assumption that premenstrual complaints are primarily biological in origin has led some researchers to suggest that modification of a woman's attitude towards menstruation and the role of stress in the premenstrual phase might produce a more effective and lasting therapeutic response (Sommer, 1973; Parlee, 1974; Koeske & Koeske, 1975). Some workers (Rodin, 1976) argue that women who learn to expect alterations in their physical and psychological functioning in the premenstruum perform better than women who do not know about premenstrual tension and who, therefore, have nothing to which they can attribute the decrease in efficiency, the changes in mood, and the various physical experiences when they occur. However, others argue that encouraging women to attribute psychological and physical discomforts to speculative internal biological abnormalities may merely lead to further feelings of poor self-esteem and inferiority on the part of the afflicted woman and may reduce her ability and motivation to change undesirable factors operating in her environment (Valins & Nisbett, 1971). To date, however, no study of the therapeutic efficacy of providing information concerning the possible nature and extent of the premenstrual syndrome or of altering women's attitudes to premenstrual symptoms has been reported, while such studies of psychotherapy as have been reported (Rees, 1953; Fortin *et al.*, 1958) have been equivocal.

Given the paucity of evidence favouring any of the established treatments of premenstrual symptoms, therapeutic pessimism or even nihilism might seem indicated. Yet the high placebo response in this condition reported in a number of double-blind controlled trials (Clare, 1979) suggests that such pessimism is misplaced.

ILLUSTRATIVE CASE HISTORY

The patient was a 35-year-old married woman who presented with depression, irritability, mild headaches, and feeling bloated during the 10 days or so preceding her menstrual periods. Her husband confirmed the patient's account and attributed all manner of domestic and marital difficulties to his wife's 'hormonal problems'. A brief history revealed that the symptoms had become noticeable when the patient discontinued an oral contraceptive some three years earlier and tended to become worse when the patient felt particularly under stress. It was also noted that following the births of her two children, the patient had been briefly but clinically depressed. Before commencing treatment, the patient was encouraged to complete a daily symptom-rating diary (Taylor, 1979), examination of the completed version revealing definite premenstrual irritability and headaches, but depression, though worse premenstrually, was none the less present at other times during the menstrual cycle. The patient was started on pyridoxine 50 mg twice daily while further clarification of her depressive symptomatology was undertaken. A pathological early childhood dominated by a highly critical, sarcastic, and cold father emerged, as did the fact that the patient's husband regarded his wife as a neurotic and rather inept person with limited abilities and strengths. The patient made a little response to pyridoxine and progesterone suppositories were added. Considerable improvement occurred but the patient began to complain of break-through bleeding, nausea, and headaches which eased on discontinuation of the progesterone. The substitution of spironolactone 50 mg twice daily maintained the improvement in her premenstruum, while supportive guidance and reassurance in a series of short out-patient consultations, several of which also involved her husband, led to a gain in self-esteem and a more decisive and confident attitude towards her role as housewife and mother. Eventually, the patient took a part-time job as a secretary and 12 months after first attending began to phase out her drugs on the grounds that she could now cope with such premenstrual changes as she still experienced. Her husband's attitude was still largely critical but the patient coped much more effectively.

This case-history illustrates the importance of approaching the problem of premenstrual complaint on a broad front. Unravelling the relationship between premenstrual complaining and marital problems can be very difficult; in many cases, however, it is somewhat irrelevant, for effective treatment requires that both be tackled. It is not unusual to find a history of hormonal sensitivity as revealed by post-partum depression, and improvement (or deterioration) with oral contraceptive use. At the present time, the evidence in favour of the main physical treatments derived from proper double-blind, placebo controlled trials, suggests that none is unequivocally superior to placebo but the response rate is in excess of 75 per cent. A reasonable approach is to commence with pyridoxine, which is safe and well tolerated, to continue with a synthetic progestogen or natural progesterone if response to the vitamin is insufficient or disappointing and to switch to a psychotropic drug if it becomes clear that the psychological symptoms are less clearly premenstrually linked and more likely to be manifestations of an underlying depressive illness. If the premenstrual symptoms are predominantly related to suspected fluid retention (such as subjective feelings of bloatedness or even frank weight gain) a diuretic, preferably spironolactone, may be tried. In the event that premenstrual breast tenderness is severe it may be worth trying bromocriptine but it is as well to proceed cautiously with the dose for many afflicted women tolerate side-effects badly.

Finally, this is a condition in which the anecdotal reports of treatments which patients themselves have tried and found effective abound. Relaxation, avoidance of coffee during the premenstruum, acupuncture, massage and physical exercise have all been recommended as helpful (Lever *et al.*, 1979) and it is certainly a clinical impression that a positive therapeutic approach, based on reassurance, sympathy, and attention to psychological and social factors as well as physical symptoms, brings positive therapeutic rewards in the majority of cases.

8.6
Endocrine disorders

J. R. W. CHRISTIE BROWN

Reliable modern hormone assay techniques and advances in understanding of the endocrine system have given a new lease of life to investigations of the relationship between endocrine states and psychological ones. Earlier work was marred by the lack of such methods, by a lack of sophistication in unravelling complex relationships and by an undue reliance on unsupported speculation. Nevertheless, the same themes attract renewed interest now as they have for many years. These themes include the relationship between hormones and various aspects of personality development including intelligence, psychological gender, sexual orientation, and sexual activity; the relationship between hormone changes at epochs of life such as puberty, pregnancy, and the menopause, and also the changes of the menstrual cycle, and psychological changes; the significance of psychological changes in endocrine disease and finally the significance of hormonal changes in psychiatric illness. What has become clear is that few, if any, of these possible relationships are simple ones and recent research has often raised more questions than it has answered. A good example of these difficulties is given by the investigations of premenstrual tension, a syndrome which at first glance should provide a relatively simple example of psychological and endocrine relationships; as it has turned out, there are problems of epidemiology and case selection, as well as in trying to disentangle far from simple putative relationships between variable psychological

changes and changes in the levels of a number of hormones over different time scales (van Keep & Utian, 1981) (and see also chapter 8.5 of this volume).

Many of the matters raised in these introductory remarks will be covered in other sections of the *Handbook*. In this section two main issues will be considered. The first issue is the occurrence of neurotic symptoms in specific association with endocrine disorders, and it can be said at once that such symptoms do occur. The association of endocrine disorders and more severe psychiatric disturbances which can be characterized as functional and organic psychoses will not be dealt with here.

The neurotic symptoms which do occur in endocrine disorders do not do so singly but in groups or syndromes. Indeed, Bleuler (1967) has described an 'endocrine psychosyndrome' in which normal drives and motivations are impaired, which he claims to be a feature of a wide range of endocrine disorders, but this idea has not been widely accepted because the syndrome is so broadly described as to be hard to distinguish from simply feeling ill. In some cases the neurotic syndromes accompanying endocrine disorder are indistinguishable from such neuroses occurring as primary psychiatric illness and in the clinical setting the endocrine disorder is diagnosed by recognizing its own specific features; in other cases the neurotic syndrome has characteristic features that will suggest the endocrine diagnosis if the history is carefully taken.

Both from the clinical and academic points of view, a number of questions have to be asked about any association between an endocrine and a neurotic disorder. First, is the association coincidental? Secondly, are the neurotic symptoms provoked or are pre-existing ones exacerbated in a general way by the experience of having a physical illness, particularly if that illness has not been properly diagnosed? This point is perversely illustrated by the case of a 32-year-old philosopher who presented to a physician with neurotic depression and was incorrectly diagnosed as having Addison's disease: his subsequent reading of medical texts profoundly deepened his depression which was successfully treated by investigating his endocrine status and showing that he did not have Addison's disease. More commonly and more to the point one comes across patients in whom an endocrine diagnosis has been missed for a long time and who have therefore been subjected to much unnecessary distress. Finally, there is the question of whether the endocrine changes are a necessary cause of the neurotic symptoms, a question most often answered by observing what happens when the endocrine disorder is treated.

There remains one question, which is whether a neurotic disposition, neurotic symptoms, or life stresses play a part in causing endocrine disorder, and this is the second main issue to be considered here. This issue of 'psychogenesis' is clearly one of great interest but has deliberately been placed second because it largely remains in a methodological fog. The majority of the studies in this area have failed to overcome the difficulty of producing reliable assessment of pre-morbid disposition compared with properly selected controls or to show that stressful life events have occurred in excess of chance expectation and independently of the endocrine disorder being studied.

Four endocrine disorders, hyperthyroidism, Cushing's syndrome, hyperparathyroidism, and secondary amenorrhoea will now be discussed to illustrate and expand the general points that have been made.

Hyperthyroidism

There is no conclusive evidence as to whether emotional instability is a precursor of hyperthyroidism or whether the condition may be precipitated by stress. The only wise conclusion is that both factors may operate at least in some cases (Lishman, 1978).

Neurotic symptoms are, by contrast, found in most cases. Restlessness, anxiety, emotional lability, disturbed sleep, and impaired concentration are among the commonest presenting symptoms and it is well recognized that the condition may be incorrectly diagnosed as a simple anxiety state. Less often there may be depression and occasionally apathy. Careful investigation may show that there are minor cognitive deficits (Whybrow *et al.*, 1969). It seems, however, that a careful history will usually prevent mistakes being made. Apart from physical signs that may be present, the most useful discriminating symptoms are intolerance of heat and increased appetite despite weight loss. Indeed, clinical pathologists have complained that the clinical diagnosis of hyperthyroidism is made too readily and that a large number of unnecessary laboratory investigations are carried out (White & Walmsley, 1978), presumably because patients with simple anxiety neuroses are not examined thoroughly enough.

As far as the neurotic symptoms associated with hyperthyroidism are concerned, there is a close relationship between them and the metabolic state. Exacerbations of the hyperthyroidism make them worse and they clear up when it is effectively treated except in cases where the association is essentially coincidental.

Cushing's syndrome

The term Cushing's syndrome is here taken to cover cases in which excess cortisol is produced as a result of primary adrenal over-activity (tumours), or adrenal over-activity secondary to oversecretion of ACTH by the pituitary (sometimes due to adenoma), or from an ectopic site (non-pituitary tumours). It has been said that the onset of Cushing's syndrome may follow psychological stress but there is no convincing evidence on this point. It has long been claimed that there was a strong association between Cushing's syndrome and depression, which was found in up to 80 per cent of cases. The depression itself was reported as indistinguishable from primary depression and ranging from the relatively mild and neurotic presentation to the severe and psychotic. Some of the earlier work has been criticized because the cases were selected because of the association itself, but more recent studies of a series of consecutive cases of Cushing's syndrome not selected for psychiatric disturbance have confirmed the earlier work. Cohen (1980) in a series of 29 patients found a 'distinct affective disorder' in 86 per cent and that this association was strongest in cases of adrenal hyperplasia. Jeffcoate and co-workers (1979) in a series of 40 patients found depressive states in 55 per cent but discovered no particular association with one form of Cushing's syndrome. Both studies showed that the depression cleared when the endocrine disorder was treated, except in those few cases with a history of depression definitely antedating the Cushing's syndrome. Kelly and co-worker (1980) included a control group and a group of Cushing's patients in their study and again concluded that there was a specific association between the active endocrine disease and depression.

This association is of particular interest because there are endocrine changes in primary depressive states very similar to those found in Cushing's Syndrome. From the Cushing patients it can be argued that the depression is secondary to the endocrine changes: where the depressed patients are concerned it is as yet far from clear whether the endocrine changes are secondary to the depression.

Hyperparathyroidism

There is nothing to suggest that psychogenesis is important in this rare disorder, which will be considered simply because of its instructive association with neurotic symptomatology. It is also known to produce organic psychoses in more severely affected cases.

In primary hyperparathyroidism a secreting parathyroid adenoma causes raised serum calcium, lowered serum phosphate, hypercalciuria, and bone rarefaction. The direct physical symptoms and signs related to bone pain, renal stones, and abdominal disturbances often pass unrecognized as indicators of the disorder, and the very common symptoms of minor mood disturbance, apathy, fatigue, and impaired concentration may lead to a diagnosis of primary neurotic disturbance. It is a condition *par excellence* in which a failure to make the correct diagnosis subjects the patient to needless suffering and exacerbates any direct effect the metabolic changes may have on the psychological state.

Interesting changes follow parathyroidectomy, which causes a rapid fall in serum calcium initially to subnormal levels. It has been shown (Christie Brown, 1968) that at the time of this fall there is an increase in minor depressive symptoms and also a significant impairment on learning tests unlikely to have been caused by the mood disturbance. The cognitive impairment is not great enough to be picked up at an ordinary clinical interview, and it is quite possible that minor but significant degrees of intellectual impairment pass unrecognized in many endocrine and metabolic disorders.

Secondary amenorrhoea

There is a well known association between secondary amenorrhoea and psychiatric disorder, particularly with schizophrenia and anorexia nervosa. In the former case drug treatment may play some part, and in the latter amenorrhoea is a defining characteristic of the syndrome. In this section, however, only the concept of psychogenesis will be examined as secondary amenorrhoea provides the clearest example of an endocrine disturbance precipitated by an actually or potentially stressful life change.

Anecdotal literature, and life itself, abound with accounts best summed up in 1898 by Alexander Simpson who said that many cases of amenorrhoea were caused by 'a fright, a disappointment and a fit of passion'. More systematic studies have shown that transient amenorrhoea occurs in a proportion of women subjected to stress, the rates varying with the severity of the stress. Thus rates of 10–30 per cent have been reported in women taking up the religious life or joining the army (Drew & Stifel, 1968; Drillien, 1946). Christie Brown (1972) studied a group of 63 nurses entering their training and followed up for five months; 11 per cent missed one or more periods, and 61 per cent showed an increase in menstrual irregularity but none developed enduring secondary amenorrhoea. Those who showed any of these alterations in menstrual pattern were significantly heavier in relation to their height than those whose menstruation did not alter. It seems then to be clearly established that life change or stress can disturb menstruation but that the significance of this mechanism in amenorrhoea of six months duration is not so clear. The delineation of subtypes of secondary amenorrhoea, including those associated with pituitary micro-adenomata and hyperprolactinaemia/galactorrhoea has dampened enthusiasm for the relevance of life stresses. However, Christie Brown (1972) showed that independent life stresses were significantly more common just before the onset of the disorder in a group of patients with secondary amenorrhoea than in a control group. The importance of these mechanisms remains: unfortunately their identification has not led on to any treatment of established success based on psychological methods.

8.7

Skin disorders and dermatitis artefacta

GERALD F. M. RUSSELL

Views range widely regarding the role of emotional upheaval in diseases of the skin:

If they (emotional factors) are ignored the effective management of at least 40 per cent of the patients attending departments of dermatology is impossible. (Rook & Wilkinson, 1968)

Shuster (1981) speaks of

the psychosomatic myth:

. . . I would not expect treating the mind would improve the rash: and that is why we haven't seen improvement from years of mindbinding drugs and psychotherapy. We can now forget this treatment if we simply treat the skin effectively, the psychological cloud will lift as quickly as the tele-weatherman's plastic symbols.

Shuster's position is an extreme one, but he stresses that skin diseases, though they rarely kill, create much misery. He points out that facial acne in the young gives rise to a poor 'self-image'. Simple treatment of the skin alone with benzoyl peroxide gel improves the acne in over half the patients: at the same time 'self-image' is restored as measured by a form of repertory grid (Shuster, 1981). Skin lesions which are unsightly or disfiguring may be deleterious to the emotional development of a child at an early stage by influencing the attitude of his mother toward him (Rook & Wilkinson, 1968), later on by causing other children to shun him.

Disorders of the skin influenced by psychological factors

There is commendable hesitation on the part of experts in ascribing a 'psychogenesis' to skin diseases. This is the only position to take while we remain ignorant of the causes of many dermatoses, the mechanisms whereby emotional upheavals may influence the skin and the individual nature of a patient's vulnerability. Nor is it known whether there is an increased association between skin disease on the one hand, and mental illness, personality disorder, and preceding stressful life-events on the other. In his review of the relevant studies, Whitlock (1976) points out the lack of matched control groups and the overriding effects of patient self-selection.

In spite of these limitations a study by Kenyon (1962) gave an indication of certain psychological features of patients with skin disorders. In a psychiatric survey of a random sample of 100 out-patients attending a dermatological hospital, he detected 14 patients who merited a psychiatric diagnosis – a neurotic syndrome in 12 and endogenous depression in two. These 14 patients were identified by psychiatric interview following a screening procedure using the Maudsley Personality Inventory, patients with a high neuroticism score being selected for interview. Yet the group of 100 patients, taken as a whole, did not differ significantly from normal in their mean scores for neuroticism. About a quarter of the patients described a special stress during the six months prior to the onset of their dermatoses, but the significance of this finding is uncertain.

Classification according to 'psychogenesis'

Whitlock (1976) modifies a list put forward by Rook and Wilkinson (1968) in which the degree of the psychological contribution to the dermatoses is ranked in descending order of importance.

(1) *Skin disorders wholly attributable to the patient's psychological disturbance.* Under this heading come *dermatitis artefacta* and *trichotillomania* (hair-pulling tics). The perplexing problems raised by dermatitis artefacta will be discussed in the second half of this article.

In a different category are the patients described by Cotterill (1981) as examples of 'dermatological non-disease': they are preoccupied with skin complaints but, on examination, have little or no evidence of a skin disorder. The symptoms are most commonly referred to the face, scalp and perineum. There is frequently a disturbance of body image (*dysmorpho-phobia*) and a depressive illness may be present. *Delusions of parasitosis* may be a feature of mono-symptomatic hypochondriacal psychosis (see volume 3).

(2) *Dermatoses partly of other origin but aggravated by self-inflicted trauma.* These are *lichen simplex* (scratching), *acné excoriée* ('picking' of the lesions), and *acne necrotica* (possibly scratching).

(3) *Skin disorders frequently provoked or perpetuated by emotional factors or where tension or depression intensify itching and cause aggravation through scratching.* They are *anogenital pruritis* and *general pruritis*. *Hyperhidrosis* and *excessive blushing* commonly arise from emotional precipitants.

(a) Anogenital pruritis. Whitlock (1976) relates that at one time sexual conflict was deemed to play an important role in anogenital pruritis simply because of the emotional connotations of this area of the body. It was even considered that pruritis and scratching were a source of conscious sexual gratification. He points out, however, that a high proportion of patients had a family history of allergy, and had themselves suffered from eczema of other parts of the body. The perianal and genital skin is particularly liable to give rise to the sensations of itching, burning, and pain, which are likely to be aggravated by local vasodilatation and sweating. Emotional tension and fatigue accentuate and prolong itching. The itch – scratch cycle is set up with resulting thickening (lichenification) of the skin. Macalpine (1953) reported on a 40-year-old man suffering from pruritis ani who had scratched through seven pairs of trousers in two years. The disorder in most patients starts with a major or minor lesion of a localized kind giving rise to recurrent bouts of itching and scratching. Emotional disturbances can induce the physiological changes in the skin which precipitate and aggravate the itch – scratch sequence. Pruritis ani is commonly associated with sexual difficulties, constipation and abuse of laxatives. Macalpine views the disorder as a form of hypochondriasis.

(b) Generalized pruritis. Most writers take the view that psychogenic pruritis is uncommon. Nevertheless, many patients display increased tension, depression and insomnia, and the treatment of the psychological disorder may provide marked relief from the itching.

(4) *Dermatoses in which emotional predisposing, precipitating, or perpetuating factors are often implicated.* Authors differ as to which skin disorders come under this heading, though there is most agreement about *eczema* and *atopic dermatitis*. *Seborrhoeic dermatitis, urticaria*, and *pompholyx* may be included.

Atopic dermatitis is assumed to be of multiple aetiology with psychological factors ascribed a significant role. Other causal factors include an increased liability to form reagin antibodies and a greater susceptibility (genetically determined) to certain diseases such as asthma and hay fever. In addition to allergic factors, infection, climate, and other variables may contribute to the attacks of itching and inflammation of the skin. Among these, psychological influences may lead to vasomotor and sweat changes, and contribute to the allergic responses, thus augmenting the patient's innate tendency to itching, and eczema formation. In some patients the scratching may have the characteristics of a conditioned response to emotionally disturbing events. The itching which is of prime importance may be due to the liberation in the skin of hormonal substances known to cause this symptom, and which may well be initiated by emotional arousal (Whitlock, 1976).

(5) *Dermatoses in which emotional factors are only occasionally implicated.* This is a group of dermatoses in which emotional factors are generally exonerated from playing any role, but in the occasional patient they may be suspected of precipitating an attack or causing an exacerbation of the skin lesions. In this category are listed *psoriasis, lichen planus, alopecia areata, vitiligo, aphthosis* and *herpes simplex* (Rook & Wilkinson, 1968). Alopecia areata is the main disorder, in which its onset or extension is said occasionally to follow acute emotional stress (Ebling & Rook, 1968).

Treatment of skin disorders accompanied by psychological disturbance

The recognition that an individual patient's skin disorder is associated with an emotional disturbance should not detract from applying the standard methods of dermatological treatment, as in the example given by Shuster (1981), of young patients with acne treated with benzoyl peroxide gel, who consequently improve in their self-regard. When the psychiatrist collaborates with the dermatologist and aims at helping the patient to adjust to his life problems, Menninger's sound advice should be borne in mind:

The more or less homespun psychotherapy of the dermatologist is often more efficacious than the more scientifically ordered psychotherapy of the psychiatrist for the simple reason that the latter is apt to conceive of a more radical and revolutionary change in the patient's personality structure. (Menninger, 1947)

Especially in patients complaining of severe itching of the skin, symptomatic treatment should be attempted including the relief of insomnia with a safe hypnotic. In patients in whom there is an association between depression and pruritis, this symptom may be cleared with the appropriate treatment for depression (Edwards, 1954).

Dermatitis artefacta

Definition

Dermatitis artefacta is a skin disorder which the patient secretly inflicts on himself and for which he seeks medical attention. It differs from the excoriations of neurotic patients who scratch or pick their skin in order to relieve itching or inner tension, or to obtain gratification.

Aetiology

Dermatitis artefacta affects particularly young, unmarried women. It may occasionally occur in men whose motives are more transparently those of escaping from an unpleasant situation or securing financial compensation. More commonly, and especially in women, the motives are obscure. The associated personality disorder may escape detection because there is no overt behavioural disturbance; social adjustment at first sight is adequate, and the patient may appear courageous and long-suffering. The patient's reluctance to accept psychological investigation may conceal the severity of the personality disorder, which is most often of an immature or hysterical type. Because of this reluctance and massive denial on the part of the patient it is difficult to understand the motivation and the degree to which it is unconscious. But the self-injuries are repeated with such frequency and deception that their performance cannot easily be attributed to a state of dissociation such as occurs in hypnosis or an hysterical trance. Gillespie referred to the patient's adoption of the sick role:

> The patient . . . is committed to make his illness the main topic of his life: while the charitable assistance, whether in money or solicitous attention that he receives becomes his modus vivendi. (Gillespie, 1938)

Clinical Features

The diagnosis of dermatitis artefacta is made in the first instance by a physician, dermatologist, or surgeon, who recognizes from his experience that the skin lesions do not conform in their appearance to those which occur in natural skin diseases. This impression can be dissected into the discrete features of self-inflicted lesions as described by Stokes and Garner (1929). The lesions tend to be destructive – an ulcer, erosion, denudation, or gangrene. The last is particularly suspicious when confined to the skin without involving deep subcutaneous tissues. If the lesion is an ulcer, the remaining skin appears normal almost to the edge of the injured tissue. Individual lesions may be of unusual shape, square or triangular, and the lesions may be grouped in too regular a pattern – gridiron, spiral, or crisscross.

The formation of new crops of lesions after the patient has been left unobserved, or their first display in the morning, is suggestive. The diagnosis may unfortunately be delayed until several ineffectual surgical operations have been attempted. Prosser Thomas (1937) described a nursing student who began with gangrene of the left little finger and underwent 33 amputations aimed at arresting successive spread to the left hand and arm, until the arm was amputated up to the scapula.

It may be possible to prove that the patient is causing the injuries herself by securing a confession, or detecting her in the act. A search of her belongings after admission to hospital may reveal the method used. Acids, alkalis, and other chemicals may be applied to burn the skin; needles, scissors, and other mechanical means are less common; some patients use a hypodermic syringe to inject aspirin or faecal material under the skin.

Having established the self-inflicted nature of the skin injuries, exploration of the patient's psychiatric disorder and elucidation of her motivation remain daunting tasks. She will often object to seeing a psychiatrist, staunchly defending her position that she is physically ill. She may have strong allies among members of her family or in her general practitioner. If the patient allows a psychiatric examination, it may be possible to establish the presence of an hysterical personality disorder. What may have struck her relatives and doctors as remarkable stoicism in the face of suffering, becomes more clearly understood as 'belle indifférence'. There may have been previous episodes of aphonia, urinary retention, paralysis, or fainting attacks. Less often there is a history of earlier periods of depression. The diagnosis is compatible with a superior intelligence and high social achievement. The life situation contributing to the self-injuries varies from patient to patient. She may wish to win sympathy or compensation: there may be a disturbance within the family (death or desertion of a parent, or excessive responsibility in the home). Psychosexual development may remain immature. Often the underlying motivation is obscure and it is necessary to postulate unconscious factors (Brown, 1938).

ILLUSTRATIVE CASE HISTORY

This 46-year-old lady had been admitted to hospital for the sixth time in 12 years,. The skin of the whole of the dorsum of her left forearm was covered with raised crusted lesions exuding large amounts of pus (see Fig. 8.7.1). Her ring finger had been amputated 9 years previously. The patient said that the trouble began when she knocked a wart on her ring finger while picking up a prescription from her general practitioner's desk. The GP curetted out the wart but the wound became infected and never healed. The amputation of the finger was deemed necessary because the whole finger was covered with masses of 'warts'. Sepsis gradually spread up the forearm over the course of months. The patient attributed her latest deterioration to the district nurse's failure to change the dressings regularly. On admission she declared blandly that her arm would never heal and clearly required amputation.

During the course of the psychiatric interview the patient gave the impression of inappropriate stoicism and emphasized how she could dig the garden and decorate the house in spite of her arm oozing with pus. She denied any worries. She mentioned that she had married at 24 but she and her husband had separated after one year. Even more significant were the omissions from her history which were filled in by her GP. The couple she called her parents were her aunt and uncle who had adopted her after her mother's death during the delivery. It also transpired that the patient was prone to dramatic fainting attacks and had previously developed an hysterical paraplegia. The GP had established that she was still virgo intacta. In contrast with her medical history, she had an excellent work record and had been employed by the same firm for 30 years.

The patient's arm was found to have linear scratch marks near the elbow. It was treated with Eusol and liquid paraffin and left uncovered. The skin healed rapidly. The patient was discharged from hospital and agreed to attend for psychiatric treatment as an outpatient. The dermatologist in charge advised that the patient should not be confronted abruptly with the diagnosis of self-inflicted lesions. Interviews were unproductive and she voiced criticism of the treatment she had received. She reluctantly agreed to her brother and sister being interviewed: they expressed admiration for her courage and noted that she had improved while her adoptive mother had been admitted to hospital for a hysterectomy. After three months her skin broke down again. It was considered that a sufficiently good therapeutic relationship had been established to confront her with the facts of her self-injuries, while expressing sympathy for all her past and current difficulties. She failed to keep her next psychiatric appointment. Follow-up by the dermatologist during the next seven years enabled symptomatic treatment to be provided when new skin lesions appeared over the left arm, right leg, and right eye. She also developed a transient right-sided hysterical hemiparesis.

Treatment and prognosis

It is most important to make the correct diagnosis of self-inflicted skin lesions. Inappropriate

Fig. 8.7.1. Clinical photograph: left forearm of a 46-year-old woman showing extensive purulent and crusted lesions due to self-inflicted injuries and infection. Reproduced by kind permission of Dr C.D. Calnan and Dr D.A. Burns.

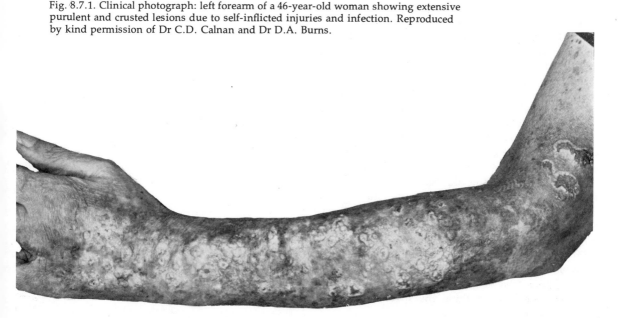

forms of treatment will thus be avoided, including the crippling effects of surgical amputations.

Having established that the lesions are self-induced, the question arises whether the patient should be confronted with the facts. Expert opinion differs on this issue. Hollender and Abram (1973) suggest that confrontation sometimes produces a salutary effect and cessation of self-injury. Others are more cautious and say that direct confrontation with the patient or relatives leads to the interruption of treatment (Brown, 1938; Sneddon & Sneddon, 1975). This was the experience with the patient described in the case history. The risk is that the patient will seek another doctor prepared to treat her as suffering from physical illness. Zaidens (1951) cautions that it is bad therapy to unmask the patient without first encouraging her and 'building her up psychologically'. The best approach is that of Lyell (1972) who advises the maintenance of confidence between the patient and her doctor: he should somehow indicate that he 'knows' without saying so, and that he remains sympathetic. This is the approach usually adopted by the dermatologist who will admit the patient to hospital and induce healing by providing constant nursing observation, occluding the injured area efficiently with elastoplast or plaster of Paris, or immobilizing the offending arm by splinting. The dermatologist will often try persuading the patient to see his psychiatrist colleague, although the view may be held that the psychiatrist is of little help (Calnan, 1980).

If the patient accepts psychiatric treatment, the aim will be to elicit her trust and avoid appearing as an adversary, or as a detective (Hollender & Abram, 1973). Patience is needed in overcoming the patient's formidable defences and elucidating her conflicts. Brown (1938) describes in detail the psychotherapy of a patient with the aid of hypnosis and the study of her dreams: he succeeded in eliciting masochistic ruminations. Gillespie (1938) gives an account of the successful therapy of a young woman who had given up work to nurse her invalid mother. She confessed that she had inflicted the skin lesions herself, and in the course of therapy further admitted to a secret resentment towards her mother. She had compulsive fears that she would kill her mother and assuaged her guilt by digging into the skin of her own forearm with scissors. The treatment was successful, the lesions healed rapidly and she made a good adjustment.

In contrast with these therapeutic successes many patients refuse psychiatric help or resist treatment when it is attempted. It is best then for the dermatologist to continue supervising the patient, avoiding what she might construe as threatening, and applying symptomatic treatment as the need arises.

In a thorough follow-up study, Sneddon and Sneddon (1975) traced 33 out of 43 patients previously diagnosed as suffering from dermatitis artefacta. Thirteen patients continued to produce lesions or were severely disabled in other ways, an average of some 12 years after the onset of symptoms. Twenty had recovered. The authors conclude that the prognosis is relatively poor: recovery seemed to occur when the patient's circumstances changed rather than as a result of treatment.

8.8
Hypochondriasis

ISSY PILOWSKY

Definition, psychopathology, classification, aetiology

Hypochondriasis is a form of abnormal illness behaviour (dysnosognosia) in which the individual experiences and manifests a degree of concern over his state of health, which is out of proportion to the amount considered appropriate to the degree of objective evidence for the presence of disease (Pilowsky, 1978).

There has been a good deal of controversy over the psychopathological status of hypochondriasis. This is not surprising since the abnormal attitude to health can take the form of a phobia, an obsession, a delusion, or an overvalued idea (morbid preoccupation). Furthermore, it is often not possible, even after the most painstaking phenomenological analysis of the patient's experience, to decide whether the patient may be said to be deluded, preoccupied, or phobic. Indeed, in some patients shifts occur from one psychopathological form to another, over extended periods of observation. In clinical practice, however, it is important to distinguish between hypochondriacal states in which reality testing is severely impaired and the patient may be said to be deluded, and those in which this is not the case. The delusional forms may be part of a depressive psychosis, schizophrenia, or a monosymptomatic hypochondriacal psychosis, and will not be discussed here in detail (see vol. 3, chaps. 1–5, 16, 17). The non-delusional forms usually take the form of a phobia or a morbid preoccupation and much less often an obsession.

When the hypochondriacal reaction presents as a phobia, the patient has fears of diseases which may befall him, such as a heart attack or a stroke. In his calmer moments, the patient will acknowledge the irrational nature of these fears and accept the role played by psychological stressors in their production.

The patient with a hypochondriacal preoccupation is not concerned about diseases to which he might fall victim in the future, but rather with the meaning of the symptoms of which he is currently aware. He reports spending considerable time in concerned thought over the various disease states which his symptoms might be due to. In the rarely encountered obsessional form of hypochondriasis the patient experiences thoughts of disease which he regards as ego alien and attempts to banish, but in severe forms he may repeatedly seek examination and reassurance.

A few researchers have attempted to clarify the nosological and psychopatholotical status of hypochondriasis but, as yet, no clear agreement has been reached.

Kenyon (1964) studied the case notes of Maudsley patients, comparing those diagnosed as primary hypochondriasis with those diagnosed as secondary. He concluded that no differences emerged between the two groups, although an examination of his data suggests that there might have been some. His studies suffered from the obvious flaw, however, that the diagnosis had been made by a number of psychiatrists, and there is no guarantee that they used similar criteria for primary and secondary hypochondriasis.

In a personally conducted study in Sheffield, 66 patients were diagnosed as primary hypochondriasis and 81 as secondary (Pilowsky, 1970). The findings differed from those of Kenyon in that the 'secondary' group tended to have a shorter history at referral, to be more likely to have made a suicidal attempt, and to be treated with ECT and antidepressants. They were also more often described as 'anxiety prone' personalities, apt to express fears of illness, and many had been treated with minor tranquillizers. While these findings may possibly have been influenced by the bias of the investigator, they do suggest that hypochondriacal reactions are usefully regarded as an independent syndrome. Certainly, in the case of males, this dichotomy had prognostic significance; it was found that at follow-up, 51.4 per cent of the primary group described their symptoms as unremitting and continuous, while only 16.7 per cent of the secondary group did so.

Approaching the question in a different way, Pilowsky (1967) and Bianchi (1973) used factor analysis in an attempt to clarify the nature of hypochondriasis.

In the first study, a 14-item self-administered questionnaire was given to 200 psychiatric patients half of whom exhibited hypochondriacal features in their illness (Pilowsky, 1967). Their responses were submitted to a principal component analysis with rotation. Three factors emerged which were labelled: (a) bodily preoccupation, (b) disease phobia, and (c) a factor which is briefly described as 'disease conviction' and reflects the form of hypochondriasis characterized by 'a firm conviction of the presence of serious pathology accompanied by a paranoid attitude to relatives and medical personnel which may, at times, be considered psychotic'.

Bianchi (1973) carried out a personal study of 119 psychiatric in-patients manifesting various forms of abnormal illness behaviour of the disease-affirming type, such as disease phobia, disease conviction, bodily preoccupation, and psychogenic pain. Information reflecting psychopathology, personality, parental features, and pain and sensation sensitivity was included in a principal component analysis, which produced five meaningful hypochondriacal configurations. These included a syndrome characterized by psychogenic pain, somatic preoccupation, 'unnecessary operations' and being female, family illness, low sensation threshold, 'life defeats', and a poor prognosis. In the male counterpart, a hypochondriacal premorbid personality took the place of 'unnecessary operations'. The female constellation bears a clear resemblance to that described as 'hysteria' by Perley and Guze (1962), but Bianchi preferred the term 'hypochondriacal neurosis'. Two patterns of disease phobia emerged. In one case the phobia was associated with anxiety and depression; in the other with inhibitions of anger and childhood exposure to maternal solicitude. The fifth pattern was one of disease conviction associated with paranoid feelings and also exposure to maternal over-solicitude. On the basis of his studies overall, Bianchi (1973) concluded that disease phobia is associated with a low sensation threshold, over-exposure to family illness, and current anxiety.

The studies cited are consistent with clinical experience which suggests that abnormal attitudes to illness may be conceptualized in terms of the experience of bodily sensations, the subjective attitude to the possibliity of illness and one's own health, and the response to the reassurance provided by doctors. It is not surprising, therefore, that hypochondriacal neuroses have been defined in terms of the 'multitude' of symptoms, the fears of disease, the preoccupation with health related matters, the tendency to complaints, and the lack of response to reassurance. This last feature is of particular interest since medical writers appear to have been more intemperate in their description of these patients than any other. Alvarez (1944), for example, advised that one 'should try to get them out of the office as quickly as possible because the time they take up is spent to no good purpose'. Gehring (1932) wrote that 'in the meantime I am suffering like a she-elephant in the pangs of childbirth for I am confronted by a hypochondriac'.

There is probably no other group of patients which has been referred to in this way, publicly or privately, and it is interesting to consider that the hypochondriacal individual, by his non-acceptance of advice and the critical questioning of doctors, confronts physicians as individuals and the health services as a whole with their most searching and difficult test, since in the last analysis the definitive diagnosis is totally dependent on the nature of the patient's response to the doctor's behaviour, which must therefore be seen to be appropriate by some generally accepted standard.

It is difficult to estimate the prevalence of hypochondriacal reactions. As independent syndromes, they are probably uncommon; about 1 – 2 per cent of populations of psychiatric patients. But estimates of hypochondriasis associated with other psychiatric illness vary from 12 to 45 per cent. Interestingly in the Manhattan survey, Langner and Michael (1963) found 'hypochondriasis' in 25 per cent of their sample.

Hypochondriacal reactions occur in both sexes and all ages, but appear to predominate in the middle and later years. In addition, they appear commoner in lower socio-economic status groups, an observation which may have something to do with the fact that bodily complaints represent a more ready access to the sick role in manual workers than do complaints relating to emotional distress. In addition, the question as to whether symptoms are being consciously exaggerated is often raised where compensation is an issue and may lead to referral for a psychiatric opinion where such a course might not otherwise be considered (see chap. 6.2 and 6.3 of this volume).

Socio-cultural factors may certainly play a part in determining the vocabulary chosen for communicating distress, however, it is not always easy to tease out ethnic from occupational, language, and other influences (Pilowsky & Spence, 1977). In settings where large migrant communities exist, it would seem most important that doctors use interpreters where necessary, that they acquire some knowledge of their patients' cultures, and that, even when they share their patients' ethnic background, they do not fall prey to the dangers of self-stereotyping. It is not an uncommon experience to find doctors making sweeping generalizations about fellow countrymen who happen to originate from a different social class or geographical region. Similarly, one sometimes wonders whether the urban doctor needs an interpreter when interviewing a rural patient!

Psycho-dynamic aspects

Psycho-analysts have paid relatively scant attention to hypochondriacal reactions presumably due to the fact that they have not been regarded as suitable for psycho-analytic treatment. Freud himself focused on the bodily complaints and sensations which he considered were due to undischarged libido. Later writers, however, emphasized the shifts of attention, or displacement from objects to the body. In other words, the body or parts of the body image with special significance for the individual become the target for concerns and fears rather than specific persons or situations. In the same way as a fear of one's own impulses may be expressed as a phobia of animals, it may also be expressed as a fear of disease, that is, of being attacked or destroyed by one's own body.

Alexander (1949) described the presence of three major psycho-dynamic components in the genesis of hypochondriasis, (a) withdrawal of interest from objects to self, (b) a need for punishment based on guilt feelings, and (c) a displacement of anxiety. He considers that an increased narcissism is present in hypochondriacal patients due to frustration of the wish to be loved. This leads to hostility, anxiety, and guilt with a need for suffering to assuage the guilt. Thus hypochondriasis allows a relatively guilt-free withdrawal into the sick role while simultaneously permitting the communication of disguised and not-so-disguised hostility towards others and, in partic-

ular, the medical profession, by the persistent presentation of complaints despite the efforts of others to do what they believe to be appropriate.

Diagnosis

The diagnosis of hypochondriacal reactions is difficult because the essential features tend to unfold in the course of the development of the doctor – patient interaction, and may only be fully apparent after a number of treatment transactions, when the patient can be seen to be following an anomalous course. Characteristically, it is in the 'negotiation phase' of the doctor – patient interaction that the hypochondriacal illness becomes clear, since the patient is not really able to negotiate, in that he is unable to reach agreement with the doctor as to the nature of his illness, except for short periods. Indeed, he cannot be reassured and asks for further investigations and treatments.

The phenomenology of hypochondriacal syndromes discussed earlier is central to their diagnosis and their differentiation from other illnesses which can present with hypochondriacal features. These include schizophrenia, depressive psychosis, and early dementia.

It should be emphasized that the diagnosis can only be made definitively after the patient has been fully assessed both physically and psychosocially, and an appraisal of the situation in language he is able to comprehend has been presented to him.

Management

As can be appreciated, hypochondriacal states are multifaceted in their nature and a great many patients show a mixture of features which make a clear-cut diagnosis difficult. In terms of explaining, understanding, and treating hypochondriasis, it is more important to elucidate the various dimensions of the illness and devise therapies which respond to all the elements of the disorder.

It is important that the diagnosis of a hypochondriacal reaction should be made as early as possible so that inappropriate investigations and treatments can be avoided. However, the detection of a hypochondriacal neurosis tends to be more difficult when the phobic component predominates, since the patient may be inhibited about expressing his fears. It may be that the patient hesitates to communicate his fears for fear of having them confirmed, or anticipates criticism for behaving irrationally. Often both concerns are based on the feeling that the illness is a punishment for some wrong-doing. On the other hand, the patient who is preoccupied with illness rarely hesitates to convey his worries about his health and his dissatisfaction with treatment.

CASE HISTORY 1

A 35-year-old woman attended her general practitioner complaining of palpitations and headaches which had troubled her for two months. She worried constantly that she might develop a brain tumour or suffer a stroke or heart attack. Physical examination revealed no abnormality, but it was not possible to reassure her completely.

She was a woman who had always been anxious and as a child was considered 'anaemic'. She was married with two young children, and in order to supplement the family income had taken a job as a petrol pump attendant. At her work she had become emotionally involved with a salesman who visited regularly. She was extremely worried about this because she feared that her husband, whom she described as an intensely jealous man, would kill them both if he found them out.

About a month before her illness began, the salesman abruptly ended their affair, and she was both upset and relieved. He stopped visiting her garage, but she could not help hoping that he might appear. Her first attack of palpitations and headache occurred when he finally did call for petrol one day but made no attempt to re-establish their relationship and treated her rather formally.

She was seen for psychotherapy at weekly, and then fortnightly, intervals over a period of three months. She was able to ventilate her feelings about her marriage and display appropriate affect. Her physical concerns gradually receded and after three months she was functioning well, although still liable to occasional fears over her health when stressed. Throughout her illness, she remained able to work.

Hypochondriacal patients inevitably cause doctors to feel inadequate, helpless, guilty, frustrated and angry. Unless the doctor has an understanding of the reasons for the patient's hypochondriasis, he will have the greatest difficulty coping with these feelings and will not be able to manage the patient satisfactorily.

It is usually the case that a therapeutic alliance is more readily established with the phobic patient than the preoccupied patient, since the former is often able, at least intermittently, to regard his fears as irrational even to the point of being able to joke about them.

In managing the patient it is useful to make a distinction between the illness experience, illness statements and illness behaviours. Thus a patient who makes illness statements may manifest very few illness behaviours and may indeed be leading a reasonably active and productive life. This distinction underscores the need to accept the patient's use of hypochondriasis as a coping strategy or psychological defence, albeit maladaptive. Once this is understood it will be appreciated that the doctor must convey his acceptance of the defensive strategy and the fact that he will not demand that it be dismantled willy-nilly. The simplest way to indicate this acceptance is to listen attentively to the patient's illness statements, that is, complaints and symptoms. This usually means that each interview begins with a discussion of the patient's fears and concerns and may sometimes lead to a physical examination or special investigation. The doctor should not do these to set the patient's mind at ease, but because the clinical picture requires them to be done. There should never be a concern that by so doing the doctor will reinforce the abnormal illness behaviour. This will only happen if the carrying out of physical examinations constitutes the only way in which concern and interest in the patient is demonstrated.

It is a regular clinical experience that most hypochondriacal patients do not go on complaining in physical terms if they are encouraged to say all they wish to say at the outset of the interview. Indeed, after a few minutes they will stop and are prepared to discuss other aspects of their life situation.

On what basis may a psychiatrist enter into a therapeutic contract with a hypochondriacal patient? Perhaps the most workable approach is for patient and doctor to accept that since the former's fears and concerns have not been confirmed, and it has not been possible to establish any indications for physical therapeutic intervention, it is reasonable for them both to see the illness as one with physical and emotional aspects, both of which require monitoring and management. Indeed, some patients find it far easier to conceptualize their emotional problems as consequences of their physical discomforts, and on that basis are prepared to discuss life problems in the same way as a patient with demonstrable physical pathology might be.

Given this type of agreement, hypochondriacal patients can be treated with supportive or brief psycho-dynamically orientated psychotherapy.

It is important to bear in mind the role played by the patient's family in relation to the illness. The family's response to hypochondriasis may oscillate between excessive encouragement of the patient's illness behaviour on one hand, and hostile rejection of his complaints on the other. On rare occasions a *folie à deux* may develop between a patient and a spouse, with both convinced that serious disease exists (On even rarer occasions such a shared psychosis may develop between a patient and a doctor who then defends the patient's position against other physicians.)

Wherever appropriate and practicable, the therapist should involve the family in treatment. This may take the form of conjoint sessions in which marital problems are dealt with, or the spouse is advised as to the most appropriate way to respond to the patient's complaints. Children should be helped to understand that their parents' complaints are neither their fault nor their responsibility. It is usually also necessary to explain to family members that the patient may have a mixture of physical and psychological problems, each affecting the other.

It is useful to explain the overall management to the patient and spouse in a conjoint session at an early stage. It should be emphasized that the patient should try as much as possible to direct complaints to the doctor and to no one else. Many hypochondriacal patients have good insight into the fact that their complaint behaviour may upset and exhaust their relatives and, indeed, alienate them. They will, on occasion, ask the doctor what they should do when a relative asks them how they are feeling because they fear that their behaviour may lead others to abandon them. At a conscious level, they are often able to see the logic of advice to reserve their symptoms for the doctor, but it is easier for them and their spouses to follow this course if it has been presented and explained to them in a conjoint interview.

CASE HISTORY 2

A 55-year-old foreman in a textile factory was admitted to a medical ward after complaining of chest pain for a month. No physical abnormalities were found.

At interview, he described fears of having a heart attack for about one month with frequent chest pains. Two friends had recently suffered infarcts and one had died.

The patient was married, with three children who lived away from home. Three months before his admission, he had entered into a sexual relationship with one of the young women whom he supervised. One week before, it had been announced that staff would have to be dismissed. The woman had come to him and threatened to tell his wife about their relationship unless he ensured that she was not dismissed.

It was striking that once having been able to talk openly about these problems, the patient felt much relieved and returned to work. He did not take up the offer of further treatment.

CASE HISTORY 3

The patient, a typist aged 34 years, said 'I've got a stupid idea that I will probably die of cancer'. This had been present for two years. During the six months before her fears began, a number of people known to her had died of cancer.

She was the third of four children and had married her first husband at 19 years of age. The marriage was unhappy and she divorced her husband after he had been violent to her. She had a 14-year-old daughter of the union. She remarried at 29 years, and although happy with her husband, always felt guilty because, as a Roman Catholic, she should not have been divorced. She was terrified of falling pregnant and also reported phobias of the dark and enclosed spaces.

She was treated with psychotherapy and chlordiazepoxide, but her fears persisted. She attended a psychotherapeutic group with some benefit. At no stage of her illness did she stop working, and two years after her first presentation, she reported feeling well although she experienced occasional fears.

Prognosis

In a follow-up study of 147 hypochondriacal patients (Pilowsky, 1968), over an average of 31 months, it was found that 48.3 per cent had a good outcome with hypochondriacal symptoms absent or only occasionally present, and work capacity essentially unimpaired; 27.8 per cent had a fair outcome with hypochondriasis still a prominent feature, but very little impairment of capacity for work. A poor outcome was found in 23.8 per cent of patients with symptoms constantly present and severe impairment of work capacity. It was observed that the presence of anxiety and depression predicted a good outcome. Two clinical patterns were associated with a poor outcome. These consisted of older men who showed feelings of resentment, resistance to reassurance with no response to ECT, and younger women with hysterical personalities who had seen a variety of physicians and surgeons before being referred for psychiatric help.

These findings indicate that the prognosis for hypochondriasis is not as gloomy as often thought, particularly if diagnosed early, that is, before many inappropriate physical therapies have been administered. Even though patients may not be able to relinquish their hypochondriacal defences completely, they may, none the less, function well in most areas and at the very least be able to avoid submitting themselves to unnecessary, time-consuming, and expensive treatments and investigations.

8.9
Sick role and illness behaviour in children

LIONEL HERSOV

It is now clear from the large body of literature on the psychosocial and social determinants of health and disease, that disorders of bodily function are not the only criteria for deciding whether or not an individual regards himself as ill, is considered to be ill, is referred to the medical services, or is admitted to hospital (Kessel & Shepherd 1965; Mechanic, 1962; Kellner, 1963). It is estimated that 70 per cent to 90 per cent of all self-recognized episodes of sickness are managed outside the medical care system (Zola, 1972) and Kleinman and co-workers (1978) consider that contemporary medical practice has become increasingly discordant with public expectations. Nowadays it is necessary to examine systematically the social, psychological, and physiological determinants of health and disease against the background of daily life to 'understand the influences of a variety of norms, values, fears and expected rewards and punishments on how a symptomatic person behaves' (Mechanic, 1962).

The concept of the sick role was first put forward in 1952 by the sociologist Talcott Parsons and has since influenced medical sociology in general, and studies of sick people in particular. Parsons argues that being 'sick' is a special role in society as well as a medical condition, and there are expectations associated with the role. Sick people are exempted from certain social obligations, for example, going to work, or in the case of a child, going to school, and also from the responsibility for the state they are in, or for

getting well. It is assumed that they need help, that they want to get well, that they will seek help, accept it, and co-operate in treatment. The illness is legitimized by medical sanction, or by close relatives and other influential people, and the 'good' patients do what the doctor tells them and so depend on his authority. The patient and his family respond to the illness in socially patterned ways which have often been learned in childhood. There is also an obligation to use the privileged position of the sick role for as short a time as possible and to 'want to get well'. However, the rewards are sometimes so great, as Parsons notes, that 'the privileges and exemptions of the sick role may become objects of a secondary gain which the patient is positively motivated, usually unconsciously, to secure or to retain. The problem, therefore, of the balance of motivations to recover, becomes of first importance'.

This behaviour can be strongly reinforced by the reactions of people around the patient, particularly in children who have learned from earlier experience of illness that they will be treated in a special way (for example, kept at home from school by an over-anxious mother when the child complains of feeling ill). The concept of sick role includes not only the behaviour of the sick person but also the responses of people in the environment including physicians and, in the case of children, parents and other family members. Parsons' (1952) description of role relationships between patient and doctor includes the family as acting on and modifying the relationship, 'the solidarity of the family imposes a very strong pressure on the healthy members to see that the sick one gets the best possible care'.

Parson's sick role formulation has been criticized on several grounds (Twaddle, 1972) as applying only to a limited range of illnesses and not covering, in particular, stigmatized illnesses which often carry an assumption of responsibility for their onset. The concept of 'illness behaviour' (Mechanic & Volkart, 1961) permits the shift from broad societal roles to individual behaviour with reference to the experience of illness, and has more practical relevance to the clinical approach. By illness behaviour is meant 'the ways in which given symptoms may be differentially perceived, evaluated and acted (or not acted) upon by different kinds of persons' (Mechanic, 1962). The emphasis on differential behaviour applies not only to the person with symptoms but to all the other people involved in the illness situation. This is particularly so when children become ill, since most of the contact with medical services and almost all other illness behaviour is initiated by other persons. Much has been written about sick children's psychological needs, behaviour, and treatment (Freud, 1952; Bergmann, 1965) but less is known of their parents' attitudes and behaviour (Robinson, 1972). However, illness is still a personal event even for children in families, and stoical children will make light of their symptoms while others will ask quickly for help (Mechanic, 1964). There are social and cultural differences in responses to illness as well as other influences, such as earlier experience of illness and the way children are trained in different families to respond to and deal with symptoms. In this sense, part of illness behaviour is learned behaviour. Campbell (1978) has shown that children's reports of how they act when ill are clearly tied to age and sex roles as well as to parental socio-economic status. A 'spartan' orientation is characteristic of older children, boys, and children of parents with higher socio-economic status.

Most 'illness behaviour' is on the basis of recognized disease but a large amount arises from fear of diseases which, however minor, act as stresses in themselves. It is very likely that where there are problems of uncertainty over diagnosis there may be added stress. In addition, substantial amounts of illness behaviour are generated by the advantages of the invalid role (Kendell, 1974) which ensures attention and concern as well as the avoidance of anxiety-provoking situations.

Pilowsky (1969) has gone further by advancing the notion of 'abnormal illness behaviour', in which there is a persisting inappropriate or maladaptive mode of perceiving, evaluating, and acting in relation to one's own state of health (see chapter 8.2, 8.8 in the present volume). This occurs in spite of the doctor providing the patient with what, to a physician, is a reasonably lucid explanation of the nature of the sufferer's illness. Present-day physicians too often make diagnoses, offer explanations of symptoms, and treat patients in terms of *diseases,* whereas patients suffer from *illnesses,* that is, altered states of personal awareness, discomfort, and impairment of social function (Kleinman *et al.,* 1978), which are disregarded by physicians who look upon the disease as the disorder. In the case of a sick child the parents' response to what they are told by a doctor may be inappropriate or they may become confused by contradictory or changing explanations and inconsistent management. Their own uncertainty and anxiety may

be conveyed to their sick child thus heightening his own fears that he is suffering from an unknown or dangerous condition, so that he maintains his 'abnormal illness behaviour' long beyond the time when recovery should have occurred, according to the natural history of the disorder and the expectations of his doctor.

Dubowitz and Hersov (1976) drew attention to a number of children presenting with undiagnosed disorders of gait in which it appeared that the abnormality of motor function had followed on an initial organic illness. When the children were seen in hospital for a second opinion it was difficult to discern whether the presenting symptoms and signs reflected the persistence of the original disorder or were due to what would commonly be called psychogenic or functional overlay. Five children were described, 3 boys aged between 10 and 12 years and 2 girls aged 12 and 13 years respectively, all showing disorders of motor function, either inability to walk or bizarre gait. All 5 had associated complaints of muscle pain and tenderness in the lower limbs and in one there was gross loss of normal motor function. In four cases the initial illness presented with gastro-intestinal upset or pyrexia together with complaints of muscle or joint pain. All the children were investigated, in several cases at more than one hospital, with consistently negative findings and there was no objective evidence of a viral illness or encephalitis. Two of the children had been subjected to enforced bed-rest and even immobilization. In all cases the referral to a postgraduate teaching hospital was a last-ditch effort after several months of ineffective treatment. The 'experts' were under pressure to find the answer and restore the children to health.

The usual procedure in such cases is to repeat the earlier investigations, often with considerable distress to patient and family but with little gain in understanding. As Creak (1969) has written: 'In children, hysterical symptoms command both sympathy and unrewarding investigations which eventually fail to clarify and so prolong the clinical picture'. Too often the search for a disease to explain the symptoms, and the disregard of the important social and psychological factors maintaining the illness, create additional problems by confirming the fears of patient and parents.

It has been suggested that it is more fruitful to ask *why* children behave in this way rather than *what* is the matter with them. This requires a different approach from the usual one of substituting the label of 'hysteria' or 'hysterical overlay' for an organic diagnosis, calling in the psychiatrist, and expecting him to cope with the problem. Instead, a combined approach by paediatricians and psychiatrists, together with all the other professional disciplines in hospital involved with the child and family, is more effective. The notion of abnormal illness behaviour allows clinicians to set up hypotheses as to how the behaviour arose and is maintained, and to test these out by a plan of management to alter it. Dubowitz and Hersov (1976) have set out the essentials of effective management as follows, (1) to stop further investigations beyond the minimum which may be needed to assure the physician ther there is no residual structural abnormality; (2) to institute without delay a management programme of overall rehabilitation by involving the psychiatric team from the outset; this ensures a full assessment of social and psychological stresses at home, in school, and arising from earlier illness experience; (3) the objective is to assist the child to relinquish his illness behaviour and to alter the parents' perception of their child from that of a chronic invalid to that of a potentially healthy and normally developing youngster. The outcome in all the cases reported was uniformly good and subsequent cases managed in this fashion have also responded well. The following case history will illustrate this style of management.

CASE HISTORY

A 10-year-old boy developed a sore throat soon after taking part in a sponsored distance swim. Congested tonsils were found and penicillin was prescribed by the GP with initial improvement but followed by a recurrence of symptoms 6 days later. Additional complaints of stomach-ache led to the suspicion of a viral illness, resulting in a hospital visit for a blood test which proved negative. The boy became increasingly weak, listless, and lethargic but retained a good appetite and his usual interest in watching TV and reading.

A pathologist was called to the home for a further blood test and the GP offered the diagnosis of a possible encephalitis, described as 'inflammation of brain membranes', to the boy's parents in his presence and hearing. The family were told that 'it would take 6 –18 months to clear completely'. A neurologist then examined the boy at home and he was admitted to hospital with suspected tuberculous meningitis. He remained in hospital for 3 weeks during which 'psychogenic overlay' was diagnosed because of negative tests, including a normal EEG and lumbar puncture. A psychiatrist was called in who insisted on full motor activity but this was difficult to achieve because the boy shuffled along, seemingly unable to walk properly or raise his head at first. He was discharged home 'well' with instructions to parents to treat him as 'well' and 'normal'. Within a fortnight at home he had regressed to his former state of apathetic weakness but, in addition, appeared unable

to walk upstairs unless carried by his father. By now both parents were thoroughly puzzled and alarmed. He was therefore readmitted to hospital where a repeat of the early tests proved negative. On this admission he was more emotionally upset, drowsy and withdrawn, and physically weak. Subacute sclerosing panencephalitis was suspected, explained to his parents as 'a virus left over from earlier measles' which needed very sophisticated investigations, and the boy was transferred to a second hospital with the appropriate facilities. On examination he was drowsy, withdrawn, speaking only in a whisper, with full but weak limb movement and normal reflexes apart from intermittent upgoing toes to plantar stimulation. A further lumbar puncture was negative, as were tests for measles antibodies and other viral studies. The possibility of a cerebral tumour was eliminated. A final authoritative statement was given to boy and parents that there was no disease to account for his symptoms. However, the boy still remained 'ill': depressed, withdrawn and unresponsive with fluctuating abnormal neurological signs which were regarded as induced. A psychiatric interview elicited little information except that the boy, who spoke only in a whisper, said that he had 'encephalitis' by which he understood 'a brain disease'. He resisted all attempts at mobilization, insisted on being transported in a wheelchair or carried, was aggressive to his parents and staff, but enjoyed daily visits and many gifts from parents and siblings. Both parents had begun to change their opinion that he was dangerously diseased to thinking that he might be maintaining his 'illness' for reasons which they could not discern. In the previous hospital the only explanation, other than that of serious disease, had been that of 'nerves', and this was accompanied by the offer of psychiatric intervention, which made little sense to them.

The hypothesis was set up that this was an instance of 'abnormal illness behaviour' following a real minor illness which had been maintained by traditional medical-type investigation and treatment and parental beliefs that the boy was dangerously ill from an undiagnosable disease. It was predicted that if management could focus on providing rewarding responses to healthy normal behaviour the boy would gradually give up the inappropriate behaviour and return to health. The psychiatric team and attending paediatricians decided to manage the boy on a paediatric ward.

Nursing staff, physiotherapists, teachers, ward attendants, and paediatricians were given a detailed formulation of the psychological and social mechanisms involved and the importance of not responding to symptoms but to the overall behaviour. They agreed to the treatment plan even though the boy was not ill in the formal sense to which they were accustomed. The family were also given a detailed explanation of the mechanisms responsible for their son's behaviour since the onset of illness two months earlier, and the importance of their own contribution to the management plan was emphasized. The boy's mother in particular expressed great relief from earlier confusion and uncertainty, understood very well the aims of the treatment, and offered full co-operation which she maintained throughout.

A treatment programme was set in motion with the agreement of all ward staff which eliminated any further investigations, daily temperature, enquiry about symptoms, and responses to complaints of weakness. Instead, a programme of rehabilitation with graded goals offering an 'escape with honour' was established, with the emphasis on a positive response by ward staff and parents to any improvement in motor function, and attempts at normal speech and normal activity. The patient's family were told what to do during visiting times and later on at weekends at home. Goals of treatment were to get the boy (a) out of bed; (b) walking normally in all respects; (c) riding a bicycle in the hospital gymnasium and eventually at home; (d) going swimming; (e) return to school; (f) speaking in a normal tone of voice instead of a whisper. A step-by-step programme was set in motion with social rewards for normal speech and activities in ward and school, and no response for dependent helpless behaviour or whispering. Progress was slow but sustained and the initial scepticism of the ward staff was replaced by pleasure at their success in reaching treatment goals without the customary means of investigation, medication, or operation. The boy eventually returned home fully recovered and has remained so 5 years after discharge from hospital.

The essence of this approach is the effective collaboration of paediatric and psychiatric teams. The details of treatment are familiar to a psychiatrist but not easy for physicians to accept, trained as they are in the disease – illness dichotomy and needing to change their view of a patient from someone with a disease to someone who can become a therapeutic ally (Kleinman *et al.*, 1978). The psychiatrist's consultation-liason role on a paediatric ward is a crucial part of management. It should include helping the paediatricians to work with families and learning that illness behaviour can be viewed in different ways, not only as possible symbolic manifestations of unconscious conflict, but as operant behaviour acting on the environment to produce secondary gains which maintain or even strengthen the symptoms. They include attention from family, doctors, nurses, and other patients, and the avoidance of situations which arouse anxiety. A behavioural modification approach can be allied with a psychotherapeutic approach in the treatment of adults as well as children (Mrazek, 1976).

The dilemma of the physician faced with this sort of clinical problem is well described by Sir George Pickering (1974):

> To pronounce that a patient has no organic disease and that the symptoms are those of a psychoneurosis or that the patient is not so sick as he or she thinks and should do more for himself or herself requires more courage and determination than any other decision that I know in medicine . . . It is an issue most doctors like to avoid and it demands the highest degree of professional skill.

9
Sexual disturbances and deviation

9.1
Sexual problems
JOHN BANCROFT

Sexual relationships, like many other aspects of people's lives, vary from the highly successful to the complete failures. There are probably few couples who do not experience at least temporary difficulties at some stage in their sex lives. Having a sexual problem is not therefore an all-or-nothing matter, and the decision to seek help for such problems will not be determined simply by their severity. Difficulties in discussing the subject with a professional helper, scarcity of suitable help and the social stigma attached to such treatment are also important. Some couples find it easier to present with a sexual problem, which they see as a physical illness than to admit they have interpersonal difficulties.

The incidence of sexual problems
Not surprisingly, we have scant information on the true incidence of sexual problems. In Kinsey's study of male sexuality, 1.6 per cent of his sample had 'reached more or less permanent erectile impotence'. This was strongly related to age; by the age of 70, 27 per cent were in this category (Kinsey *et al.*, 1948). Thirty-five per cent of his male subjects reported incidental erectile failure (that is, occasional, or due to understandable and temporary causes) and in 7.1 per cent the problem was 'more than incidental' (as reported by Gebhard & Johnson, 1979).

In females, most attention has been given to difficulty in experiencing orgasm. Kinsey and his colleagues in their study of women found that the proportion capable of orgasm increased steadily with age until by the mid-thirties 90 per cent were capable of orgasm (Kinsey *et al.*, 1953). Other studies have given figures for orgasmic difficulties that range from 5 per cent (Fisher, 1973) to 15 per cent (Hunt, 1974) though the criteria were not necessarily the same.

The extent to which people who experience sexual dysfunctions are dissatisfied with their sexual relationships has received less attention. In one recent study (Franks *et al.*, 1978), dissatisfaction with sexual relationship was more closely associated with other types of difficulty (for example, poor communication, inability to relax, low sexual interest) than with sexual dysfunction *per se*.

One of the few recent studies to achieve satisfactory population sampling was carried out in Holland, using a recently developed Sexual Experience Scale (Frenken, 1976): 250 men and 250 women, all married and less than 50 years old, representing an 85 per cent acceptance rate, provided a good sample of 'broad middle-class' Dutch men and women. Twenty-six per cent of men and 43 per cent of women indicated problems with enjoyment and arousal, with a further 9 per cent of women expressing actual aversion. Twelve per cent of men and 33 per cent of women indicated difficulty or dissatisfaction with orgasm, a further 5 per cent of women being anorgasmic. Such figures suggest that large numbers of individuals are dissatisfied sexually, of which a very small proportion seek help.

In Edinburgh, 1000 women attending a family planning clinic were given a questionnaire; 750 completed it. Twelve per cent of the respondents said they had a sexual problem, 8 per cent were uncertain. This population was predominantly middle-class and the majority (60 per cent) were single. The mean age was 27 years (Dickerson, Begg & Warner, unpublished data). Lack of sexual interest rather than specific sexual dysfunction was the best predictor of those who acknowledged a problem.

The relevance of social class

The association between lower social class and sexual problems or dissatisfaction has been found in a number of studies though it is the working-class female more than the male who appears to be at a disadvantage (Kinsey *et al.*, 1953; Chesser, 1956; Rainwater, 1966). Kinsey and co-workers (1948) found that working-class men were more likely to accept rapid ejaculation during intercourse. Rainwater (1966)

linked dissatisfaction to the degree of 'segregation' in the marriage, that is, when husband and wife have little shared interest and activity. Schmidt (1977) pointed out that this is a characteristic not so much of the working classes in general, but of the 'unstable working class', who suffer lack of regular and secure employment, have no vocational training, and who live in slum areas. He found little difference between the 'stable' working class and middle class in his German sample. Social-class factors are nevertheless of great importance, not only in influencing attitudes to sexuality and marriage but in affecting the acceptability and relevance of current methods of sex therapy. The basis of equality and reciprocal pleasure that is assumed in counselling is often difficult for the working-class man to accept. His sense of masculinity is often more dependent on the traditional 'double standard' sexual ethic, than is the case with middle class men.

The clinical presentation of sexual problems

In spite of the obvious importance of these interpersonal and 'non-genital' factors to common sexual problems, the clinical literature has tended to focus on genital or orgasmic responses. Recently there has been growing acknowledgement amongst sex therapists of the importance of other factors in working towards a method of classification that has clinical relevance.

Bancroft & Coles (1976) categorized a consecutive series of 200 patients attending a sexual problems clinic in the United Kingdom. They found that for women 'general unresponsiveness', that is, inability to enjoy lovemaking, or lack of any sexual desire, was by far the largest category (63 per cent). Only 18 per cent complained principally of orgasmic dysfunction and 12 per cent of vaginismus. Similar findings were reported by Mears (1978) from a larger sample of family planning clinic referrals. There is a striking difference between men and women and the way that they present their problems. Men predominantly complain of erectile or ejaculatory problems. Although complaints of low sexual interest appear to be increasing they are still in the minority and complaints of 'lack of enjoyment' are unusual. Women complain predominantly of 'loss of interest' or 'lack of enjoyment'. Complaints of orgasmic difficulty and vaginismus are infrequent by comparison. Women therefore emphasize the subjective quality of their sexual experience more than its physiological efficiency. Whereas for the male, erection is necessary for vaginal intercourse, women can get by with impaired genital response even if their enjoyment is impaired. But they may experience pain as a consequence, and pain is therefore a much more important problem for the woman than it is for the man. Sex role stereotypes also encourage men to judge their performance in physical terms and women to look more for interpersonal criteria of success. A third and probably crucial factor is related to age differences. Clinical populations consistently show that male presenters are older than female presenters. This age difference is almost entirely attributable to the 'erectile failure' group. This raises the possibility that physical factors related to ageing may underly many erectile problems.

Aetiological factors
The psychosomatic circle
Psychological factors influence our reactions to erotic stimuli and subsequently our physiological responses. In turn, our perception of these responses and the sensations accompanying them will further affect the system, either positively, when we are excited by our own enjoyment, or negatively, when we are made apprehensive by our apparent failure. The system therefore reverberates, positively, leading to increasing arousal and eventually orgasm, or negatively, leading to increasing failure. We can call this the 'psychosomatic circle of sex'. Breaking into the circle at specific points enables us to identify particular types of problem or pathology. Thus, studying the physiological mechanisms of erection may reveal impairment of vascular responses or their neural control, as in diabetics. Focusing on specific sexual beliefs may reveal negative psychological influences and so on. But only if we replace these specific factors into the total system, can we get their effects into perspective. For example, one man may develop minor impairment of erection due to slight peripheral arteriopathy or drug effect. He may take little notice of it, and his sexual relationship may be more or less unimpaired. The same degree of impairment in a man who for other reasons is sensitive about his sexual performance or insecure in his sexual relationship may cause repercussions in the system that lead to complete erectile failure. Conversely, a specific negative belief or value about the undesirability of women being highly sexually aroused or abandoned may be identified as the principal cause of orgasmic difficulty or unresponsiveness in one woman, and yet be found in another woman who

has no difficulty responding sexually (Fisher, 1973). The universal tendency to see problems as either psychologically or physically determined is never as misleading as it is in this field.

With this point very much in our minds, let us look at some of the factors that may interfere at specific points in the psychosomatic circle.

Physical factors in the male
Interference with normal erectile mechanisms may result from peripheral vascular disease, and in some cases this may be the only obvious manifestation of such disease. Erection normally becomes less efficient with advancing age. The reasons for this ageing process are not clear, but if it involves deterioration in the efficiency of the specialized valvular mechanisms that appear to be involved in normal erection, then more extreme forms of the same aging process may lead to significant erectile problems. Interference with the neural control of these vascular mechanisms, as in diabetes mellitus may also cause problems. Impairment of erotic sensory pathways resulting from disease or injury to peripheral nerves or spinal tracts, may also interfere with normal sexual response.

Side-effects of drugs are an important cause of sexual dysfunction, though in most instances the pharmacology is not understood, in particular whether the effects are peripheral or central. Drugs involved in lowering blood pressure are commonly implicated. Antidepressants present special problems, as depressive states are often associated with impaired sexual interest and antidepressants may produce both sexual improvement because of the alteration of mood and deterioration because of the other pharmacological effects (Beaumont, 1979). Androgen deficiency and hyperprolactinaemia, if severe enough, lead to loss of sexual interest and an inability to ejaculate (Skakkebaek et al., 1980). Peyronie's disease, a form of vasculitis of obscure aetiology, leads to interference with erectile mechanisms in the corpora cavernosa resulting in asymmetrical, and often painful erection, or if more severe, erectile failure. Cerebral pathology has a very unpredictable association with sexual dysfunction, though temporal lobe epilepsy is associated with a loss of sexual interest and arousability.

Local causes of pain in the penis, particularly from retraction of the foreskin (for example, balanitis) may inhibit sexual response.

Physical factors in the female

In the female enjoyable intercourse requires tumescence and lubrication of the vulva and vagina. Failure of such vaginal responses is likely to result in pain or discomfort when penile entry is attempted. Such discomfort effectively inhibits any further sexual response and serves to perpetuate the problem. Psychological inhibition is probably the commonest cause of failure of the vaginal response and the consequent discomfort. Evidence of arterial disease or peripheral neurological disease as important causes of dysfunction in women is lacking. The incidence of sexual dysfunction in female diabetics, though varying from study to study, does not appear to be as high as in male diabetics. Common local causes include vaginal infections and vaginal atrophy associated with oestrogen deficiency (for example, in postmenopausal, oophorectomized, or lactating women). Apart from this local effect, the role of hormone deficiency in causing female dysfunction is still uncertain (Bancroft, 1980a). Scarring or webs of skin that result from perineal tears, episiotomies, or inadequate posterior vaginal repairs may cause painful intercourse. Deep pain may be associated with pelvic pathology.

Psychological factors

Sexual problems are commonly accompanied by feelings of anxiety, tension, guilt, or anger. Whereas it is far from clear that sexual dysfunction is a direct consequence of these emotional states, it is reasonable to assume that they at least share a common cause (Bancroft, 1980a). Treatment aimed at alleviating the emotional disturbance is thus quite likely to improve the sexual response. Let us therefore consider some common reasons for these emotional reactions.

Misunderstanding and ignorance. Simple lack of basic knowledge about sexual anatomy and response can seriously impair an individual's self-confidence and lead to anxiety when sexual activity is attempted. But it is not unusual for individuals to use 'ignorance' as a cover for other difficulties, such as fear or guilt, that they find more difficult to reveal, either to themselves or to others.

Misleading assumptions about what is 'normal' and hence desirable are also widespread, resulting in self-imposed pressures which spoil sexual enjoyment. The belief that mutual orgasm is the 'proper' end to lovemaking, and that normal women

experience orgasm from vaginal intercourse alone, are two common examples.

'Bad feelings' about sex. Sexual pleasure may be regarded as wrong (and hence to be concealed if not avoided); only exciting if occurring in an illicit relationship; disgusting (perhaps reflecting an approach-avoidance conflict or, alternatively, fastidiousness about bodily cleanliness) or a threat to self-control. Those who see sex as acceptable only as an expression of affection and romantic love, may be disturbed by the high levels of sexual excitement as orgasm approaches. Such excitement is difficult to reconcile with a romantic concept of love, and orgasm itself is very much an individual experience, unlike the earlier and later stages of love-making. Sexual intercourse may be feared as painful or dangerous, often for women a self-fulfilling prophesy because of the vaginismus or vaginal dryness that such apprehension may produce. Fear of pregnancy was obviously the commonest and most reasonable fear before the days of effective fertility control. Sometimes these various fears have a phobic quality which may reflect a disposition to neurotic anxiety. But at other times, the apparent sexual threat is maintained in spite of reassuring experiences or information, because of other emotional benefits that result; so-called 'secondary gain'. Thus a phobia of vaginal entry may be used to protect an individual from the threat of an 'adult' sexual relationship and the responsibilities that this entails.

Low self-esteem. Feelings of discomfort with one's body-shape or physical appearance are not conducive to good sex, and affect many women who tend to rely on their physical appearance for their self-esteem. Men are commonly concerned about the size of their penis, and feel inadequate if they believe it to be small. Other reasons for low self-esteem may also have sexual repercussions. Low self-esteem is a characteristic of depressed states and depression may affect sexuality in other as yet obscure ways.

Relationship problems. Resentment and insecurity are two emotions that arise in sexual relationships and predictably produce sexual repercussions. Often the two emotions feed on one another. Of particular significance is chronic unresolved resentment. It is surprising how often couples fail to recognize the link between some long-standing feeling of hurt or resentment and problems in their sexual relationship. Communication in general is of fundamental importance and interpersonal problems that should otherwise be transient may become chronic because of poor communication.

In attempting to understand such interpersonal conflict, we have to consider not only 'here and now' causes of resentment and insecurity, but also the earlier factors in the individual's experience that have determined how such issues are coped with. Many learn to hide their anger or bottle it up, regarding open expression of emotion as undesirable. Often this reflects difficult attitudes to anger that prevailed in their families. The particular needs that an individual has in order to feel emotionally secure are also influenced by early experiences. In Fisher's (1973) study of female orgasm, the only characteristic that distinguished between women of high and low orgasmic attainment was in the latter a tendency to fear loss of close relationships linked with an earlier detached relationship with their fathers.

The 'here and now' problems that challenge a relationship include differing expectations of marriage and in particular conflict over assumed roles for men and women, an area that is of increasing importance in marital discord. Where more traditional expectations are shared, sex is often seen by the woman as 'her side of the bargain' in return for the emotional and material security she expects from her husband. Failure on his part may lead to her withdrawing her sexual contribution to the detriment of both. Failure of the husband to acknowledge the considerable difficulty that confronts the young mother with pre-school children and to provide appropriate support is another cause of resentment which is often compounded by the woman's sense of personal failure and loss of self-esteem in those circumstances.

At various stages during the life of a marriage each partner has to contend with crises in his or her personal development. Women may react adversely to the effects of ageing on their physical attractiveness or fertility; men may be undermined by failure or decline in their careers. Either may revert to extramarital affairs or flirtations in an attempt to bolster their flagging self-esteem, and as a consequence provoke feelings of insecurity and resentment in their partners.

Unsuitable circumstances. The importance of mundane factors such as lack of privacy or comfortable surroundings for lovemaking should not be under-

estimated. It can be of overriding importance among the less affluent. Pressures at work, and consequent fatigue, take their sexual toll of the affluent and poor alike, as the enhancing effect of a holiday so often confirms.

In general, it is difficult to associate particular types of sexual dysfunction with specific psychological factors. Men with premature ejaculation may be more prone to neurotic anxiety and those with retarded ejaculation to general inhibition. Vaginismus is often associated with neurotic personality problems. But these associations are weak. The form that a sexual dysfunction takes is probably determined more by the physiological vulnerability or earlier autonomic conditioning of that individual than by any specific psychological precipitants.

Assessment of patients with sexual problems

When confronted with an individual or couple complaining of a sexual problem, what are the objectives of the initial assessment interview? First, one has to consider the possibility of a medical cause which is curable or reversible by medical means. Secondly, if medical treatment is not indicated or is not sufficient to solve the problem, we have to decide whether limited advice and reassurance will be sufficient, or whether more concerted professional help is required, for example, a course of sexual counselling.

The initial interview

In the initial assessment interview, the following points should therefore be covered.

(1) Establish the nature of the sexual problem. Often the referral is misleading, the problem may not be sexual or may be relatively trivial. Not infrequently, the nature of the problem turns out to be quite different from that presented by the patient, or important aspects of the problem are omitted from the patient's account (for example, premature ejaculation of the partner in a woman complaining of orgasmic difficulties).

(2) How do the individual or couple feel about the problem? At this stage it may become apparent that one partner has lost interest in continuing the relationship and is seeking official approval that there is nothing that can be done to improve it.

(3) The therapist should respond appropriately to the expectations of the patient. If the patient believes that the problem is a physical one, an extra

effort should be made in discussing the evidence for and against such an explanation. In the process, the therapist should show that he knows what he is doing and is aware of the various alternatives. In general, the assessor is aiming to establish rapport that will help the patient or couple to approach treatment in a positive way.

(4) Take an adequate history of the individual's current physical health and past illnesses of possible relevance. In particular, careful note should be made of the drugs which are currently being used and which might interfere with sexual response or interest.

(5) Explain the nature of the treatment that is being offered, emphasizing the extent to which the onus for change and the need for the necessary commitment lie with the patient.

(6) Check on practical issues which may affect treatment (that is, whether suitable contraception is being used, whether the time is going to be available, not only for attending treatment sessions week by week but for a reasonably clear run free from interruptions such as change of job, moving house, and so forth). This adds further emphasis to the commitment that is required.

(7) Offer treatment and leave the patient or couple to make the decision whether to accept it. Often with a couple it is sensible to ask them to report back with a decision, having gone away to discuss it together and to consider fully the implications.

In making an offer of treatment it is important to consider whether sexual counselling is the most appropriate form. General marital counselling may be indicated when there is marked hostility between the couple or ambivalence in one or other partner about the continuation of the marriage or the wish to improve the sexual relationship. In some instances when the sexual difficulties are secondary to basic personality problems, individual long-term psychotherapy may be regarded as more appropriate.

Depression often poses problems to the clinician at this stage. Sexual counselling requires the active collaboration of the individual or couple if it is to succeed. If someone is too depressed, then this collaboration may be too difficult for them. On the other hand, depression is often a reaction to an unhappy marital or interpersonal situation and tackling that problem directly may be much more effective in improving the depressed mood and encouraging hopefulness than treating the depressed person as sick. A judgement therefore has to be made

whether the treatment of the depression should precede sex therapy.

Apart from these possible exclusion criteria, it is difficult to judge the likely outcome of sex therapy or to refuse treatment on rational grounds. Sometimes the most unlikely cases respond dramatically and vice versa. Probably the best indicator of a useful response lies in the reaction of the patient or couple to the first three or four sessions of treatment. Hence, if there are doubts about the suitability for treatment, it is appropriate to offer a 'limited contract' on the understanding that if there is no sign of progress at the end of a few sessions, the treatment will stop.

In practice, it is the patients themselves who most often make the decision about treatment, the therapist first having made clear what the treatment involves. This has the additional advantage of emphasizing the educational rather than the curative nature of sexual counselling and hence the need for the patient to accept in an adult fashion responsibility for the decision to proceed.

Physical examination

The indications for physical examination present one of the most important unresolved problems in the clinical management of sexual difficulties. There are two main issues; first, should physical examination be carried out routinely and of both partners? Secondly, should the physical examination always be done before counselling starts? It is uncertain what the cost-effectiveness of routine examination would be and the problem is complicated by the fact that a large proportion of sexual counsellors are not medically qualified. The primary need is for the recognition of the 'treatable' medical conditions (for example, acute vaginal infections, drug side-effects, and so on). The majority of physical causes of sexual dysfunction are unfortunately of an irreversible kind (for example, autonomic neuropathy or peripheral vascular disease) and the same sort of counselling approach is required in such cases to improve the sexual relationship or to make the best of the limitations imposed by the physical condition. It is arguable whether sexual problem clinics should be seen as places for screening pathology which is not directly relevant to the treatment of the sexual problem, but obviously recognition of medical conditions presenting as a sexual problem (for example, early diabetes mellitus) is important. A further complicating factor is the fear of physical examination, particularly in women with vaginismus. Ironically, this is the one form of sexual dysfunction which can be properly identified by means of physical examination. Nevertheless, it is important to build up the necessary trust and confidence in the therapist before confronting the patient with what is to her such a threatening procedure.

In general, there is a clear need for operational research on this important issue, but in the meantime there are some common-sense guidelines to follow.

(1) Sexual counselling should not be carried out in isolation from medical diagnostic facilities. Either patients should have received adequate physical screening (for example, by the general practitioner) before referral or a medical member of the clinic team should be available to carry out examinations when necessary.

(2) In multidisciplinary teams, some selection of the initial assessor should be based on the likely need for physical assessment. In doing so the following points should be considered.

(a) Age; above the age of 50 the likelihood of associated physical problems increases in both men and women.

(b) Pain; complaint of pain or discomfort during intercourse should always lead to physical examination.

(c) Evidence of recent physical illness or treatment. Non-medical assessors should check for such factors in their interview and ask a medical colleague to carry out a physical examination if there are any such indications.

(3) Vaginal examination in women with vaginismus should be delayed until an appropriate stage in treatment.

(4) Physical examination of either the male or the female should be seen as a valuable opportunity to learn about the patients' feelings and attitudes towards their bodies. Much clinically relevant material, apart from the direct results of the physical examination, will become apparent to the sensitive and perceptive examiner.

(5) Physical examination of males should routinely check the heart and blood pressure. Apart from obvious genital abnormalities, evidence of hypogonadism should be looked for (that is, small testes, deficient body hair, eunuchoid body proportions, gynaecomastia). In uncircumcised men, retraction of the foreskin should be checked. The penis should be palpated for indurated plaques (that is, Peyronie's disease). Evidence of deficient peripheral circulation and neurological abnormalities of the legs should be looked for.

In women, apart from a general check of the cardio-vascular system, particular care should be taken during genital examination to look for areas of local tenderness, both superficial and deep, and for evidence of vaginal atrophy or inflammation. The position of the cervix should be checked – is it low, is the uterus retroverted?

Laboratory investigations

Routine checking of urine for glucose is probably justified in men with erectile problems or delayed or altered ejaculation. Plasma testosterone and gonadotrophins should be measured when there is clinical evidence of hypogonadism or in the case of men over 50 in whom testicular failure may not be accompanied by obvious clinical signs. If low testosterone levels are found, plasma prolactin should be checked. Other investigations are obviously determined by clinical findings. As yet, it is difficult to base rational hormone therapy in the female on the results of laboratory tests except in the cases of clear cut endocrine disorder. Cytology of the vaginal epithelium may give indications for local oestrogen therapy, particularly in post-menopausal or post-oopherectomy women.

The distinction between organic and psychogenic dysfunction

Due to the advent of surgical methods of treatment for erectile impotence, particularly those, such as penile implants, which by providing a prosthetic erection determine that normal erection is no longer possible, it is obviously of some importance to distinguish between irreversible organic causes and the psychogenic ones which may respond to psychological methods. Considerable interest has been shown in the measurement of nocturnal erection for this purpose (Schiavi, 1979). The assumption is that the occurrence of 'normal' nocturnal erections (usually associated with REM sleep) is evidence of the psychogenic nature of the erectile problem and vice versa. This procedure is in fact being used to select patients for surgical treatment. But until its diagnostic validity has been properly established it is unjustified to use irreversible surgical procedures before a conservative policy involving adequate counselling has been tried.

Attention is also being paid to the angiographic investigation of impotence (Ginestie & Romieu, 1978) and it is claimed that a high proportion of men with impotence have some degree of obstruction of the blood supply to the erectile tissues. More research will be needed before these procedures can be regarded as part of the normal investigation.

The principles of sexual counselling

Methods of psychological treatment used for sexual problems reflect the full range of the psychotherapies, including long-term psycho-analysis and behaviour modification based on strict operant principles. In the past ten years, however, the major increase in sex therapy has been greatly influenced by Masters and Johnson (1970) and conforms to the style best described as behavioural psychotherapy. It is this approach which will be described here. Some consideration will also be given to non-psychological methods of treatment, though at present they play a small part by comparison.

The essence of behavioural psychotherapy is a combination of 'doing' and 'understanding', that is, getting patients to try things and helping them to understand the difficulties they have in carrying them out. The framework of therapy and the structure of the therapy session can therefore be summarized as follows:

(1) Set appropriate behavioural assignments ('homework'; the 'behavioural component').
(2) Examine the patient's attempts to carry out those assignments.
(3) As a result, identify those obstacles (attitudes, fears or other feelings) that underlie the difficulties encountered.
(4) Help the patient to modify or reduce those obstacles so that the behaviours can be carried out successfully (the 'psychotherapeutic component').
(5) Set the next appropriate behavioural assignments.

The particular strength of this combination is that the setting of relevant target behaviours is a rapidly effective way of uncovering the crucial interpersonal or intrapersonal problems that underlie these obstacles and have to be dealt with. Such an approach is a combination of behavioural change and discovery. The therapist can reasonably assume that relevant material will emerge during the course of treatment – it is not necessary to elicit all the information during the initial assessment. This means that there need be no delay in getting the patient actively involved and started on the behavioural programme, providing that appropriate assignments suggest

themselves. Let us look more closely at the components of treatment.

The behavioural component

Whereas in general, the specific behavioural assignments are chosen to suit a particular case, they are also influenced by whether the emphasis is on the couple or the individual, and if the former, whether it is the 'relationship' or the 'sexual performance' that receives primary attention. Let us, to start with, consider couple therapy, as this is both the most commonly used form of treatment and in many respects the easiest to apply. Sex therapists working with couples vary in their principal objectives. Many, including this author, focus primarily on the relationship. Thus the initial assignments concern the couple's method of communication during love-making, both verbally and physically and their ability to protect and assert themselves, and to make each other feel secure. The early 'sensate focus' stages advocated by Masters & Johnson (1970) are particularly effective in this respect. The couple are asked to accept limits on their love-making and to avoid any direct genital contact. They are encouraged to take time to touch one another anywhere except the genital areas. Initially the objective of the 'toucher' is to find ways of enjoying touching; the person being touched simply has to protect himself or herself against anything that is unpleasant. Later, the 'toucher' aims to give pleasure as well, and relies on indication from the partner as to what or where is enjoyable to the touch. Subsequently genital touching is incorporated following the same principles. Such assignments rapidly reveal problems of resentment in the couple, feelings of insecurity or lack of trust (for example, can the partner be trusted to keep to the limits?) and negative feelings relating to taking the initiative or experiencing pleasure without first giving pleasure.

When a couple is able to deal with a particular behavioural stage with no difficulty, they move on to the next stage without delay. On the other hand, behavioural progress may be halted for some time while crucial interpersonal or intrapersonal conflicts are resolved. The therapist who focuses on the relationship may thus use the 'sensate focus' assignments in a relatively standardized way at the beginning of a course of counselling, regardless of the nature of the specific sexual problem. Couples' reactions to these assignments, however, will obviously vary and have to be dealt with in an individualistic manner. As treatment proceeds, so the behavioural tasks become more tailor-made and specific techniques for dealing with premature ejaculation, vaginismus, and other specific dysfunctions are incorporated into the programme. Often the most important issues are dealt with even before genital touching is attempted. In other cases, the main problems only arise at this later genital stage, when fears of sexual arousal or loss of control and 'performance anxiety' are commonly encountered.

With the individual, presenting without a partner, there is no opportunity to focus on the 'sexual relationship' within treatment and hence a similar standardized start is inappropriate. But it is often relevant to focus on the individual's relationship with his or her own body, and assignments closely akin to 'sensate focus' but involving the one person are often useful. Frequently they need to be combined with other specific behavioural tasks and for this purpose a more detailed behavioural analysis may be needed before suitable assignments are identified.

CASE HISTORY

As an example, a 32-year-old man recently presented complaining of inability to ejaculate in the vagina. He had been married for 11 years to a woman who had never permitted vaginal entry – they had enjoyed mutual petting to orgasm. He left his wife two years previously, formed a relationship with a younger girl who enjoyed vaginal intercourse but the patient found himself only able to ejaculate outside the vagina. By the time he attended the clinic, this relationship had ended. Questioning revealed firstly that during masturbation, he never imagined vaginal intercourse, only petting. This raised the possibility that intravaginal ejaculation was threatening to him, even in imagination. He was asked to modify or 'shape' his fantasies (Bancroft, 1977) to incorporate images of vaginal intercourse and he was able to do this without difficulty. Further questioning indicated that in order to achieve orgasm during masturbation, he required very vigorous penile stimulation. As soon as he entered the vagina, the intensity of stimulation necessarily dropped. He was therefore advised to practise masturbating with gradual reduction of intensity of stimulation in order to slowly 'unlearn' the habit which was incompatible with normal intercourse. Because the intensity of stimulation required suggested a prevailing degree of psychological inhibition, he was also given individual 'sensate focus' instructions in order to become more relaxed with his own body and sexual responses.

Whether a suitable behavioural task can be identified for the individual patient varies from case to case and consequently individual counselling is more difficult from both treatment and outcome points of view. The possibility of group treatment in such cases will be considered later.

The psychotherapeutic component

In some cases, the setting of appropriate behavioural tasks is all that the therapist is required to do for improvement to occur. The reasons for this are usually not clear but the reduction of 'performance anxiety', the increased sense of security with the partner that follows the setting of defined limits, the information and education that inevitably accompany such behavioural analysis and goal setting, the enhanced sexual response that may follow a novel approach and the 'permission' of the therapist that explicitly or implicitly accompanies the instructions may all play a part.

In the majority of cases, whether individual or couple, difficulties will be experienced at some stage in carrying out a specific behavioural task. The psychotherapeutic skills of the therapist then become important. It is at this point that the inexperienced therapist is likely to flounder. Whereas there is no theoretical model which adequately accounts for what happens at this stage in successful counselling, it is still possible to define principles of action for the therapist to follow. These can be considered under two heads – (1) facilitating the patient's understanding of the specific difficulties encountered, and (2) taking active steps to help the patient resolve those difficulties.

(1) *Facilitating understanding.* Reaching an understanding of why one has difficulty carrying out a particular task is often followed by a reduction in that difficulty. Although in every-day problem solving this is usually a matter of recognizing a better way of going about things, in psychotherapy the explanation for the improvement that follows 'insight' is less obvious. Perhaps the most likely explanation is that the new understanding leads to a reappraisal of the problem and the beliefs and values associated with it. A female patient was finding that during her lovemaking sessions, she would start to become aroused and then rather suddenly 'switch off' and be incapable of any further response. After repeated experiences of this kind and continuing consideration of why this might be so, she eventually recalled that during her childhood she had the habit of masturbating to orgasm whenever she had been naughty and received punishment or criticism. She realized that the link between the sexual excitement and 'naughtiness' had made it difficult for her to incorporate her sexual response into the good and loving relationship she

had with her husband. Following this insight, the 'switching off' process ceased and she became orgasmic during intercourse. Having identified a cause for her difficulty, she was able to reappraise it in adult rather than childhood terms. This is an example of what cognitive therapists call 'cognitive re-structuring'. Such reappraisal is likely to continue covertly and between treatment sessions. But what can the therapist do to facilitate it?

(i) Setting further appropriate behavioural goals may help to focus on the specific problem. Identifying the difference between one's reactions to two subtly different tasks may be particularly helpful. Why, for example, is it possible for a woman to become aroused when her partner initiates the session, but difficult when she initiates it herself? Why is it difficult to show her partner how she would like to be touched, but easy to show what she finds unpleasant?

(ii) Encourage examination and description (labelling) of the feelings experienced at the time of the behavioural difficulty.

(iii) Encourage the patient to produce an explanation himself. The therapist should start to produce his own list of possibilities as soon as the difficulty is encountered and look for evidence to support a given possibility. But it is probably more effective if the patients can produce the best explanation themselves rather than have it provided by the therapist. Initially, it may be helpful to expose the patient to the same difficulty by repeating the homework assignments until it becomes obvious that there is a 'need to understand'. This need should then be stated explicitly and the patient encouraged to produce his or her own list of possible explanations and test them out. If this does not succeed, a Socratic method of questioning may be used in which the therapist, having a particular possibility in mind, questions the patient in such a way as to increase the likelihood that the patient will consider that possibility. As a last resort, explanations can be offered by the therapist, preferably giving a number of alternative possibilities so that the patient can still choose which is the most appropriate. The 'cognitive re-structuring' that follows is facilitated by the clarification of the precise difficulty and the correct labelling of the associated feelings. The therapist may further influence the process by authorization of the 'correct' interpretation as well as by implicit permission for alternative ways of thinking or responding.

The problem may, however, remain unchanged or incompletely resolved after such insight. Further steps then need to be taken.

(2) *Helping with the resolution of the problem.* The active steps taken by the therapist can be considered under four headings:

(i) *Making explicit the patient's commitments to specific changes.* At the outset, goals of treatment are usually vague, particularly if the emphasis is on improving the quality of the sexual relationship rather than the efficiency of the sexual performance. But as treatment proceeds and specific obstacles are encountered, it becomes necessary to establish whether or not the patient or couple want to overcome these particular obstacles or problems. Thus if a woman has difficulty in touching her partner's penis, is this something she wishes to overcome? Is the 'resistance' regarded by the patient as a nuisance (that is, 'ego-alien') or is it consistent wih his or her value system (that is, 'ego-syntonic') and not something that ought to be changed? Obtaining explicit commitment of this kind is the next appropriate step in counselling.

(ii) *Set further appropriate behavioural steps* specifically designed to overcome the resistance. Often the difficulty reflects fear of a 'phobic' kind. It is then appropriate to recommend a graded or hierarchical approach. Thus the woman reluctant to touch her partner's penis may be encouraged to do so initially for a very short period. A woman who fears anything entering her vagina may be encouraged to insert her finger a short distance and for a short time. In general, this approach involves the use of small steps which do not overwhelm the patient with anxiety, and the encouragement to 'stay with' the anxious feelings, rather than avoid them, until they start to decline.

(iii) *Reality – confrontation.* When the patient indicates no wish to overcome a particular resistance (that is, the 'ego-syntonic' reaction), the therapist has to judge the extent to which this will genuinely obstruct the course of treatment. This problem commonly arises in relation to masturbation; the therapist may recommend self-stimulation or individual 'sensate focus' as appropriate behavioural assignments, and not infrequently the patient refuses on the grounds that such behaviour is unacceptable. If the patient asserts that he or she came for help with the sexual relationship with his or her partner and not with their individual sexual feelings, then the therapist should look for alternative routes to reach that goal. If, on the other hand, the patient regards genital touching of any kind as unacceptable, then the therapist can justifiably point out that such a view is incompatible with the patient's stated objectives. Not infrequently, the therapist is confronted with a difficult decision, whether to accept the patient's values or challenge them for the sake of treatment (Bancroft, 1980c).

Often there is a need to confront patients with the inconsistencies between their beliefs or expectations and their actions. Such reality testing may involve providing factual information to challenge their beliefs (for example, the common belief that 'normal' women experience orgasm from vaginal intercourse alone, which may make it difficult for a woman to accept or enjoy direct clitoral stimulation). The permission-giving role of the therapist involves confronting the patient with inconsistencies between their values and the therapist's. Obviously for this to be effective, the therapist needs to have earned respect and to be seen in a positive light by the patient.

(iv) *Facilitating the expression and communication of affect.* As indicated earlier, there is commonly a link between sexual dysfunction and negative emotional reactions. Part of the process of understanding the difficulty is the correct labelling of these associated affects. Frequently, the affect stems from interpersonal problems, for example, security or resentment towards the partner. Few therapists would disagree that such feelings when unexpressed, or misunderstood by the partner, serve to keep the problem going. Thus an important function of the therapist is to facilitate their expression in addition to helping the partner understand them. Often the difficulties in doing so reflect the long-established attitudes to dealing with anger that the individuals have brought into the relationship; the belief that it is wrong to show anger or fear, that the relationship may be put into jeopardy by doing so. The therapist therefore has three tasks – first, to educate the couple in the adverse effects that unexpressed and misunderstood feelings produce in close relationships and in the healthy use of appropriate methods of expression; secondly, to help the couple to recognize specific instances when such feelings are arising and being inappropriately dealt with, that is, 'feedback'; thirdly, helping them to work out satisfactory ways of expressing and communicating their feelings.

CASE HISTORY

A couple presented with sexual problems. For some time their relationship had become strained because of chronic resentment on the wife's part that her husband was withdrawing into a world of his own and spending very little time with her. She at the time was concerned about her inability to conceive and felt that her husband, who was several years younger than she was and was keen to have children, was losing interest in her because of her infertility. He felt that she was becoming emotionally overdemanding and unreasonable and coped with this by withdrawing. Much of the communications that did occur involved critical and undermining comments in both directions. The first objective of the therapist was to help the couple to understand how each of their individual patterns of coping had aggravated the other, she with the tendency to become overdemanding and he with the need to withdraw. In each case failure to understand why the other one was reacting in that particular way led to resentment and further over-reaction. The likely consequence of this pattern on other aspects of their relationship, particularly the sexual, was then explained and the importance of expressing one's feeling of hurt clearly so that they were not misunderstood was emphasized. This was the 'educational component' based on the historical evidence. As counselling continued, they were then given specific indication of when such miscommunication was happening, during the counselling session itself and also on the basis of the weekly reports. This was the 'feedback' component. In each such instance the therapist discussed with them alternative ways of reacting that would be more effective and encouraged them to use these on the next appropriate occasion.

Other general principles of treatment

Throughout treatment, the therapist should strive to keep 'in touch' with how the patient or couple are feeling about the treatment. This is particularly important in the early stages when doubts about the appropriateness or acceptability of the specific treatment method may be experienced by the patient, though not expressed because of the wish to appear co-operative or respectful to the therapist. Frequently, however, the point of a specific instruction (for example, imposing a ban on genital touching and intercourse) is not understood by one or other of the couple. This may show itself in various subtle ways; apparent ambivalence about carrying out the assignment, evidence of weakening commitment to making or keeping appointments, turning up late, and so on. The therapist is advised to assume that the rationale for the behavioural steps is not properly understood or accepted the first time it is given. Regular checks should be made. It should be emphasized to the couple that treatment does not rely on magic, but rather on good psychological common sense. Hence, it is the therapist's responsibility to explain his approach in terms that are comprehensible to the patient. This gives permission to the patient to express doubts or scepticism and at the same time underlines the educational rather than the curative nature of the counselling. Not only should the therapist explain why particular assignments are given, but he should take trouble to ensure that the patient or couple have some understanding of why improvement does occur, so that should they run into further difficulties in the future they can apply the same principles without recourse to professional help.

Common doubts expressed by patients include the feeling that the behaviour programme is too clinical or too standardized. Certainly, the therapist should avoid going through a routine failing to respond to the needs of the particular case.

When working with couples, a special effort is often needed to maintain a reasonable balance in dealing with the two partners. It is all too easy to concentrate on one partner, giving the impression of 'ganging-up' on the other, or alternatively leaving the other to feel neglected. A partner may also collude with the therapist to foster this neglect so that he or she can maintain the role of being 'uninvolved'.

The basic theme of security in the sexual relationship is emphasized in the early stages by the authoritative setting of limits by the therapist. It should be remembered that this 'externalization' of control has to be gradually reversed so that by the end of treatment the couple have taken back the responsibility and have demonstrated to each other that they are capable of setting and keeping to limits when necessary. Only then will the feelings of safety continue beyond the end of treatment.

Practical considerations

Masters and Johnson (1970) have relied on intensive treatment programmes lasting two to three weeks requiring the couple to attend the therapists daily, living isolated from their normal every-day pressures. The advantage of this isolation (which is also experienced by many couples when they go on holiday) is countered by the need to integrate their improved method of relating into their normal busy lives when they finally return home. It may be that the advantages outweigh the disadvantages, but in most clinical settings this intensive form of treatment is not practical. Out-patient attendance on a weekly basis or less often is more usual. As yet, there are no firm grounds for determining the frequency of treatment sessions. One study failed to find any differ-

ence in outcome between weekly and monthly counselling sessions (Carney et al., 1978). But it makes good sense to start with weekly sessions until the therapist has established a working relationship with the couple and then vary the timing according to their needs. It is probably desirable to tail off treatment in the later stages so that the couple have plenty of time to assert their independence of the therapist before finally terminating treatment. When regular and frequent counselling sessions are stopped abruptly, there is often a tendency for the couple to lapse into inactivity as though they needed the incentive of regular attendance. This is particularly so when there is still scope and need for further improvement.

Other treatment approaches
Group therapy

Increasing interest is being shown in group methods for treating sexual problems. The basic approach is that used with couple and individual therapy; members of the group are given homework assignments and report back to the group. The main difference is in the use of the 'peer group', rather than of the therapist, to give 'permission' and to confront the patient with reality. Most attention has been paid to groups of individuals – particularly unresponsive or anorgasmic women (for example, Barbach, 1974) and to a lesser extent men without partners (Zilbergeld, 1975). Some therapists have used groups of couples (Kaplan et al., 1974; Leiblum et al., 1976). Evaluation of these methods is still minimal but the indications are that with some selection, group methods may be as effective as individual or couple therapy (Golden et al., 1978).

Drug therapy

Although there is a widespread tendency for doctors to use drug treatment whenever possible, there is still very little evidence to support such use in treating sexual disorders. Claims have been made for the value of monoamine oxidase inhibitors and certain tricyclic antidepressants in treating premature ejaculation, but the evidence still lacks conviction. Unless it can be shown that improvement in ejaculatory control continues after withdrawing the drug, it would be difficult to justify their use instead of appropriate counselling.

The therapeutic role of hormones still awaits clarification. Though, in the male, sexual problems associated with frank androgen deficiency are likely to benefit from androgen replacement, the female continues to present a riddle in this respect (Bancroft, 1980b). A recent study demonstrated apparent benefits from combining androgens and counselling in sexually unresponsive women (Carney *et al.*, 1978), but replication is required.

Other methods

At the present time, we are seeing a resurgence of interest in surgical methods of treatment, particularly for erectile impotence. Penile splints are now being used quite widely in the US (Renshaw, 1980) and surgical revascularization of the corpus cavernosum is receiving increasing attention (Michal, 1978). The proper indications for these methods await to be demonstrated.

The use of sex aids deserve some consideration. Riley & Riley (1978) reported better results in the treatment of female orgasmic dysfunction when vibrators were combined with counselling. It seems sensible to use them as potential supplements to, rather than substitutes for, the basic counselling approach.

Conclusions

Whilst much of the optimism about the treatability of sexual problems that has accompanied the new wave of sex therapy may turn out to be exaggerated, there seems little doubt that effective methods of counselling are being used more and more widely. Doctors and other health professionals can no longer justify turning a blind eye to sexual problems, and there is more to be gained than the resolution of these problems. Our understanding of psychosomatic principles is being enhanced by progress in the field, but there is much still to be learnt. In the past, the field of human sexuality has suffered from being regarded as a scientific 'soft option'. There is need for a special combination of scientific rigour and sensitive enlightened humanity.

9.2
Homosexuality

JOHN BANCROFT

There are two obvious ways in which homosexual relationships differ from heterosexual. First, they will not bear children and secondly, in most cultures, they will be subjected to social stigma. There may be other differences which will be considered later, but before proceeding, it is important to emphasize the extent to which social attitudes have confounded scientific or medical opinion on the subject. Thus, theories of causation have often been influenced by the wish to absolve the homosexual of responsibility for his state. Evidence that homosexual preferences can be altered by treatment may be exaggerated by those who believe in the desirability of suppressing homosexuality or rejected by those who are protecting the rights of an individual to continue in a homosexual life-style without any moral obligation to change or seek treatment. Dispassionate objectivity in this field is hard to find and it is with this qualification that the available evidence will be summarized in this section.

Although homosexual behaviour, particularly of the male variety, has been legally proscribed in most Western societies 'decriminalization' has occurred in many countries in recent years. In Scandinavia, Holland, Belgium, and France, homosexual behaviour between consenting adults has been legally acceptable for some time. In 1962, Illinois was the first American state to legalize homosexuality, several other states following suit. The law was changed in England in 1967. In Scotland, all forms of male

homosexuality remain proscribed though prosecutions are unusual if 'privacy' is maintained and the 'age of consent' is not breached. In the majority of countries, the law does not specifically concern itself with female homosexuality. In spite of the 'decriminalization', however, legal discrimination persists in various forms. In England and most States of the U.S., the age of consent is higher (that is, 21) for homosexual than for heterosexual relationships (that is, 16). Although men may solicit women, they may not solicit other men. 'Privacy' is defined in a much more restrictive sense for homosexual than for heterosexual acts. Penalties are more severe than for the equivalent heterosexual offence. Any form of homosexuality is illegal for members of the armed forces or merchant navy (Freeman, 1979).

The reason for this universality of social stigma amongst civilized societies is not clear. It is linked to repressive attitudes to sexuality in general and it is notable that those countries with the least negative attitudes to homosexuality, for example, Scandinavia and Holland, are those with long traditions of relative sexual permissiveness. Ford and Beach (1952) reported that a sizeable proportion of the primitive societies that they studied tolerated or accepted homosexuality. These were usually the generally permissive societies and it was apparently unusual, from the rather limited evidence that is available, to find exclusive homosexuality in these groups. Homosexuality was usually accepted as an alternative or transitional form of sexual behaviour.

Attempts to understand the origins of the stigma have considered the following societal mechanisms: hostility to minority groups and their use for 'scape goating'; the assumed link between sexual abnormality and other forms of antisocial behaviour; the offence against 'nature' (or God) and more precisely the rejection of non-procreative sex. Homosexuality may be seen as a threat to established 'norms' of behaviour, particularly as they relate to socially defined gender roles. Much of the hostility towards homosexuals is linked to the stereotypes of the effeminate male and the 'butch' female. On a more individual basis, 'reaction formation' by those who consciously or unconsciously fear a homosexual component in themselves, is often considered to be important. The church and the medical profession have both played very active roles in sustaining these negative social attitudes (Bancroft, 1974). Perhaps the church has shown an institutional form of 'reaction formation' as it has struggled over the centuries with the homosexual potential of its clerics (Bullough, 1976).

The incidence of homosexuality

For reasons that should now be obvious, it is difficult, if not impossible, to establish the true incidence of homosexual behaviour. As Gagnon and Simon (1973) point out, it is less important to be precise about the figures than it is to demonstrate that very large numbers are involved. Part of the problem lies in distinguishing between homosexual acts and homosexual individuals. From most points of view, the latter is more important. Regardless of the frequency or even the occurrence of homosexual activity, whether an individual regards himself or is regarded by others as 'a homosexual' will have an enormous impact on his life, through his career, his circle of friends, and possibly his psychological well-being.

The available evidence of incidence relates to behaviour rather than identity. The most important source is from Kinsey and his colleagues. Their original figures have been re-analysed in view of the disproportionate number of subjects with criminal records who have a particularly high incidence of homosexual activity. Gagnon and Simon (1973), as a result of this re-analysis, reached the following conclusions. They concentrated on a group of 2900 young men, at college between 1938 and 1950, the majority being under 30 at the time they were interviewed. They regarded this as the most representative subgroup of the Kinsey sample. Thirty per cent of this group had been involved in a homosexual experience in which one or other person had attained orgasm. The large majority of these experiences had occurred in adolescence, more than half before the age of 15. This left about 3 per cent with extensive homosexual as well as heterosexual histories beyond adolescence and 3 per cent with exclusive homosexual histories. A similar re-analysis of the female data showed that only 6 per cent (as compared with 30 per cent of the men) had undergone at least one homosexual experience including a mere 2 per cent who had had a significant amount of homosexual experience and an additional 1 per cent or less who were exclusively homosexual. Later large scale studies of men have reported around 1 per cent exclusive homosexuality and 1–3 per cent bisexuality, though these were not representative samples (Hunt, 1974; Pietropinto & Simenauer, 1977). Whether we are talking about 1 per cent or 10 per cent, we are considering large numbers of people.

The determinants of sexual identity, that is, whether an individual considers himself to be homosexual, heterosexual, or bisexual, are complex. Many engage in homosexual activity of a casual or impersonal kind, whilst maintaining a heterosexual relationship or front (Humphreys, 1970). For those who are prepared to declare their homosexual interest, there is a selection of homosexual subcultures which vary in the extent to which members can conceal their homosexuality (Hooker, 1967). But in the more open homosexual or gay world there is often a degree of intolerance of bisexuality, particularly amongst men. Of those acknowledging homosexual interest, women are more likely than men to consider themselves as bisexual (Bell & Weinberg, 1978). For many individuals, sexual identity is an evolving and sometimes fluctuating issue, depending on recent experiences. There is a 'threshold effect' – once you have 'come out' there are powerful social forces both in the 'gay' and 'straight' world that keep you there. But later experiences may still occur and cause the individual to reconsider his or her sexual identity (Blumstein & Schwartz, 1976).

The origins of homosexual preferences

Normal sexual development involves the coming together of the three main components of our sexuality; sexual responsiveness, formation and maintenance of emotional dyadic relationships and 'gender identity' (that is, sense of maleness or femaleness). Through childhood these remain relatively detached from one another. Around puberty we normally start to incorporate our sexual responsiveness into our relationships with other people and in so doing begin to establish our sexual preferences. At the same time, the nature of these sexualized relationships influences our gender identity and vice versa. Why it is that the majority of people sexualize relationships with members of the opposite sex is not properly understood. It is difficult to avoid the conclusion that social learning plays a major part. There are a wide variety of factors which may push us away from or pull us towards a particular type of relationship. A fundamental, and as yet unanswered, question is whether there is 'equipotentiality' for this social learning. In other words, is there a 'preparedness to learn' either homosexual or heterosexual preferences, and if so is it a result of earlier learning, say during infancy as many psycho-analysts would have us believe, or determined by innate characteristics? The search for genetic factors reveals a substantially higher concordance for homosexuality amongst monozygotic than dizygotic twins (Heston & Shields, 1968). But this may simply mean that genetic similarity increases the likelihood of responding to environmental influences in a *similar* way rather than in a *particular* way. Attempts to find hormonal characteristics of homosexuals that might suggest an innate basis have also been inconclusive and usually ill-conceived (Bancroft, 1978). Of interest has been the finding that some homosexual men have a hypothalamic response to oestrogen provocation which is suggestive of a female type 'positive feedback' (Dörner *et al.*, 1975). Have their brains therefore been hormonally 'feminized' in utero? Apart from doubts about the validity of Dörner's findings, his conclusions are based on the origins of positive feedback in lower mammals which do not appear to be relevant to primates or man. If however Dörner's findings are replicated, whatever the explanation, there may be some grounds for linking such hypothalamic mechanisms to gender identity development. As has already been mentioned, gender identity should not be equated with sexual preference but the two are interrelated. There is now increasing evidence that effeminate boys are likely to develop homosexual preferences when they reach adulthood (Green, 1980; Zuger, 1978) and a sizeable proportion of adult homosexuals recall evidence of effeminacy in their childhood (Whitam, 1977). It is possible, though as yet unproven, that genetic or other innate factors could influence such gender identity development and thus, indirectly, sexual preferences. But we can only find evidence of cross-gender identity in a minority of homosexuals and it does occur, though in a much smaller proportion, in the histories of heterosexuals also.

Gender identity could therefore be an important contributory factor but not a sufficient explanation for homosexual preference. It is nevertheless a useful starting point for discussing the complex and varied social learning that may be involved. In this respect we need to consider not only gender identity of a cross-gender type (that is, a boy feeling or behaving in a feminine way) but also the lack of confidence in one's assigned gender that may be fostered by such influences as an absent or emasculating father, an over-protective mother, physical disability, or genital abnormalities during development. Any of these features in a boy could have the following effects.

(1) Make him unattractive to the opposite sex or undermine his self-confidence in relating to them

so that attempts at heterosexual contact are likely to be unrewarding or even punishing.

(2) Make him attractive to other males who seek 'unmasculine' partners but aren't attracted to or can't cope with females.

(3) Motivate an escape from the competitiveness of the male world where he is likely to fail. An alternative is the homosexual world where there are different criteria for gender success (Hooker, 1967).

In a comparable way, we can consider the possible consequences of development of sexual anxiety or guilt, particularly in relation to the opposite sex. Such negative feelings are often learnt during childhood, possibly as a result of incestuous feelings or experiences, or alternatively the consequences of a sexually repressive environment in the home. Such anxiety may act as a 'push' factor away from heterosexual relationships. For those who have had problems in their dyadic relationships, particularly lacking a secure relationship with one or other parent, sexual relationships may offer them an alternative. Thus if a boy has been deprived of a good relationship with his father, a close relationship with another male may have special appeal.

In addition to the variety of factors that combine in leading us to our earlier sexual experiences, we also have to consider the social 'polarizing' forces that affect us once those initial experiences have occurred. In our particular society (but not in many others) we are strongly encouraged to believe that we are either homosexual or heterosexual. A homosexual experience is therefore seen as evidence of one's homosexual identity and subsequent heterosexual experiences then become less likely or, if attempted, become affected by lack of confidence.

It thus seems possible, and in my view most likely, that both heterosexual and homosexual preferences are determined by processes of a similar kind, though working in different directions. At present there is no reason to believe that these processes are different for the two sexes. The exclusiveness of sexual preference may be related to the polarizing social attitudes which are characteristic of a sexually repressive society.

Personality characteristics of homosexuals

Much misunderstanding stems from the prevailing stereotypes of the homosexual. I have already commented on the stereotype of the effeminate male or 'butch' lesbian and the fact that only a minority of homosexuals manifest such cross-gender behaviour. It is also commonly assumed that homosexuals are neurotic and unhappy. What basis is there for this popular image? Most of the evidence that might support such a view has come from studies of homosexuals attending psychiatric clinics. Schofield (1965) and others have shown that psychiatrically disturbed homosexual men have more in common with psychiatrically disturbed heterosexuals than with other homosexuals. It is therefore important that we do not rely on clinical populations for building up our picture of the homosexual in general. The best evidence is from the recent large scale studies of Weinberg and Williams (1974) and Bell and Weinberg (1978) from the Kinsey Institute. They did find a higher incidence of loneliness, lower self-acceptance, depression, and suicidal ideas in their male and female homosexuals compared with heterosexual controls. This was reflected in a higher incidence not only of previous suicidal attempts but also of seeking professional help. But it is important to stress that these problems were confined to a minority of the homosexuals and most were well adapted and happy. Siegelman (1972, 1978) found that although his homosexuals were more neurotic than his controls, this was accounted for by those with evidence of gender identity disturbance, thus adding further importance to gender identity development. Thus it seems reasonable to conclude that being a homosexual does carry certain problems but for most these can be satisfactorily overcome. How much of the difficulty is a result of the social stigma associated with homosexuality is difficult to say but it is likely to be a substantial proportion. This gives some validity to the decision of the American Psychiatric Association in 1974 to remove homosexuality from their list of diagnoses and replace it with 'sexual orientation disturbance' that is, those people who have problems adapting to a homosexual identity. Homosexuality *per se* has officially lost its medical status as an illness and the majority of doctors would now probably agree, though psycho-analysts persist in regarding it as pathological.

Other stereotypes concern the sexual behaviour of homosexuals, that they conform to heterosexual-type roles (being either sexually dominant or submissive) and are promiscuous. Although there are some homosexuals who are relatively exclusive in their choice of sexual activity (for example, always being the 'insertor' or 'insertee' during anal intercourse or fellatio), the large majority are much more flexible, responding to the needs of their partner in a way which is often lacking in heterosexual couples (Masters & Johnson, 1979). In some instances, the

particular pattern of sexual activity is neurotically determined, such as the compulsive fellator who seems to gain some boost to his self-esteem by fellating masculine men (Hoffman, 1968) but these patterns are not typical of homosexuals in general. Similar patterns abound in the heterosexual world and in such cases are not regarded as representative of heterosexuality.

Promiscuity amongst homosexuals is a more complex issue. Undoubtedly many male homosexuals experience sex with a large number of partners, to an extent which is rare in the heterosexual world. This does not seem to be the case with lesbians and one is left with the distinct possibility that the observed promiscuity is more to do with being male than being homosexual. In the heterosexual world, the promiscuous tendencies of the male are tempered by his more monogamous female partner. But added to this is the fact that society actively discourages stable homosexual relationships whereas it does just the opposite for the heterosexual pair.

Bell & Weinberg (1978), by means of factor analysis, arrived at a typology of relationships in the homosexual world. The 'close-coupled' pair is comparable to the happily married and faithful heterosexual couple. The 'open-couple' maintain a reasonably stable friendship with a fair amount of 'extra-marital' sexuality. The males in this category seem to cope better with this life style than do lesbians, reflecting the sex difference discussed above. The 'functionals' were not in stable relationships but enjoyed a wide variety of partners. They were younger and more highly sexed than the average. Once again, the males in this group had less problems than the females. The 'dysfunctionals' conformed to the stereotype of the 'unhappy homosexual', with recurring problems in their sexual relationships, often involving sexual dysfunction or discomfort with their homosexual identity. The 'asexuals', having low sexual interest, were more inclined to lead solitary existences. The proportions of males and females in each category are shown in Table 9.2.1. It should now be clear that the common stereotypes of the homosexual are not only misleading but tell us more about the attitudes of the heterosexual world than about the homosexuals themselves.

Helping the homosexual
The help homosexuals are likely to receive is strongly influenced by the attitudes of professionals

to homosexuality. Many homosexuals find that whatever their problems (medical or psychological) a heterosexual doctor is likely to attribute them in some way to their homosexual life-style. This must discourage attempts to obtain help. In Masters & Johnson's (1979) study of homosexuality, more than half approaching them for help had sought treatment for their sexual problems previously and of these about three-quarters had been refused help, many more than once.

There are now more doctors and health professionals interested in helping homosexuals in a relatively unbiased way but there is still a reluctance in the homosexual community to take up such help unless the professional is also homosexual.

Problems faced by homosexuals can be simply categorized as follows:

(1) Interpersonal (non-sexual) problems in homosexual relationships. To a large extent these are similar to those in heterosexual relationships and require the same sort of help.

(2) Sexual dysfunction in homosexual relationships. Once again, the treatment approach is basically similar to that described in the previous chapter (Masters & Johnston, 1979).

(3) Depression or other psychological difficulties in accepting homosexual identity or the social stigma associated with it. Here the person needs the type of counselling used for members of any stigmatized minority group; helping to distinguish between intrapersonal and interpersonal conflicts, attributing guilt in an appropriate way and learning to manage one's identity in public.

(4) Dissatisfaction with the homosexual role and desire for a heterosexual lifestyle, or some of its accompaniments such as bearing children. Until quite recently, when homosexuality was more likely to be viewed as an 'illness', such people were usually offered treatment aimed at suppressing their homosexual feelings, either by drugs or psychological methods such as aversion therapy. Over the past 10 years it has become apparent that not only are such negative procedures ineffective for such purposes, but it is more efficacious as well as ethically more acceptable to help such people to explore alternatives to homosexuality – in other words, to add to their behavioural repertoire rather than subtract from it (Bancroft, 1974). Even help of that kind remains ethically controversial, but most therapists would feel that an individual should be allowed and hence be helped to explore heterosexual relationships if he or she really wants to (see Bancroft (1980) for fuller discussion). How successful professional help of this kind is likely to be is difficult to judge. Masters & Johnson (1979) reported relatively good results with homosexuals who came to them with a potential heterosexual partner prepared to co-operate in couple therapy of the kind described in the previous chapter. Obviously, in such cases the important first step has already been taken before coming to the therapist and the outcome is therefore relatively hopeful. But there are a variety of other ways, mainly based on simple common-sense counselling about heterosexual skills and relationships which can be used with an individual without a suitable partner (Bancroft, 1977). In such cases, the eventual success in establishing a rewarding heterosexual relationship must be very uncertain at the outset, emphasizing the importance of maintaining and if necessary enhancing homosexuality as an alternative. The therapist in offering such help is proclaiming, in contrast to the prevailing social attitudes, that the quality of a sexual relationship is more important than the gender of the participants.

Table 9.2.1. *Typology of homosexuality* (*Bell & Weinberg, 1978*)

	Males ($n = 686$) %	Females ($n = 293$) %
'Close-coupled'	10	28
'Open-coupled'	18	17
Functional	15	10
Dysfunctional	12	5
Asexual	16	11
Unclassifiable	29	28
	100	100

9.3
Transvestism, transsexualism, and exhibitionism

A. WAKELING

Transvestism and transsexualism
Introduction

There is little doubt that in recent years changes in social attitudes have led to a more tolerant and less inhibited approach to sexuality. Currently there is more open and more informed discussion, and a growing awareness of the enormous diversity of sexuality and sexual behaviour between and within different societies. The crucial role of social and cultural factors in the shaping of sexual expression, particularly those aspects that are deemed masculine or feminine, is now well recognized. In recent years many of the basic assumptions about sexually dimorphic behaviour have been questioned and we have witnessed deliberate attempts on the part of many social groups to blur the previously well-demarcated modes of behaviour, conventions, and styles of dress between males and females. The desire of some men and women completely to adopt the cross-gender role has been recognized since antiquity. It is however, only in recent times that medical science has developed to the point whereby these desires can be partially realized by surgical or medical intervention. This has led to a greater awareness of cross-gender problems and an increasing demand for surgical transformation to the opposite sex.

In this climate two terms, transvestism and transsexualism, one old, the other relatively new, have gained currency. Although they are frequently used interchangeably they have distinct meanings.

Transvestism may be defined as the propensity to wear clothes appropriate to the opposite sex; it is technically the description of a behaviour. Transsexualism is a syndrome characterized by a disturbance of gender identity where there is a strongly held conviction that true gender is misrepresented by anatomical sex. It is related to transvestism only in the cross-dressing behaviour.

Aetiology

There is a profound lack of precise knowledge regarding the factors involved in the derivation of sexual behaviour. The determinants of gender identity, gender role behaviour, sexual preference, and sexual behaviour are still largely unknown (Wakeling, 1979).

Specific aetiological theories of sexual deviation have been promulgated from both psychoanalytic and learning theory. Psycho-analytic formulations focus on the importance of early infantile experiences such as pre-oedipal and oedipal conflicts and see sexual deviation as a defence against infantile castration fears. Rosen (1979a) and Stoller (1979) give detailed accounts of the psycho-analytic theory of sexual deviation, including transvestism and transsexualism.

Learning theory explanations of the genesis of sexual deviation emphasize the importance of events associated with the onset of sexual behaviour at puberty or during adolescence and the role of masturbation to deviant phantasies (Maguire *et al.*, 1965). Whilst such theoretical formulations are of interest, particularly if they generate testable hypotheses, they would appear to be too simplistic to account for the enormous complexities and variations of deviant sexual behaviour. Because of the lack of precise knowledge, the causes of any specific sexual deviation should be viewed in a multifactorial framework. It is prudent in the clinical situation to allow for a number of possible causal factors each contributing to a varying degree to the aetiology and to anticipate that different factors may operate at different strengths in different individuals with the same clinical condition. Specific genetic and constitutional factors, including perhaps the early hormonal environment may predispose towards the development of certain forms of sexual deviation. Early life experiences and relationships with parents, particularly the mother, will play a part in shaping psychosexual development, gender identity and gender role behaviour, and patterns of sexual preference. The experiences in relationships with both parents and peers during puberty and particularly at the time of first sexual experiences exert an influence in confirming a young person's sexual identity and behaviour (Erikson, 1968). It is possible that a complex variety of constitutional factors and early life experiences may predispose an individual to sexually deviant behaviour but that given favourable adolescent experiences with his peer group, a normal adjustment will occur. Conversely, adverse sexual circumstance during adolescence may tip the balance the other way with the onset of deviant behaviour. Whether this then continues will depend upon a whole host of factors which include the personality attributes of the individual, his attitude towards the behaviour, and the various rewards and contingencies associated with that behaviour. Once a pattern of sexual arousal and gratification is established during adolescence the tendency is towards persistence throughout life.

Transvestism

Transvestism occurs in a number of different conditions. It may occur as a manifestation of homosexuality: an effeminate homosexual on occasions may dress and effectively pass as a woman. It occurs in some individuals with severe psychotic illness associated with gross disturbance of psychosexual behaviour. It can present as a transient phenomenon in otherwise normal adolescents or adults. It occasionally develops in association with temporal lobe disease (Blumer, 1969). However, the largest and clinically most important group comprises those individuals whose cross-dressing is fetishistic. This is fetishistic transvestism and Stoller (1971) has suggested that the term transvestite should be confined to this group and this convention will be adopted here.

Fetishistic transvestism (transvestites)

The central characteristic of this disorder is that opposite sex clothes assume a fetishistic quality and cross-dressing is associated with sexual arousal and orgasm. Greenacre (1979) has succinctly defined fetishism as the obligatory use of some non-genital object as part of the sexual act without which culmination cannot be achieved. The object chosen, the fetish, may be some other body part, some article of clothing or an apparently impersonal object. In most cases the object needs to be touched or smelled or seen during or in preparation for the sexual act whether this is masturbatory or some form of intercourse. In fetishistic transvestism the cross gender clothes clearly assume the quality of the fetish.

General classification. This disorder is almost entirely confined to men. When women cross-dress it is seldom for the purposes of sexual excitement or gratification. There are three broad and overlapping groups of transvestites. First, there are those who are excited by a single female garment, typically panties, stockings, silk underwear, a brassiere, or a few such garments, and these remain fairly consistent throughout. These garments may be worn intermittently to produce sexual arousal as a prelude to masturbation or they may have to be worn to allow heterosexual intercourse to occur. In some individuals the garments are worn continuously beneath normal male clothing. The texture, style, appearance, or even the smell of the garments often have important significance to the transvestite. The second group comprises those in whom there is a gradual development of the desire to be completely cross-dressed and to pretend to be women for short periods of time that may encompass just minutes or may extend for a few hours. This complete cross-dressing is typically associated with genital excitement and sexual gratification. It may, however, in some individuals assume with the passage of time an anxiety- or tension-reducing function. In the third group the desire to completely cross-dress extends further as such individuals learn to pass skilfully as women and spend extended periods living as women. These transvestites often acquire extensive female wardrobes and are usually very concerned to imitate, down to minute details of dress and make-up, specific female fashions of the day. Some develop dual identities which may be startlingly different and which may be kept strictly apart. Typically, such a transvestite wants to pass as a woman when cross-dressed, but does not want to be a woman. Some element of sexual arousal is usually generated by the cross-dressing and successfully passing as a woman. The awareness of his penis beneath the women's clothing he is wearing is often a powerful source of excitement for such a transvestite. In some, however, there is a gradual diminution of the overtly sexual gratification element, and the desire to be a woman and not just to pass as a woman begins to crystallize. The gradual development of a transsexual condition may thus occur.

Further clinical features. The cross-dressing usually starts during puberty or adolescence. It may start in an intermittent way earlier than this and very occasionally begins in middle life. In retrospect, transvestites usually say that the cross-dressing started out of curiosity and that the first time a female garment was put on there was an immediate sense of excitement and arousal culminating in masturbation and orgasm. The experience is usually more intense than any previous sexual arousal and assumes all the qualities of a key experience. It is then repeated and continues to be secretly indulged whenever there is opportunity. The original experience may be further elaborated through masturbatory fantasies. The behaviour is often resisted for long periods because of strong feelings of guilt which may at times be overridden by the intense gratification afforded by the cross-dressing. The association with shame and guilt may continue, leading to considerable distress. For many transvestites, however, the fetishistic cross-dressing becomes an important part of their lives which they often manage to keep secret. Once established the behaviour tends to persist but may fluctuate in its expression. There is a tendency for the cross-dressing activities to decline with age, but in some individuals age changes lead to loss of control and the expression of more indiscriminate behaviour. In some transvestites the cross-dressing comes to assume with time an anxiety-reducing function and may be indulged in excessively during periods of stress or marked life change.

Fetishistic transvestism occurs principally in heterosexual men. Most transvestites are married and have children and prefer women as sexual partners in reality and in phantasy (Prince & Bentler, 1972). Their overt behaviour is that of typical male heterosexuals. Outwardly they lead normal sex lives, and many keep their vicarious sexual activity secret from their wives and partners. Great difficulties may occur in the relationship when their behaviour comes to notice.

Incidence. There is no specific knowledge of the incidence of fetishistic transvestism. In its minor form it is generally considered to be widespread, and perhaps the commonest sexual deviation after homosexuality. Most transvestites never come to the attention of either the medical profession or the law. They are not overrepresented in any one social or economic group and are apparently represented in all walks of life. (Prince & Bentler, 1972).

Treatment. Only a few transvestites ever seek advice or help from a doctor. There is in general a low moti-

vation for treatment or change because of the gratification associated with the behaviour. In addition, many transvestites do have a relatively normally heterosexual component to their lives running in parallel to their circumscribed transvestism. An understanding of the reasons for medical referral thus assumes importance. Some patients come to notice through the courts when they have been apprehended stealing female garments from a washing-line or a shop. Some seek help because of distress caused by mounting obligatory urges to cross-dress during periods of stress. Advice may be sought when a hitherto unsuspecting partner learns of the transvestism. In this context the transvestite is urged by the partner to seek help and cure, and the relationship is placed under great stress. In other cases a partner may have been fully aware and accepting of the cross-dressing which becomes a focus of dissatisfaction only when the relationship is strained for other reasons. Others come to notice because of changes occurring under the impact of primary physical or psychiatric disorder, often during middle or late life. A disorder of mood may be associated both with changes in sexual behaviour and in attitudes towards it. Any illness that impairs cerebral functioning may lower self-control, allowing the expression of more indiscriminate behaviour. This can occur at the onset of a dementia process or in association with cerebrovascular disease, epilepsy, alcohol dependence, or cardiovascular disease.

Treatment will thus be based on a full psychiatric, physical, and personal appraisal of the individual, including a detailed sexual history. The nature, development, and the factors that influence the expression of the transvestism, its meaning to the individual, and its impact on his own life and that of his family should be scrutinized. The factors related to the request for help must be fully ascertained.

The patients seeking help in general look for understanding, support or counselling rather than radical cure or change, although a cure is often pressed for by a partner or the family. It is perhaps this low motivation that accounts, in part, for the fact that prolonged psycho-dynamically-orientated psychotherapy or psycho-analysis has proved ineffective in these patients (Stoller, 1979).

Initially, any primary physical or psychiatric disorder should be treated. In individuals where the deviant sexual behaviour occurs as one aspect of a profound disorder of personality the general supportive, directive, and educational measures appropriate to such patients are utilized. It is helpful in these cases to attempt to increase self-control, and this will entail repeated examination with the patient of those events and circumstances which appear to trigger off deviant acts. Focusing in such a way on these precipitating events and working out with the patient more appropriate ways of coping with them can be beneficial. In some patients with marked personality limitations some increase in self-control might be all that can be achieved. In others approaches aimed at improving social skills and facilitating those elements of more appropriate sexual functioning that may be present should be considered (Bancroft, 1977).

For many patients it is important to include the partner in any treatment approach. This usually involves examining ways in which increased understanding and tolerance by the partner can help in the control and containment of the deviant behaviour. These approaches require tact and patience and the doctor usually has to settle for limited aims and goals. For instance, transvestism when carried out in private could be regarded as harmless and some understanding and acceptance of a limited form of cross-dressing within the home by the partner may bring about changes for the better. Acceptable compromises and limited changes can often be achieved.

In recent years some success in the treatment of transvestism has been achieved by behaviour therapy using aversive methods. So far, however, only small groups of patients have been treated and the follow-up periods have been relatively brief. Gelder and Marks (1969) showed that these treatments are most effective when the cross-dressing is entirely fetishistic, and are relatively ineffective in the presence of transsexual elements. Although experience of behaviour therapy in transvestism is limited it is worth considering in those fetishistic transvestites with no transsexual elements who have a genuine motivation for change and some normal heterosexual functioning.

CASE HISTORY

This patient illustrates the gradual transition from simple transvestism to complete cross-dressing. He presented first at the age of 66 at the instigation of his wife.

The patient comes from a middle-class professional family and is the eldest of five siblings. He was an active healthy child who achieved well at school and went on to University to take a Law Degree. After a period in the Royal Navy he married and had a successful career as a solicitor, achieving some eminence in his local law society. Two years prior to presentation he had retired and moved from Lon-

don with his wife to live in a coastal resort. His cross-dressing had started just prior to puberty with wearing secretly his sister's and mother's undergarments. This induced intense sexual excitement and was continued intermittently throughout his school and university life. From the age of 20 his cross-dressing gradually progressed until in his early twenties he was completely cross-dressing and possessed his own female wardrobe. At the time of his marriage he was regularly cross-dressing secretly at home and was only able to confide in his wife after marriage. She was initially shocked but in the early years of their marriage he was able to keep his behaviour largely away from her notice. However, gradually over the years he developed the desire to spend longer periods cross-dressed and would sit at home wearing a gown with wig and makeup. As this process continued the overt sexual gratification subsided and gave way to an urge to go out and pass in his own community as a woman. He did this for a number of years, going out only at night at enormous professional risk.

He was always rather timid and passive sexually and had a low sex drive. Sexual intercourse was infrequent throughout marriage and was usually initiated by his wife. They had two children who grew up normally and completely unaware of his cross-dressing. There was never any confusion of gender identity and he had no desire to attract men or to enter into any sexual relationship with them. He experienced a marked sense of achievement and satisfaction at passing successfully as a woman on his nocturnal excursions.

Following retirement the patient felt increasingly less able to control his urges to cross-dress. He was bored and restless and had started to drink alcohol in the day time and spend much of the day cross-dressed. Just prior to referral he had started for the first time to go out cross-dressed during the day time and had been questioned and almost recognized by one of his neighbours. His wife urged him to seek help at this time.

When seen the patient was adamant that he did not want to give up cross-dressing, as he regarded it as an important and enjoyable constituent of his life. However, he recognized that in his new environment control and secrecy were more difficult to achieve. The problems were discussed in a number of joint interviews with his wife who was prepared to accept a limited amount of cross-dressing at home but could not accept his going out cross-dressed. He was encouraged initially to take up some kind of activity during the day and to control his drinking. With help he found a part-time administrative post related to the law and in this context was able to curtail his drinking. With his wife's agreement a contract was then established whereby he was allowed to completely cross-dress on three evenings a week and to sleep dressed as a woman but was not allowed to go out of the flat cross-dressed. They both found this tolerable and the patient gradually felt he had regained control. Nevertheless he periodically experienced powerful urges to pass as a woman outside which he has managed to control over the last 2 years. The couple remain in contact and during periods of stress find joint interviews helpful.

Transsexualism

The central characteristic of the transsexual syndrome is intense gender dissatisfaction. Transsexuals have an inner conviction of belonging to the sex opposite to that represented by their anatomy and take active steps to live continuously in the opposite sex role. To this end they pursue sex conversion surgery and not only want to pass as members of the opposite sex physically but to be accepted by the community as such.

Clinical features. There is, as in all sexual disorders, a continuum of gender identity disturbance and some overlap with other conditions. Nonetheless a clinical differentiation between primary and secondary transsexualism is usefully made.

The primary transsexual is born anatomically normal and assigned to the appropriate sex. However from early childhood at a time when gender behaviour first appears there is the preferential development of behaviour appropriate to the opposite sex. For the male transsexual there is typically a lack of aggressiveness and an early display of effeminate behaviour. He begins to act as he were a girl with preference for girls' games and toys and the association with girls rather than boys. He will tend to adopt feminine modes of speech, dress and behaviour. In retrospect the transsexual will recall wanting to be a girl from an early age. He is, however, almost invariably treated by his family as a boy and is dressed and goes to school appropriately. At school he is often withdrawn and does not participate in physical games and play, and is usually regarded as soft and effeminate. There is intense distress at the onset of puberty and the outward physical manifestation of masculinity. By this time there are acute awareness of being different from other boys and strong secret longings to be a girl. He views his developing male genitalia with repugnance. In adolescence, sex drive is low and masturbation seldom occurs. Attempts may be made at this time to achieve a homosexual adjustment. This is soon given up as the transsexual is repelled by any sexual interest in him as a male. He gradually seeks employment in occupations more appropriate to women. There will usually be marked difficulties in achieving satisfactory relationships and problems with his family typically become manifest. The transsexual is painfully aware of living a lie and of having to conceal from others what he regards as his true identity. By late adolescence he will often have sought help with a view to sex reassignment and by this time he may well have learned to dress and pass appropriately as a woman.

In the primary male transsexual there is no development of masculine heterosexual behaviour. He never achieves the feeling that masculinity is valuable and there is no development of male genital sexuality. He is not homosexual and expresses preference for heterosexual men as partners: those who will want him as a woman not as a man. There is no fetishistic aspect to the cross-dressing. Primary female transsexualism, although less common, is essentially similar. In this condition there is an intense identification with masculine gender and gender role, and a lack of any real development of feminine heterosexual behaviour.

Secondary transsexuals, in contrast to primary transsexuals, develop some sex-appropriate identity and genital sexuality. They may develop for years in an outwardly normal way and some marry and have children. They usually report, however, in retrospect, that from the time of puberty or adolescence they were aware of an impulse or feeling towards being of the opposite sex. Typically there is an increasing urge to the cross-gender identity and cross-dressing behaviour develops. Subsequent evolution is varied and a homosexual or transvestite solution may be sought or develop. There is then a gradual crystallization of the transsexual state. For the male the desire to be a woman intensifies and there is a growing repugnance towards all aspects of masculinity. Masculine, erotic homosexual, and transvestite urges are all apparently submerged and sexual and civil reassignment as a woman is sought. These cases may be present in the third or fourth decade and can pose considerable diagnostic problems as there is clearly some merging with the categories of homosexuality and transvestism.

Incidence. The prevalence of transsexualism is difficult to establish. The syndrome is not common and there are difficulties of diagnosis because of overlap of secondary cases with other sexual deviations. Two epidemiological surveys, however, one from Sweden (Wålinder, 1968) and one from England (Hoenig & Kenna, 1974) demonstrated similar prevalence rates. The English figures were 1 in 34,000 for males and 1 in 108,000 for females. There is no firm evidence to suggest over-representation in any particular social class.

Differential diagnosis. Disorders other than transsexualism may manifest in part with gender disturbance, leading to a request for sex conversion surgery and sex reassignment. Adolescents with psychosexual problems or homosexual desires, schizophrenics with gender confusion, individuals with schizoid personality disorders, or those with chaotic personality structure may all occasionally present in this way. Homosexuals occasionally request sex reassignment in order to rationalize a relationship between two men. A transvestite may decide impulsively that sex conversion surgery will resolve the confusion and dilemma associated with living out two separate lives.

A systematic psychiatric history and full sexual history, together with proper evaluation of the mental state, will identify those individuals with psychotic illnesses or severe disorders of personality. Individuals who are predominantly transvestite will have retained elements of genital sexuality with some positive valuation of the male genitalia. The homosexual male, although he may cross-dress, will continue to identify with the homosexual milieu and will have a desire for erection and ejaculation during homosexual intercourse. Sex conversion surgery is contra-indicated in all these cases. Some individuals with the transsexual syndrome will show a number of abnormal personality traits and may lead very disordered and chaotic lives. In these transsexuals with coexisting severe disorder of personality surgery is also inappropriate.

Treatment. The goal of the transsexual is for civil and surgical sex reassignment. This is not cure but essentially a form of rehabilitation. Attempts by all forms of orthodox psychiatric treatments to bring about cure, that is, the acquisition of or return to a congruous masculine or feminine heterosexual adjustment, have proved singularly ineffective. Transsexuals characteristically refuse treatments other than sex reassignment, often threatening suicide or self-injury if their requests are not met. Sex conversion surgery for transsexuals remains a contentious treatment (Meyer & Reter, 1979) and its availability is limited. The dilemma is that although a transsexual may achieve a more satisfying life adaptation by living in the cross-gender role short of full sex conversion, he will continue to press vigorously and persistently for sex conversion surgery, despite all difficulties and possible complications.

In those cases where an initial diagnosis of transsexualism is made it is necessary to ascertain that the individual can live satisfyingly and with appropriate behavioural adaptation in the cross-gender role before a final diagnosis is reached and before the possibility of surgery is considered. This trial period should continue for at least two years. During this time the transsexual lives and works within the cross-gender identity. Civil status is changed and hormonal treatment is instituted. An appropriate regime for the male transsexual is either diethyl-stilboestrol 0.25–0.50 mg daily or ethinyl-oestradiol 0.02–0.05 mg daily together with medroxyprogesterone acetate 2.5 mg daily if breast development is insufficient with oestrogens alone. For female transsexuals testosterone oenanthate 200–400 mg every three to four weeks is given by intramuscular injection. These regimes usually allow the full assumption of the male or female role with reversibility of the biological changes if the hormones are stopped. However some male transsexuals will seek removal of facial hair by electrolysis to enable them to pass easily as females, and some female transsexuals may require mastectomy to resemble males anatomically.

To assume a full cross-gender role, and to live, work, and develop all the behavioural skills necessary for satisfactory adaptation is demanding. All the varied difficulties and complications of changing sex are experienced and have to be overcome. During this period the physician's role is essentially one of monitoring progress regularly and giving practical help where necessary. No commitments to surgery should be made. It is when faced with adapting in this way that those individuals with some ambivalence about conversion become discouraged by all the difficulties and voluntarily stop living in the cross-gender role. Others, particularly those who have retained some elements of genital sexuality or some fetishistic behaviour, will also give up the transsexual role during this period. A number of these patients will then continue to exist in a role somewhere between the sexes. Others will oscillate from one gender to the other, while some will achieve adjustment as either homosexuals or transvestites. Many will continue to press for sex-conversion surgery which is of course contra-indicated in patients who are not complete transsexuals. It is important to make this clear to the individual while continuing to offer such support and help as is acceptable.

For those individuals who complete a satisfactory trial period sex conversion surgery can be considered. These patients will have demonstrated that they can live satisfying lives with appropriate behavioural adaptation in the cross-gender role. To qualify for any surgical procedure the individual should be over 21 years, single, and supported in his request by at least one member of his family. Moreover he should have a sound personality structure. Previous antisocial and psychopathic behaviour contra-indicate surgical intervention. Serious depression or psychosis during the trial period is also a contra-indication to surgery. The individual should be of at least average intelligence and of a body configuration acceptable for the chosen gender. Surgical technique has now advanced to the point where cosmetically satisfactory and functional genitalia can be constructed for such patients. A number of follow-up studies have indicated benefit from these procedures, but experience is still insufficient to allow firm conclusions to be drawn (see Meyer & Reter, 1979). For those rigorously selected patients who come to surgery, adequate pre- and post-surgical counselling for the individual and his family is necessary (see Money & Walker, 1977). An account of the surgical procedures is given by Edgerton and Meyer, (1973). Continuing evaluation of surgically treated patients is essential in this field. So far, few surgically treated patients have been followed up into late life. The long-term psychiatric and physical consequences of surgical intervention are yet to be evaluated. Thus, although it is extremely difficult to resist the patients' pressure it is clear that agreement to sex-conversion surgery should be made only after lengthy and detailed investigation and knowledge of the individual transsexual.

Abnormal gender behaviour in childhood. There is much retrospective evidence and some limited direct evidence from prospective studies (see Green, 1977) linking atypical gender role behaviour during childhood with the acquisition of atypical sexual behaviour in adult life. Almost all primary transsexuals report cross-gender behaviour and cross-dressing during childhood. In addition, the retrospective accounts of many adult transvestites date the onset of cross-dressing behaviour to before the onset of puberty (Prince & Bentler, 1972). Persistent cross-gender behaviour and cross-dressing during childhood should therefore be viewed seriously. It might be that active intervention at this stage will hold out the best hope for the prevention of these sexual disorders which are so resistant to treatment once they are established in adult life.

Green (1977) and Stoller (1979) have described treatment programmes for children showing persistent atypical sexual behaviour. The primary goals of treatment for these children are to enable them to develop behaviour appropriate for their sex and to establish a positive and pleasurable anticipation of an appropriate adult sex role. If the child is a male he should have a male therapist with whom to identify; the family must also be included actively in the treatment programme. Parents are helped to identify and actively discourage feminine behaviour and to encourage and promote masculine behaviour. Close attention to family attitudes and interaction is important as by the time the child comes to treatment the family may be encouraging the atypical behaviour in a variety of subtle and often covert ways. Attempts should be made to promote a close father–son relationship, as typically feminine boys are alienated from their fathers. Close counselling of father may be necessary in order to include him fully, and joint activities with father are encouraged to promote a more positive male identification. On the wider front parents are helped to find appropriate peer-group experiences and interests for their son. Parents often discourage male peer-group activities when their son is effeminate and retiring: a change of school may be necessary to institute a new set of peer relationships.

Such treatment programmes are essentially pragmatic and their effectiveness has yet to be established. The importance of further research in this area cannot be overestimated.

ILLUSTRATIVE CASE HISTORY: PATIENT 1

This patient, now aged 24, is an example of primary male transsexualism.

He was born in Ceylon and is the eldest of three siblings. Shortly after the patient's birth his parents, who are both Hindu, came to England where his mother has worked regularly as a school teacher. His father, a barrister, has held numerous administrative posts abroad and has spent little time with the family in England.

According to his mother, the patient's early life and development were normal. He was however a little slower at school than his siblings and was regarded as somewhat shy, unathletic, and lonely. His gender difficulties first came to notice at the age of 16 when he was admitted to hospital after swallowing sulphuric acid at school. In the context of this episode of self-injury he first openly discussed his conflict and wrote to his mother directing her to the private diary he had kept for some years.

At 16 he was an articulate but shy and softly spoken young man, slim and attractive in appearance and retiring in manner. There was a definite female quality to his behaviour which was subdued rather than flamboyant. He described feeling from the age of 6 that he would like to be a girl and from the age of 10 that he really was a girl and desperately wanted to live as one. From the age of 11 he kept a private diary recording his thoughts and feelings. Thereafter he had become increasingly distressed as physical development as a male occurred throughout puberty and he became acutely upset when he had to start to shave. He had never worn female clothes but in attempting to conceal his developing maleness by wearing 'unisex' clothes and growing his hair long he had come into conflict with his parents. He was intensely preoccupied with the desire to become a woman but could see no solution to his dilemma. He had a low libido and denied any experience of masturbation and had no homosexual inclinations. He was found to be a physically normal post-pubertal male of average intelligence.

His parents were both shocked by his revelations and vehemently refused any suggestions that consideration be given to his living as a female. During the next 18 months he was engaged in intensive psychotherapy while being encouraged to continue to live as a male and to attend college. This was a very unhappy period as he found it increasingly difficult to identify himself as a male at college and eventually he refused to attend, spending much time locked in his room at home. He eventually terminated psychotherapy and continued to insist that he would like help to enable him to live as a woman and to proceed to sex reassignment surgery.

His father then took him to India where he was to be working for a year, on the assumption that a period in primarily male company would be beneficial. However this proved unhelpful and led to complete estrangement from his father. He returned home and again spent much time alone in his room. Following a series of threats to kill himself he was readmitted to hospital at the age of 19. At this time his mother very reluctantly agreed to allow him to try to adjust in a female role. Over a period of 2–3 months in hospital he started to dress and live as a woman. He made this transition easily, his appearance, movement, and behaviour allowing him to pass readily as a woman. He was prescribed female hormones and received electrolysis to remove facial hair. The previous history of dependence on his parents and his apparent psychosocial immaturity suggested that he might experience difficulty in adapting to the demands of his new situation. However, he was soon able to lead, for the first time, an independent life and he has worked successfully and continuously as a saleswoman. On discharge from hospital his mother refused any contact with him. He continued to press for surgery complaining that without this he was unable to develop other than superficial relationships with men. After two years living as a woman, sex reassignment surgery was carried out 2 years ago. The patient insists that this has been helpful but continues to experience difficulty in making lasting relationships with either men or women. During the last year there has been a reconciliation with his mother.

ILLUSTRATIVE CASE HISTORY: PATIENT 2

This patient, now aged 41, is an example of secondary male transsexualism. He presented at the age of 31 with a request for 'sex change' surgery after previously having lived as a heterosexual and a homosexual.

He comes from a working class background. His parents were divorced when he was aged 9 and his father had spent little time in the family home before that. He has a brother 13 years older with whom he has had little contact. During childhood there was no conscious recognition of gender disturbance and he saw himself as a normal male. However, during adolescence he was distressed on becoming aware of his sexual preference for men rather than women. He initially felt guilty and ashamed and there were two minor episodes of self-injury. He gradually became reconciled to his homosexuality although at that time he was never able to accept it completely. He led an active sex life as a homosexual until at the age of 24 he married in an attempt to establish himself as a heterosexual. Initially there were no difficulties in his new sexual role and the couple had twin children. However, after 2 years of marriage he reverted to homosexuality and subsequently left his wife.

At 29 he met his current partner, an avowed homosexual of the same age, when they started to live together. They had an active and mutually enjoyable sexual relationship, with the patient usually taking the passive sex role. In the context of this relationship the patient started to experience a subjective sense of femininity.

When seen at the age of 31 he described the gradual development over the previous year of the feeling that he was becoming increasingly feminine and had persistent notions that he wanted to live as a woman.

There was no evidence of formal psychiatric disorder or drug or alcohol abuse and he had a stable work record and a circle of homosexual friends. There were some suggestions of stress in his relationship with his partner who was unhappy about the patient's avowed intention of sexual transformation.

The patient was then engaged in regular psychotherapy during the next two years. Throughout this period he continued to live with his partner, but the transsexual notions persisted and became more dominating. He felt he was becoming more and more female and started to cross-dress occasionally at home, with feelings of relief and self-fulfilment. At the end of this period he decided to live as a woman. Sexual contact with his partner ceased and the patient had started to view his own genitalia with repugnance. Gradually, over a period of six months, he changed his mode of dress, adopting unisex clothes and letting his hair grow so that he was able eventually to pass as either a man or woman depending upon the circumstances. He then felt confident enough to live entirely as a woman and he moved with his partner to a new neighbourhood where they lived as man and wife. He was able to pass acceptably as a woman and with his partner's support pressed for surgery. This was refused but female hormones were prescribed regularly during this period. After 2 years his partner left him and started to live again as an unattached homosexual. Shortly after this the patient ceased living as a woman, moved again, and lived alone as a single, rather effeminate male. Three years ago the patient and his former partner came together again and re-established their former relationship. The patient has been living entirely as a woman since then and continues to press for surgical transformation.

Exhibitionism

Definition. Exhibitionism is a pattern of behaviour which can be defined narrowly as an act of genital exposure to someone of the opposite sex who has not requested such a display. The term exhibitionist is confined to those for whom such genital display serves as a source of sexual excitement or pleasure in itself: the exposure being the sole sexual aim. Exhibitionists are thus distinguished from those who expose themselves to express a desire for intercourse or masturbation and those whose exposure is a prelude to sexual assault. They are also distinguished from paedophiles who may expose themselves to children as part of a general immature personal and sexual contact with them.

Indecent exposure is a legal term used to define an offence. An exposer is someone who is convicted of, or at risk from, conviction for indecent exposure. Radzinowicz (1957) has shown that the great majority of exposers are exhibitionists.

Incidence and forensic aspects. There are no specific figures available for the prevalence of exhibitionism in the general population. However, the fact that indecent exposure is the commonest type of sexual offence committed by adults suggests that it is not uncommon. Forensic studies (Radzinowicz, 1957; Mohr, Turner & Jerry, 1964; Gebhard, 1965) have demonstrated that genital exposure is exclusively a male offence, usually committed by men under forty, with the highest proportion being in their twenties. The majority of convicted exposers have a good prognosis, in that up to 80 per cent are never reconvicted after their first offence. This suggests that the trauma of a court appearance may be a sufficient stimulus to enable these individuals to control their urges subsequently. However, for those convicted a second time there is a high risk of persistent recidivism. The prognosis is worse when there is exposure to children, when the offender has had previous convictions for non-sexual offences, and when there is evidence of severe disorder of personality. However, the recidivist exposer is generally more a social nuisance than a menace, in that although his prognosis is poor in relation to his exposing he seldom progresses to more serious or violent sexual offences (Rooth, 1971). Nevertheless it should be borne in mind that this progression has been documented in a few cases (Gibbens *et al.*, 1977).

General classification. Exhibitionists are usually of normal intelligence and are not confined to any one social or occupational group. Two general groups are recognized clinically (Rosen, 1979b). The largest comprises those of relatively blameless personality but who are generally timid, shy, unassertive, and sexually inhibited. They are usually sensitive, touchy, easily upset, and discouraged by life's vicissitudes. Many are immature in appearance and behaviour and the tendency is towards underachievement. They often resist their impulses to expose: exhibitionist acts usually follow some sexual or social trauma or disappointment or minor humiliation. Following the act they feel guilty, humiliated, and ashamed of their behaviour. The second group are those with more serious personality disorder. They are much less inhibited and often have marked psychopathic traits associated with poor impulse control. Individuals in this group are more likely to have other sexual deviations, psychiatric disorders and a history of non-sexual crime. The recidivist offenders usually come from this group.

Further clinical features. Early sexual development is usually unremarkable, with a normal onset of puberty. However, from this time there is often continuing conflict and uncertainty about potency, masculinity, and physical appearance. Difficulties in establishing heterosexual relationships are encountered and sexual timidity and hesitancy develop. Many exhibitionists marry but their sexual lives are usually unsatisfactory: impotence, premature ejaculation, and a ready retreat into sexual phantasy and masturbation are common. The marriages, however, often to older partners, are usually surprisingly stable.

Exhibitionism typically starts in the late teens or early twenties. The behaviour usually begins after a period of mounting impulses to expose, associated with a period of increasing life stress. In others it can start without prior warning, apparently fortuitously. For example a youth may be masturbating in a state of high arousal when a woman happens to pass and see him, and he may then deliberately expose to her on impulse. Yet others start deliberately after feeling humiliated by a female partner, or after some other personally wounding sexual encounter. The specific circumstances of the first exposure usually become highly charged with sexual excitement and this helps to establish an habitual pattern of exposing. Enormous risks are then taken in repeating the act and this may occur with mounting recklessness until it is terminated by police arrest. As these episodes are typically associated with increasing life stress or depression of mood or physical illness there is often relief at being apprehended.

For the exhibitionist the essential components of the act are that the penis should be seen by the female and that she should respond in a shocked or horrified way. There is a tendency for the exhibitionist to expose in a premeditated way in a specific place and at a specific time to a female with specific characteristics in an almost fetishistic way. He typically has no desire for intercourse or intent to harm his victim or make any contact with her. The act concludes when the penis has been seen and the exhibitionist rushes off to masturbate, immediately or later, to the memory of the scene. The act itself has a powerful and complex meaning to exhibitionists (Rooth, 1971).

Aetiology. There are no specific data available about aetiology and the comments about the derivation of abnormal sexual behaviour outlined earlier under transvestism and transsexualism have general application. The most comprehensive theories are those derived from psycho-analysis and these are well outlined by Rosen (1979b).

Treatment. Individuals are referred for psychiatric treatment either prior to conviction or more commonly from the courts following conviction. First-time offenders are often referred even though the court appearance appears to be an effective deterrent in itself for most of them. The small group of recidivist offenders pose the greatest therapeutic problems.

A good prognosis is indicated for those patients with a reasonably stable personality who have achieved some elements of mature heterosexual functioning. A general psychiatric approach is appropriate to the treatment of such patients where, within a therapeutic alliance, the doctor attempts to utilize what strengths the patient has to encourage self-reliance and autonomy, and to encourage positive change. Emphasis is placed on understanding those factors which prevent the full expression of healthy sexual behaviour rather than suppressing the unwanted behaviour. Understanding the ways by which frustration and inability to express angry feelings may lead to exposing is often important. Focusing with the patient on such precipitating events and examining possible alternative styles of behaviour can be helpful. Attempts are made to increase understanding of the nature of the relationship to the patient's partner, particularly those aspects related to

the themes of dominance and submission. A sympathetic and understanding partner who is willing to co-operate can be very helpful in this general approach. Specific treatment to control excess anxiety and to stabilize mood may be appropriate. There may be a need to alter environmental circumstances, and a skilled social worker can be an important adjunct to treatment. In some patients behavioural treatments such as systematic desensitization to the heterosexual situation may form part of the overall treatment approach. Such a general clinical psychiatric approach can be very rewarding in a proportion of patients.

A poor prognosis is indicated by severe disorder of personality associated with poor impulse control and lack of development of adequate heterosexual relationships. Patients in this group tend to offend persistently and it is clear that long prison sentences provide no answer to these problems. These individuals require more specialized help and pose a considerable therapeutic problem. The two main approaches to treatment are group psychotherapy and behaviour therapy. Group psychotherapy approaches have been reported to be successful in some of these patients (see Rosen, 1979b). Experience suggests that such treatment should be carried out in a group containing people with similar problems and should continue for a minimum period of six months. In some of these impulsive repetitive exhibitionists the chemical suppression of sexual behaviour for a period may allow the individual to become more accessible to psychotherapeutic intervention. The drug of choice is cyproterone acetate which is an anti-androgen and suppresses hormonally determined sexual behaviour without producing feminization (see Wakeling, 1977, 1979). The normal treatment regime is an initial daily dose of 100 mg until libido has been decreased and inhibited followed by a daily maintenance dose of 25–50 mg.

In recent years there have been a few reports of exhibitionists being successfully treated by behaviour therapy. Systematic desensitization, electric aversion therapy, and self regulation techniques have all been shown to be effective, albeit in a small number of patients and with short periods of follow-up (Rooth and Marks, 1974). Although experience in this field is limited, these techniques do hold out the possibility of rapid control of unwanted behaviour. If available they should be offered to persistent offenders unresponsive to other approaches.

9.4
Incest (child referred to psychiatrist) (See also chapter 12.2)

SULA WOLFF

Incest is an emotive topic. To highlight this, a clinical illustration precedes the more general discussion.

A CASE REPORT

An intelligent and charming 15-year-old came to a child psychiatrist with her somewhat mannish mother because of their violent conflict over the girl's association with a young, delinquent man who had recently left his wife and child. Two months previously the patient's father had left home because of local gossip over a theft from his employer.

This father, dominated by his mother in childhood, had met his more intelligent wife, the patient's mother, through their joint interest in ballroom dancing. He was the better dancer. Twelve years after their marriage he lost his job, began night work, started home brewing and drinking by day. The mother became critical and sexually unresponsive. It was at this time, when his daughter was ten, that he began to make sexual advances to her just short of intercourse. When she was thirteen this behaviour ceased and only then did she inform her mother. The mother became even more distant from her husband, he continued to drink and finally, after the theft, left home.

The mother disclosed the incestuous relationship between husband and daughter with much hesitation, worried that it might have to be reported to the police. She blamed herself for what had happened. Of her daughter she said 'She wouldn't go with him and I never knew why. From ten years onwards I used to wonder why she didn't go and she didn't want to be alone with him . . . I've thought about it for two years. I just wish I could have done something to spare her this.'

The mother used the current crisis over the boy-friend, whom the patient insisted she would marry as soon as she was of age, to contact her husband. Her greatest wish was to re-establish their former, better relationship, to get him off alcohol, and have him rejoin the family. This she succeeded in doing and only later did she reveal that her own father had been a police sergeant who saw things in terms of black and white, whom she and her brother often deceived about their childish misdeeds and who was always reprimanding her brother. 'Policemen', she said, 'see such a lot of bad. Once a person's bad they watch him and nothing he does is ever good . . . My father has a way, when you do something wrong, of making you feel that size (one inch) and it doesn't do anything for anyone's morale.' It became clear that she had decided to manage things differently. Symbolically she would act like the understanding father she had always longed for.

Commentary

This case illustrates the subjective explanatory links between experiences within the family of origin and subsequent life decisions. The 15-year-old girl chose a boy-friend whose predicament resembled her father's. The mother chose a husband with whom she could identify and for whom she could be as she had wanted her father to be towards herself in childhood. He in turn put his wife into a position of power over himself, resembling that of his mother when he was a boy.

The management of this case was simplified by the father's initial absence from home, the girl's age, and the fact that there had been no incestuous activities for two years. No special care arrangements were needed and the question of legal procedures involving the girl in giving evidence against her father never arose. The emotional damage to the patient had been done. It was increased because she blamed herself for her parents' deteriorating marriage after her revelations to her mother. She was helped by her mother's eventual success in re-establishing the marriage, and psychiatric treatment was aimed to support the mother in her efforts.

The patient paradoxically accepted that it was illegal for her to have intercourse with her boy friend while under age. By the time she was 16 they had parted. But she then embarked on a series of superficial relationships which her mother saw as a reaction to her past excessive intimacy with her father. The law relating to the age of consent had protected this rather impulsive girl from an early marriage unlikely to succeed. The law relating to incest had failed to protect her and her father from a pathological relationship likely to have profound effects on her adult sexual adjustment. The fact that legal procedures could be avoided protected the girl from more guilt and preserved the family intact, safeguarding 1979), and the legal implications have been discussed

(Scottish Law Commission, 1980)and treatment approaches described (Mrazek & Kempe, 1981).

Review of the literature

Incest has recently been reviewed (Bluglass, 1979), treatment approaches described (Mrazek & Kempe, 1981) and the legal implications discussed (Scottish Law Commission, 1980).

There are no adequate, controlled studies of the antecedents and consequences of incest involving children. Incest has most often been studied by examining offenders before the court or after conviction in prison. The established characteristics of this group of sex offenders (Gebhard *et al.*, 1965) are not particularly helpful in clinical practice. On the other hand useful summaries of clinical experience often lack acceptable scientific method. Weinberg (1955) found that sisters reported brothers more often than daughters accused fathers, suggesting that incest between siblings is less shocking than between parents and children. In this study, offending fathers had often themselves been reared by violent fathers and tended to be single or widowed. Oldest daughters were the commonest victims, and affected families often had a marginal socio-economic adjustment. Peters (1976) examined child victims of sexual assault, including incest, and makes three helpful points. While sexual offences against a child by a stranger unite the family, incest does not. If the father is the offender, the mother vacillates between believing and protecting her child and loyalty to her husband. Fathers as a rule deny sexual approaches to their children (some may occur in states of altered consciousness) using massive psychological defences, and mothers tend to feel that if they believe their child they will have to disown their husband, perhaps even report him to the police. Serious psychological harm can be done to children if no one believes them, dismissing their accounts of paternal behaviour as fantasy (not only have they been seduced, they are now distanced even more from their mothers). Cowie and colleagues (1968) report incest experiences in a number of female runaways. Promiscuity and lesbianism are possible later consequences.

Meiselman (1978) reviews the literature and reports on a comparison between patients attending a psychiatric clinic run by a commercial firm for its employees who revealed incest at some stage in their lives, and a control group of similar patients who did not. Brother/sister incest although thought to be commoner, was in fact less common than father/daughter incest in this group of disturbed adults, and mother/son incest was rarest. Women seduced in early childhood were more disturbed than those seduced later. As in Weinberg's study, poverty and very poor fathering in the offending father's childhood were common. Some offending fathers were extremely dominant, moralistic, and intrusive. Unemployment with much father–daughter contact in the home and alcoholism were other features.

In this study adult patients who had experienced incest had more marital conflicts, more sexual difficulties, and more physical symptoms than other patients, but it was not possible to evaluate separately the effects of incest and of the pathological family functioning which had preceded and followed these events.

A comparison of women who had had incest with their fathers in childhood and women whose fathers had been merely seductive showed that the first group more often ran away in adolescence, attempted suicide, and had early pregnancies. The incestuous fathers were more often violent and their wives more often were chronically sick or disabled (Herman & Hirschman, 1981).

Clinical Management

In child and adolescent psychiatry treatment of incest in a family is based on a number of principles, which are akin to those used in the management of non-accidental injury.

(1) The clinician needs to accept that the events reported to him actually took place. At once children feel understood and less isolated. He needs to be aware that older children are likely to accept some responsibility for the events and to have considerable guilt feelings.

(2) The next task is to protect the referred child and any other children at risk from further sexual advances without taking any action that would be destructive to other members of the family, including the offender, and of the family as a whole.

(3) While siblings can often face up to their own incest behaviour, parents can rarely do so. Family interviews are often difficult because fathers tend to be totally resistive. It is usually the non-offending partner (that is, most often the mother) who is the pivot in treatment.

(4) She can contribute most by either not permitting husband and child ever to be alone together or by allowing the children at risk to be taken into the care of the local authority social services depart-

ment. If she can accept the child's statements without rejecting her husband or reporting him to the police, she will not only have protected him from experiences likely to increase his personality deterioration but she will also have protected the child from having to give evidence against her father and from sharing the responsibility for the break up of the family.

In practice, many cases are referred when the police are already involved. The child victim may have talked to neighbours who alerted the police; the mother may have contacted the police directly; or she may have approached a local authority social worker who has responsibilities to society as well as to the individual client and may have considered it her duty to inform the police. Child psychiatrists can even be helpful at this stage by offering to provide a psychiatric report on the father to his solicitor, by protecting the child from having to give evidence in open court, and by ensuring, with the help of social services departments, that there are adequate safeguards to protect the child and any other children at risk from further sexual advances.

(5) What is less certain is how affected children can be protected from deviant personality development as a result of their early seduction, their abnormal family relationships, and their inevitable loss of respect for their father.

Brother/sister incest

Sexual activities between siblings are very common in early childhood but persisting sexual activities in middle childhood and adolescence and full intercourse are rare. Psychiatrists who see children and adolescents that have had such experiences usually find a background of family neglect and lack of affectionate care. Sexual activities between non-related children and adolescents occur in poorly run boarding schools and residential children's homes. Between siblings they take place when either both parents or single parents managing a family alone have serious personality deficits, for example, associated with mental deficiency, schizophrenia, or alcoholism. Children turn to each other for physical comfort, for the relief of boredom and for secret, mutual (sexualized) expressions of outrage against the parents.

10
Alcoholism, drug dependence, gambling

10.1
Childhood antecedents of alcoholism and drug dependence

P. T. d'ORBÁN

Although abnormal personality development and neurotic symptoms may render patients vulnerable to dependence on drugs or alcohol, there is no characteristic 'addiction-prone' personality and a variety of both social and psychological factors contribute to the development of dependence. When a drug is widely used and socially accepted (as is the case with alcohol) many individuals without serious psychopathology may become dependent on it. By contrast, with socially prohibited drugs personality anomalies play a more important role in the genesis of dependence. However, the patterns of psychological disturbance in childhood which predispose to alcoholism or drug dependence in adult life are not specifically predictive of the dependency syndromes. Similar adverse patterns may occur also in the backgrounds of patients with personality disorders who do not become dependent on drugs or alcohol. Social and environmental factors operating in adolescence and adult life play a crucial role in the development of dependence. Among these factors are exposure to drugs or alcohol, availability, peer group pressures, and the social context of drinking or drug use. Some environmental factors also operate in childhood. Parental example influences attitudes to drugs and alcohol and instils norms of drinking behaviour. For example, McCord and McCord, (1960) noted parental disagreement on drinking attitudes and parental conflicts about drinking in families of children who later became alcoholics. A study of young Irish and

English drinkers suggests that parental attitudes towards alcohol as perceived by their children are an important determinant of ethnic differences in drinking behaviour (O'Connor, 1978). Similarly, illicit drug use by adolescents is in part related to their perception of parental use of psycho-active drugs or alcohol (Kandel, 1974).

Childhood antecedents of alcoholism

In established alcoholics Kessel and Walton (1974) describe several personality patterns. Passive, immature, dependent personalities are said to have strong oral dependency needs and are overattached to their mothers. Self-indulgent personalities have overprotective parents; as adults they seem unable to tolerate frustration and crave continuous gratification. The self-punitive often have over-strict or rejecting parents; they are unable to express hostility and appear to use alcohol in a self-destructive way to relieve tension. However, some of the personality traits attributed to alcoholics may be the consequences of their dependence rather than causative factors. Prospective studies have failed to confirm such childhood attributes as passivity, overdependence, oral tendencies, neurotic traits, or parental overprotection. On the contrary, evidence from these studies suggests that alcoholics as children are more self-assertive and aggressive than passive or dependent. In a 20-year follow-up of boys from the Cambridge–Somerville Youth Study, McCord and McCord (1960) found that boys who developed alcoholism were characterized in childhood by self-confident, aggressive behaviour and the absence of childhood fears and inferiority feelings. Parental conflict, inconsistent maternal affection, maternal resentment of her role in the family, parental escapist reaction to crisis, and paternal rejection and punitiveness were some of the significant features in the families of alcoholics compared with controls.

More recent studies suggest that childhood conduct disorder predisposes to alcoholism. In the Oakland Growth Study (Jones, 1968) boys who subsequently became problem drinkers were undercontrolled and rebellious in childhood. Robins (1966) in a 30-year follow-up of children seen at a child guidance clinic found that those who became alcoholics were characterized in childhood by antisocial rather than neurotic symptoms. They had poor school performance and high rates of truancy, theft, and running away from home. The childhood behaviour of the potential alcoholic resembled that of the potential sociopathic personality. Their family backgrounds were also similar, with high rates of parental separation or divorce, fathers who drank to excess, and siblings who were frequently antisocial. Studies of adoptees have also shown a significant correlation between childhood conduct disorder and subsequent alcoholism (Goodwin et al., 1975; Cadoret & Gath, 1978). Alcoholism in the adoptee was associated with a history of alcoholism in the biological parent, suggesting that genetic factors may be more important than childhood family environment.

In recent years there has been an increase in the incidence of alcoholism and alcohol-related problems in young people. Young alcoholics generally display marked personality disturbance; they show significantly more antisocial behaviour than those with a late onset (Foulds & Hassall, 1969; Schuckit, Rimmer, Reich & Winokur, 1970) and they more often have disturbed family backgrounds. Glatt (1974) noted that adolescent alcoholics frequently experience emotional deprivation and psychological trauma in childhood. There is often a history of heavy drinking by one parent and dominance by the other, difficulties in sexual adjustment, and antisocial behaviour or social withdrawal.

(See also vol. 2, Chap. 14.)

Childhood antecedents of drug dependence

Many studies of young drug abusers or addicts have found a high incidence of personality disorder associated with family disruption and antisocial behaviour predating drug use. However, it should be borne in mind that these studies are retrospective and that they deal with subjects identified in a particular setting such as treatment clinics, penal institutions, or circumscribed communities. The findings from studies of such groups are not necessarily applicable to middle-aged therapeutic addicts who develop drug dependence during the course of medical treatment, nor to addicts in other societies where drug dependence is endemic and widespread, for example in Iran (Mehryar & Moharreri, 1978). There are also rapid changes in the patterns of drug abuse and the characteristics of addicts and the findings have to be seen in their historical context. Although young drug abusers and addicts in Britain are a heterogeneous group and stereotypes should be avoided, they commonly have disturbed family backgrounds with a high incidence of parental separation, divorce, illegitimacy, and poor family discipline. Educational under-achievement and an unstable work record are characteristic. Female opiate addicts show a high incidence of disturbed psychosexual development with homosexual orientation (d'Orbán, 1970). A significant proportion of opiate addicts have a history of convictions prior to drug use (Wiepert, d'Orbán & Bewley, 1979). The relationship between drug abuse and delinquency is parallel rather than causative, with common underlying factors leading to both forms of behaviour (d'Orbán, 1973). Studies of delinquent adolescent drug abusers in remand homes suggest that the degree of their involvement with drugs is proportional to the severity of their personality disorder and adverse childhood background (Scott & Willcox, 1965; Noble, 1970). Although young drug takers in the community show much less biographical disturbance, here, too, those who are most committed to drug use have more adverse backgrounds (Plant, 1975). Adolescents who both abuse drugs and have a history of a juvenile court appearance, whether for delinquency or for being in need of care, are especially vulnerable to future progression to more serious drug involvement (Noble & Barnes, 1971).

An important conclusion which emerges from studies of the antecedents of both alcoholism and other types of drug dependence is that the young patient is particularly likely to have a disturbed family background, prior antisocial behaviour, and serious maladjustment. Any treatment plan should take account of these problems.

10.2
Drug dependence
P. T. d'ORBÁN

Definitions

From the point of view of their pharmacological action, drugs of dependence are classified as narcotic analgesics, CNS depressants, stimulants, and hallucinogens. There has been much discussion of terminology in the field of drug dependence but the definitions of the WHO Expert Committee on Drug Dependence (WHO, 1974) have now been generally accepted. *Drug abuse* is defined as persistent or excessive drug use unrelated to or inconsistent with acceptable medical practice. *Drug dependence* is defined as a state, psychic and sometimes also physical, characterized by behavioural and other responses which always include a compulsion to take a drug on a continuous or periodic basis in order to experience its psychic effects, and sometimes to avoid the discomfort of its absence. The characteristics of dependence vary with different drugs and the type of dependence must be specified. In morphine, alcohol-barbiturate, and amphetamine dependence, *physical dependence* may occur and is characterized by a specific withdrawal syndrome when consumption of the drug is abruptly stopped or substantially reduced. Other drugs produce only *psychological dependence*, defined as a drive to repeat drug consumption in order to produce pleasure or avoid discomfort. Psychological dependence postulates conscious awareness of drug use. Thus physical dependence may occasionally occur without psychological dependence, for example in the new-born children of opiate-dependent mothers or in patients treated with opiates who are unaware of the nature of their treatment. The physiological mechanisms underlying tolerance and dependence are discussed in volume 2, chapter 15. However, as the WHO definition implies, drug dependence is essentially a psychic rather than a physiological phenomenon.

Psychological aspects of dependence

A characteristic that drugs of dependence have in common is that they reduce anxiety or alter mood in a way which is experienced as desirable or pleasurable. For the psychologically dependent individual the effects produced by a drug become necessary to maintain an optimal state of well-being (Jaffe, 1975). Psychological motives for initiating and continuing drug use include self-medication for anxiety and depression, recreational or hedonistic use, or the desire to experience altered states of consciousness in a search for self-knowledge or spiritual experience. The pharmacological action of drugs is modified by psychological factors and there is considerable individual variation in response to psycho-active drugs. Drug effects are influenced by the personality of the user and his mental set: his attitude to drugs, his motives for taking them, and his mood and expectations. Thus it is not surprising that placebo effects are common, especially in young drug abusers; the expectation of a 'high' can produce a stimulant effect from a pharmacologically inert substance or even from a major tranquillizer. Psychological dependence may vary in degree from an intermittent and mild desire to take cannabis or LSD, to the strong craving and compulsive drug use of the established opiate addict. When psychological dependence is severe, preoccupation with drug-seeking and drug-taking may lead to deterioration of moral standards and impairment of inter-personal relationships and social adjustment.

Social factors

Drug effects are also influenced by the social setting in which the drug is taken. For example, smoking cannabis or drinking alcohol by oneself may have little euphoriant effect, whereas the same dosage taken in a social situation among friends may produce a pleasant experience. Similarly, adverse reactions to LSD are less likely to occur in the presence of a friend who is an experienced user. Social influences are especially significant in initiating drug use in a non-medical context; the commonest examples are the influence of peer groups in starting to smoke or to drink alcohol. Taking illicit drugs may be an expression of disaffection with conventional social norms. There is some evidence that the use of cannabis among students occurs in this context (Kosviner, Hawks & Webb, 1974). For the rootless, emotionally disturbed adolescent drug-taking may provide a means of escape from his problems and a path to acceptance in a drug-using subculture which bestows social rewards for drug use and a sense of identity as a drug user or a 'junkie'.

CASE HISTORY

Drug abuse as a solution to the disturbed adolescent's search for identity is illustrated by a patient aged 23 from an unhappy family background. He was a lonely, shy, insecure boy, who truanted at school and mixed with older delinquent boys, accompanying them on shop-lifting sprees. At 14 he started smoking cannabis, grew his hair long, and wanted to become a hippy. At 16 he started taking amphetamines, barbiturates, and alcohol and wanted to join the Hell's Angels. He had no motor cycle and no friends belonging to this group but he tattooed himself with the name of an imaginary Hell's Angels chapter and wore appropriate clothing. At 18 he started injecting barbiturates, amphetamines, and later heroin. He was unable to obtain regular supplies of heroin and did not become physically dependent, but his only ambition in life was to become a heroin addict and to be registered as such at a drug dependence clinic. Thus he went through a series of phases as a juvenile delinquent, hippy, Hell's Angel, and junkie, and used drugs regarded as appropriate to these roles, hoping to gain acceptance in a group. He failed in all of them and he is now a solitary drifter and an incipient alcoholic.

Dependence as learned behaviour

Neither the social and psychological factors that initiate drug use nor physiological factors can by themselves adequately explain the compulsive feature of severe dependence, its lasting nature, and the phenomenon of relapse after prolonged periods of abstinence. Learning theory has made a useful contribution to understanding the processes of initiation, continued use, and the interplay of psychological, social, and physiological factors that perpetuate dependence (Wikler, 1975). The initial drug experience may be pleasurable, neutral, or often (as with opiates or tobacco), unpleasant. Social reinforcement through acquisition of companionship or status, or pharmacological reinforcement through euphoriant or anxiolytic effects help to establish a pattern of repetitive drug use. If physical dependence develops the person learns to take the drug to suppress withdrawal symptoms and the relief of symptoms then reinforces continued drug use. Eventually drugs are used to anticipate withdrawal symptoms before their actual onset, as an anticipatory avoidance reaction. Even with drugs that do not cause physical dependence, psychic discomfort becomes a stimulant to further drug consumption. Drug use may then become a generalized conditioned response to unpleasant psychic states of tension, anxiety, or boredom. Relapse after prolonged abstinence can be precipitated by environmental cues that have become associated with drug use. In such situations withdrawal symptoms may occur as a conditioned response in addicts who have been abstinent for prolonged periods. Conditioning to injections (becoming a 'needle freak') is well recognized by many addicts who feel they are more addicted to the process of intravenous injection than to any particular drug.

Clinical features
Drug dependence in adolescents

Experimentation with drugs is usually a transient event in adolescence and the great majority give up taking drugs. Progression from relatively harmless experimentation to habitual abuse and dependence is symptomatic of maturational delay and emotional disturbance. The clinical observation that serious adolescent drug abusers show marked emotional immaturity is supported by controlled studies using the MMPI (Brook, Kaplun & Whitehead, 1974). Their immaturity makes them especially ill-equipped to deal with the stresses of adolescence. A smaller but more obviously disturbed group suffer from depressive mood swings, with feelings of failure, emptiness, and low self-esteem; they lead an unstable, drifting existence and seek oblivion in drugs such as barbiturates with apparent indifference to the consequences.

The rapid changes in patterns of adolescent drug abuse reflect the availability of drugs from illicit sources or from prescribing by doctors. At such times small localized epidemics of abuse occur among young people, for example opiate abuse in a West Country town (James, 1973) or solvent abuse in Lanarkshire (Oliver & Watson, 1977). Opiate dependence in adolescents has remained a limited problem and Home Office statistics show a progressive decline in the number of notified opiate addicts aged under 20, from a peak of 764 in 1968 to 34 in 1980. Offences involving controlled drugs have also shown a marked decrease in this age group. However, it is possible that the recent increase in heroin supplies will in future again lead to an increase in the number of adolescent opiate addicts. The prevalence of adolescent amphetamine abuse has also declined as a result of legislative controls and more cautious prescribing, although there is some abuse of illicitly manufactured amphetamines. Of medically prescribed drugs barbiturates and sedatives are the most frequently abused. Among drug-dependent individuals identified in London casualty departments Ghodse (1977) found that barbiturates were the main problem, but in addition a wide range of non-barbiturate hypnotics and minor tranquillizers were abused, often in combination with alcohol. A high incidence of multidrug abuse was noted, and many had obtained their drugs from illicit sources. The management of barbiturate abuse and drug overdosage in young people is discussed in volume 2, chapter 15.

There is less awareness of the abuse of drugs that are available without prescription and are therefore readily accessible to adolescents. They include caffeine tablets ('Pro-Plus'), proprietary asthma remedies ('Do-Do' tablets containing ephedrine and caffeine) and cough syrups ('Phensedyl' containing ephedrine and codeine). The preparations containing caffeine and ephedrine are taken for their stimulant effects, but mild physical dependence of the opiate type may occur in those who take large amounts of codeine. The author has encountered several adolescents seriously dependent on 'Phensedyl' and a boy who developed an amphetamine-like psychosis on 'Do-Do' tablets.

The inhalation of glues and volatile solvents has attracted more attention (see volume 2, chapter 15). The substances used include a variety of readily available household products. Adhesives are the most popular and generally contain toluene; nail-varnish removers contain acetone, lighter fuels contain butane, and dry cleaning fluids and aerosols contain halogenated hydrocarbons; petrol-sniffing has also been described. Solvent inhalation is usually a group activity predominantly of boys aged 12 to 16. In the small minority who continue into their late teens or early twenties sniffing has usually become a means of escape from emotional problems rather than a recreational activity, and they develop psychological dependence. Physical dependence can occur on toluene but it is not a significant feature. However, habitual abusers of glues containing toluene develop marked tolerance and may use large quantities. The usual method of use is to smear adhesive inside a plastic bag which is then held over the face and intermittently inhaled; liquid solvents are inhaled directly or from a saturated cloth. The immediate effects are euphoria, intoxication, and perceptual disturbances, followed by drowsiness and stupor if inhalation is continued. The harmful effects usually arise from intoxicated behaviour but there is also a risk of suffocation from the plastic bag. Manufacturers rarely specify the composition of their products but if necessary information can be obtained from Poison Centres. Fortunately, toluene which is the most widely used substance is relatively non-toxic although weight loss, mild anaemia, renal abnormalities, polyneuropathy (Goto *et al.*, 1974), and several cases of encephalopathy (King *et al.*, 1981) have been reported. Cleaning fluids containing trichloroethane and aerosols containing fluorohydrocarbons are far more dangerous and carry a significant risk of sudden death from cardiac arrest (Bass, 1970).

CASE HISTORY

Some of the problems associated with severe solvent-dependence are illustrated by a boy aged 17. He was the youngest child of elderly, rigid parents and grew up in an atmosphere of family discord. A brother and a sister became delinquent and another brother became a heroin addict and died at 21 from an overdose. The patient had an IQ of 115 but his scholastic performance was poor and he was eventually excluded from school for sniffing glue. His first contact with glue was through making Airfix models and he started sniffing at the age of 12. By the age of 13 he was sniffing glue regularly on the school playground and all his friends were also glue-sniffers. From 14 to 16 he had numerous juvenile court appearances for car theft and burglary, activities which he found exciting and which relieved his boredom. During this period his glue sniffing diminished but when his delinquent behaviour temporarily ceased he again started heavy glue sniffing. He used a half pint tin of 'Evostick' daily, sometimes mixing it with petrol, sniffing alone in his room continuously for 4 to 8 hours during the evening and night and sleeping during the day. He suffered a marked loss of weight and became hostile, irritable, and occasionally violent, smashing his furniture or assaulting his girlfriend. He developed ideas of reference and paranoid ideas about being chased by policemen. He was unable to sustain any relationships and became increasingly solitary and withdrawn; two girl-friends left him because of violent behaviour when he was intoxicated with glue. Despite a variety of treatment approaches he repeatedly relapsed. When last seen at the age of 20 he was facing a charge of burglary and still using glue. An unusual feature was that he did not escalate to the abuse of other drugs or alcohol. His glue-sniffing and delinquency initially seemed to some extent interchangeable and shared a common element of risk-taking behaviour providing excitement and relief from boredom and tension, but by his late teens glue-sniffing came to dominate his life.

Clinical features determined by personality and social adjustment

Some of the symptoms and the psychiatric complications (for example amphetamine or cocaine psychosis) are specific to a drug and related to its pharmacological action. However, the clinical features of dependence are determined more by the patient's premorbid personality and social adjustment than by the specific drugs on which he is dependent. The mode of initiation into drug use provides a broad distinction between two psychosocial patterns of dependence. *Therapeutic addicts* who become dependent on prescribed drugs tend to be middle-aged, females predominate, and their prior social adjustment is relatively stable. The onset is related to illness or to an adverse life-event for which they seek medical help and their dependence develops in the course of treatment. They use drugs as a means of coping with insomnia, anxiety, inadequacy, or depression. They attempt to conceal their dependence and their drug use is solitary and secretive. *Non-therapeutic addicts* are a contrasting group who take illicit drugs and their dependence is unrelated to medical treatment. They are predominantly young males and are initiated into drug use through association with other drug users. They commence taking drugs for recreational or hedonistic motives. Those who progress to serious dependence are usually unstable personalities and show antisocial behaviour and other features of personality disorder rather than neurotic symptoms. They are nearly always multiple drug-users and the clinician should be alert to the possibility that they may be simultaneously dependent on more than one drug, for example opiates and barbiturates. They sometimes progress to intravenous drug use. They associate with other addicts and tend to form a subculture with a distinctive life-style. However, it should be emphasized that these are generalized descriptions and that in practice there is considerable variation and overlap in these patterns. Chronic opiate dependence of non-therapeutic origin is compatible with stable social functioning (Stimson, 1972). Conversely, some therapeutic addicts may have severe personality instability prior to drug use while others may gradually develop deterioration of social functioning and moral standards as a result of chronic dependence.

CASE HISTORY

An example of such deterioration was shown by a woman of upper social class origin and previously stable personality who at the age of 27 was prescribed heroin for intractable headaches following a minor head injury in a road accident. For the next 23 years she became dependent on heroin and later also on amphetamines. She developed physical complications from intravenous injections and her health deteriorated. She attended a drug dependence clinic where she started mixing with young non-therapeutic addicts and over the years she became a well-known figure on the London 'drug scene', selling part of her large heroin prescription to help support herself. At the age of 50 she was sent to prison for selling drugs. During her sentence she was withdrawn from drugs, her health improved, and she made a remarkable recovery. However, she relapsed again after leaving prison.

Specific types of dependence

Patients suffering from drug dependence show an interesting interaction between the personality features and problems of social adjustment which render them vulnerable, neurotic symptoms such as anxiety or depression which may lead them to drug use, the psychological effects of the drugs themselves and finally the consequences of drug dependence on their mental state, social functioning and health. The psychological effects of individual drugs and the physiological aspects of specific dependence and withdrawal syndromes are described in volume 2, chapter 15. The emphasis in the present section is on case histories illustrating the clinical picture that results from the interplay of personality, psychological, and social factors in different types of dependence.

Opiate dependence. (See also vol. 2, chap. 15.) Chronic dependence on opiates and the differences between therapeutic and non-therapeutic opiate addicts are exemplified by the following two patients.

CASE HISTORY

A haemophiliac aged 30 requested treatment for his dependence on dihydrocodeine (DF 118) tablets. He came from a stable home background but because of his illness he had an overprotected upbringing with frequent hospital admissions and a special boarding school education. His personality was shy, anxious, dependent, and introverted. At the age of 20 he was treated for depression after the failure of a business venture and an unhappy love-affair. The following year he had frequent bleeding episodes and was prescribed dihydrocodeine as an analgesic but he found that it also helped to alleviate his anxiety and depression and he gradually increased his dosage. However, he remained unaware of his dependence for 2 years, when he first experienced withdrawal symptoms on running out of tablets. By that time his bleeding episodes were infrequent and he realized that he was taking dihydrocodeine more for its euphoriant than for its analgesic effects. He made several unsuccessful attempts at drug withdrawal but repeatedly

relapsed. His relapses were precipitated by the stresses of another unhappy relationship with a girl-friend and his difficulties in finding suitable employment. His daily dosage increased to 40–50 tablets. On one occasion he forged a prescription to obtain increased supplies and was put on probation. He became increasingly withdrawn, introverted, and lacking in drive and felt that drugs were dominating his life. He was admitted for drug withdrawal; when off drugs his symptoms of depression and depersonalization became more marked but responded to antidepressants. However, some months later he again started taking dihydrocodeine, gradually increasing to 25 tablets daily, and he is likely to require readmission. This patient's use of other drugs (alcohol and cannabis) was minimal and he never escalated to other opiates. He remained an oral drug-user despite being used to intravenous self-injection of cryoprecipitate for his haemophilia. His case illustrates the role of personality inadequacy, neurotic symptoms, and chronic physical illness in the genesis of dependence on a prescribed drug.

CASE HISTORY

A contrasting picture of non-therapeutic opiate dependence is presented by a female patient aged 28. Her parents met when they were both patients in a psychiatric hospital. The father deserted the home when she was aged 4; the mother, an artist, formed several further liaisons and had 3 further children. The patient was neglected and frequently beaten by her mother who favoured the younger children. At the age of 8 she ran away from home and was taken into care. She attended boarding-schools for maladjusted children and had no further contact with her family. At 17 she worked as a secretary for a brief period but has not been employed since. She married at 18 when she was already in advanced pregnancy and left London. Her husband ill-treated her and they separated when she was 21. Her drug abuse commenced at the age of 15 with chlorodyne 'to calm her nerves'. At 16 she inhaled solvents regularly and smoked cannabis. She first injected methadone at 16, obtaining her drugs from a boy-friend who was attending a drug-dependence clinic. At 17 she took amphetamines, barbiturates, Mandrax, and LSD in addition to methadone. She then stopped using drugs because of her pregnancy and remained off drugs for 3 years until the break-up of her marriage. She was distressed at her husband gaining custody of their child and at 21 she returned to London and started taking drugs again. Since then she has led a drifting, unstable existence. She formed a liaison with an addict who supplied her with heroin and she became re-addicted. Their relationship ended when he was sent to prison for armed robbery of a pharmacy. She then obtained heroin, methadone, and occasionally morphine on the black market, supporting herself by drug dealing or casual prostitution. She also got dipipanone (Diconal) from a general practitioner, crushing the tablets and injecting them. She continued to take barbiturates and amphetamines sporadically. She has not worked for years, lives in temporary squats, and all her friends are addicts. Her health has deteriorated: at various times she suffered from hepatitis, septicaemia, abscesses from injecting in her femoral veins and feet, and venereal infection. Since the age of 16 she has had 7 convictions for theft, cheque frauds, and possession of drugs and has served several prison sentences.

Until a year ago she adamantly refused all offers of treatment, preferring to remain on the illicit market, but she has now started attending a drug-dependence clinic and is on methadone maintenance. This patient's primary dependence is on opiates: her preferred drug is heroin but when unable to obtain this she takes other opiates such as methadone, morphine or dipipanone. She concurrently abuses other drugs. Underlying her drug dependence she has a severe personality disorder consequent on a broken home and parental rejection. She was a battered child who became a battered wife. When off drugs she has marked lability of mood with episodic tension, depression, and self-mutilation, often without any obvious precipitant. Drug-taking as an attempt to suppress these symptoms seems an important factor in her chronic dependence. She has a poor self-image and cannot form any relationships other than those dictated by her need to obtain drugs. Her chaotic lifestyle may yet improve but she is likely to require long-term treatment and social support. Her case is not untypical of female opiate addicts attending London drug-dependence clinics.

Amphetamine dependence. (See also vol. 2, chap. 15.) The differences between therapeutic and non-therapeutic addicts are seen also in amphetamine dependence. The clinical picture is modified by the specific psychological effects and psychiatric complications of amphetamines. The characteristic symptoms of amphetamine abuse are euphoria, increased energy, restlessness, irritability, insomnia, anorexia, and weight loss. Amphetamine psychosis is more common in non-therapeutic addicts and the symptoms vary from transient paranoid delusional ideas accompanied by fear ('the horrors') which are of brief duration and are rapidly followed by insight, to a more prolonged illness closely mimicking acute paranoid schizophrenia. Helpful distinguishing features from schizophrenia are a history of amphetamine abuse, the finding of amphetamines in the urine, the absence of thought disorder and inappropriate affect, and the characteristic content of the delusions, which are usually frightening. The delusions are often related to the illicit nature of the patient's drug use or other illegal activities and centre on persecution by the police, the so called 'police paranoia'. For example, the patient with adolescent identity problems described on page 361 developed an amphetamine psychosis shortly after a homosexual experience with a young boy. He believed that the police, gangsters and Hell's Angels were spying on him and chasing him and he heard passers-by calling him a junkie and a child molester. The delusions may have a vivid, terrifying and dream-like quality: at a time when heart-transplants were much in the news a woman arrested for disorderly behav-

iour and put in a police van believed that the police had kidnapped her and were transporting her not to the police station but to the hospital to become a heart-donor in a transplant operation.

The pattern of amphetamine use also tends to differ in therapeutic and non-therapeutic addicts. While middle-aged women who become dependent after being prescribed amphetamines for weight reduction or depression manage to cope on regular small doses for prolonged periods, non-therapeutic addicts, particularly intravenous users, tend to have cyclical periods of amphetamine use lasting for some days or weeks with rapidly escalating dosage. As the unpleasant effects (irritability, restlessness, stereotyped activity and paranoid symptoms accompanied by fear) supervene they discontinue the drug and there follows a period of prolonged sleep, lethargy, and depression. This may lead to restarting amphetamines, thus initiating another cycle. Antisocial and aggressive behaviour tends to occur particularly during the end-phase of the cycle when drug use is at its height and it is often related to paranoid symptoms.

Barbiturate dependence. (See also vol. 2, chap. 15.) Barbiturate-dependent patients also tend to show the distinct psychosocial patterns of therapeutic and non-therapeutic dependence. The specific drug effects include drowsiness, confusion, and neurological symptoms such as dysarthria, nystagmus, and ataxia. Intoxication leads to defective judgement, disinhibition, or aggressive behaviour. The recognition of physical dependence is important because of the risk of epileptic convulsions and delirium associated with abrupt withdrawal. Symptoms of intoxication and a history of withdrawal convulsions are found more often in non-therapeutic addicts who take variable doses. Therapeutic dependence on regular doses may be difficult to recognize if the patient conceals his drug use. Characteristically the mental state tends to fluctuate, often rapidly; for example the patient may alternate between periods of muddled euphoria or maudlin depression. Tension, irritability, and anxiety induced by barbiturate dependence may be mistaken for the symptoms of an anxiety state for which the drug was originally prescribed and the patient himself is usually unaware of the reason for the worsening of his symptoms and demands more drugs to alleviate them.

CASE HISTORY
A patient with a paranoid personality disorder associated with severe tension and phobic anxiety was prescribed

amylobarbitone and became dependent on it for years. He became increasingly tense, aggressive, paranoid, and depressed, and his phobic symptoms became disabling. He insistently demanded more drugs from his general practitioner, took chloral hydrate (prescribed as a hypnotic) during the day-time and drank alcohol in an attempt to relieve his symptoms. A crisis necessitating admission afforded the opportunity to withdraw him from barbiturates and his anxiety and tension improved; he eventually responded well to antidepressants and desensitization for his residual phobic symptoms. His case also illustrates the tendency for barbiturate addicts to abuse alcohol and other hypno-sedatives.

Lysergic acid diethylamide. (See also vol. 2, chap. 15.) The use of LSD rarely comes to medical attention unless psychiatric complications arise. 'Bad trips' may take the form of acute psychotic or non-psychotic adverse reactions. Acute psychotic reactions are characterised by intense terror, paranoid delusions, hallucinations, or sometimes catatonic features or profound depression. In acute non-psychotic adverse reactions the person experiences tension, anxiety, fear, unpleasant illusions, depression, and depersonalization. While both these reactions are usually of brief duration they may merge into more prolonged states of psychosis or depersonalization. Such prolonged adverse reactions occur more often in predisposed individuals but they are also seen in patients without serious pre-existing psychopathology.

CASE HISTORY

A 20-year-old university student was an experienced LSD user. He had one previous 'bad trip' 3 years before, but no history of psychiatric illness. On a visit to friends at another university he took LSD after which he experienced frightening illusions and a feeling of omnipotence in which he felt he could control external events. During this period he attempted to steal and drive a car. His perceptual disturbances ceased after 24 hours but he then developed a schizophrenic-like illness with thought disorder, thought broadcasting, pseudo-philosophical preoccupations, and marked perplexity. He thought his lecturers were persecuting him and making personal allusions to him in their lectures. His symptoms subsided spontaneously 6 months after the acute reaction without specific treatment.

An interesting phenomenon is the 'flashback' experience, a spontaneous recurrence of LSD effects occurring months or even a year after the last LSD use. It may be precipitated by other drugs (especially cannabis) and occurs more often in heavy LSD takers. The phenomenon has also been described with cannabis. Flashback experiences are unexpected and although they are mostly transient and mild, at times they may be frightening and unpleasant: there are occasional reports of suicidal attempts or driving accidents attributed to a flashback. The causation of flashbacks is unknown; both biochemical and psychological explanations have been suggested.

Benzodiazepines. (See also vol. 2, chap. 15.) Dependence on benzodiazepines has been recently reviewed by Tyrer (1980). Physical dependence on high dosages with epileptic convulsions on abrupt withdrawal has been recognized for some time and is similar to dependence of the barbiturate-alcohol type. Recent evidence suggests that a high proportion of patients on therapeutic dosage also develop a mild abstinence syndrome with anxiety, depression, depersonalization, insomnia, muscular twitching, and perceptual disturbances. Psychological dependence is shown by many patients who remain on long-term treatment and find it difficult to discontinue benzodiazepines. Young multiple drug abusers now often take benzodiazepines but as the euphoriant and intoxicating effects they seek are relatively mild with this group of drugs, they tend to use them only as a substitute for their preferred drugs and take benzodiazepines in an irregular fashion. Regular use and consequent dependence occurs almost exclusively in the course of medical treatment and these patients resemble therapeutic addicts to other drugs.

CASE HISTORY

An example is a 34-year-old woman from a broken home with an unsettled childhood. She was a dependent, anxious girl with low self-esteem. At 18 she formed an insecure liaison with a married man and had three illegitimate children who were adopted. Her fourth pregnancy was terminated and she then developed feelings of guilt, anxiety, and mild depression and was prescribed diazepam. Over the next 10 years she gradually increased her dosage to 150 mg daily. Later she was also prescribed Distalgesic (containing dextropropoxyphene) for headaches, eventually taking 25 tablets daily. When her anxiety led to over-eating she was put on diethylpropion (Tenuate). She obtained these drugs simultaneously from different doctors and was convicted three times for forging prescriptions. After a court appearance she tried to discontinue diazepam abruptly and developed epileptic convulsions. She eventually responded well to phenelzine and supportive psychotherapy. Her case illustrates that inadequate personalities with chronic neurotic symptoms are at risk of dependence on a variety of drugs and that benzodiazepine dependence may coexist with dependence on minor analgesics, appetite suppressants, or other hypno-sedatives.

Physical complications

Physical complications may arise with most drugs of dependence due to overdosage or accidental injuries associated with intoxication. The pathogenic effects of specific drugs include the carcinogenic effects of tobacco, the cytotoxic effects of alcohol on the liver and CNS, the toxic effects of some solvents and nephrotoxic analgesics (see volume 2, chapter 15), and ulceration of the nasal mucosa in chronic cocaine sniffers due to localized vasoconstriction. Barbiturates may cause adverse drug interactions (for example with anticoagulants). With these exceptions, there is at present no evidence that the commonly used drugs cause any irreversible pathological changes and most of the serious physical complications of drug dependence result from the method of drug use rather than the physiological effects of drugs. An example is the risk of suffocation from plastic bags in solvent inhalers. The most frequent source of serious complications is self-injection. The injection of drugs manufactured for oral use, for example barbiturate preparations, dipipanone (Diconal) and methylphenidate (Ritalin) gives rise to necrotic ulceration or thrombophlebitis. The additives in these preparations, and adulterants such as talc or cornstarch present in illicit drugs may cause pulmonary microembolisms. The commonest complications arise from unsterile injections leading to local infections, (abscesses, thrombophlebitis, or gangrene) and systemic infections (septicaemia, hepatitis, endocarditis, and pulmonary or renal disease). The morbidity and mortality of injecting opiate addicts is well documented and reviewed in volume 2, chapter 15.

Management and treatment
Diagnostic assessment
Establishing the diagnosis of drug dependence presents a number of clinical problems and both the physical and the psychological aspects of dependence require assessment.

The history may be unreliable as patients who seek a prescription may exaggerate their drug use while others conceal it. Multi-drug users have a variable pattern of drug use or take illicit drugs of uncertain composition which makes it especially difficult to assess their physical dependence on specific drugs. Particular attention should be paid to eliciting withdrawal symptoms which confirm physical dependence. In order to evaluate the truthfulness of the patient's account the clinician has to be familiar with the effects, tolerance, and abstinence syndromes of specific drugs described in volume 2, chapter 15, especially the opiates and barbiturates. Since patients may simultaneously use a variety of opiates, it is useful to know their dosage equivalents in order to assess total opiate use in terms of heroin or methadone. The patient's psychological dependence and commitment to drug use also require careful appraisal and his life-style serves as a useful pointer. Enquiry should be made about his social contacts with other drug users, his sources of income, his expenditure on drugs and the ways in which they are procured. Familiarity with the 'drug scene' will help the clinician to judge the truthfulness of the history given by the patient.

Physical examination may reveal signs of an abstinence syndrome or physical complications. In addicts who inject themselves the history should be compared with objective evidence of needle and track marks, although some patients may attempt to simulate injection marks. The examination should include possible unusual injection sites such as the feet, legs, and groins.

Urine analysis gives no quantitative information about the dosage of drugs taken and a single positive test may only provide evidence of sporadic use. A finding of 3 positive urines over a period of 10 to 14 days is reasonable confirmatory evidence of dependence (Gardner & Connell, 1970).

Information should also be obtained from independent sources whenever possible, including the family, the general practitioner, and other treatment agencies with whom the patient has had previous contact. When there is a history of delinquency the patient may be known to the probation service or to a prison medical officer. If opiate dependence is suspected enquiry should also be made to the Home Office Drugs Branch, as the patient may have been previously notified from other sources or may already be under treatment elsewhere. In Britain notification of addiction to cocaine and opiates is required by regulations under the Misuse of Drugs Act 1971; details of the procedure are outlined in a Guide to the Act (DHSS, 1977).

Motivation for treatment
Motivation is a key factor in treatment but it can be deceptive and changeable. Often the patient at first may seem anxious to relinquish drugs but is unable to sustain his motivation when he is admitted for drug withdrawal. Treatment goals should be realistic and aim at the optimum that can be achieved for the individual patient at any given time. With chronic addicts treatment may initially have to be limited to simple goals such as the reduction of drug consumption, the treatment of physical complications and practical help with social problems. At the same time

the therapist should take a long-term view and patiently persist with the gradual building of motivation towards a change in life-style and eventual abstinence. The natural history of drug dependence and of the underlying personality disorder has to be taken into account. Winick (1962) suggests that there is a tendency to mature out of addiction with increasing age, and a similar process of improvement often occurs in antisocial personality disorders (Robins 1966). At an early stage of his addiction career the patient may show little motivation for treatment but as the adverse consequences of his dependence become increasingly stressful he may try to give up drugs. The transition from dependence to abstinence is rarely a clear-cut change and most patients make a series of attempts to relinquish drugs before they can achieve lasting abstinence. Motives for abstinence include difficulty in procuring drugs, court pressures, a threat to a significant relationship, physical complications, pregnancy, and often merely weariness with the effort involved in sustaining the lifestyle of an addict. A long-term supportive relationship will provide the therapist with an opportunity to exploit these events. With patients who have failed to respond to treatment at an earlier stage intervention may yet become effective later when it can reinforce and encourage the process of maturation.

Although drug dependence is often a chronic illness, long-term follow-up studies provide some justification for maintaining therapeutic optimism. A recent follow-up study of a representative sample of injecting heroin addicts treated at London drug-dependence clinics in 1969 showed that 7 years later over a third of the patients had stopped using opiates and had changed their life-style. There was no evidence that they had transferred their previous dependence on opiates to alcohol or other drugs. A comparison of abstainers with continued users found no useful predictors of abstinence, except that those who eventually relinquished drugs were younger and had a shorter period of heroin use prior to treatment (Oppenheimer, Stimson & Thorley, 1979). The difficulty in identifying prognostic factors is in keeping with other research evidence and with the clinical experience that even very disturbed addicts may unexpectedly achieve abstinence.

Drug withdrawal

The specific methods of withdrawal are described in volume 2, chapter 15. Many patients prefer to attempt out-patient withdrawal and this may be feasible with those who retain some social stability. However, patients who are physically dependent on barbiturates and other hypno-sedatives should be withdrawn in hospital. Some severely disturbed multi-drug users are so disorganized and at risk of overdosage that only in-patient detoxification is possible and at times this may require short-term admission under the Mental Health Act. Although there is no evidence that prolonged institutional treatment is effective in the treatment of drug dependence, short-term admission may be life-saving. An experimental hostel has recently been opened in London for drug abusers referred from casualty departments, where patients can be admitted voluntarily for detoxification and arrangements made for more long-term rehabilitation. Whatever the method of withdrawal or the setting in which it occurs, during the early abstinence phase the patient requires support and the opportunity to discuss and explore his underlying problems. Anxiety, depression, irritability, and insomnia occur after withdrawal of all dependency-producing drugs. Drug treatment of these post-withdrawal symptoms carries the risk of substituting dependence on another drug. Drugs such as chlormethiazole or benzodiazepines should only be used for a limited period and phenothiazines are preferable for the treatment of tension and anxiety associated with withdrawal. Depressive symptoms usually remit spontaneously and antidepressants are rarely necessary.

Maintenance treatment

For opiate addicts who are unmotivated to undergo immediate withdrawal a period of maintenance treatment may be a more realistic approach. With short-acting opiates such as heroin or morphine frequent drug use is necessary and alternate euphoria and withdrawal symptoms tend to increase the addict's preoccupation with drug use. By contrast, methadone has a more prolonged action and a single dose suppresses withdrawal symptoms and maintains the addict in physiological balance for over 24 hours. Because it is effective orally and exhibits cross-dependence with other opiates it is the drug of choice for maintenance treatment or for gradual opiate withdrawal. Oral methadone maintenance has been used extensively in the United States. In Britain long-term maintenence is not usually a deliberate objective and gradual weaning from drugs is attempted, though in practice some patients remain on methadone for an indefinite period. The technique of methadone maintenance is described in volume 2, chapter 15. Methadone maintenance should be used only in a specialized clinic where prescribing is but one element in treatment and can be combined with supportive psychotherapy, social work support, and access to a wide range of rehabilitation facilities. The decision to prescribe methadone should only be taken after careful assessment and not be rushed. The hope of weaning a patient from the black market into a therapeutic relationship and increased social stability must be balanced against the risks of converting a drug abuser into a physically dependent addict, or of prolonging dependence in a patient who would otherwise have given up drugs. It is also difficult to identify the type of patient who is likely to benefit from maintenance, but they tend to be those who show some potential for achieving social stability. Blumberg and co-workers (1974) noted that at the London drug-dependence clinics those who were accepted for treatment and given a prescription for opiates were less involved in criminal activity, had better employment records, and were less likely to abuse additional non-opiate drugs than those who were not given a prescription.

Amphetamines and barbiturates are unsuitable drugs for maintenance and it is doubtful whether any but a very small minority of psychologically dependent, socially stable middle-aged patients should be prescribed these drugs in limited quantities.

Strict control of prescribing is an essential aspect of treatment. When other psycho-active drugs such as benzodiazepines, hypnotics, or antidepressants are prescribed to addicts or to patients at risk of dependence, all prescribing should be taken over by one doctor. The prescribing role should be clarified between the psychiatrist, the patient, and his general practitioner. This helps to avoid escalation of dosage, the prescribing of additional drugs, and manipulation or deception. If the patient is seen at less than weekly intervals post-dated weekly prescriptions will help the patient to avoid using up his supply of drugs before the next prescription is due, as so often happens when he is given several weeks' supply at a time. For maintenance opiate prescribing at drug-dependence clinics a special prescription form is used and drugs are dispensed daily by arrangement with the pharmacist.

Rehabilitation

The cardinal feature of successful rehabilitation is to help the patient to find effective substitutes for drugs. Rehabilitation should begin when the patient first makes contact. It involves a variety of professions and the need for co-ordination and team work is obvious. Practical help with accommodation and employment are often the initial needs; vocational training, further education, and a change in environment may be more long-term objectives. Contact with the family should be established when possible but often family disturbance is so severe that reconciliation cannot be achieved. Rather than returning to his family or spouse the young addict may achieve a better adjustment by finding new relationships with non-addicts, or a more tolerant environmment in a therapeutic community or a half-way house.

Therapeutic communities

Many therapeutic communities for addicts are modelled on the Phoenix House programme which provides a structured, authoritarian, and hierarchical regime based on a system of sanctions and rewards. The programme includes group therapy, education, and work assignments; the addict is encouraged to assume a position of responsibility in the community and eventually to become involved in the treatment of other addicts. The outcome for the first 100 admissions to Phoenix House in London has been reviewed by Ogborne & Melotte (1977) and resembles the results found in similar programmes elsewhere (Smart, 1976). Although less than 10 per cent of admissions complete the programme, about one-third of all admissions improve and become abstinent or only sporadic users. Improvement, including reduction in criminal activity, is related to length of stay (De Leon et al., 1972, 1973). Other therapeutic communities do not aim at such a radical restructuring of the personality and have a more tolerant regime, sometimes with a religious bias. Suitability of the particular programme for the individual patient has to be considered, but all require the patient to be drug free before entry and prior in-patient drug withdrawal may be necessary.

Psychotherapy

Psychotherapy is an essential component of a multidimensional approach to treatment and rehabilitation. Social factors play such an important role in drug dependence that psycho-dynamically orientated individual psychotherapy is of little value (Harding, 1975). In therapeutic communities various forms of group therapy have evolved using techniques of confrontation, confession, and catharsis. Limits and controls are set and the importance of commitment to the community is emphasized. Supportive psychotherapy is used in most other settings. In supportive psychotherapy with addicts treatment should focus on the here and now situation. Environmental manipulation, practical help and a consistent and directive approach are more helpful than traditional detachment.

Drug dependence viewed as a life-style or as a symptom of neurosis or personality disorder implies that treatment must concern itself not merely with abstinence but with remodelling of the patient's self-image and his social adaptation; success will depend more on his ability to discover a satisfying alternative to his addiction than on any specific method of treatment.

10.3
Alcoholism
GRIFFITH EDWARDS

Introduction

Alcoholism treatment is today in a state of transition. This chapter seeks to reflect some of the changes in understanding which research has been forcing. In such circumstances it would be premature to expect any absolute consensus to have emerged on the clinical approach to alcoholism, but a number of texts provide discussion of different perspectives (Glatt, 1970; Hore, 1976; Madden, 1979; Mendelson & Mello, 1979; Cutting, 1979; Edwards & Grant, 1980).

There has been a loss of faith in the intensive interventions and prolonged in-patient stays which have traditionally been seen as constituting 'good treatment' (Orford & Edwards, 1977). The focus of interest is switching toward the efficacy of simpler interventions and the influence of the immediate patient–therapist interaction. Treatment is seen as having to be in alliance with 'natural history'. There is a growing awareness, too, that any clinical alcoholic population is likely to be very heterogeneous, with no one approach suitable for every person. The special problem of the woman alcoholic is receiving increased attention (Camberwell Council on Alcoholism, 1980), and when the patient is in this chapter for brevity referred to as 'he', the meaning should of course always be read as 'he' or 'she'.

In Britain the organization of National Health Service treatment has, up to now, centred on specialized regional alcoholism treatment units. The future direction which the work of these units will take is much under debate (Shaw *et al.*, 1978), with a recent DHSS report recommending a more community-based approach and the establishment of community alcoholism teams (DHSS, 1978). Treatment within the penal service has always been restricted by resources, but the role of the probation service is certainly important.

Briefly to signpost this chapter, it is organized in terms of the following sections. The chapter starts with a discussion of definitions in this area, followed by presentation of two short illustrative case examples. Aetiology, natural history, and epidemiology are dealt with in sequence. A reminder is entered on the need for thorough physical examination, and a note given on special problems in mental state examination. Reflecting a belief in the importance of thorough assessment not only for information-gathering but as a basis of therapy, a section deals with assessment at length. The next section then discusses a minimal or basic approach to treatment, with emphasis on the belief that so far as possible, one should not escalate beyond this simple way of proceeding. The following section deals, though, with common ancillary treatments and general reasons which may arise for going beyond the minimum. Underlying or complicating psychiatric conditions are then discussed, which between them give rise to a set of questions of considerable but often neglected clinical importance. A short note is given on forensic implications of alcoholism.

Definitions

The postwar years have been marked by much debate as to the meaning to be given the word 'alcoholism'. A widely quoted definition was that put forward in 1952 by WHO:

> Alcoholics are those excessive drinkers whose dependence on alcohol has attained such a degree that they show a noticeable mental disturbance or an interference with their mental and bodily health, their interpersonal relations and their smooth social and economic functioning; or who show the prodromal signs of such developments.

This definition is cast in very general terms, and the key concepts which it employs remain undefined.

It has long been recognized that not all abnormal drinking falls into one pattern, and attempts have therefore been made to *typologize* alcoholism. Here the most influential suggestion was that made by Jellinek (1960) who proposed that alcoholism could be broken down into at least five species:

Alpha
Excessive drinking without physiological dependence (excessive non-addictive drinking)
Beta
Excessive drinking leading simply to tissue damage
Gamma
Addictive drinking with 'loss of control': the typical alcoholism of Anglo-Saxon countries
Delta
Addictive drinking with 'inability to abstain': the typical alcoholism of France and generally of wine-drinking countries
Epsilon
Bout drinking or classical 'dipsomania'

The definitions given above are only a paraphrase of the original and carefully argued exposition. Jellinek's terminology has passed into very general usage, and in particular the phrase 'gamma alcoholism' seems on occasion to be used as loosely synonymous with 'the disease of alcoholism', 'real alcoholism' or 'the alcoholism of AA'.

An alternative formulation suggests that rather than there being a multiplicity of true subtypes, drinking behaviour can be moulded by a range of *pathoplastic* factors (personal, cultural, and social), so as to give rise to a wide range of possible presentations. Such an approach would, for instance, argue that Jellinek's gamma and delta alcoholism are not in any fundamental sense distinct 'species', but presentations determined by the pathoplastic influence of relative degrees of alcohol availability and social moulding of drinking behaviour, or by underlying personality.

A recent WHO formulation (Edwards *et al.*, 1977) suggests that a *core syndrome of alcohol dependence* can be identified, which exists in degrees rather than being an all-or-none phenomenon, and with a presentation which will then indeed be much influenced by the type of pathoplastic factors which have been discussed above. As for the essential nature of alcohol dependence, we are clearly to an extent dressing up old ideas in new words, and the concept of a dependence syndrome is closely allied to old ideas of 'addiction'. The meaning which is currently being given to the dependence concept is, however, far more subtle than older 'addiction' formulations, and the latest WHO report on this topic talks of 'dependence residing within a system' (WHO, 1981). Alcohol dependence can, this report argues, only be understood as a psychosocial-biological phenomenon, with behaviour governed by the interaction of multiple determinants. There is though growing evidence (Hodgson *et al.*, 1978) to support a model which proposes that the repeated experience of alcohol withdrawal symptoms and repeated engagement in withdrawal relief drinking, may constitute a crucially important learning process which can move the individual from 'drinking too much' to 'alcohol dependence'. Clinical characteristics of the dependence syndrome are discussed further below (p. 375).

The 1977 WHO formulation (Edwards *et al.*, 1977) then goes on to suggest that in addition to the notion of a *dependence syndrome*, the idea of an *alcohol-related problem* (disability) is also required. A person suffering from dependence will in practice inevitably suffer from disabilities. But it is quite possible for someone to experience serious alcohol-related problems without being dependent. This last statement is an important corrective to a sometimes apparent previous medical tendency to see only the advanced case of 'alcohol addiction' as important, while dismissing patients who had not entered that sort of phase as not being 'real alcoholics', and as therefore not constituting suitable cases for treatment.

If we accept this two-part WHO approach (dependence and problems) as a good practical basis for clinical work, where does this leave the word 'alcoholism' itself? There is no doubt that this word will remain in circulation and that many different people will use the term in various different ways. So varied indeed are the likely ways in which this word is employed that it seems best to accord it a purposely loose and generic meaning, as implying 'any sort of more or less severe problem with alcohol, whether or not dependence is involved'. That is the sense in which we will employ the word in this chapter.

Two typical case presentations

These two brief case histories are presented as illustrating the usefulness of thinking clinically in terms of the two dimensions of alcohol-related problems and the dependence syndrome.

A woman with problems. This 34-year-old woman whose husband had deserted her, was living with six children in temporary accommodation. She was referred to a hospital out-patient clinic by a social worker who reported that her client was 'drinking a lot of wine'. Initial assessment revealed that the patient was consuming up to two bottles of cheap wine on two or three days each week, that when intoxicated she

had broken her wrist, that she had fought with a neighbour when drunk, and that even this degree of drinking was embarrassing her financial situation. She was taking a lot of valium.

To make alcohol the centre of this woman's problems would be absurd, but to dismiss the damaging emergence of drinking as an added complication in her life situation would be equally unwise.

A man with dependence and several alcohol-related problems. A 50-year-old executive leading a successful but fraught life was referred to a psychiatrist after a routine medical check had revealed an enlarged liver, and he had admitted that he 'probably drank too much'. The history then given was of gradually escalating drinking, which had been at the level of about one to one-and-a-half bottles of whisky virtually every day for the previous five years. Over the last twelve months he had experienced morning withdrawal symptoms, and was keeping a bottle in his briefcase for a morning drink on the commuter train. He had lost his driving license and his marriage was endangered.

Assessment and treatment skills (and sympathies) must contain the range of cases portrayed by these two cases, and a host of other presentations besides. It is obviously absurd to think in terms of stereotyped 'alcoholism', or stereotyped treatment.

Aetiology of alcoholism

The causes of alcoholism are an extension of the personal and social determinants of the drinking of alcohol. If we want to know why some people drink too much (in a way which creates problems or leads to dependence), we have first to ask why people drink. If one graphs out a population's alcohol consumption, a smooth unimodal curve is obtained with a long low upper tail, strongly suggesting a multifactorial explanation of drinking rather than one explanation for 'normal drinking', with a second explanation needed for an extreme (Ledermann, 1956).

What then are the multiple determinants of drinking, and of heavier drinking? It is convenient to group the key factors under two headings – environmental and personal – although, in practice, one is always dealing with interactive effects.

Under the environmental heading can, for instance, be placed the influence of *real price*: if alcohol is in real terms cheaper, a society will drink more, and people with greater disposable income will on average drink more heavily. Licensing and control of sales outlets may, in this regard, be public health measures (Bruun *et al.*, 1975). People in certain jobs are exposed to greater drinking pressures (Plant &

Hore, 1980), and hence the elevated risks of alcoholism among barmen, journalists, salesmen, actors and entertainers, and so on (people with a tendency to heavy drinking may also be attracted to professions which offer drinking opportunities). Life stresses, negative life events, and personal loss may move someone into heavy drinking. A mass of subtle socio-cultural influences are also operating: men drink more than women in most cultures, the Scots drink more than the English, and the Catholics more than the Jews (Pittman & Snyder, 1962). Social disruption and rapid socio-economic change are often associated with the breakdown of traditional informal controls, and hence the problems with alcohol that are being experienced in many parts of the Third World (Edwards, 1980).

As for the personal factors in the equation, there is evidence that genetic predisposition may in some instances be important (Goodwin *et al.*, 1974; Shields, 1977). The child's modelling on a heavy drinking parent must also contribute to familial incidence. No specific 'alcoholic personality' has been demonstrated, but a variety of personality traits may predispose to drinking – the person who is insensitive to social controls and expectations, the person who is anxious or uneasy in his self-image, or the person who simply enjoys company and exhilaration. Psycho-dynamic processes certainly also need to be understood. The relevance of underlying mental illness is discussed in a later section of this chapter (p. 379). But what needs to be stressed here is that alcoholism does not necessarily predicate gross psychopathology.

The implications for clinical work of this brief review of social and personal determinants of drinking must be clear. Each patient must require a separate analysis of what for him (or for her), is the unique network of determinants, and this information must then speak to the planning of the treatment regime.

Natural history

What happens to people with drinking problems over time must be very dependent on the sample which is chosen and on the cultural setting. The excessive mortality rate on follow-up of clinical alcoholism population is one fact which is starkly established: among males the excess mortality over age-corrected expectation is about 2.7 to 1 and among females 3.1 to 1 (Nicholls *et al.*, 1974).

An important question in natural history studies has been whether alcoholism is likely to show any fixed pattern of progression over time, and any constant ordering of symptoms. Jellinek's description of 'the phases of alcoholism' (Jellinek, 1946) was very influential and was interpreted as favouring a disease theory, but was not well supported by later work (Orford & Hawker, 1974): there are probably many different patterns of natural history rather than any one fixed march. Another question relating to natural history is whether alcoholics return to normal drinking (Davies, 1962): again, the answer must rest on what is meant by 'alcoholics'. In any heterogenous population of patients with drinking problems, it is probable that there will be some who succeed in returning to controlled drinking, but it seems less likely that the heavily dependent person can do so (see discussion of treatment goals, p. 376). We need in fact much more information on lifetime drinking careers, rather than rely only on perspectives limited to the usual 1–2 year hospital treatment studies (Vaillant, 1979; Polich *et al.*, 1980).

Epidemiology

Estimates of prevalence must be dependent on definition of what is to be counted, and, given the varied meanings that have been attached to the term *alcoholism*, it is unsurprising that estimates of alcoholism prevalence have shown similarly wide variation. At least three different epidemiological approaches have been employed:

(1) Direct house-to-house surveys, with operational definition of a 'problem drinker' in terms of a count of symptoms. A survey of this type in London suggested that 6 per cent of men and 1 per cent of women had experienced, over a twelve-month period, serious difficulties because of their drinking (Edwards *et al.*, 1973). The male:female ratio has undoubtedly narrowed over recent years, there being an increased problem rate among women.

(2) The 'reporting agency' technique, where all relevant 'agents and agencies', such as general practitioners, hospitals, and social agencies within a locality, are asked to tally their cases over a period (Edwards *et al.*, 1973).

(3) The previous two approaches have the attraction of operating close to the field, but in practice are expensive and subject to many errors. Some alcoholism epidemiologists have therefore preferred to work with seemingly 'harder data', even if the relationship between these data and what is clinically meant by alcoholism is problematical. For instance, much recent work has concentrated on the

epidemiology of the cirrhosis death rate, as an indirect indicator of 'alcoholism' (Schmidt, 1977).

The physical complications of alcoholism

The physical complications which may arise as the result of direct tissue damage, malnutrition, and vitamin deficiency, biochemical disturbance, or trauma, are legion. The psychiatrist should therefore never overlook the importance of a full physical assessment of the patient with a drinking problem. These complications include: varieties of brain damage (see p. 380), optic atrophy, and the subdural haematoma resulting from a drunken fall, peripheral neuritis, myositis, cancers of the mouth and oesophagus, carditis and disorders of cardiac rhythm, pneumonia, lung abscess, and pulmonary tuberculosis, hepatitis, fatty liver, cirrhosis and hepatoma, pancreatitis, peptic ulceration, anaemia and disorders of clotting, hyperlipaemia, hypoglycaemia, electrolyte imbalance, varieties of vitamin deficiency, a rare disorder of bone, impotence, gout, and finally every variety of trauma that may present in a casualty department. Foetal damage (the foetal alcoholism syndrome) has also been reported.

Mental state examination

The mental state examination is basically the same as that for any other psychiatric patient. There are however certain additional points that can be usefully borne in mind:

(1) Mental state examination is not of much value when the patient is intoxicated, and may have to be in some ways provisional until the patient has completely recovered from withdrawal – seemingly severe anxiety and depression may prove to be transient. Cognitive functioning may recover over weeks or months, so that a gloomy initial assessment may be premature.

(2) The assessment of 'previous personality' may be very difficult if much of the patient's adult life has been overlaid by excessive drinking. A very different picture may emerge with sobriety, and the promiscuous application of a secondary diagnosis of 'personality disorder' should be resisted.

(3) Very careful assessment should however be made for a range of possible underlying or accompanying mental disorders (see p. 379).

Assessment

The assessment of a patient with a drinking problem must include as groundwork the complete routine psychiatric and physical assessments, together with appropriate investigations. Special assessment has then to be made of the patient's drinking problem. The clinical skill lies not only in knowing what to ask, but also in knowing how to ask questions in a way which is likely to win the patient's openness and co-operation.

The extent to which patients with drinking problems are likely to be dishonest is easily exaggerated – the degree of trust which can be won from someone who feels himself threatened and disgraced must as ever be dependent in large measure on the skill of the interviewer. Nevertheless, patients will be met who conceal or minimize aspects of their drinking history, or even engage in massive denial. A history from an independent informant should therefore, whenever possible, be obtained.

Taking the view that a behavioural perspective is not an alternative to any other way of looking at a problem, but properly inherent in any analysis of behaviour, it may often be useful to identify the apparent cueing for a particular individual's drinking. In response to what cues will drinking occur, and what set of cues are then likely to suggest excessive drinking or the termination of drinking? Analysis of the 'typical heavy drinking day' may be made in these terms, but it can also be useful to analyse the conditions in which the drinking may be more controlled.

As regards psycho-dynamic perspective, much the same may be said – the attempt to understand the psycho-dynamic meaning of the patient's drinking must be inherent in the whole interview rather than an entirely separate exercise.

The headings below then provide a framework for major aspects of the drinking enquiry:

(1) *'The typical heavy drinking day'*. Rather than ask the patient a general question about how much he drinks in a day, it is better tactics to get him to reconstruct the drinking of a recent *typical heavy drinking day* (Caetano et al., 1978), relating the enquiry to a specific point in time such as 'yesterday' or 'before you went on holiday'. Questioning starts with enquiry as to what time the patient wakes up, how he feels when he wakes up, what time he takes the first drink, the quantity of that first drink, the perceived reasons for that drink, and then an hour-by-hour reconstruction of the day's drinking and the circumstances of each drink. The summated picture of total quantity drunk is likely to be very different from

what usually emerges from casual questioning along the lines of 'How much do you drink in a day?'. Moreover, the drinking is given its meaning and context.

(2) *Dependence syndrome.* The aim is to determine whether the patient is exhibiting the dependence syndrome and if so, the degree of dependence (Edwards & Gross, 1976; Hodgson *et al.*, 1978; Stockwell *et al.*, 1979). Symptoms which have to be covered include experience of *withdrawal symptoms,* with separate enquiry into tremor, sweating, nausea, and mood disturbance. For each of these symptoms skilled questioning has to be directed at intensity, frequency, and historical duration – crude recording of 'yes' or 'no' will miss all the clinical subtlety. Here, for instance, are two ways of asking about tremor.

First:
>   *Doctor* Do you ever get the morning shakes?
>   *Patient* No.

Or, alternatively and much better:
>   *Doctor* Do you ever find your hands are at all unsteady in the morning?
>   *Patient* A bit unsteady perhaps, but not what you would call the shakes.
>   *Doctor* Can you shave in the morning?
>   *Patient* I use an electric razor – I wouldn't like to try a wet shave.
>   *Doctor* Are your hands steady when you're holding your first cup of tea?
>   *Patient* I'll spill a bit in the saucer.
>   *Doctor* How long has it been like that?
>   *Patient* Not long, really. I suppose it was just after Christmas I first noticed that sort of thing, less than a year certainly.

The clumsy approach misses the important information that during the previous twelve months the patient had begun to show early but definite signs of the dependence syndrome.

Careful questioning is similarly needed on the symptoms which help to delineate the other elements of the syndrome, and its degrees. *Withdrawal relief drinking* may be so established that the patient has to take a large swig from a bottle of spirits before getting out of bed, or it may be a matter simply of his knowing that the first drink at morning opening time is eagerly awaited and needed to 'put him straight'. The touchstone is indeed the patient's awareness that alcohol relieves his withdrawal symptoms – he will know the time-interval between the drink and the relief, and the quantity of alcohol required. *Subjective awareness* of dependence may be difficult for the patient to put into language and yet

be central to his experience. At the extreme, his drinking and the next drink pervade his thoughts, and he will describe classical 'loss of control' – when he drinks he will go on drinking to intoxication despite any initial resolves. *Narrowing of the repertoire* implies that as the patient becomes more severely dependent, his drinking pattern will become increasingly stereotyped: he will drink in a time-tabled fashion, weekdays and weekends. *Salience* of drink-seeking over other drives becomes apparent – drinking becomes more important than affection of family, social reputation, or health. *Heightened tolerance* to alcohol is a prerequisite of development of dependence, but in later stages tolerance may be lost, and the patient becomes easily and embarrassingly drunk. *Reinstatement* of dependence after a period of abstinence will be more rapid the greater the severity of the previous dependence. The assessment of the dependence syndrome is completed by a consideration of the *coherence* of the story which has been given. The severity of the different symptoms should be in step. If this is not the case then the patient is being less than frank or, more probably, the history has been clumsily taken. Additional factors though need to be explored as possibly complicating the presentation: the heavy use of benzodiazepines may, for instance, partially suppress withdrawal symptoms or the need for relief drinking, while early morning depressive symptoms may be confused with affective symptoms of withdrawal.

(3) *The personal drinking history.* It is useful to reconstruct the patient's drinking history in terms of the sequence of influences and events which have shaped his drinking, levels of drinking, and periods of abstinence, consequences of drinking, perceptions of drink being a problem, and his help-seeking.

(4) *Troubles with drinking.* Some of the information will probably have emerged already under other sections of questioning, but a focused point must be retained in the interviewing for specific questioning on potential areas of trouble. Under the heading of *social problems* enquiry should be made as to impact on the family, work history, debts, and criminal involvement. *Physical problems* which must be considered involve the possible impact of excessive drinking on nearly every system of the body. Accidents should also always be on this list. *Mental health problems* include alcoholic blackouts, which may be more fragmentary or block amnesias. This is also a convenient place to ask about certain syndromes which are

related to dependence: hypnagogic hallucinations, subacute hallucinatory states, delirium tremens, alcoholic hallucinosis, and alcohol withdrawal fits. Evidence of alcohol-related brain damage will, of course, be picked up in the course of general assessment of mental state or by special investigations (Ron, 1979).

(5) *Motivation and the profit-and-loss of drinking.* To phrase the question in the usual way as to 'whether the patient is motivated or not', is to show blindness to the patient's essential predicament. In all probability he is highly ambivalent, and both wants to go on drinking, and to stop or ameliorate his drinking (Orford, 1976). Assessment therefore implies the drawing-up with this patient of a kind of profit-and-loss account related to continuance of his present style of drinking, rather than questioning of a sort which seems to imply that the only acceptable answers are those which will involve denial of the reality of the predicament. It may often be best therefore to start by purposively counteracting any expectations that the doctor only wants to hear a bogus statement that drinking is seen by the patient as unmitigated evil, and invite him to give an account of what for him is 'good about drinking'. This may, for instance, immediately indicate the relative importance for this patient of alcohol as a drug which relieves apprehension of affective distress, as a substance which provides an agreeable 'high state', as a drug which eases sociability or aids self-assertion. It may alternatively be clear that a major attraction of drinking is the social setting and the companionship – the patient finds it hard to envisage life without the pub.

Exploration of the debit side means enquiry into how the *patient himself* weighs the significance of this or that consequence of his drinking, or potential threat of his drinking. For one patient it may be loss of health which is of paramount importance, for another, the threatened break-up of the marriage, and so on.

The minimal approach to treatment

In this section an outline will be given of a minimal approach to treatment, while in the following section circumstances will be discussed which may propose the need to go beyond these basics. The treatment philosophy inherent in this two-stage approach is again the belief that much that has previously been deemed the non-specific element in treatment comes to the fore as the very essence of the helping process. And this belief is coupled with an insistence that the patient should not be overtreated, with dangers of iatrogenic learnt helplessness.

Aiding reappraisal

It is here that the whole process of assessment starts to be turned to therapeutic ends. The assessment which has been gone through in the previous section has to be *shared* between doctor and patient, rather than just remaining something for the case notes. By the doctor tentatively offering an interpretation of this or that aspect of the patient's experience and amending these views in the light of the patient's positive engagement in the discussion, an agreed formulation of the nature and extent of the drinking problem (in context) is worked towards. What is in fact being invited is a cognitive restructuring by the patient of the nature of his predicament, the surrender of denials and defences, and the design as it were of a map of understanding which can be helpfully used in finding a way forward. Attention must in particular be given at this stage to discussion of the degree of the patient's dependence, the criteria on which this diagnosis is being based, and the personal implications of such a diagnosis.

Aiding decision-making

It is then the therapist's task on the basis of the information which has been shared and discussed, and the understandings which have been built, to sense the stage which the patient's ambivalence has allowed him to reach on any decision making, and to aid in a re-adjustment of that ambivalence. The threats inherent in drinking may need sympathetically to be re-explored (within subareas), and the patient's negative feelings towards a life without (or with less) alcohol empathetically discussed and rationally met. The degree of success which the doctor can expect to achieve in this persuasional role must depend on his perceived credibility as an informant and his ability to move by small steps.

Turning decisions into goals

If the patient has been able to make some broad decisions as to what he is going to do about his drinking (and his life), the next stage is that of helping him to interpret those decisions in terms of specific short-term and long-term goals, in each of a number of areas. These areas are likely to include the marriage, the parental role, finances, work, and leisure. Such a simple matter as getting the house painted or the garden in order or taking the children to a football match, may be set as usefully attainable achievements. But important though it is to agree with the patient a vision of what has to be accomplished which embraces much else besides, the drinking goal is also vital. At the end of these discussions there must have been a clear formulation on the drinking. The most usual question to be determined is whether the patient takes abstinence as his goal, or aims at more controlled drinking.

Although the criteria on which confidently to answer that question are not at present fully determined, some provisional guidelines can be spelled out as follows. The patient will do best to aim at abstinence if any one of the following criteria is fulfilled:

(1) if he wants so to do (for instance, if he is firmly committed to an AA ethic).

(2) if further drinking or occasional lapse into uncontrolled drinking carries serious danger of disastrous consequences such as further tissue damage, or violent acting-out. Rationally it must, though, be admitted that espousing the *goal* of abstinence (as opposed to its achievement) by no means guarantees a reduction in such threat.

(3) if the treatment of underlying or accompanying conditions (for example, depressive illness) requires abstinence at least in the short- or medium-term.

(4) if the patient shows symptoms of a well-established dependence syndrome.

(5) if the patient has aimed at controlled drinking and been given help with that goal, but has failed.

The criteria which would suggest the feasibility of a controlled drinking goal can be worked out on the basis of opposites to this check-list. In practice, matters are often not as clear-cut as any neat check-list would suggest. For instance, the patient may show definite symptoms of the dependence syndrome, but it can be a difficult judgement whether the syndrome is so far advanced as to make controlled drinking unlikely. It may be reasonable in such circumstances to go along with the patient who desires controlled drinking on a sort of experimental basis, with the patient and doctor together monitoring its feasibility.

Setting up the expectation of self-responsibility and conferring hope

It is easy for the patient with a drinking problem to leave the consultation in a state of perplexity on the central question of who is now responsible for what aspects of that patient's future. At worst, he may accidentally have been given the confusing message that he is a 'sick alcoholic' whose sickness excuses his behaviour, at the precise moment when what would in fact most benefit him is a restoration of the sense of autonomy and self-responsibility. The importance and subtlety of the set and expectations which evolve from the therapeutic encounter cannot here be left to chance but need to be brought out into the open and talked about. On this basis there can be discussion of how the patient is himself to work toward his goals, and the detailed strategies he will employ (Litman *et al.*, 1979).

This is not, though, a matter to be handled negatively or with implications of rejection. The message is one of confidence in the possibility of the patient's helping himself, and, properly put across, this is a message which can confer self-esteem and help.

Review and reporting

There can be no fixed rule as to how often the patient should be seen at follow-up, but the tendency in the past has certainly been to give more frequent appointments than is necessary. Indeed, there is a case for arguing that, with many patients, after the initial assessment and goal-setting no further appointments should be offered at all, thus confirming the patient's own responsibility (Orford & Edwards, 1977).

In other instances, it may be useful to ask the patient back for spaced appointments, with the expectation given that these sessions are for review and reporting of progress, rather than for continuing or major 'treatment'.

Detoxification

The majority of patients will be able to withdraw from alcohol in an out-patient setting. Indications for in-patient admission for detoxification include a previous history of delirium tremens or withdrawal fits, or findings from the present assessment to suggest a severe degree of dependence and hence the risk of a major withdrawal experience.

Out-patient withdrawal should be accomplished with the minimal medication possible, and it is a bad practice to give a large supply of drugs to a patient who is still drinking. Many patients will require no medication at all, while others may be helped by a dose of up to 10 mg chlordiazepoxide or 500 mg chlormethiazole initially up to three or four times per day in diminishing doses for 5–7 days.

Treatment of major withdrawal states on an in-patient basis may require larger drug doses (Schuckit, 1979). See also vol 2, chap. 14.

The family perspective

Whatever the origins of the excessive drinking, it inevitably becomes in time a 'family problem' and is then a behaviour embedded in the family dynamics. Stereotypes of 'the alcoholic wife' are not well-supported by the research literature (Orford, 1975) and the implications of the drinking have to be looked at in each marriage separately. The coping-style which the spouse is employing can usefully be analysed (Orford & Guthrie, 1976). The possible needs of the children must not be forgotten (Wilson & Orford, 1978). It is, though, inappropriate and again an over-escalation of treatment to suppose that wherever there is a drinking problem, formal marital or family therapy is indicated.

The treatment setting

The treatment of patients with drinking problems should usually be accomplished in an out-patient setting (Edwards & Guthrie, 1967). Indications for ward admission may include detoxification of the severely dependent patient, assessment and treatment of concomitant psychiatric conditions, or life-saving intervention.

Common treatment ancillaries and reasons for going beyond the basic approach.

What has been emphasized in the previous section is the view that the essential treatment of alcohol problems resides in the interchange between doctor and patient rather than in elaborate and special therapies. However, a number of ancillaries to the basic approach deserve note and clinical circumstances in which it may in any case be necessary to go beyond the minimum also deserve consideration.

Common ancillaries to the basic approach

(1) *Alcoholics Anonymous.* AA provides a very valuable example of a self-help organization and every psychiatrist should acquaint himself with its manner of working (Robinson, 1979).

AA is firmly committed to an abstinence goal, so it is usually inappropriate to refer a patient who is aiming at controlled drinking. But with that proviso there is much to be said for referring every patient with a drinking problem to AA, if he is seeking

abstinence. By no means every such patient will successfully affiliate to AA, but the message should be given that it is in the patient's own best interests to attend at least a few AA meetings so that he himself may determine whether these meetings help him. A-Anon is a similarly useful organization for the families of alcoholics.

(2) *Psychotherapy.* The approach which is being commended in this chapter relies heavily on the exploitation of psychological understanding and the use of a relationship. But in many centres, the help given puts heavy emphasis on formal psychotherapy, most usually in terms of some variety of case work, group therapy, or family therapy. Hypnosis has also had its vogue. The objective evidence for the efficacy of the near routine deployment of psychotherapy for alcoholism is, however, unpersuasive.

(3) *Behaviour therapy.* Aversion therapy for alcoholism provided one of the earliest examples of behaviour therapy in any area. Despite striking initial claims, classical aversion with apomorphine or emetine has largely fallen into disrepute. Over the last decade or so, a great deal of work has, however, been done on application of a variety of other behavioural approaches to alcoholism, and there is growing evidence for their utility in certain circumstances (Nathan et al., 1978).

(4) *Deterrent drugs.* Disulfiram (Antabuse) and citrated calcium carbimide (Abstem) are drugs which interfere with the metabolic breakdown of alcohol, and produce an acute and unpleasant reaction. There is still no conclusive indication as to their true place in clinical practice. A provisional view might be that these drugs may be of value for some patients who believe in them. Dangers and side effects should not, though, be neglected.

Reasons for going beyond the minimum

(1) *Skid Row and the vagrant alcoholic.* The alcoholic who is completely lacking in social support and caught up in the Skid Row way of life often requires special help if he is to have a base of sufficient stability from which to make a recovery (Cook, 1975; Otto & Orford, 1978). Special hostels and 'shop front' community facilities have been developed to this end.

(2) *The specially problematic case.* Every clinical service must be familiar with the seemingly intractable alcoholic – the patient who is destroying him-

self, causing enormous distress to his family, and also straining the goodwill of treatment staff. The temptations include outright rejection but more often a haphazard escalation of treatment effort takes place – a further admission, or more drugs or more psychotherapy. What is often much to be advised is a calm and detailed reassessment of the case and the reformulation of agreed goals and methods for their achievement.

Underlying and accompanying psychiatric conditions

Before considering some individual psychiatric conditions, it is useful to state some general principles. Excessive drinking frequently coexists with other psychiatric problems, and a careful general assessment is therefore always indicated. The diagnostic work may be very difficult to complete when there is suspicion of underlying or accompanying illness and the patient is still drinking. Admission simply for diagnosis may therefore be indicated. The prior treatment of an underlying mental condition may also be vital to dealing with the drinking, while a confused therapeutic approach with no clear priorities and too much prescribing of drugs to a still drinking patient is a recipe for wasted time or even disaster. The discussion which follows on specific conditions is essentially just a variation of these themes: depression will be taken first as providing a good example and one of great clinical importance.

Depression

The recurrent challenge is that of being faced yet again by an alcoholic patient who is miserable, and who is perhaps even threatening suicide. On the one hand, the clinician will be aware that true depressive illness and alcoholism frequently coexist and that suicide among alcoholics is appallingly common (Nicholls *et al.*, 1974) On the other hand, he will know that depressive illness can in such patients be overdiagnosed, with a labile disturbance of mood, a common feature of intoxication.

(1) The classical biological features of depressive illness are likely to be so confused by the impact of drinking, that an orthodox symptomatological approach to diagnosis is of limited value – every severely dependent alcoholic will, for instance, experience morning withdrawal symptoms which may confusingly suggest diurnal variation.

(2) The history therefore becomes of prime diagnostic importance. A clear history of recurrent depressive illness or of depressive illness leading to purposive self-medication with alcohol may stand out clearly, despite the overlay of drinking.

(3) Antidepressants should not be given in an ill-thought-out therapeutic experiment, to the alcoholic who is still drinking. Antidepressant medication in such circumstances seldom produces benefit, even if the patient is seriously ill with depression.

(4) It is worth while trying on an out-patient basis to get the patient off drinking, and then, after withdrawal is complete, reassessing the question of depression.

(5) If in any serious doubt, it is best to play safe and admit the patient for detoxification and assessment in a safe setting.

Not infrequently the diagnostic problem remains puzzling even when the patient is off alcohol, and in alcoholism work one comes across atypical cases of very chronic depressive illness – the woman who, for instance, appears to have suffered from a never fully remitted illness following a puerperal depression experienced ten years earlier, and whose excessive drinking originated in this setting.

Hypomania

Patients with hypomanic illness may drink excessively, either as a consequence of a general carefree disinhibition, or because of an unpleasant element of anxiety in this mood disturbance which is relieved by drinking.

Schizophrenia

As alcoholism is a very common condition and schizophrenia a relatively common disorder, it is not surprising that the two diagnoses should sometimes coexist. Whether their coincidence is greater or less than would be expected by chance is unknown. In general, a patient suffering from schizophrenia may find alcohol an unattractive drug: the experience of intoxication may be threateningly unwelcome and sensed as imperilling a tenuous adjustment. Some schizophrenics may, though, be drawn toward drinking as a means of relieving accompanying affective distress, and the schizophrenic who gravitates towards Skid Row may add drink to his other problems as part of this disorganized way of life. The differential diagnosis between schizophrenia and alcoholic hallucinosis can often not be made while a patient is drinking, and it is frequently necessary to admit the patient for observation over a period of weeks.

Brain damage

Brain damage is, of course, widely recognized as a potential consequence of excessive drinking. What is not sufficiently realised is that a drinking problem may evolve as a result of brain damage. A cerebral tumour may present as 'alcoholism'. Excessive drinking may be a sequel of head injury in a young person, or occur following a cerebrovascular accident or consequent on a dementing process. Sometimes there is a circularity: drinking damages the brain, and the brain-damaged alcoholic drinks with ever lessening control.

Phobic states and anxiety

Patients suffering from situational phobias may drink to cope with their anxiety. In such circumstances alcohol may be viewed by the patient as an almost indispensable medicine. The best course of action is then to admit the patient, and when detoxification is complete treat the phobic condition behaviourally. Sometimes, though, a surprise is in store, and once the patient is off alcohol the previous seemingly severe phobic symptoms fade away. It appears therefore that drinking may not only relieve phobic anxiety but also, on occasion, paradoxically exacerbate such disabilities, perhaps because chronic subacute experience of alcohol withdrawal raises the basal level of anxiety. Social phobia may also be a contributory cause of excessive drinking, in which case detoxification followed by vigorous treatment of the underlying condition is again indicated.

Patients with drinking problems may be found who exhibit all levels of free-floating anxiety, from the mildly incommoding to the near crippling. Use of the ordinary range of sedative–depressant drugs is contra-indicated, for there is a risk that dependence on these drugs will be substituted for dependence on alcohol. A common-sense emphasis on 'learning to live with it' and on finding other strategies for coping or the use of relaxation training is the best approach, but where symptoms are very severe there may be an indication for beta blocker drugs, such as propanalol.

Personality

The quest for 'the' alcoholic personality has properly been abandoned. Drinking problems may occur in the setting of any type of personality and clinically what is important is to attempt an accurate and sympathetic appraisal of the strengths and vulnerabilities of the particular individual rather than retreat to stereotypes.

Sexual problems

Such problems are not infrequently associated with excessive drinking. Careful enquiry into sexual orientation should therefore always be made, and appropriate help given. It is also important routinely to ask about the possibility of more serious sexual problems rather than to 'forget' this area of questioning because of one's own inhibitions. Impotence is a well-known consequence of excessive drinking: the patient will be helped by knowing that partial or complete recovery often takes place when drinking stops.

The possibility of underlying sexual problems in women deserves note, particularly because these are rather easily overlooked by the male therapist.

Pathological jealousy

This condition is classically described as a consequence of excessive drinking, with speculation that it may be associated with alcohol-induced impotence. Adequate studies are in fact lacking, but it seems likely that in many instances the jealousy has been a prior and very long-standing problem, with alcohol then used to relieve the associated anxiety. When this is the chain of events, it may be found that if the patient can be helped to give up drinking although the jealousy will still remain, the drunken and unrestrained (and perhaps violent) expressions of jealousy may be brought more under control.

Forensic implications

Many people who commit an offence are drunk at the time of the incident, but it remains notoriously difficult to establish causality. A survey of men in one London prison showed that 56 per cent of those serving a sentence of less than 3 months had a drinking problem, and excessive drinking undoubtedly contributes to the social instability of the petty offender or recidivist who makes up so large a sector of the prison population (Edwards *et al.*, 1971).

The psychiatrist is sometimes asked to give a court opinion in such cases. Despite the sense of weary despair that this kind of story often engenders there are possibilities of worthwhile help, and if drink is got out of the equation a radical change in social adjustment may be seen.

The psychiatrist is much more likely to be asked for an opinion when drink is involved in violent crime or murder: one Scottish series showed that 47 per cent of murderers were intoxicated at the time of the killings (Gillies, 1965). The response of the court in such instances is always uncertain and drunkenness itself is of course no defence, but if diminished responsibility can be pleaded, a murder charge may be reduced to manslaughter. Mania *a potu* (pathological intoxication), is probably not a real clinical entity (Coid, 1979).

Specialism and generalism

There is a continuing place for the psychiatrist who gives at least some of his time to specialized work with alcoholism, and who provides support to non-specialists who deal with these problems. But it is important to stress that today the general psychiatrist should be willing to learn much more about alcoholism and develop the confidence to deal with the majority of these patients without any specialist referral.

10.4
The impact of alcoholic parents on their children
SULA WOLFF

The literature

Even social drinking in pregnancy can result in spontaneous abortion (*Lancet*, 1980). Excessive drinking in pregnancy can lead to malnutrition in the mother; to intra-uterine and post-natal growth retardation of the baby; to congenital abnormalities; to neonatal irritability; and to developmental delays (Smithells, 1979).

There is evidence from adoption studies for a genetic component to the intergenerational transmission of alcoholism. Adopted sons whose biological parents were hospitalized for alcoholism, like their non-adopted brothers, had higher rates of alcoholism, of alcohol-related problems, and divorce than children of other parents (Goodwin *et al.*, 1973, 1974). Adopted men who became alcoholic, more often had alcoholic natural parents than adopted men who did not, whereas the rate of alcoholism among their adoptive parents was not excessive (Bohman, 1978). There were too few adopted alcoholic women for analysis. What precisely is inherited, a low physical tolerance of alcohol, a proclivity to develop physical dependence on alcohol, or predisposition to heavy drinking, is not known.

The suggestion that psychological and social processes are unimportant in the transmission of alcoholism (Goodwin *et al.*, 1974) is not borne out by clinical experience (where parental alcoholism is a common feature both of male alcoholics and of their wives) nor by a number of studies of the drinking patterns and attitudes towards alcohol of young people.

Comparative studies of children of alcoholics have tended to focus on attitudes to drink and later drinking behaviour. The results are conflicting. Hawker (1978) suggests that children adopt their parents' patterns of drinking and abstinence, while a study comparing English and Irish young people (O'Connor, 1978) found English parents to be more casual and permissive in relation to their children's alcohol consumption but Irish children, although drinking less, to be in more trouble over drinking than the English.

A series of imaginative studies investigating how Glasgow children of different ages view drink and drinking showed that very young children have mildly positive attitudes to drink, that these give way to considerable criticism of drink and drunkenness between six and ten years (when children are exceptionally conforming to adult teaching), but that at adolescence peer-group influences predominate, drinkers are given status, and seen as both tough and sociable (Jahoda & Crammond, 1972; Davies & Stacey, 1972). The attitudes of young children to alcohol are a function of a complex interplay of forces including parent models, other sources of authority, and the public media. In two small extreme groups of these children parental-role models were found to be very important: two-thirds of the six- to ten-year-old children who mentioned heavy drinking in their own homes thought that they themselves would drink when older, while two-thirds of those who said that their parents never drank thought that they would not drink in later life either. Unfortunately, in the study of adolescents, parental drinking patterns were not asked about.

Plant (1979) has demonstrated that drinking behaviour is at least in part socially determined, for example by employment in the distillery trade. Certainly, excessive weekend drinking with associated domestic violence is much more common in Britain in unskilled working-class families. Affected fathers often have other features of sociopathy and the high association with psychiatric disorder, especially conduct disorder and subsequent sociopathy in the sons, is likely to be mediated by a cluster of interrelated processes. Nylander (1960) compared children aged 4–12 years whose fathers had obvious alcoholism with controls. Divorce or separation had occurred in 28 per cent of the first group but in only 4 per cent of the second. While attendances at child guidance clinics were similar in the two groups, teachers identified almost five times more children of alcoholics as disturbed. Many symptoms, especially anxiety and depression, were commoner in both sons and daughters of alcoholics. But among children admitted to a psychiatric unit whose fathers were alcoholic, two-thirds were boys and many were over 12 years of age.

Clinical practice

In child psychiatric practice in the UK, a common pattern is the association of early aggressive behaviour and later delinquency in boys whose fathers are excessive, weekend drinkers, violent to their wives and sometimes their children. Often the mother had married her husband when both were very young, in rebellion against the maternal grandmother; by the time of referral the mother may have left the father but now reads into her son's behaviour all the bad characteristics of her husband. She expects self-control from the child before he can manage this, warns him repeatedly of the consequences of disobedience, fails to intervene physically before accidents or fights occur, and punishes him repeatedly both for his misdeeds and for displays of temper. In the genesis of the child's conduct disorder, often accompanied by high levels of anxiety and low self-esteem, the influence of the father's frightening role model is likely to be no more important than the mother's hostile attitudes to her husband and son. His fear is that he will become aggressive and damaging like his father and cast out by his mother. Repeatedly, he engages in behaviour (for example, wandering, stealing, soiling, smearing faeces, fighting) which tests out the limits of safety. Such children see themselves as unlovable; they tend to be defensive and often express their anger indirectly.

In some cases, excessive drinking and violence on the part of the father is matched by basic affection for him and all the children on the part of a masochistic wife. The anxiety level of the children, boys and girls, is high but the behavioural difficulties, often taking the form of aggressive behaviour, may be confined to the school setting.

Jacob, a large boy with average ability and educational attainments, was ten on admission to an assessment centre because of violent behaviour at school. His first school excluded him for 'viciously' attacking children and teacher; he could not be contained in a small school for the maladjusted; and had just been excluded again from an ordinary primary school.

The mother, a large, emotionally labile woman who sat embracing her son throughout the interview, had been the oldest of eleven children, of average intelligence but illiterate and with poor self-esteem. After a young sister was burnt to death when she herself was 15, she left home to become a prostitute. She cohabited steadily, had two children both privately fostered, drank excessively and was often, although briefly, in prison.

Jacob's father, her second cohabitee, was alcohol addicted. The parents fought regularly when drunk and both made a series of suicide attempts. When seen alone, *Jacob* mentioned his great fear of getting into fights and also that when he was seven he had fallen into a river and would have drowned had he not been rescued by a passer-by. He worried greatly about his parents and, when residential schooling was discussed, he said 'my ma would go barmy if she weren't allowed to see me. She's the only one I've got . . . if my parents split up, it will break up my dad. I care about him as well as my mum.'

One of the most stressful and potentially dangerous situations is when the alcoholic father also has a *delusional jealousy syndrome*. The family members are often tied to each other with considerable affection but outbursts of extreme violence can occur and the children involved, boys and girls, in great conflict between their affection for their father and their terror at his behaviour, can have a variety of presenting symptoms: psychoneurotic, psychosomatic, emotional, or antisocial.

When, more rarely, it is *the mother* who *is alcoholic*, the children's development is at risk not only because of conflicting emotions and inadequate parental role models but because even basic physical care and protection are now lacking within the home.

An alcoholic and drug-addicted mother left her three-year-old, *Susan*, alone with the similarly disabled father. At the age of ten the child recalled how she had thought the red pills he was eating were sweets. He told her that he loved her and her mother before, as she then thought, he fell asleep. When neighbours entered the house she had been alone with his dead body for three days.

Now she is excessively talkative and demanding in her small children's home, has outbursts of rage which distress her and her housemother, and plays repetitive, sadistic, teacher–pupil games. She loves her mother but is terrified of growing up to be like her and feels guilty because of these fears. The memory of her father's death is still vivid in her mind.

Jason was adopted in infancy. His adoptive father died of a heart attack when he was 3. His adoptive mother, the oldest of a large Catholic family, never close to her own mother, now became a bout drinker. She was a highly competent woman who moved around the world with Jason from one responsible post to another. The child was often alone with her when she was drunk. She would get him to go out to buy whisky for her and at times he found himself locked out of the house. Twice he was raped by a houseboy and

on one of these occasions his usually very gentle mother beat him severely.

At interview, Jason was very fidgety, anxious, and with a marked tic. Like the two children described above, he too knew that his mother really loved him and he too was relatively undefended, remembering the traumatic events of his life vividly and in detail. He mentioned his mother having an operation for 'bleeding down below'. He accepted most readily the phrase that when his mother drank she was 'not herself'. He said she was 'like another person (then), she couldn't keep her balance.' She allowed the cat to die and once 'when I came home from school the doors were locked and I shouted through the letterbox and she was like somebody else at the time and I shouted and she paid no attention and she said she was coming but she never did. I sat on a chair and my uncle came up and took me out with my three cousins.'

In school he had written a letter to a girl full of sexual allusions. He said he thought sexual things were 'dirty like, say, kissing. I find it dirty when a boy kisses a girl.' He never wants to marry.

All three children required long-term auxiliary care. Jacob went into a community home, Susan was in a small family group home, and Jason went to a residential school for maladjusted children. What the long term effects on their personality development will be of their shocking life experiences at an age at which they could not cope with the anxieties aroused, is not yet known.

What is clearly demonstrated is that excessive drinking and alcoholism can prevent even affectionate parents from providing the essentials of child care and, especially when there is no healthy parent, exposes the children to serious and recurring dangers.

10.5
Gambling

E. MORAN

Introduction and definitions

Gambling may be defined as an activity involving two or more persons in which some property, usually referred to as the stake, is transferred between the people concerned so that some gain at the expense of others. The result of this is dependent on the outcome of a risky or uncertain situation, which may be natural or contrived for the purpose. Participation in this activity can be avoided and is typically pursued in an active fashion, often for reasons unrelated to the property staked.

Since gambling involves risk-taking which provides the experience of thrill, it is an activity which is very popular but usually not taken to excess, leading to little harm in the majority of cases. Some gamble much more than the average and in addition are able to make a livelihood out of this. These professional gamblers are successful because their gambling is carefully planned and deliberate, frequently involving horse-race and greyhound-race betting, concerning which they usually have special sources of information not available to ordinary people.

In contrast to these professional gamblers, there are others whose excessive gambling leads to adverse financial, social and psychological consequences for themselves and their families. This condition is referred to as compulsive or pathological gambling. Although both these terms have been used interchangeably, the latter is more satisfactory since the condition does not arise from a true obsessive-compulsive disorder.

Incidence and prevalence

In general, the activity of gambling has pejorative overtones. Because of this and the fact that detailed surveys have not been performed, the full extent of the activity is unknown. The last concerted attempt to assess its incidence was by the last Royal Commission on Gambling (HMSO, 1978). It concluded in its Final Report in 1978 that in the UK, £7100 million was staked on gambling in 1976. This rose to £8000 million in 1977. Just over 10 per cent of this was actually spent or lost by gamblers, providing the profits and covering the expenses of the promoters as well as the takings of the Inland Revenue. The remainder was regained by gamblers and subsequently restaked, emphasizing that gambling money goes round and round. If one includes minor forms of gambling, such as an occasional bet or buying a raffle or lottery ticket, 39 million people, or 94 per cent of the adult population (aged 18 years and over) gamble at some time or other, with 39 per cent doing so regularly. However, regular gambling is above the national average of 39 per cent in the following categories: men, persons aged 45 to 64 years, manual workers, and those living in the North, North West, West Midlands and Greater London. The limited, more detailed statistics available about gambling in the UK have recently been collated by the Home Office (HMSO, 1980).

A survey conducted by the US Commission on the Review of the National Policy toward Gambling (1976) showed that 61 per cent of the adult US population (about 88 million people) participated in some form of gambling. Among these people, there were about 19 million who gambled only with friends in a social setting, leaving about 69 million people or 48 per cent of the adult population who patronized some form of legal or illegal commercial gambling. Only 11 per cent of the adult population gambled illegally and the overwhelming majority who did so also patronized one or more of the legal varieties of gambling.

As far as pathological gambling is concerned, a survey in licensed betting offices concluded that there were over 80 000 pathological gamblers in the UK involved in horse-race and greyhound-race betting (Dickerson, 1974). While it is known that this is the most common form of gambling and that most likely to become pathological, there is no reliable information about the incidence of pathological gambling in other types of gambling, such as gaming which is particularly liable to be taken to excess. The US Commission on the Review of the National Policy toward Gambling (1976) estimated that approximately 0.77

per cent of the adult population could be classified as 'probable compulsive gamblers' and an additional 2.33 per cent could be considered 'potential compulsive gamblers'. In Nevada where most gambling is legal, the incidence of compulsive gambling appeared to be significantly higher. On the basis of interviews with 296 Nevada residents, it was projected that 2.62 per cent of the Nevada population were 'probable compulsive gamblers' with an additional 2.35 per cent 'potential compulsive gamblers'. According to surveys of British prisons and reception centres, up to 10 per cent of their populations are pathological gamblers (Royal College of Psychiatrists, 1977).

Aetiological factors

As with many other activities, there is wide variation in the intensity of gambling within a given population. At one extreme, there are a number of individuals who abstain completely, at the other there are some who gamble excessively, while the majority contain their gambling within moderate bounds.

Social pressures

There is increasing evidence that pathological gambling is often a manifestation of excessive participation as a consequence of social pressures (Royal College of Psychiatrists, 1977; Moran, 1979). In these circumstances the condition occurs as an exaggeration of normal mechanisms responsible for gambling. Among the latter, the transfer of property which is referred to as the stake, is an essential part of the gambling contract. Since, at the present time, money is the usual stake, it is often assumed that the motivation underlying the gambling must be related only to this. It is true that in some cases, especially the professional gambler, the gambling is *for* money and the object is to win the stake. Much more frequently however, the stake is no more than a means to an end. The money is a token which is used to purchase something else, such as excitement, amusement, comfort. Consequently, it is a mistake for us to focus exclusively on the financial aspects of gambling, and fail to appreciate the psychological and social factors which enter into its motivation.

It has long been recognized that the experience of risk is thrilling and may therefore be pleasurable. Furthermore, if the uncertainty continues for a limited time, as in the case of gambling, the feelings of tension which are associated with it, are relieved when the uncertainty ends. The beneficial effects of this experience were recognized by the ancient Greeks, who referred to it as catharsis. It seems that it is this element which makes gambling so attractive in the majority of cases. This is well illustrated by those gambling facilities referred to as amusement arcades in which, as the name implies, amusement can be purchased. This highlights the fact that by the very nature of the gambling contract, the activity is a social one. Indeed the most common organization of gambling involves the gambling industry which is usually the other party to the contract. Obviously, in gambling as in any other commercial enterprise, those who provide the facilities expect to make a profit. However, this can occur only at the expense of the gambler. Therefore, devices introduced to increase the proprietor's profits will inevitably do so by inciting people to gamble more or gamble excessively. This is compounded by the general assumption that some of the financial proceeds from gambling should be made available for other purposes. An example of this is the betting levy in the UK which is used to subsidize horse-racing. Another example is the principle behind lotteries.

Psychological factors

In the presence of social pressures, predisposed individuals are propelled towards pathological gambling. Some of the factors involved in this predisposition are as follows:

(1) *Morbid risk-taking.* Since gambling is a type of risk-taking, it lends itself to be used by those who, for reasons related to their personality, have a high need for risk. The pathological gambler appears to be such a person. It is probably more accurate to see him as one who spends large amounts of money on the intangible commodity of risk in a manner analogous to that of the antique collector who derives pleasure from purchasing expensive antiques. The main difference is that whereas the antique is tangible and the collector has something to show for the money he has spent, the subjective experience of risk is fleeting and therefore may easily pass unnoticed.

This propensity to take risks shows itself in other morbid ways such as attempted suicide. A survey of pathological gamblers has shown that the incidence of attempted suicide is about eight times the expected rate (Moran, 1970b).

(2) *Other personality factors.* The study of the personality characteristics associated with pathological gambling has been mainly psycho-analytic in orientation. Freud (1928) suggested that gambling resembled masturbation and was a substitute for it. This occurred in the context of unresolved oedipal diffi-

culties, where the gambling was a means of self-punishment to expiate the sense of guilt. Others have suggested that the problem arises from an unconscious desire to lose because of a deep-seated urge to produce situations in which the gambler feels unjustly treated. This self-punishment arises from a psychological mechanism referred to as 'psychic masochism' (Bergler, 1970).

(3) *Processes of learning.* Gambling with its winnings and losses provides an opportunity for operant conditioning. The most effective schedule encouraging gambling is one of intermittent reinforcement (wins) in which the number of wins varies from time to time. This produces a stable and persistent response, the long-term net gain or loss being almost irrelevant. This unpredictable contingency of reinforcement is exploited by the gambling industry. Within this setting, a large win at a critical period of development in adolescence seems to produce the predisposition to pathological gambling. This sequence has been referred to as 'beginner's luck' and is related to other superstitious notions common in gambling (Moran, 1975).

Apart from the winnings and losses, the gambling situation itself may affect learning. As far as the random processes inherent in gambling are concerned, all participants, even a total failure, stand on an equal footing. This may be the only circumstance in which some individuals have this experience and may therefore provide a means of avoiding pathological anxiety in the presence of feelings of inferiority. Gambling may thus be a conditioned avoidance reaction to anxiety and a sense of inadequacy.

(4) *Mental disorder.* Pathological gambling may occur in the context of any mental disorder. However, it is most commonly associated with depression. More usually, a neurotic type of depression occurs after a bout of heavy gambling with large losses. Alternatively, the depression may be primary, with gambling arising as a response to the symptoms of tension or as a self-destructive expiation of feelings of guilt symptomatic of depression. This latter situation is similar to alcoholism and shop-lifting occurring as part of the depressive syndrome.

Pathological gambling may be a manifestation of the broader disorder of psychopathy or may be associated with excessive use of alcohol.

In addition, those whose gambling has become pathological may experience loss of control similar to that found in psychological dependence on alcohol.

There is thus a state of psychological dependence on gambling (Moran, 1970a; Wray & Dickerson, 1981).

Clinical features

Pathological gambling can usually be recognized by the presence of any of the following:

(1) Concern on the part of the gambler or the family about the amount of gambling which is considered to be excessive.

(2) The presence of an overpowering urge to gamble so that the person concerned may be intermittently or continuously preoccupied with thoughts of gambling: this is usually associated with the subjective experience of tension which is found to be relieved only by further gambling.

(3) The gambler's subjective experience of an inability to control the amount, once gambling has started, in spite of the realization that damage is resulting from this.

(4) Various disturbances for the gambler and family because of a felt need for the activity. Among possible consequences are the following:
(a) Financial disturbances such as debt and shortage.
(b) Social disturbances such as loss of employment and friends, running away from home, eviction, criminality, imprisonment, marital problems, divorce, and behaviour disorders in the children of the family.
(c) Psychological disturbances such as depression and attempted suicide.

In general, pathological gambling is most easily recognized in men. This seems to be due to the fact that for various social reasons, horse-race and greyhound-race betting and gaming are more frequently patronized by men. These types of gambling have a high turnover of money and therefore the consequences of excess become evident more quickly. On the other hand, women are more likely to gamble on bingo or football pools. These do not involve such large sums of money and when excessive gambling occurs the presentation is much more subtle, with disturbances in the social sphere rather than through the accumulation of large debts.

While pathological gambling is seen at all ages, an increasing number of young people have recently found themselves in difficulties as a result of fruit-machine gambling and horse-race and greyhound-race betting.

ILLUSTRATIVE CASE HISTORY

A 45-year-old married man who was an insurance clerk, was admitted to hospital after a drug overdose. He had accumulated debts of £7000 and was about to be evicted from his home because the rent had not been paid for several months. These financial difficulties had occurred as a result of horse-race and dog betting. After years of quarrelling, his wife had threatened to commence divorce proceedings after another bout of heavy gambling.

His early background was dominated by heavy gambling. Whilst still a small boy, he used to accompany his father to the race-course and was often sent by his paternal grandmother to place bets with the street bookmaker. In his early 'teens, he placed his own first bet on a horse and vividly recalled how he won £5 on a stake of one shilling. After this he gambled intermittently, his stakes never being more than a shilling or two. When he was aged 20 years, he married a woman who was a few years his senior. She soon showed herself to be a rather aggressive, demanding person who knew about his gambling but, at that time, did not consider it to be a problem. Indeed, she often accompanied him to the local greyhound stadium, when they were first married. After the birth of the first child, his gambling increased but the debts which accumulated were paid off by his mother.

In the early 1960s, following the liberalization of the gambling laws, a licensed betting office was opened near the insurance office where he was working. Initially he and a friend regularly called into the betting office in the lunch hour. Although his friend soon lost interest, he continued to go there regularly because he found that he was 'very lucky'. Unfortunately, the wins did not continue for long. Since he appeared to have a great facility for persuading other people to lend him money, he managed to cover his increasing losses. Subsequently, he spent longer periods in the betting office. He found the racing commentary heightened the sense of excitement he felt when placing his bets just before the 'off'. He also began to find that if he did not have money for gambling, he would become increasingly tense and this would only be relieved by placing a bet. Not infrequently, he would lose and then found that he had a strong urge to place further bets. This 'chasing' of his losses would continue until he had no more money to hand and could get no further credit. At these times, he would dread the thought of further betting since he was aware that he was unable to control his gambling. However, it would not be long before the craving returned, resulting in further gambling. At other times, particularly when he was abroad on holiday, the urge to gamble would temporarily leave him. Over the years, his gambling gradually increased, resulting in an accumulation of problems and culminating in the disturbance which led to his admission to hospital.

After discharge from hospital, the patient was referred for psychiatric assessment. There was no evidence of mental illness and, apart from the serious gambling problem and its consequences, there were no significant abnormalities. He and his wife were seen separately and jointly. In the course of these interviews, marital counselling was provided and arrangements agreed whereby the husband's income was paid direct to his wife, who would control the finances and provide an allowance to cover his limited expenses. This arrangement was to continue for the foreseeable future. In addition, the couple were encouraged to draw up a detailed inventory of the debts and the regular financial outgoings, as well as the income. They were

advised to discuss a realistic repayment scheme with the creditors. Further discussions took place when they were urged to modify their life-style in order to stimulate joint interests, such as social outings, visits to clubs and cinemas, with a view to making new friends who were not involved in gambling. They succeeded in building up family-orientated activities such as shopping expeditions and weekend visits. They became active members of Gamblers Anonymous.

Two years later, he had not gambled again and was still paying off his debts. The family relationships had improved considerably.

Management and treatment

The first thing that needs to be recognized when dealing with the problem of pathological gambling is that it involves more than just the activity of gambling. Quite apart from the effects of this pursuit, it involves a whole way of life which has many ramifications. The limited notion of treatment as applied to illness is therefore not applicable: what is required is management of various aspects of the life of the person concerned and rehabilitation. It often requires a multidisciplinary team approach, with help from the social worker and the psychologist.

Assessment of the problem

It is essential to obtain a detailed history concerning the disorder. It needs to be recognized quite early that pathological gambling is a form of behaviour for which there is more than one possible explanation. This point should be emphasized quite strongly at the beginning of the assessment. Both the gambler and his family often look for simple explanations and solutions, but they need to understand that the disorder arises out of a complex of various factors.

It is particularly important to have information about the following:

(1) *Present gambling*. Precise details are required about the type, amount and location of the gambling activity. In relation to the amount of gambling, the amount of time devoted to it may be as important as the amount of money spent.

(2) *Previous gambling*. A detailed history of the development of the gambling problem is required, in particular the first contact with any form of gambling early in life as well as details of the first occasion when the individual himself gambled. It is important to have as much detail as possible about circumstances and life-events associated with changes in the gambling behaviour.

Since the situation in which the gambler finds himself is often highly complex and even frankly chaotic, it may assist him to produce a coherent history of the development of his condition. This may be done by asking him to provide a written chronological account which can subsequently be used as the basis of discussion and amplification.

As part of the assessment, it is important to attempt to obtain some indication of the person's motivation. Many gamblers seek help to assist them with the problems that flow from their excessive gambling, without appearing to accept the need even to restrict their gambling. Indeed, many of these gamblers readily admit that they enjoy the gambling and are only seeking advice because relatives have insisted they should do so, or because of impending legal proceedings for some misdemeanour due to the excessive gambling. Such people are difficult to help.

Counselling on the nature of the problem

On the basis of the information obtained during the course of the assessment, there needs to be some detailed discussion with the gambler and the spouse, both individually and jointly, concerning the significance of the facts that have been ascertained. In particular, it is important to discuss details of the nature of the gambling activity, drawing attention to some of the snares involved such as the exaggerated ideas of the importance of skill and the subtle ways in which excessive participation can occur. It is amazing how many hardened gamblers are often very ignorant about the real facts involved in the activity of gambling.

As part of the counselling process, there needs to be some discussion of the whole procedure of habit-formation and the development of loss of control. This then leads on to the suggestion for at least a period of total abstinence from all gambling. Since most gamblers derive some satisfaction from gambling, it is often unrealistic at this early stage to advise them to stop gambling in any form for the rest of their lives. It is, therefore, wise to suggest a period of total abstinence for six months initially and then to review the situation. Controlled gambling as a treatment goal has been found to be effective (Dickerson & Weeks, 1979).

Financial problems

The most common reason for pathological gamblers to seek help is because of mounting debts and their consequences. It is therefore important to obtain a detailed statement of these debts as well as an inventory of the income and outgoings of the gambler and his family. In terms of this information the gambler needs to be encouraged to draft a realistic plan of repayment. Since the debts are often considerable, the repayments may have to continue over many years. This can obviously only be achieved by encouraging the gambler to discuss the whole matter with the creditors involved. However, it is important that the repayments should be consistent with the person's regular income and circumstances. There is a considerable danger that in the first flush of enthusiasm, unrealistic repayments will be contemplated which may lead to temptations to gamble in order to maintain them.

Excessive gambling is usually associated with a disturbed appreciation of the value of money. Because of this and the continued temptation to gamble, it is probably wise for the family finances to be controlled by the gambler's spouse, at least for some time. Regular income from wages or salaries should be paid into a bank account over which the spouse has sole control. In time, as the period of abstinence from gambling continues, the gambler needs to become gradually more involved in working jointly with the spouse in controlling the family finances.

Social help

The gambler and the spouse need to be encouraged to review the whole organization of their social life. In particular they need to consider how they spend their spare time, what friends they cultivate and what interests they have. It is often within specific settings that incitements to gambling occurred in the past and the gambler and the spouse need to make very careful arrangements to avoid future temptations. This may be easier to achieve by helping them to draw up a joint contract which spells out in detail those types of behaviour to be avoided as well as those to be encouraged.

The help of the organization of Gamblers Anonymous can be invaluable. Gamblers Anonymous is a form of self-help for pathological gamblers which is organized in the form of local groups which meet regularly. As well as meetings for gamblers, there are also separate ones for their spouses. Quite apart from the valuable work done in the group setting, Gamblers Anonymous provides a valuable means of establishing alternative social contacts to those that went with the excessive gambling. Indeed in some pathological gamblers, Gamblers Anonymous is the vehicle through which all the necessary forms of help can be provided. Even if this is not always the case, Gamblers Anonymous still provides a valuable form of help and support for the individual and the family.

Psychological and physical forms of treatment

Reference has already been made to the need to discuss attitudes to gambling in particular, and to life in general. In certain cases there may be special neurotic problems which may be amenable to more complex forms of psychotherapy. Furthermore, there are often serious marital problems which may be primary or secondary. In either case, marital casework may be an important aspect of the help to be provided.

Attempts have been made to deal with pathological gambling by means of behaviour therapy. In particular, aversion treatment has been used (Seager, 1970). The results have not been very encouraging since, although excessive gambling will usually cease on this form of treatment, the relapse rate is fairly high. Furthermore, it requires specialized facilities.

Coexisting mental illness such as depression will need treatment, including the use of antidepressant drugs.

Prevention

Pathological gambling in the majority of cases can be seen to be a condition arising out of faulty habits established as a result of social pressures. The full effect of health education on the activity of gambling has yet to be realized. However, an impact will only be achieved if gambling is part of a broader educational approach concerning other types of behaviour, such as that used by Moran, J. (1979). Since the incidence of pathological gambling is partly determined by facilities for gambling and the pressures to encourage excess, public policy on gambling obviously plays an important role in its prevention.

Prognosis

Although detailed follow-up studies have so far not been performed, clinical experience indicates that the prognosis of pathological gambling is very variable. In general, further episodes of heavy gambling occur after shorter or longer intervals. This is in large measure due to the persistence of strong social pressures. However, important elements determining a successful prognosis are the integrity of the personality of the gambler as well as the social support provided by the people immediately surrounding him, such as his family, friends, and employer.

PART IV
Personality disorders

11
Sociopathic personality

11.1
The childhood origins of delinquency and antisocial behaviour

D. J. WEST

Identification and prognosis of 'antisociality'

Delinquency and antisocial behaviour commonly originate in childhood. They are most frequently detected among the lower strata of society and among materially and educationally deprived families, especially where there are more children than can be properly managed. Often the children, especially the boys, appear to be following a family tradition of criminality. A raised incidence of almost any social problem one can name – broken or discordant marriage, erratic employment, welfare dependency, alcoholism, prostitution – occurs in the families from which recidivist delinquents originate.

These observations are differently interpreted by sociologists and clinicians. The former tend to regard much anti-establishment attitude and conduct as a normal response to social pressures and subcultural traditions, the latter tend to emphasize the deficits and peculiarities of antisocial individuals that may be produced or aggravated by circumstances of social deprivation. This difference in approach is of more than academic interest. If delinquency is a healthy reaction to intolerable conditions the psychiatrist who tries to 'adjust' the social rebel to his circumstances may be doing a disservice both to the individual and to the cause of social justice.

The clinical practitioner has to resolve this issue each time he is faced with complaints of misbehaviour, and has to assess whether or no they signify a serious deviation from standards appropriate to the client's age and social situation. Psychiatrists have not always been successful in setting aside their own value systems and cultural expectations when assessing clients from a different generation and background. The unscientific pronouncements that used to be made about the dire mental effects of youthful masturbation illustrate this. Of course, mistakes can be made through underestimating as well as overestimating the significance of behavioural peculiarities. Although thieving and other acts defined as delinquent are extremely common among young persons, youthful delinquency cannot always be dismissed as psychiatrically unimportant.

Psychiatrists are concerned with the social maladjustment evident among persistent delinquents, not with their delinquent acts *per se*, many of which are trivial, opportunistic, and situationally induced. Juvenile courts are called upon to deal with many minor incidents of no relevance to mental health. Commonplace illegal acts by adults, such as tax evasion, minor motoring offences, or pilfering small articles from work are not thought to be psychiatrically significant, and there is no reason why rule-breaking by children should necessarily indicate disorder. A certain amount of nonconformity is expected of children, especially of boys, who come under pressure from their peers to prove their courage by going along with delinquent escapades. They are less restricted than adults, who have more reason to fear loss of reputation and career prospects if they are caught. The criminal justice system, which is responsible for attaching the official label 'delinquent', usually does so on the basis of proved acts of theft, since this is easy to define and deal with in a legal context. The psychiatrist is concerned with antisociality in a broader sense, including all behaviour that is deviant, disruptive, unduly impulsive, or aggressive and maladaptive to the individual as well as harmful to others.

Misbehaviour is a matter of degree. When sufficiently frequent to lead to repeated court appearances, or to be perceived by teachers and parents as problematic and warranting referral to a psychiatrist, this already differentiates the individual from the majority of his social peers. The results of self-report delinquency studies show that the majority of normal youngsters engage in a surprising amount of delinquency, and that only a small fraction of delinquent incidents come to official notice (Hood & Sparks, 1970). However, these studies have also shown that the admission of unusually frequent or serious misconduct in response to self-report questionnaires is associated with having or subsequently acquiring an official conviction record (Farrington, 1979). The recidivist delinquent is in fact a deviant among his social peers. At school, even in so-called delinquent neighbourhoods, such children are recognized by classmates as trouble-makers and tend to be unpopular (West & Farrington, 1973). Just as depressive symptoms, according to quality and severity, can be a sign of a 'normal' grief response, a temporary reactive illness, or a major psychotic breakdown, so can delinquent behaviour, according to degree, signify normal assertiveness, temporary social maladjustment or a malignant personality disorder.

In a survey carried out by the Cambridge Institute of Criminology of a sample of normal males recruited from schools in a working class neighbourhood in London, it emerged that a fifth of them acquired a criminal record for offences committed as juveniles under 17, and over a third were convicted for offences up to the 24th birthday (West & Farrington, 1977). Obviously, such large proportions of the male population cannot be regarded as psychiatrically disordered. All the same, even those juveniles who had no more than one official finding of guilt were found to differ to a statistically significant degree from their non-delinquent schoolfellows on important social variables. For instance, they were more likely than others to have been identified as troublesome at an early age by their teachers and to have come from large-sized, low-income families in which a parent or sibling already had a criminal record. Recidivist delinquents, however, were much more sharply distinguished from their peers in all these respects, and, although few of them were in fact referred, it would have been reasonable to regard their recidivism as reason enough for psychiatric screening.

Among males the incidence of criminal convictions declines rapidly after eighteen, so that even amongst those classed as recidivists at that age many are not subsequently reconvicted. In the Cambridge study only a quarter of the delinquents were classed as persistent recidivists, with multiple convictions extending beyond the nineteenth birthday, and only about a sixth were persisting offenders at age 24. This is why delinquency is often referred to as a self-limiting disease. Nevertheless, the pattern of youthful convictions is a useful prognostic indicator. The larger the number of juvenile convictions and the younger the age at first conviction the more likely is the individual's conviction career to persist into adult life. It is said that nothing predicts behaviour so well as behaviour. Certainly the number of previous convictions usually predicts future reconvictions better than social or psychological data, although it is also true that adverse family circumstances contribute significantly to the likelihood of persistent antisociality.

Delinquents referred to clinics are necessarily a biased group, already picked out as maladjusted, but surveys of less selected samples confirm that young recidivists at large, even though they may never have been near a psychiatrist, often manifest a constellation of deviant attitudes and behaviour that amounts to personality disorder. In the Cambridge study, by means of extended interviews at age eighteen, it was found that, in addition to the behaviour leading to criminal convictions (which was mostly thieving in one form or another) a majority of young recidivists (48 out of 62), compared with only a small minority of nondelinquents (42 out of 288) manifested at least four out of a list of eleven 'antisocial' characteristics. The list included gambling, driving after drinking, immoderate smoking, sexual promiscuity, unstable work record, anti-establishment attitudes, involvement in acts of violence, unconstructive use of leisure, association with antisocial groups, use of prohibited drugs, and having oneself tattooed. Furthermore, as a predictor of reconvictions in the future, the impulsive, hedonistic personality reflected in this 'antisociality' assessment proved to be as effective as the record of previous convictions for predicting reconvictions later on (Osborn & West, 1978). Whereas most delinquents became much less 'antisocial' and more like non-delinquents as they reached the age of 24, those who continued in delinquent careers retained their socially deviant characteristics and frequently failed to provide satisfactorily for the children they fathered.

Aggressive and antisocial acts may begin in childhood as an understandable and apparently healthy response to erratic parental discipline or frustrating social conditions, but this can develop into such an all-embracing and socially inappropriate pattern of behaviour that the youngster's education, employment, and personal relationships are permanently blighted. Martin Roth (1972) has argued very persuasively that persistent delinquents whose antisocial behaviour pervades their whole life style are not just ordinary members of the under-privileged sections of society or persons with an unpopular scale of values. They exhibit a definable syndrome that would bring them into conflict in any society. The syndrome 'has a characteristic sex distribution, age at onset, family history of similar symptoms and disorders, and family constellations and influences that show a considerable measure of consistency in their course and outcome.' The syndrome manifests in varying degree of severity, 'Terms such as "sociopath" and "psychopath" merely refer to points along this continuum. . .'

Typically, the antisocial youngster displays a constellation of maladaptive features that may include any of the following:

(1) Aggressiveness, manifest in defiance of parents and authorities, destructiveness, quarrels and fights with peers, cruelty and bullying, disgruntled and resentful attitudes, fierce temper, and intolerance of frustration.

(2) Failure to acquire social skills, manifest in carelessness and slovenliness, poor educational attainment in comparison with measured intelligence, clumsiness and uncooperativeness in team efforts, restlessness and inattentiveness in school, and frequent absences from class. Tasks calling for patience and sustained mental effort are particularly poorly performed. Teachers perceive these children as lazy and insufficiently motivated.

(3) Nonconformity to social rules, manifest in thieving, vandalism, driving away vehicles, reckless risk taking, truancy, drug and alcohol use, precocious sexual behaviour or misconduct, running away from home, and stopping out at night.

(4) Failure in personal relationships, manifest in chronic conflicts with parents, distrustfulness towards other adults, a restriction of friendships to other antisocial characters and unwillingness to participate in organized leisure activities.

(5) Incorrigibility, manifest in hostile reactions to discipline, stubbornness, unresponsiveness to punishment, and lack of guilt or remorse.

Most cases of antisociality are so closely linked with adverse social situations that it becomes unprofitable to try to distinguish the psychiatric from the social component. In the minority of cases in which the youngsters come from stable parental homes that appear to be psychologically sound and of good social standards, one looks for abnormalities in the child himself, such as cognitive deficits or neurological impairments. More often, however, one finds evidence of covert family conflict, or subtle forms of emotional rejection, that have interfered with the normal disciplining and socializing processes. Anti-sociality developing in backgrounds of this type, where there is great contrast between the behaviour of the troublesome youngster and the standards adhered to by other members of the family, is particularly liable to be accompanied by anxiety, guilt feelings, ambivalent attitudes, and neurotic symptoms.

The antisociality syndrome usually begins under the age of ten and becomes fully developed well before adolescence. If present to any marked degree it carries a serious prognosis. In her follow-up study of 500 guild guidance clients, traced and interviewed after an interval of 30 years, Robins (1966) found that adult pathology was much more likely to follow from childhood antisociality than from childhood neurosis. Children who had been referred for predominantly neurotic complaints, such as phobias, nervous habits, sleep disturbance, enuresis, and psychosomatic complaints were no more likely to become neurotic adults than were a control group made up of schoolfellows of the clinic patients. Among those with a significant constellation of antisocial symptoms in childhood (6 or more items), a third became sociopathic adults compared with only 2 per cent of the control children. Referral for antisociality in childhood was a precursor of many forms of disturbance, such as problem drinking, social alienation, dependence on welfare, suicide, unsatisfactory army service, and psychiatric hospitalizations. Over half of the antisociality referrals were destined to be divorced and 43 per cent of the males to be imprisoned. Even so, there was a noticeable improvement with age in many cases, especially in the decade 30 to 40, when the grosser threats to the life and property of others tended to diminish. Although severe and lasting, the disturbance was not necessarily immutable.

Robins (1966) was investigating a particularly deprived and deviant sample. Her gloomy prognosis holds true only where the syndrome is very pervasive and unreactive to circumstances. There are better prospects for children who are aggressive at home but not at school, for those whose behaviour improves during temporary fostering, and for those capable of attaching themselves to at least one non-threatening adult. Criminological experience highlights the cumulative effects of an array of adverse circumstances in childhood, so that those who have experienced the very worst family and social backgrounds are the ones most likely to continue a disorganized and criminal life-style into their adult years. Glueck and Glueck (1959), who conducted several large-scale and long-term studies of delinquent careers, used to claim that assessment of family circumstances during infancy, or even at birth, could be used as a reliable predictor of delinquency in later life. This holds true only for extreme cases. Prediction based on early background variables is limited to the identification of groups with a varying statistical risk of becoming delinquent (Wadsworth, 1979). The outcome in an individual case is always to some extent uncertain. Children are not mere passive victims of circumstance, they do not all react in the same way, and there are many influences outside the home, at school or elsewhere, that affect their behaviour.

Aetiology

The search for a single cause is futile. The antisociality 'syndrome', which takes varied forms and occurs in all degrees of severity, is the end result of complex psychobiological interactions in which individual and environmental variables both play their part.

Learning theorists seek explanations of the impulsiveness, untamed aggression and incorrigibility of antisocial characters in terms of a failure to acquire the patterns of restraint necessary for harmonious social living. The failure can often be traced to circumstances inimical to social learning. The normal processes of socialization, which are at their most critical phase in infancy and early childhood, are thought to depend upon consistent conditioning, the presence of adequate behavioural models, and an environment in which the child feels secure, develops strong bonds of affection towards the parents, readily identifies with their ideas, and feels anxious and guilty if he deviates in thought or deed (Trasler, 1973). Among children from deprived and disorderly homes, where the essential requirements for social learning are lacking, the incidence of antisociality is very high. The hindrances to learning that are most commonly observed include parental discord that often leads to separation and the break-up of the home, neglect and lack of supervision so that children grow up 'on the streets', harsh or erratic or carelessly lax discipline, occasional physical abuse, actual or threatened rejection by parents, criminality or alcoholism or personality disorder in the parents, and periods spent away in children's homes or with parent substitutes. Exposure to blatantly unsatisfactory parental behaviour and lack of care seems to be the predominant cause of many cases of antisociality.

In his psycho-dynamic theory of the origin of antisocial character disorder Bowlby (1951), following psycho-analytic tradition, stressed the importance of the earliest years of development and regarded as crucial to normal development the uninterrupted maintainance of an affectionate and close maternal bond in babyhood. Subsequent research (Rutter, 1972) suggests that events in the later years of childhood, and the behaviour of the father as well as the mother, are also important factors in the genesis of antisociality. Repeated insults appear more damaging than any single trauma, such as a temporary separation from the mother. Moreover, separation often occurs in a context of family upset or discord, so that its effects are hard to distinguish from those of other sources of disturbance. In her follow-up of boys originally 'identified as potential delinquents McCord (1978a) concluded that parental instability was a most powerful factor in the genesis of delinquency, but that the presence of just one stable and affectionate parent, especially if unhampered by the simultaneous presence of a hostile marriage partner, could go a long way to protect the child.

Recent Danish adoption studies (Hutchings & Mednick, 1977) have revived interest in the possibility that vulnerability to delinquency and antisociality may have an appreciable genetic component. Among adopted sons, criminality in their biological fathers appears to have a greater influence upon the likelihood of their becoming delinquents than does criminality in their adopting fathers. An adoption study carried out in Sweden yielded rather more equivocal results (Bohman, 1978). The association between criminality in male adoptees and criminality in their biological fathers was apparent only where, as was often the case, paternal criminality was associated with alcoholism.

It is difficult to draw firm conclusions from adoption studies because they all suffer from the difficulty that adoption agencies do not allocate children at random, so that some of the correlations reported could be spurious. More convincing than adoption data, the massive study of twins in a Danish national sample carried out by Christiansen (1977) confirmed the existence of an hereditary factor affecting the likelihood of acquiring a criminal record, especially a serious recidivist record such as might be expected to reflect the presence of the antisociality syndrome. The effects reported in this study were, however, much smaller than earlier and less methodologically sophisticated surveys had suggested. Moreover, it

cannot be emphasized too often that the demonstration of some hereditary predisposition does not explain the mechanism of transmission or pinpoint the anomalies that underlie the deviant behaviour.

Environmental and family pressures appear to be the main determinants of antisociality, but these factors interact with the characteristics of the individual child. Intellectual deficits, neurological impairments, and temperamental peculiarities, all of which may have some genetic component, may make a child difficult to socialize. Through the stress they cause to their parents by feeding problems, sleep disturbance, fretfulness, crying, delayed sphincter control, retarded speech, or general unresponsiveness such children may generate an unfavourable environment for themselves.

That physical disabilities make some contribution to the development of antisociality and delinquency was shown by Stott (1966), author of a teachers' questionnaire for identifying troublesome and maladjusted children. He studied a large sample of delinquent boys on probation in Glasgow and showed that, corresponding with increasing degrees of maladjustment, there were significant increases in the incidence of deviant stature, physical defects (such as squint, spasticity, and congenital deformities), poor eyesight, and a history of hospitalization in infancy. It is well known that physical disorders involving the brain, such as chorea, cerebral palsy, and viral encephalitis may lead to childhood behaviour disorders (Freeman *et al.*, 1965; Slater & Roth, 1969). In their Isle of Wight survey Rutter and co-workers (1970) found a very significantly raised prevalence of psychiatric disorder among epileptic schoolchildren. The connection between all these disorders and antisociality is complicated by the fact that they all tend to occur more often in socially disadvantaged segments of the population. Moreover, children with these disorders are much more likely to develop antisocial reactions if they are exposed to influences similar to those which produce antisociality in the physically normal.

Minimal or subclinical brain damage is sometimes advanced as a cause of behaviour disorders, especially when the usual environmental causes are not in evidence. The phenomenon of behaviour disturbance following brain injury is well recognized (Shaffer *et al.*, 1975). Behavioural sequelae may persist in the absence of physical signs, which is presumably caused by subclinical damage. There is good evidence for intellectual deficit and behaviour disorder being sometimes the result of substantial brain damage during birth. Beyond this, researches have unearthed associations between perinatal disorders, including prematurity, and subsequent behaviour disorder in children who do not necessarily display any neurological signs to verify the presence of brain damage (Knoblock & Pasamanick, 1966). Such findings lend support to the subclinical brain damage theory, but many of the reported associations could be explained in other ways, in terms of intervening variables such as family size, poverty, area of residence, or choice of hospital for the birth, all of which are statistically associated with both the level of perinatal disorders and the incidence of antisocial behaviour. The results of some English surveys (West, 1969; Davie et al., 1972) suggest that there is no substantial relationship between the generality of behaviour disorder and the commoner forms of perinatal disorder.

Difficulties at least as great stand in the way of a completely convincing demonstration of the connection – much publicized in recent years – between high serum-levels of lead, probably produced by atmospheric pollution, and behaviour disorder and intellectual impairment in children (Rutter, 1980; Gregory & Mohan, 1977). Some of the apparent deficits in children with high lead-levels in their blood may be explicable in terms of concomitant social factors such as poor education (Ratcliffe, 1977). There is, however, some evidence that medication to reduce lead levels in affected children will reduce hyperkinesis when there are no other causes for the symptom (David et al., 1976).

The concept of minimal brain damage has some practical application in the diagnosis of the hyperkinetic syndrome of childhood. As described by Wender and Eisenberg in the USA (1974), the important features are overactivity, restlessness, fidgeting, short attention span and difficulties in concentration, aggressiveness and emotional lability, poor impulse control, learning problems not attributable to generalized intellectual impairment, discord between child and parents, clumsiness and poor performance on tests of psychomotor co-ordination, variability of performance on different cognitive tests, and a high prevalence of 'soft' neurological signs, notably non-specific EEG abnormalities, clumsiness, and speech disorder. Follow-up studies suggest that the restlessness improves with age but that the antisocial traits are liable to persist into adulthood.

British clinicians have tended to be more conservative than their American counterparts in the use made of the diagnosis of hyperkinesis. They usually limit the term to cases in which over-activity is pervasive and accompanied by demonstrably erratic cognitive functioning or mental retardation and by neurological abnormalities detectable on examination. Otherwise there is hardly anything to distinguish the hyperkinetic syndrome from ordinary conduct disorder. Recent British research (Sandberg, Rutter & Taylor, 1978) casts doubt upon the validity of the broader concept of a hyperkinetic syndrome, given the low intercorrelations between the component symptoms, but the link between the key feature of over-activity and behaviour disturbance is not disputed. Despite justified scepticism on the status of the syndrome the concept is useful in practice since some cases so diagnosed improve remarkably with drugs of the amphetamine type. That this should lessen misconduct by increasing conditionability and so facilitating socialization is to be expected according to Eysenck's explanation of antisociality (Eysenck, 1977). The problem of the hyperkinetic child is one that merits more sustained attention and research than it has so far received in view of the considerable theoretical and practical issues to be resolved (Cantwell, 1977). In dealing with the over-active, behaviour-disordered child in practice, as in other cases where neurological disorder is present or suspected, psychosocial measures are at least as necessary as in the case of the troublesome but apparently neurologically intact child.

In addition to the identification of definite medical pathology, attempts have been made to establish statistical differences between same-sexed populations of delinquents and non-delinquents along dimensions of normal variability. Personality traits (for example, neurotic extraversion), physique (mesomorphy), intelligence, and speed of conditioning (in passive avoidance learning) have all been measured and are said to be relevant, but the results are of academic rather than clinical interest. The correlations are low and the small variations from the norm to be expected in an individual case (about 5 points of IQ for example) is of little prognostic value.

Aggressiveness, whether measured by attitude tests, low frustration tolerance, or self-report of real life confrontations, is probably the psychological trait most clearly linked with antisociality. It is stable over time and has predictive value for the likelihood of reconviction among delinquent populations (West & Farrington, 1977) It could be that inherited vulnerability to antisociality, manifest via this trait, is mediated by the reactivity of the autonomic processes that underlie deviant emotionality. On the other hand, there is no doubt that culture and training are of great importance in the development of uninhibitedly aggressive personalities. More research is needed to distinguish between types of aggression, such as the over-reactive anger of the explosive temperament, the chronically hostile and suspicious stance of the paranoid personality, and the relatively unemotional conduct of the person who has learned to use violence 'instrumentally' to obtain material or psychological advantage (Berkowitz, 1969). At present it remains unclear which varieties of aggression are the most important components of the antisociality syndrome.

Treatment

Antisocial behaviour and delinquency is inseparable from the social context in which it occurs. Treatment must often take the form of social and educational intervention rather than specifically medical or psychiatric measures. Co-operation between disciplines and between systems, for instance between hospital services, social services, local authority community homes, and Home Office penal establishments, is highly desirable, though extremely difficult to achieve across administrative and financial barriers.

The common forms of intervention have rarely been shown to be beneficial. One of the most ambitious schemes for prevention ever mounted, the Cambridge–Somerville Youth Study in Boston, recruited a large sample of boys, many of whom were considered to be at grave risk of becoming confirmed delinquents. They were arranged in matched pairs, according to age, delinquency-prone histories, and other criteria. One member of each pair was allocated to a control group, the other to an active treatment programme that lasted five years. Thirty years after the termination of treatment the criminal and social histories of 253 treated individuals and their 253 'matched mates' were compared. Those receiving treatment had been tutored, given friendly (big brother) counsel, introduced to youth facilities, and provided with medical assistance. Many recalled their counsellors warmly and were convinced that they had been helped and steered away from a delinquent life style. Objectively evaluated, however, the differences between the treated and the untreated groups were small, and nearly all to the disadvantage of the

treated group, which included more recidivist offenders, more men with alcohol problems, and a larger number with a history of mental illness (McCord, 1978b).

This result is merely a particularly striking example of a general trend. Two influential reviews of the outcome of treatments for offenders, one American (Martinson *et al.*, 1976) and one British (Brody, 1976), both came to the conclusion, that nothing seems to work. No matter at what stage the treatment effort is mounted – preventive or rehabilitative – and no matter what form the treatment programme takes – intensive supervision and counselling as an out-patient or on probation, individual psychotherapy, residential therapeutic community, or traditional penal regime – the result is the same, no demonstrable effect upon the clients' subsequent conviction rates.

These negative reports have been influential, especially in the United States, in discouraging rehabilitative programmes for offenders and curtailing or abolishing systems of supervision on parole. Treatment is seen as costly and ineffectual and an unjustifiable infringement of the offender's right to be regarded as responsible for his actions and punishable only in proportion to the gravity of his offence.

In spite of current fashions the maligned 'treatment ideology' is unlikely to disappear, any more than the practice of psychotherapy disappeared under the onslaught of critical evaluation (Rachman, 1973). Some therapists argue that they are concerned with maladjustment rather than rule-breaking and that the benefits of treatment are better measured in terms of improved social competence, raised self-esteem, and the absence of dysthymic symptoms than by conviction statistics. If a client returns to a social milieu in which offending is inseparable from his way of life then reconvictions do not necessarily imply psychological malaise. It may be, therefore, that some delinquents can become better adjusted without giving up crime, but as a general rule persisting delinquency reflects a constellation of disturbances. It would be an odd result, and one very disappointing to the community at large, if treatments intended to curtail delinquency improved everything else except delinquency.

Although the benefits of treatment should be expected, eventually, to reveal themselves in reduced convictions the effect may be delayed by social pressures or obscured by the inefficiency of conviction statistics as a measure of behaviour. The high level of undetected offences means that each conviction includes a large element of chance. Moreover, crude conviction counts do not adequately reflect changes in the seriousness or frequency of offending and do not allow for the special surveillance to which those known as ex-offenders may be subjected.

A likely reason for the failure of many treatment projects, especially those taking place in the confines of penal establishments, is that the impact of the therapy is slight in comparison with the total effect of the institutional regime. McClintock and Bottoms (1973), who followed up a sample of youths who had been exposed to a new programme of counselling and individual attention in Dover Borstal, found no change in reconviction rates, but remarked upon the difficulty of implementing radical modifications in a traditional institutional setting and noted a strong tendency to revert to old ways. The demands of security and the authoritarian attitudes of custodial staff can easily undermine attempts to apply therapeutic principles. Quay (1977), in a re-evaluation of a group counselling project in Californian prisons (which had been cited by Martinson and colleagues (1976) as a prime example of the ineffectiveness of treatment) was able to point to many indications of superficiality, poor training, insincere commitment, and coercive pressures which were more than enough to account for the lack of benefit observed.

After making all possible allowances for inefficiencies in application and evaluation, it must be admitted that the results of treatments designed to change antisocial habits have been disappointing. Older psycho-analytically oriented writings underestimated the strength of social determinants and encouraged over-optimistic expectations for the results of individual psychotherapy. Disillusionment with the psycho-dynamic approach to the control of antisocial behaviour has led to increased interest in techniques of behaviour modification, that is, the systematic manipulation of rewards and punishments according to operant conditioning principles. The method lends itself readily to objective measurement of short-term changes in behaviour, such as the reduction of aggressive incidents in institutions or, more interestingly, a reduction in disapproved behaviour among delinquents living at home with parents who have been coached in the manipulation of rewards (Alexander et al., 1976). However, as evaluative reviewers have pointed out (Emery & Marholin, 1977; Farrington, 1979) follow-up studies extending longer than a year are virtually non-existent.

The conventional psychiatric approach to antisociality in a young person is essentially eclectic. Firstly, medical history-taking and evaluation is essential for the identification of any modifiable physical conditions that may be underlying or complicating the picture. Unfortunately, diagnostic evaluation does not always point the way to effective treatment. For instance, the statistical association between non-specific EEG abnormalities and behaviour disorders does little to aid either treatment or prognosis in the majority of cases. The satisfactory control of epileptic fits does not necessarily alleviate accompanying behavioural problems.

An important minority of antisocial children are suffering from intellectual limitations or specific learning difficulties or defects of speech or expression. Remedial teaching and vocational training, and an adjustment of goals to what is reasonably attainable, will relieve tensions and improve social behaviour.

Very often the damaging secondary consequences of antisocial behaviour call for more urgent intervention than the primary causes. This is so, for example, when the immediate problem is drug addiction, rejection by school or family, commitment to delinquent associates, inappropriate sexual entanglements, or loss of rapport with conventional systems of training, work, and recreation. All these matters call for social more than psychiatric intervention. A successful treatment plan depends upon good contact with the agencies that can provide opportunities for special training and social rehabilitation.

In so far as family influences appear to be the original or continuing cause of antisocial behaviour, counselling and psychotherapy, involving both the youngster and his relatives, is the customary psychiatric response. Unfortunately, as already pointed out, treatment all too often proves ineffective. The families most in need are usually the ones least co-operative. The intensity of effort needed to rectify the effects of a lifetime of parental mishandling is often far more than a busy professional can give. The motive to change may be lacking, for however damaging antisocial behaviour may be in the long run it is often pleasurable and rewarding in the short term. Furthermore, antisocial characters can find some support from the existence of disaffected groups that profess to scorn the 'work ethic' and other values cherished by mainstream society.

These difficulties are no justification for abandoning attempts to help. A developed antisociality syndrome is a serious maladjustment and an unhappy state of affairs for society and for the family as well as for the individual concerned. Such cases should not be confused with the relatively well-socialized individuals who, at a later stage of life, discover that they can profit from dishonesty and freely choose crime as an alternative or a supplement to a legitimate occupation. The maladjusted antisocial child is 'driven' by a fatal combination of circumstances and temperament, and the fact that he is so frequently arrested and convicted is a measure of his lack of success in crime as in other aspects of life. All too often these characters find themselves in desperate need of some kind of rescue. Even if relatively little fundamental change is to be expected quickly, this does not justify professional neglect. In this country more young persons than ever before are finding their way into penal establishments and being subjected to regimes that do not even profess to be treatment-oriented. One factor contributing to this sad trend, which ought to be rectified, is the increasing unwillingness of the psychiatric services, as presently organized, to try to cope with individuals who are awkward, unruly, or disruptive.

11.2
Sociopathic (psychopathic) personality* in the adult

JOHN GUNN

Antisocial behaviour is common to all adults and is an ordinary nonpathological phenomenon. Indeed as Durkheim (1901) has emphasized, criminal acts are an integral part of all societies, 'Crime is normal because a society exempt from it is utterly impossible'. Each individual within a society shows varying degrees of traits such as honesty, aggressiveness, thoughtfulness, and altruism, and may at times find himself placed at the antisocial end of the spectrum by a given piece of behaviour. Nevertheless some individuals are more frequently and more severely antisocial than others. Indeed, it would probably be possible to place members of a society on a spectrum ranging from saintliness to sinfulness by measuring the frequency with which they break the informal and coded rules of the society. The chances are that most members of a society would fall somewhere near the centre of that spectrum.

When an individual breaks a written law then he will be dealt with by the penal system of the society concerned if he is caught and unless he can show that his behaviour was accidental, or the product of some other misfortune such as a mental illness, he will probably be punished. Most individuals in this predicament either never reoffend or only do so on a small number of other occasions. The individuals sit-

---

* Although not strictly justified on semantic grounds, the terms sociopathic and psychopathic tend to be used interchangeably. Where other authors are quoted their original term will be used.

uated at the frequently offending end of our spectrum are apparently failing to respond to the strictures of the penal system and usually derive no obvious rewards from their criminal activities. They therefore evoke curiosity as to the reasons for their particular life style and sometimes sympathy, for a good many of them appear to be in a sorry plight.

Some observers would regard these persistent offenders as automatically showing a form of personality disorder which can be labelled as psychopathic or sociopathic. However, simply applying a diagnostic label is not sufficient to indicate the presence of psychological illness. Even so the reasons for a particular individual persistently offending, in spite of punishment and the lack of reward, are of considerable scientific interest. We can consider the possible reasons for such an individual's behaviour under five broad headings, inheritance and constitution, acquired physical handicaps, learning, stress, and illness.

Origins of antisocial behaviour
Inheritance & constitution

As early as the beginning of this century investigators were intrigued by the fact that some families seemed to contribute a disproportionate number of sinners to the population. A recent review of the association between crime and disadvantage (Rutter & Madge, 1976) has shown that there is plenty of evidence that crime often does run in families. However, half a century and more of study has still not fully elucidated the mechanisms for this important finding. Constitutional theories have been popular from time to time and there is some evidence from twin studies that there is a small genetic factor in the transmission of crime from one generation to the next. This could be through particular types of personality traits or even intellectual traits (see Walker 1968a for a review) but this small genetic factor seems to be drowned by other important variables. Some researchers (Glueck & Glueck, 1956; Gibbens, 1963) have found that a mesomorphic or muscular constitution is associated with delinquency. However, nature versus nurture arguments are sterile and misleading. A given phenotype is always the product of an interaction between the genetic endowment provided at the moment of conception and the varying environments which that genotype has experienced throughout its development.

It is almost certainly thus in respect of antisocial behaviour with the behavioural and learning fac-tors playing especially important roles even though it is still not entirely clear how they operate. For example, in a recent attempt to understand the familial transmission of criminality, the common finding was noted that if one or more other members of his family have a criminal conviction, an individual has a considerably increased risk of acquiring a criminal record himself (Farrington *et al.*, 1975); however, this research did not explain how the vulnerability is transmitted from one family member to another; genetics, learning, and even selective prosecution presumably all play their part.

Physical handicaps

Troublesome offenders who get themselves locked up in prison, either because of the severity of the offence or because of the persistence of their offending show, as a group, some deviations from the general population norms in terms of their physical characteristics. In his study of Borstal lads, Gibbens (1963) found that 38 per cent of them had been rejected for military service, a rate twice that of the general population. The majority of the rejection criteria were physical problems such as defects of vision, ear, nose, and throat conditions, and tuberculosis. On the other hand in a survey of 411 London schoolboys aged 8 to 18 West and Farrington (1973) found no significant association between illness in early life and later juvenile delinquency, and there were no particular health problems noted in the survey. This contrast between prisoner populations and general populations of delinquents is important to bear in mind throughout this discussion. Medical problems of various kinds do seem to be overrepresented in prisons.

Learning

We are born with great potential but the way in which we use that potential is determined by the education (in the widest sense) that we receive. If we are born into a family of thieves then we are likely to view stealing as acceptable behaviour and are likely to acquire basic skills in larceny. This commonsense view of one possibly important factor in the background of the persistent criminal owes some allegiance to Sutherland's differential association theory (Sutherland, 1947). This theory suggests that criminal behaviour is learned from other people especially from intimates; the factors learned include techniques of committing crimes, specific motives, drives, rationalizations, and attitudes. Motives and drives are related to an acquired attitude to legal codes as favourable or unfavourable; a person becomes delinquent if he is shown better reasons for breaking the law than for keeping the law. This acquired attitude Sutherland called his principle of differential association. Recent evidence from a study of juvenile delinquents by West and Farrington (1973) suggests that this theory has some validity but is an oversimplification. The West and Farrington analysis yielded five background factors of particular significance in the genesis of delinquency: low family income, large family size, parental criminality, low intelligence, and poor parental behaviour.

West and Farrington closely examined 'poor parental behaviour'. Parents were given a global rating on this dimension by combining maternal attitude and discipline, paternal attitude and discipline, and parental conflict. Poor parental behaviour, measured in this way, correlated significantly with the children's delinquency. Perhaps this illustrates that a failure to learn 'good' social skills is as important in the genesis of antisocial behaviour as is the acquisition of 'bad' skills. The argument is that for integrated, altruistic, responsible behaviour an individual has to learn during his childhood how to assert himself in a socially acceptable manner, how to relate to others, and how to take other people's feelings into consideration when responding to his own problems. A family which does not teach these important and subtle skills is likely to produce offspring who are inconsiderate of other people's needs, who are likely to assert themselves in primitive ways, and who are likely to be defined as antisocial as a result.

In a study of 60 American families in which a child had been abused Steele and Pollock (1968) found that 'without exception' the parents had been raised in the same style which they recreated; several had experienced severe abuse in the form of physical beatings and, although a few reported 'never having had a hand laid on them', all had experienced a sense of intense continuous demand from their parents.

Stress

There is not a great deal written about the factor of stress being an immediate precipitant for criminal behaviour in the same way as it is for mental illness. This may be related to the fact that most people take it for granted. It is almost axiomatic that somebody under the stress of hunger or destitution is more likely than usual to submit to the temptation to steal. A recent study from the United States

(Masuda *et al.*, 1978) has shown that prisoners suffer an accumulation of life-change events in the years before they are imprisoned, an accumulation that reaches crisis proportions in the twelve months before incarceration.

The effects of stress on the vulnerable personality may perhaps be seen in studies such as that conducted by West (1963) when he examined the life histories of 100 recidivists, 50 of whom had significant crime-free periods in their careers. He found that the crime-free periods were associated with significant support from another person such as a parent or spouse or probation officer. Support is a very difficult concept to define but it probably depends on the reduction of anxiety and stress in one person by another.

Another way of looking at the relationship between stress and crime is to pinpoint the factors which may be associated with unusually high levels of criminal activity. A good example of an enquiry along these lines was the report of the National Advisory Commission on Civil Disorders (1968) commissioned by President Johnson after the 1967 riots in several negro areas in the United States. The Commission indicated five factors which predisposed to the riots: (1) frustrated hope, (2) an emotional climate heavy with the approval and encouragement of violence, (3) a feeling of powerlessness, (4) a new mood of self-esteem and enhanced racial pride, and (5) a view of the police as a symbol of white power, racism, and repression. They indicated that virtually every major episode of urban violence in 1967 was foreshadowed by an accumulation of unresolved negro grievances. After the riots were over the commissioners found thousands of ordinary negroes living, usually in fear, often in squalor, always discriminated against in under-privileged circumstances. The stress factors here are again self-evident and probably associated with the breakdown of law and order, and the subsequent improvement in social conditions for negroes in key American cities, such as Atlanta, has been associated with a return to calm and order.

Illness

Clearly illness is a form of stress and therefore may be non-specifically related to criminal activity in the way mentioned above. However, there is a strong belief that some illnesses, those usually associated with mental dysfunction, are particularly associated with criminal activity. No doubt this is partly related to a general fear of madness which may appear to produce uncontrollable and threatening behaviour, and partly to public knowledge of the fact that in some cases there is indeed an acting out of violent fantasies in the course of a mental illness. The famous Hadfield and McNaughton cases are well known illustrations of this (see, for example, Walker, 1968b).

Little is known about the criminality of psychiatric populations in general, although it is clear that they would have to exhibit very high levels of crime indeed to exceed the generally high level in the ordinary population (see McClintock & Avison, 1968). Some studies on the subsequent arrest rates of patients leaving mental hospitals in the United States have been done but with inconclusive results (Rappeport & Lassen, 1965; Durbin *et al.*, 1977, Sosowsky, 1978). On the other hand prisons do tend to collect an excess number of patients with mental and physical disorders. West (1963) found in a population of 100 recidivist prisoners a high level of psychiatric disturbance and 14 cases of significant physical illnesses, five of the men suffering with the effects of serious head injury. A personal survey estimated that approximately one-third of the British prison population can be regarded as psychiatric cases in the sense that they would be acceptable for outpatient treatment under the NHS (Gunn *et al.*, 1978). A previous survey (Gunn, 1978) found more men suffering from epilepsy among prisoners than would be expected from general population figures. A recent US survey has shown a similar trend (King & Young, 1978). Even when it is possible to compare a prison population with the general population fairly accurately for a specific disorder, as was the case with epilepsy, a simple cause and effect conclusion cannot be drawn. Epileptics who offend may be differentially institutionalized; a few epileptics are brain-damaged because of recklessness which also led them into crime, others are reacting bitterly to the stigma of their disorder, still others are made both epileptic and criminal by early environmental conditions.

Brain damage, such as that suffered by some epileptics is a good illustration of the way in which, on occasion, a protracted disorder may lead to persistent antisocial behaviour.

CASE HISTORY

For example there was *'Edward'*, a 39-year-old man with an apparently normal childhood in a well-integrated working class home. At the age of 29 years he was involved in a motor-cycle accident, sustaining a fractured skull which was followed by meningitis. After neurosurgical treatment he

was left with a right-sided weakness, epilepsy, and a change of personality. He attempted to return to his wife and his old job as a welder, but soon turned into an unemployed drifter, stealing frequently and sleeping either in the street or in hostels. In the ten years following his accident he was convicted of fifteen indictable offences (all for stealing) and he received a total of seven years ten months imprisonment.

Other disorders sometimes considered to be associated with antisocial behaviour are chronic psychoses and drug and alcohol abuse. As with brain damage simplistic cause and effect associations are usually wide of the mark (see Taylor, 1982, for a recent account of the relationship between schizophrenia and antisocial behaviour). Neurotic problems, however, are often considered as unconnected with crime and delinquency, yet there is no doubt that prisoner populations, for example, are highly neurotic in terms of their symptom scores on questionnaires and at interview (Gunn *et al.*, 1978). This conceptual separation of neurosis and antisocial behaviour probably depends upon two factors; first stealing, even in prison populations, is statistically unrelated to neurotic symptoms (Gunn *et al.*, 1978), and secondly, personality disorder (which many would regard as likely to lead to antisocial behaviour) is for some strange reason regarded by many as separate from the neuroses. Leaving this last large question aside it is clear that sometimes neurotic problems can lead to offending, for example, the depressed housewife drawing attention to her plight by shoplifting, and persistently antisocial individuals suffer from anxiety, depression, hypochondriasis, misplaced or excessive guilt, low self-esteem, and so on.

Sociopathic personality

Both Lewis (1974) and Pichot (1978) have described the historical developments and traditions behind the concept of psychopathic behaviour, beginning with Pinel in 1809 describing *manie sans délire*, which came into the English literature as a congenital deficiency of the moral sense (Prichard, 1835), and which has been modified by the German tradition of psychic or psychopathic inferiority. In his review Lewis examined some of the more recent attempts at definition. He says that 'the effect of reading solid blocks of this literature is disheartening; there is so much fine-spun theorising, repetitive argument and therapeutic gloom'. He points out that an inherent problem is how to agree on the range of the normal personality and on tenable criteria of mental illness. He proposes a provisional definition:

'psychopathic personality is a condition in which ingrained maladapted patterns of behaviour are recognisable by the time of adolescence or earlier, and are continuous throughout life; the personality is abnormal in the balance and quality of its components', but immediately criticizes this by pointing out that maladaptive patterns of behaviour and the balance of the components of personality are not matters of direct observation, and individual investigators would differ rather widely in judging them.

The same criticisms can surely be levelled at the criteria used by other workers. For example, the majority of the sixteen characteristics listed by Cleckley (1955) are judgemental, moralistic, and some, for example, the *absence* of suicidal behaviour, cannot be regarded as true criteria at all. He urges us to rate superficial charm, unreliability, untruthfulness, lack of remorse, 'inadequately motivated', antisocial behaviour, the *absence* of delusions, the *absence* of nervousness, and so on.

The difficulties these subjective assessments create in practice are demonstrated by the problems of reliability in making the diagnosis. Walton and Presly (1973) showed that psychiatrists do not agree very well when diagnosing different types of personality disorder and in particular they disagree about the use of the subtype sociopathy. More recently Hare and Cox (1978) have claimed that the diagnosis can be made reliably using Cleckley's check list if it is being made for research rather than clinical purposes. This tends to imply that two people working closely together can come to a working agreement about the subjective issues raised by the Cleckley criteria; however, it does not give much reassurance that validity is being approached. Indeed, validity is the central dilemma in the whole of this work. It is very difficult to think of a criterion which can be used as a measure of psychopathic disorder and which is both objective and independent of the other diagnostic criteria already used. Some interesting psychophysiological research is attempting to establish biological correlates of psychopathic disorder, diagnosed by means of the Cleckley criteria (Hare & Schalling, 1978). So far, the results of this work are inconclusive but it will surely be necessary to establish biological criteria of some kind if this diagnosis is ever to be established as anything other than subjective commentary about a selected individual's behaviour. Eysenck & Eysenck (1978) have argued that 'psychopathy . . . like most psychiatric diagnoses, is not in any conceivable sense a category . . . a dimensional approach is theoretically superior and empirically much better supported'. From their work with questionnaires these workers argue that psychopathy is in fact along a continuum between normality and psychosis.

Recently Robertson and I (Gunn & Robertson, 1976) attempted to draw out a general factor of psychopathic personality using the social diagnostic criteria listed by Robins (1966). The first problem encountered was reliability in our judgments of the social factors, and of 19 scales nine had to be dropped for this reason. The ten criteria remaining were applied to 107 prisoners referred to a special psychiatric establishment on account of their personality disorders. They failed to show much correlation between the variables and there was no general factor of psychopathy. On the other hand a more recent study by Watts and Bennett (1978), using slightly different variables but a similar technique with patients attending a psychiatric day hospital, did find some important correlations between social deviance and other variables, such as self-poisoning, care of children, social isolation, and violent behaviour, but again no overall general factor of sociopathy.

All this points to the need for caution in the use of the diagnostic category of sociopathic or psychopathic behaviour. It is clearly wrong to equate such a category with simple criminality; we have few biological criteria on which to hang any medical theory; many of the criteria used for the diagnosis are simply subjective judgements on the part of the observer; there is not much support for the idea of a single homogeneous category and even the strongest adherents to the idea of psychopathic disorder accept that it may be better understood on a dimensional model, or as a heterogeneous collection of different disorders. This being the case, it may be difficult to understand why the idea of the diagnosis dies so hard. Perhaps the reason for this is related to the importance of the diagnostic process in medicine. Walker & McCabe (1973) discuss four uses of diagnosis: explanatory, prognostic, therapeutic, and descriptive. It is often the case that information can be given in all four dimensions simultaneously by a single diagnostic term. For example, the diagnosis pernicious anaemia indicates to a doctor that a patient has a particular disorder of the blood, caused by a known vitamin deficiency, amenable to a specific treatment, and thus carrying a good prognosis. Unfortunately, the same rapid economy of communication does not apply when we use the term psychopathic personality. Indeed, very little information is communicated by this term except perhaps that the doctor using the label believes the patient to have a chronic disorder which is not psychotic and which will be manifest in some form of undesirable behaviour. To understand a patient better a receiving doctor will have to ask a lot of questions about a particular case and an expanded diagnostic formulation is essential.

An example will illustrate the argument. Mr M. was referred to hospital after he had been diagnosed as 'psychopathic disorder, and recurrent affective states'. This limited diagnosis did not transmit much information about causes or treatment. A formulation revealed the following.

A 30-year-old man began life in unhappy circumstances after his parents separated and soon ran into trouble for truancy both from school and home, stealing, and fire-raising. He developed sexual difficulties at an early age partly because of his preference for male sexual partners and partly because of an increasing need to expose himself. He has been admitted to several mental hospitals, has made many attempts to kill himself, and has set a large number of fires throughout his life. He is lonely, shy, and passionately fond of mechanical things such as bicycles, cars, machine tools. He has never been able to form a relationship lasting longer than a few months and several attempts to live with a girl failed abysmally. He is frequently depressed and sometimes elated and over-active. Fire-setting can occur during either of these mood swings.

This formulation communicates the type of information which one practitioner may require from another if he is going to undertake the management of this kind of patient. It realistically accepts that oversimplification of this type of multidimensional problem is not an effective way of achieving understanding.

Walker & McCabe (1973) do not mention the social functions of diagnosis, which include a change of social role for the patient and sometimes stigma. For example, psychopathic disorder is frequently equated with badness. A recent problem in ward management of a highly disturbed, over-active patient was alleviated at the first medical conference following the patient's admission by persuading the nurses that the diagnosis was not one of psychopathic disorder but of chronic hypomania. The patient's behaviour did not alter but one nurse volunteered 'that means this man is ill and we cannot use sanctions against him'. In many ways, the patient's behaviour fitted the descriptions of psychopathic disorder quite well and in this particular case

the aetiology of that disorder could be understood in terms of the affective disturbance. However, the change of diagnosis made a sharp difference to the social response of the caring staff to the patient. Lewis and Balla (1975) have argued strongly for the term sociopathic personality to be dropped in relation to child and adolescent patients because of the damage which can be caused by the stigma associated with this term.

Assessment and management

It follows from what has been said already that a simple label of 'personality disorder', 'sociopathy', or 'psychopathy', is not sufficient to give much guidance about the nature of the patient's problems and their management. Detailed assessment is an essential part of successful management.

Assessment

The first step is to take as full a history as possible. This may seem fairly obvious but it is surprising how often a term such as 'personality disorder' inhibits a detailed assessment, as judgements about the patient's culpability and treatability may already have been made. Yet the fullest possible history setting out the complex life events of the potential patient is particularly important with this kind of case as it is only by a clear historical understanding of what has happened in the past that one can make judgements about likely future crises and give helpful advice on how to avoid them.

The history-taking itself may require many hours spread over several fact-finding interviews (see also chapter 2 of this volume, and volume 1, chapter 9). Whenever possible, apparent facts should be checked by reference to a friend or relative. While this fact-finding is being carried out, two other important things will be going on simultaneously. First, there will be a chance for the doctor to develop some degree of rapport with the patient; secondly, an assessment of motivation for change and treatment can be made. As the assessment proceeds the possibly relevant factors should be considered under the five headings given earlier, inheritance, physical factors, learning, stress, and illness. In this way it is possible to tease out the issues, which may be amenable to professional help and to determine which type of professional advice is appropriate for each particular factor. The patient's view of his problems and their remedies is very important. It may be that the patient has totally unrealistic expectations about the nature of psychiatric assistance and the time scale in which any help can be achieved.

Management

The first step in the management of any rational patient is to come to an agreement about the problem presented and the help to be offered. This is especially important in the treatment of personality disorder. First, any misunderstandings about the nature of the disorder and its curability by psychological (?magical) means must be got out of the way. Patient and doctor should exchange ideas and come to some agreement about the important things to be remedied and the appropriate time-scale. Irremediable problems should be discussed and accepted as such by both parties. Other professionals (for example, social workers and psychologists) should be consulted and their views taken into the treatment plan. When the problems and possible lines of action have been identified it may even be helpful to write them down. However this is not always necessary; the important point is that both patient and doctor understand what goals are being aimed at, by what methods, in what period of time. Obviously, these objectives can be changed as treatment proceeds but it is very important to set realistic aims right at the beginning; in this way, achievement and reward are possible in even the most difficult cases. This setting of realistic targets is probably one of the most important aspects of treatment. For example, the socially inadequate, slightly dull, recidivist thief who turns up asking to be found a highly-paid job in a bank, has already made progress when he accepts that an industrial rehabilitation course for a semi-skilled job is more appropriate.

Quite a number of patients will come to the doctor looking for the 'I can't help myself' sick role so that they can obtain the benefits we normally accrue when we fall ill. Such a role partly deprives us of our responsibility and that can be very destructive to someone with chronic social and psychological problems. A person in that predicament has to face the fact that he and he alone can alter his circumstances. The doctor's role therefore becomes the one used for any chronic handicap: support, commitment, and encouragement towards self-determination and away from the sick role.

Once an agreement between doctor and patient has been established a programme of management is planned, at least in part. Target symptoms are tackled with ordinary remedies (for example, anxiolytics and anti-depressants), social problems are given concrete assistance (for example, help with accommodation, occupational retraining), relatives and friends are counselled; behaviour treatment, marital therapy, referral to self-help agencies may each be appropriate with particular patients. Special attention should, however, be given to techniques which are of great value in the treatment of patients with personality disorders: support, directive psychotherapy, group psychotherapy, crisis intervention.

Support

It may seem surprising that support is emphasized as a special technique. Surely every doctor gives support? Not in the sense meant here. Support is a difficult, time-consuming, irksome art. It is not necessarily best given by a doctor, indeed it is not really a medical skill but it does seem to be of great importance in assisting persistent offenders to stay out of trouble for a while (see West, 1963, and chapters 11.1 and 11.3 of the present volume). The skills involved include being able to accept unpleasant, demanding individuals, without necessarily accepting their unpleasant behaviour; patience in the face of provocative behaviour (such as turning up late for appointments); availability, even outside the formal clinic times, and commitment to a long period of treatment, perhaps lasting years. It is essential that if a therapist is going to make this kind of commitment the goals of treatment must be realistic and clearly understood, especially by the therapist, so that some rewards can be taken and constant frustration and disappointment avoided.

Directive psychotherapy

The usual emphasis in psychotherapy is on non-directive techniques, allowing the patient to air his thoughts, and receive interpretations, but no direct advice. Many antisocial patients, however, are unsophisticated and impulsive, and find such an approach irritating. Some have never had firm, reliable, helpful advice from anybody. Such patients respond well to a mildly authoritarian approach which includes direct answers to direct questions and the occasional 'I think you should do . . .' Of course not all offender patients will benefit from this style and some will require the more traditional methods, but directive psychotherapy is often worth considering with the persistent offender.

Group psychotherapy

There seems to be an established place for group techniques in respect of non-psychotic patients with antisocial personalities. Certainly it is used effectively at Grendon prison and at the Henderson hospital. A recent personal study produced some evidence that it is more effective than individual treatment amongst recidivist prisoners (Gunn *et al.*, 1978).

Crisis intervention

Crisis intervention is, like support, the kind of technique which everybody would claim to offer. Yet for it to be effective there has to be close attention to the details of each patient's life so that crises can be averted rather than dealt with after the event. For full effectiveness a therapeutic team must be prepared to carry out domiciliary visits at short notice, and to spend time dealing with employers, social security officers, and other key figures in the patient's life. It may be particularly important to admit a patient to hospital as an emergency. This has been getting increasingly difficult. In 1974 I reported three cases in my own clinic (Gunn, 1974), in each of which I was unable to admit the patient at the moment of crisis. The first, an inadequate, hypochondriacal man, was threatening both suicide and homicide. When he was not accepted for admission because he was considered a 'social' rather than a 'medical' problem he set fire to the local nurses' home. The second, an aggressive, paranoid man, attacked an old lady when he lost his lodgings. The third patient, an alcoholic, violent man, also lost his accommodation and he slid into a deep depression during which he killed himself. Since that time hospital admission decisions have become more 'democratic' with greater delays and more frequent refusals, thus reducing further the opportunity to help at the moment of crisis. To admit such patients in an emergency it is essential for the doctor looking after them to have direct access to beds, to work closely with nursing staff who should be intimately involved with the patient's care, and for the clinic ethos to accept that even social dissenters sometimes require active psychiatric intervention, including hospitalization.

It may be argued that these management techniques are not necessarily medical and need not be applied within the NHS; social service departments and voluntary bodies, for example, may provide equally good arrangements if their staff are adequately motivated and trained. Nevertheless the NHS does command important resources like hospital beds, and is thus often the best setting for the assessment and management of patients with serious and antisocial personality disorders.

Clinical examples. Three case histories may illustrate some of the points made in the text.

Patient A, a 37-year-old man referred via Alcoholics Anonymous and charged with arson. His parents separated when he was very young and he spent most of his childhood, from the age of 4 years, in residential homes. He was intelligent, but bed-wetting, plus his father's attitude, prevented him from obtaining a grammar school education. He joined the armed forces and learned electronics but began to drink heavily. His criminal record showed a series of offences of a mainly violent nature. At the time of the arson offence he had a skilled job in engineering and had recently become married although there was some evidence that his heavy drinking was throwing a strain on the marriage. He spent too much money on drink and many hours in pubs. There was a history of one episode of delirium tremens. On examination he proved to be an anxious, insecure man who saw his environment as a competitive obstacle race. He described his experience of life as showing that one should stand up for oneself. His fantasy life was preoccupied with drink. He disclosed that his offences were largely related to rage attacks which he could not control under provocation when drunk. The arson related to an incident in which he lost a fight in a pub and tried to set fire to the premises.

After some five hours of out-patient assessment spread over two months it became clear that he was well motivated to receive treatment and that his wife was supportive. On this basis a recommendation was made to the court that he should receive out-patient treatment under a probation order. The court partially accepted this advice and bound him over for five years on condition that he received some psychiatric treatment. The first objectives of treatment were to persuade him to stop drinking completely and to explore his problems psychotherapeutically. He was referred to a psychotherapy department but they advised against formal dynamic psychotherapy saying that his defences against violence and paranoia were fragile. Supportive psychotherapy was advised and this was proceeded with over the five-year period. His ability to control his drinking fluctuated from time to time but he never really abstained for long and usually, secretly, relapsed to moderate social drinking. Three major crises occurred during the course of treatment. The first was immediately after the birth of his first child. He took his wife to a pub and was involved in a fight. He was arrested for drunkenness and thus jeopardized his court order. However, in view of the otherwise satisfactory nature of his treatment, which he attended assiduously, the court took a lenient view and merely fined him for that incident. The more serious and protracted problem concerned his work. Soon after his first court case had ended he asked for a rise and became angry when rejected. His reaction was to resign from his job and attempt to set up a small electrical business of his own. This attempt coincided with the beginning of a serious economic recession and he soon found himself unemployed and in debt. The week-by-week management of his domestic and financial problems took up much time in the psychotherapy sessions, although it was still possible to discuss his changing feelings for his family. As a result of these discussions he reconciled himself to his estranged father, and took up a supportive role in relation to his alcoholic brother. Towards the end of his treatment he was charged with rape following an altercation with a work-mate who owed him some money. He threatened the man but settled for sexual intercourse with the man's girl friend. He was found not guilty.

He terminated treatment at the time specified by the court, saying that he felt he could manage on his own. The main objectives had been achieved in that he had moderated his drinking, and minimized his violence. Secondary beneficial effects were that his family flourished and that he eventually obtained a satisfactory engineering job in his previous trade. Follow-up has indicated no further problems.

Patient B, a 22-year-old single woman, was referred by a probation officer because of a moderately severe depression with suicidal ideas. She was a successful professional shoplifter who came from a family where most members had received convictions for theft and she lived in an area which was highly criminalized. She was heavily tattooed on her arms and scarred from one or two self-inflicted burns.

The depression was partly explained by the fact that her boy-friend, who was a professional robber on the run, had been found in her flat and recently re-arrested. The depression produced some suicidal ideas and considerable anorexia and weight loss. The initial aims, therefore, were to treat her depressive symptoms, support her through a very difficult period which included the trial of her boy-friend, get her to gain a little weight, and then help her re-adjust to life without the boyfriend after his inevitable long sentence. She also requested plastic surgery for her tattoos. The boy-friend was sent to prison and then failed in an appeal, and her depression did not remit for two or three years in spite of antidepressant medication. She attended out-patients regularly, however, and also established a close relationship with a probation officer. Her tattoos were removed by a series of operations. One surprising but helpful aspect of this early period was her complete renunciation of shoplifting. She began to devote her energies to looking after sick and stray animals on the one hand and aggressive burglars and thieves on the run from the police on the other. She also invested a great deal of energy in a protracted battle with her landlord over her deplorable accommodation. Her relationship with her boy-friend deteriorated as he became more violent in prison, and she found it increasingly difficult to respond to his aggressive stance towards her. However, she fought a number of battles on his behalf with the Home Office before eventually breaking off with him. By this time her depressive symptoms had improved a great deal and she was no longer underweight. Furthermore, she had obtained stable employment. Following the loss of her boy-friend she took up with one or two others, eventually selecting a highly violent man with a conviction for rape. Within weeks of marriage he began to beat her up and once again she became depressed. Some

months later she became pregnant. Several attempts to arrange joint interviews with her and her husband failed because he refused to attend. Three months into her pregnancy she also stopped attending and no further news has been heard.

This case history shows a mixture of success and failure, in that while the patient's symptoms had remitted, many of her problems had changed for the worse. The task of protecting her physically during this difficult phase was almost insurmountable, and although primary care services were alerted they were unable to offer much assistance.

Patient C, a 29-year-old man, was referred for a court report after he had been charged with indecently assaulting a small girl by fondling her genitals. He was a shy, anxious, man who for many years had been intimidated by an obsessive and overpowering father. He had run away from home as a child and was frequently bullied at school. His main problems were his almost complete inability to make satisfactory relationships of any kind with adults, a need to denigrate himself by taking demeaning jobs, and a sexual orientation towards either young children (girls more than boys) or subnormal adult women. He confessed to the charge and also told the police of some murderous fantasies including an incident during which he had put his hands around a baby's throat thinking 'it would be nice to strangle the child'. This was investigated by the police but there was no evidence they could bring into court. They also discovered in his flat some banal childish stories he had written, of a mainly erotic paedophilic kind containing aggressive and murderous ideas.

On examination, he was clearly anxious to have treatment: this was offered to the court and accepted as a condition of probation. When he was released from prison he was put on to depot oestrogens which effectively reduced his libido. (This is often too severe a treatment for paedophilia but after lengthy discussions with the patient, in which he was informed of what would happen to him, it was thought justified in view of his homicidal fantasies.) After some months his breasts began to enlarge and at about the same time he became severely depressed. He made one or two rather histrionic suicidal gestures and was admitted to hospital. The depression remitted quickly in hospital and he was then fit enough to be referred for a successful bilateral mastectomy. At this stage he was therefore without libido, normothymic, but lonely and without purpose to his life. He started to join one or two clubs to make friends, but when the probation order ended the oestrogens were stopped at his request and within a month or so he had regained his paedophilic fantasies. He was then referred to a clinical psychologist for a course of behaviour treatment which included further psychotherapy and aversion to paedophilic fantasies, but the aversion failed because his motivation was low. His desire for companionship intensified after his libido returned and he frequently advertised in newspapers for girl-friends. Eventually a feckless and semi-delinquent subnormal woman answered one of his advertisements and they fell into one another's arms. His girl-friend was the mother of a severely subnormal child whom she found very difficult to care for. She had many debts which the patient began to try to pay off for her. Warnings about the difficulties of the relationship were fruitless and they were married. As soon as they began to live together the social services department, who heard rumours of his previous history from sources unknown, attempted to separate them by putting pressure on the wife and placing the child in care. However, they remained together in a stormy relationship and fled from accommodation to accommodation, pursued by debts and social services departments. The patient also stopped attending the out-patient clinic.

This is another case history which shows a mixture of success and failure. Certainly the end result is not an ideal stable marriage, but it was clear just before he stopped attending that the relationship was more important to him than almost any degree of stress it produced. More obviously his paedophilia has been contained and the initial fear that he would slip into a paedophiliac recidivism, and possibly murder a child, seems to have been allayed, although it is difficult to predict what will happen if the current relationship breaks up. It is hoped that these three cases illustrate the main points of this chapter. Antisocial behaviour is not, in itself, a disease. Psychopathic disorder, which is the label loosely given to many people with persistent antisocial behaviour, is a confused and confusing concept. Patients who present with persistent or serious antisocial behaviour in the context of psychological and/or physical handicaps are best dealt with by a highly individual approach. This should include a detailed assessment of both function and dysfunction, followed by the provision of symptomatic relief, practical assistance with day to day problems, and long term support. Above all the patient has to be encouraged away from the sick role. Success is measured in terms of a gradual change of attitude and a gradual adjustment to reality, which will probably require a long period of supervision.

Acknowledgements. I am grateful to Dr Pamela Taylor for constructive criticism and to Mrs Maureen Bartholomew and Miss Kathy Coomes for patient secretarial assistance.

11.3
The impact of sociopathic and inadequate parents on their children (including child abuse)
SULA WOLFF

The links between parental sociopathy and psychiatric disorders of children have been repeatedly confirmed and clarified by research in the past fifteen years (Rutter & Madge, 1977 and pp. 42, chapter 1.3.1 determinants of emotional and conduct disorder in childhood, in this volume).

Shifting the focus from what holds true for groups of children and their parents to the clinical management of the individual child and his family requires the clinician to be clear about the precise nature of the parents' personality disturbance (sociopathy is not a unitary condition), in relation to the particular problems presented by the child.

Child and adolescent psychiatrists probably see more, and a wider range of, young adults with personality disorders than do general psychiatrists. In adult psychiatry, even in a service for attempted suicide or for the treatment of alcoholism, it is common practice not to accept for ongoing care, patients without formal psychiatric illnesses, especially when there are also social difficulties and the chances of effecting any enduring personality changes seem small. Child psychiatrists have exceptional opportunities for observing over time the vicissitudes of families where one or both parents are sociopathic.

A summary of research findings
In his comparative study of child psychiatric clinic attenders and children at paediatric and dental clinics, Rutter (1966) confirmed an excess of psychi-

atric hospital referral among parents of disturbed children, with a highly significant excess of personality disorder, especially sociopathy, among the latter. Wolff & Acton (1968) studied 100 primary school children referred to a psychiatric department and 100 matched controls. A structured interview was used for the psychiatric assessments of the parents. The diagnosis of sociopathy (with good interrater reliability on the basis of written interview protocols) was made when the parent had chronic interpersonal difficulties which included violence, excessive drinking, delinquency, or sexual deviation. Among the clinic attenders 17 had sociopathic mothers and 21 had sociopathic fathers, compared with three and seven respectively among the controls.

In his later studies of family influences on the development of child psychiatric disorders Rutter (1970, 1976) stressed parent behaviour, rather than psychiatric diagnosis, and in particular, overt marital discord, in the genesis of conduct disorders in boys, and in potentiating the harmful effects of other childhood stresses, such as repeated, early admissions to hospital (Quinton & Rutter, 1976). The harmful effects on children of open hostility between parents, especially violence, have been documented, for example, by Tonge and co-writers (1975) in a comparative study of problem families.

The fact that boys are more at risk than girls and specifically for conduct disorders (often associated with learning failure) suggests that one mediating process is role modelling (Tuckman & Regan, 1966; Biller, 1970). When there is domestic violence the father is usually the aggressor. When there is marital breakdown children as a rule stay with their mother. The father tends to be seen by the family and by society as the guilty partner so long as the mother looks after the children. Boys, biologically and socially programmed to love, respect and model themselves on their father, face conflicts of loyalty and damage to their self-image when the father, even if absent, is despised.

The focus on overt discord and violence between parents rather than on their personalities has been helpful in conveying a quality of family life that is pathogenic for children. But this approach underestimates the part played by enduring personality patterns, maintained presumably by underlying intrapsychic structures and processes and by mutually reinforcing social interactions with other people, in preserving individual differences and intergenerational continuities. As a result of intra-individual and interpersonal processes, the events and circumstances in early childhood can have long-lasting effects on adult behaviour, including the parenting of the next generation. Wolkind and co-workers (1977) and Hall and co-workers (1980) showed that mothers from disrupted families interacted significantly less with their 20-week-old babies than did mothers brought up continuously by their own parents. Rutter & Mrazek (1982) found significant differences in the interaction sequences between mothers and their pre-school children when the mothers had themselves been in care in childhood and when they had not. Such studies could helpfully be augmented by clinical descriptions of parental personality patterns.

Boys of sociopathic fathers are at risk of conduct disorders, and serious delinquency in childhood is highly associated with adult sociopathy in men (Robins, 1966). But what is the long-term effect on girls of parental sociopathy? Child psychiatrists see a number of mothers, daughters of sociopathic fathers and often of unaffectionate mothers, who made teen-age marriages in defiance of their parents. Their equally young husbands, sometimes already delinquent and rejected by their own mothers, then began to drink excessively, work irregularly, and, especially after the birth of the first child, become physically violent to their wives. These in turn then bring up their sons with negative expectations. Their toddlers' poor impulse control elicits not protective control, but anxious and angry exhortations and warnings, reinforced with physical punishment. Even after the father's departure, these mothers tend to foster in their children anxiety about aggression, and aggressive testing-out of the limits of safety. This then confirms their own worst fears: that their sons will turn out to be like their husbands.

Adoption and twin studies of delinquency and psychopathy (reviewed by Shields, 1976) point to a small but definite genetic component. These studies are difficult to interpret because of the unsatisfactory state of the definition, diagnosis, and subclassification of the sociopathies. What is inherited is unlikely to be a predisposition to specific behavioural acts.

Robins (1966) maintains that the transmission of sociopathy from fathers to sons, with childhood conduct-disorder mediating, is independent of social class, although both adult sociopathy and childhood antisocial behaviour correlate with low socio-economic status. But because these personality disorders are commoner in socio-economically deprived sections of the population, psychiatrists should not attribute sociopathic behaviour merely to social influences. We need to be clear also that the relationship holds only for a proportion of affected children. There is evidence that how schools and society respond to a predisposed child can powerfully affect his future behaviour (Rutter *et al.*, 1979; West & Farrington, 1977).

What protects children from the impact of parental sociopathy?

The links between parental sociopathy, childhood delinquency, and consequent sociopathy of these delinquent children are strong. Yet over half of even very seriously delinquent children do not become sociopathic in later life (Robins, 1966). The sex of the child is certainly a protective factor, girls being less a risk of overt conduct disorder and delinquency. The influence of family size has yet to be determined. Certainly the most disturbed delinquent children come from exceptionally large families especially when they are girls (Whalley *et al.*, 1978). Good intelligence has been shown to protect children from disrupted homes, for example those in residential care, against the risks of psychiatric disorder, perhaps because wider sources of satisfaction and self esteem are open for gifted children. Rutter and co-workers (1979) have demonstrated that the quality of secondary school life can safeguard children otherwise at risk of psychiatric disorder and educational failure. Perhaps most important of all, if one parent is warm and affectionate towards the child, this can counteract the pathogenic effects of marital discord and of hostility towards the child by the other (Rutter, 1976).

Sociopathic parents in child psychiatric practice

Child psychiatrists and associated social workers and psychologists are well placed to make full assessments of the personalities of the parents of children referred to them. Such a personality diagnosis is essential for accurate predictions for the future and for effective interventions.

Sociopathy on an experiential basis

The commonest personality disorders of parents of disturbed children are largely experientially induced and can be understood in terms of the parents' own childhood history (see also pp. 209 chapter 5.1.4, impact of depressed parents on their children: the Smith family). When severe they merit a label of

sociopathy, especially when there is criminality, addiction, violence, or sexual perversion, even if, as is common in women, there are also hysterical personality features. When less severe, the labels *inadequate* and *dependent personality disorder* tend to be applied. The common intercurrent complications for women are depressive illnesses and suicide attempts, and in men excessive drinking with the attendant risks of addiction, suicide attempts, and suicide. Seriously sociopathic mothers may be alcoholic, drug addicted, delinquent, or promiscuous. Seriously sociopathic fathers may have been responsible for the injury or death of another person.

Unless addiction, imprisonment, or other disasters supervene, these personality disorders improve over time and many chaotically functioning parents turn into stable grandparents. A number of less severely affected parents also respond to very long-term support.

Ian Brown* was first referred to a child psychiatry department at 5½ because of crying, temper tantrums, and aggressive behaviour at school. Throughout his life he had had numerous accidents and injuries, often a result of assaults by his father. On one occasion he remembered clearly, he was thrown out of a window. At 4 years, day care in a children's home was arranged, since the paediatrician, consulted about bedwetting, was concerned for Ian's safety within his home. The *mother*, one of ten children, was frequently admitted to children's homes because of her parents' unstable marriage. They divorced when she was 8. Her father was alcoholic and died when she was 14. Her mother, also with a drinking problem, remarried and the stepfather sexually assaulted Mrs Brown when she was 16. Mrs Brown, of good intelligence, became a qualified printer. Always sexually frigid during her marriage, she had a series of depressive illnesses with suicide attempts, often when drunk. She was still in touch with a supportive general psychiatrist. The *father*, an unemployed warehouseman, the sixth of nine children, was intelligent but explosive, and guarded about his own structurally united family. He had repeatedly assaulted Ian but treated his younger son and daughter more normally.

When first seen, Ian complained of nightmares and multiple fears and was anxious about his own aggressive impulses. While unable to control these, he was always trying to be good. These preoccupations persisted for many years. 'I don't like sleeping because I get pictures when I close my eyes . . . I dinne get peace to go to sleep.'

Following the referral, Ian's behaviour continued to deteriorate. He climbed roofs dangerously and wandered at night. The parents were quarrelling violently. A Sheriff Court established grounds for Ian's referral to a Children's Hearing as in need of compulsory measures of care, and a supervision order was made, with a condition of residence in a children's home. The placement broke down when Ian put his hands around the neck of a younger child. He was

* The name Brown is fictitious.

transferred to a small family-group home and given regular psychiatric support.

At this stage there was conflict between the psychiatric view that the parents, because of their life-long personality disorders, would not be able to change and that Ian required long-term substitute parental care, and the social work department's 'here and now' approach, in which the parents were seen not as sociopathic but as caught up by circumstances. The social workers attempted to support both Ian and his parents and to preserve family ties by regular weekend home visits for Ian.

When Ian entered the children's home, the parents became reconciled and weekend visits went well. Soon they began to ask for his return. This was deferred at first but Ian, aware of the conflict between parents and substitute care-givers, once more became aggressive in the children's home and his changing care-staff began to respond to him with increasing criticism and disapproval. Ian's improved behaviour at school now deteriorated. Because of his worsening relationships he was allowed to return to his parents. Three months later, the parents were again at odds with each other and the father resumed his attacks on Ian.

The mother attempted suicide and then requested a psychiatric hospital admission for Ian, now aged 8½. She wanted to leave her husband but resisted Ian's return to the family group home. On his admission the parents reunited again and continued to resist the child's readmission into care.

A further Children's Hearing decided that Ian should return to the family-group home and relationships with the housemother were gradually re-established. Mrs Brown left her husband for a much younger man and the two younger children were fostered by Mrs Brown's oldest sister (who had been 'like a mother' to her). The legal struggles between the parents for custody of the children were protracted and the father's visits to the younger children disrupted their relationship with their aunt. Finally the local authority assumed parental rights for all the children. The younger two were placed together in a long-term foster home, the mother maintaining contact with them and with Ian.

Ian, now 10, is a remarkably well-adjusted boy and the younger children too are not overtly disturbed. All three were of good average intelligence. They were physically attractive and with appealing temperamental traits: all were lively, open, adaptable, and sociable. While often very anxious, they were always able to communicate well with other people. Ian, unlike many children caught up in similar circumstances, has been fortunate in that the psychiatric social worker who first knew him at 5½, visited him regularly wherever he was placed. She was always perceived as someone who understood and liked him, and would try to keep him and other people safe. She was able to explain to him what was happening within and around himself (interpreting his anger in terms of understandable responses to parents he also loved and as testing out whether he himself was likeable or dangerous); and was concerned to help keep his environment as stable as possible, while maintaining positive relationships with his mother and with the changing child care staff in the children's home.

The impact of their disrupted, anxiety-laden, and often violent childhood on the adult personality patterns of all three children remains of course unknown. Plans are currently being made for long-term substitute family care for Ian.

Sociopathy on the basis of brain injury

Very rarely, fathers, previously socially integrated although perhaps with a history of predisposing childhood disadvantages, sustain a head injury or other neurological condition which leads to personality deterioration with explosive irritability and unaccountable irresponsibility and violence. Very rarely also, other parents (in clinical practice these tend to be mothers) have always been impulsive, hyperreactive, emotionally labile, and with impaired social sensitivity and responsiveness, when their past life stresses and privations are insufficient to account for this. Sometimes the mother will know she had been birth-injured, in other cases a remaining speech defect or illiteracy despite adequate intelligence will point to early cerebral dysfunction. Occasionally there are neurological abnormalities persisting from childhood.

Richard and his half-brother, *Eric*, both illegitimate, were first seen in a child psychiatry department when they were 7½ and 6 years old because of Richard's stealing, wandering, soiling, and defiance and obstinacy with his mother. The *mother*, then 27, hemiplegic following birth injury, had many hospitalizations in childhood and was teased about her calliper. She never knew her father and had a lonely childhood with her working mother. She stole and truanted. *Richard's father*, 47 and married, kept in touch with the family until he developed tuberculosis when the boys were 6½ and 5 years old. *Eric's father*, seriously delinquent, never lived with the family. The mother managed to run an orderly home during the children's early years despite poverty, but her child-rearing methods were impulsive and violent and she had twice dislocated Richard's shoulder. Her relationship with her sons deteriorated after the withdrawal from the family of Richard's father and Richard said he was trying to find him for his mother.

Psychiatric care failed to improve matters and during the next year Eric too began to soil and steal. Arrangements were made for both boys to be admitted to a residential school for maladjusted children. Two years later, however, the mother requested their return. The psychiatric clinic lost contact with the family and the education authority failed in their further attempts to provide residential education for the children.

Richard and Eric were seen again when they were 14 and 12 years old. Eric was then in an assessment centre, charged with breaking and entering and setting fire to a house, and Richard was referred after an overdose. The mother had had a third son, now 18 months old, the child of Richard's father, who had briefly returned to the family.

Richard, quick-witted and with a somewhat ingratiating manner, told the psychiatrist, weeping, about his impossible life at home: his mother fails to provide the older boys with clothes for school, forbids them to go out to play, relies on them to do the housework, encourages them to steal for her from shops and beats the baby violently unless Richard can keep him quiet. Richard recalled vividly his mother 'breaking my arm' in the past and mentioned 'a cable' that she kept at home with which to beat the children. He wanted to leave home. He told the psychiatrist of his many undiscovered thefts from shops and wished he could stop stealing.

The mother, clinically of average intelligence, was labile in mood: weeping at one moment, teasingly jolly the next. She confirmed her own extremely impulsive and also aggressive behaviour to the children frankly and without guilt. She was afraid she might seriously injure the baby. She spent most of her time at home reading crime stories. She did not want the boys to leave home. She could not look beyond her own immediate needs into the future. She was very angry about the older boys' misbehaviour and could not acknowledge that family life was not at present meeting their needs.

In this case too it was difficult to persuade the local authority social workers that the mother had a chronic and serious personality disorder on the basis of early cerebral damage and childhood privations, and that plans for the children required to be made in the expectation that their mother would not be able to modify her behaviour.

Eric was admitted to a special home for emotionally disturbed children while Richard remained at home. Social worker and health visitor called regularly to keep an eye on the baby.

Over a year later, when eleven property offences including the theft of a car were reported to the police, Richard was sent to an assessment centre and from there to a list D school (community home). The mother had by then had a further child and now at last accepted sterilization. Despite the fact that both boys were seriously retarded educationally, once away from home they adapted well to their new surroundings. It remains unclear how long they will be retained in their residential settings and the prognosis for adequate adult personality must be very guarded.

Schizoid psychopathy

Schizoid personality, encountered in a number of parents of psychiatrically referred children, is usually not severe enough to merit the label of sociopathy. But occasionally it explains permanently violent, cold or criminal parental behaviour.

Garry Collins* sustained fractured ribs and subsequently a fractured skull with subdural haematoma and generalized convulsions in his first two months of life. Assault by the father was proved at a court hearing and the child was placed under a supervision order while residing in a children's home. He was allowed to return to his parents at seven months at the parents' request and with the agreement of the psychiatrist then treating the father. At eight months the child was readmitted to hospital because of a fractured femur, the parents at court admitted to a lack of parental care and the child returned to the children's home.

* The name Collins is fictitious.

At fourteen months the family was referred to a child psychiatry department for advice to the authorities about future management. The parents wanted the child home. The mother visited him very regularly. The question was, was it safe for Garry to return home at all and, if not now, when?

The *mother*, then only 20, was the fourth of eight children from a united family. She was a part-time auxiliary nurse. She had married at 18 against her parents' wishes. She was intelligent, emotionally responsive and sensitive, conscientious, and thoughtfully concerned for her baby and her husband. From him she had tolerated much aggression and her wish always was to help him cope better. She felt sorry for him.

The *father*, 22 and unemployed, had been reared with a younger sister by a withdrawn, violent father and a mother described in one report as 'manipulative'. The father had put aspirins into his mother's face cream at 2; began stealing from his mother at 7, set fires with others at 11; was charged with malicious damage at 13; assaulted a girl at 16; and, also at 16 and for no clear reason, aimed a shotgun at six strange children who were merely passing by, shooting one through the ear.

His mother left the home with both children when Mr Collins was 16 but after a short while he returned to his father. As a boy he was of high average intelligence, literate and capable but withdrawn, sullen, friendless, and easily roused to explosive anger.

At interview the mother mentioned her feelings of depression whenever she sees friends with *their* children. She longed for Garry to come home. Sometimes she felt as if he was not her child. She tried to understand her husband. She never knew what he might do next. She tried to keep quiet to calm him down. She covereed over for him with other people. The father began the interview by saying 'I think it's a load of crap. I suppose the panel (the Scottish Children's Panel) is not a bad idea but you can see right through them. I weigh people up . . . someone's always passing the buck . . . one bloke (the minister) turned round and kept saying "now tell me what really happened" and I banged him in the mouth. I'm not bothered when I hurt people because *I* get hurt . . . I'm a violent bloke. I was brought up in a violent background.' He said he was fond of the baby 'in my own way. I'm not really fond of people'. Of his wife he said 'She's mine by law'. He described his persisting daydream, that is, his wish to buy an island and 'grow my own stuff'.

The child psychiatrist diagnosed the mother as having a mild personality disorder, passive and masochistic in type. The father was diagnosed as having schizoid psychopathy. He was insensitive to the feelings of others, callously lacking in empathy, sensitive, indeed paranoid, in relation to the motives of others, solitary and pursuing unrealistic fantasies.

Psychiatric advice was that Garry should not ever be left with the father. The children's panel did not allow the child to return home, despite the danger for later personality development of separation at his age. His mother visited him daily and undertook much of his physical care, finally leaving her husband when Garry was 2½. The father had 'lost interest', joined a pop group, and the relationship between the couple had deteriorated. Mrs. Collins took a job, rejoined her parents, her feelings for her husband slowly changed, and she began divorce proceedings. Garry made a graduated return home to her. He had a squint and there was evidence of mild developmental retardation as a result of his brain injury but his attachment to his mother did not appear to be impaired.

Clinical management

Child psychiatrists have a special responsibility for selecting treatment interventions to fit the particular needs and capabilities of each child and his family. Often they are called upon to help other professionals, social workers, psychologists, teachers, child care workers, paediatricians, and nurses, to have realistic expectations for the future and especially for the efficacy of treatment. When parents cannot change, it does not help them or their children to expect change to come about. The reverse: it can demoralize a family and create hostility between them and their aspiring helpers. This is not a nihilistic approach. Many parents, although not capable of radical change, do respond to having their difficulties understood and their responsibilities for the children shared. Moreover, a number of important prophylactic and therapeutic interventions have to be considered.

Successful treatment of a depressive illness (usually possible) or an addiction (rather less frequently achieved) can transform family life. Limitation of family size, if parents will accept this, can protect children already at risk from even greater intrafamilial stress and privation. Sociopathic parents need expert advice about contraception and sterilization and in some cases about therapeutic termination of pregnancy or adoption, if they are to have a chance of maintaining their current level of functioning.

The crises in families with one or two sociopathic parents (arising for example from suicide attempts or suicide, violence or murder, child abuse, imprisonment, debt, homelessness, and family breakdown) require a network of support if the children are to get some relief from anxiety and protection against the impact of these crises. When affected families are stable in their domicile, it is possible for social workers, teachers, health visitors, and doctors to be helpful, especially if staff turnover is slow, by providing the children with a lifeline and with supporting relationships. The need for auxiliary care must

be considered, for example, for small children in nursery schools, day nurseries, or with daily minders (specially chosen) and for older children in residential schools or homes. These measures introduce some respite from anxiety inducing events at home and provide alternative role models of adult behaviour for the children. Residential schooling is called for when the children are failing socially or educationally at school. Alternatives to family care in a children's home or foster home come up for consideration either at the parents' request, e.g. when a family is homeless or the parents consider the child's disturbed behaviour more than they can manage (that is, he is beyond their control); or at the request of social workers or police when a child is brought before a juvenile court or its equivalent, as a truant, as having committed an offence, or as being in need of care because of his parents' inability to provide adequate care and protection for him.

One of the psychiatrist's tasks is to help in deciding what measures are likely to be in the child's best long-term interest. The other is to help the child directly and the people looking after him, to cope optimally with critical life events and circumstances. The child will need opportunities for reliving ('working through') his distressing experiences and his associated feelings in play and conversation, and he requires also to have his own behaviour and emotional disturbances understood in the light of his life events and circumstances and his current stage of cognitive and emotional development. Unless a life has been lost, what is often most distressing for children is not what has happened, but that their parents were responsible for it. Here it can be helpful to convey what is generally true: that the parents had not intended the consequences of their actions. Even parents who injure their children often do so unintentionally or when in a dissociated state of consciousness. We need to be clear also that whatever helps the parents will help the child, and whatever helps the child to function better can in the end also help the parents.

At the same time, decisions about alternative, as contrasted with auxiliary, family care can never be taken lightly (to leave parents even at one's own request always constitutes a trauma) and yet they cannot be postponed if a child is to have a chance of forming new and healthier permanent attachments.

12
The 'inadequate personality'

12.1
The 'inadequate personality'
CHRISTOPHER HOWARD

Definition and clinical significance

If stripped of its evaluative connotations, the descriptive notion of inadequacy in respect of personality has the same meaning in psychiatry as it has in everyday discourse. It refers to a collection of personality characteristics which inhibit an individual from leading a fulfilling domestic, social, and working life in accordance with the normal traditions, customs, and expectations of his community. The imprecision of the definition of inadequacy in these terms is reflected in a complementary reciprocal elusiveness of exact definition for the notions of 'fulfilment' and 'normality'. However, the achievements and satisfactions of some individuals fall so far below those of members of the community as a whole that in many instances the recognition of inadequacy is not difficult. Nor need the acceptance of the concept of inadequacy be affected at the theoretical level by the existence of individuals about whose inadequacy observers might disagree.

The clinical importance of the inadequate personality cannot be overemphasized. Such individuals make frequent demands on the various helping agencies and professions in society. In the face of the most minor stresses inadequate persons may fall back on others for an inappropriate degree of support and help or contrive some excuse, often of a medical kind, to escape from a disagreeable situation. Thus they take up a great deal of the time and attention of the psychiatric services, the general medical services, and the social services. In whatever way the inadequate personality presents his difficulties, it will be imperative for the therapist or agent to identify the underlying pathology if intervention is to carry any hope of success.

This category of personality defect is perhaps even less easily definable than other forms, such as antisocial, obsessional, or hysterical personalities which are described elsewhere. Furthermore there will be much overlap between inadequate personalities and these other types.

Attempts have been made to give greater precision to the notion of inadequacy. Monro (1959) looked at the quality of inadequacy as part of a wider survey of 200 patients each of whom was rated for the presence or absence of 246 trait-terms. Examples of these trait-terms from an alphabetical list (Monro, 1954) are – absent-minded, accessible, acquisitive, adaptable, affected, and so on. 35 cluster correlations were found of which 5 seemed to correspond to different aspects of inadequacy. One such cluster is described as follows:

> This group is composed of people who make no display of feeling in relationships in which strong feelings are usually shown. Many of them avoid intimate relationships and have few or none. They deprecate the display of emotion by others. They evade danger, difficulty, adversity and pain wherever possible, and complain excessively if evasion is impossible. They express a sense of grievance, of not having what is due to them, and often wish to change their position and circumstances although no good reasons exist for so doing.

With hindsight this work may be taken to demonstrate that while inadequacy may be regarded as a quality with an objective existence it overlaps and merges imperceptibly into other aspects of both normality and abnormality and cannot be teased out into a position of sharp statistical relief. Similar conclusions can be drawn from the work of Walton and Presley (1973) who examined the relative merits of a classification of abnormal personality by clinical categories on the one hand, and through a dimensional approach on the other. 140 patients were assessed on a 46-item inventory. The data were submitted to principal components analysis and one of the four main components to emerge was the quality of submissiveness which included such items as timidity, dependency, meekness, and the avoidance of close relationships. Again there seems to be some overlap with the clinical category of inadequacy, but its existence is not substantiated in pure, readily identifiable form. This work highlighted the wide variation between psychiatrists in ascribing patients to individual clinical categories of personality while showing that there is a much higher degree of reliability in their attributing specific traits to patients.

Aetiological factors

The origins of human inadequacy are not known. Evidence of the disability is usually manifest from the onset of adult life, suggesting that it has its origin in the background and early experience of the individual, combined, in all probability, with more or less genetic predisposition. However, the disentanglement of the relative contributions of early environment and heredity in respect of inadequacy is attended by a particular lack of precise information and the same general theoretical difficulties as are found elsewhere in psychiatry. It is a common finding that inadequate individuals tend to provide inadequate homes and behave inadequately as parents. In the present state of knowledge it is therefore a reasonable assumption that environment and heredity both make their contribution. However, it is often the evolution of the circumstances of the individual's life which determines the manifestation of inadequacy in overt form. It is possible that in previous generations and other societies through the support of the extended family or the large household with its provision for total care of domestic staff, inadequate individuals were able to live their restricted and incomplete lives without ever identifying themselves as in need of extra help. The break-up of these larger networks of relationship and employment may thus have contributed to the manifestation of some forms of human inadequacy.

Mode of presentation

The mode of presentation may vary widely. The individual may attend his doctor in connection with some minor ailment, being unaware that at the same time he is seeking the less specific benefits of a close personal encounter, the interest of another person in himself, and a general atmosphere of caring and concern. Such experiences are rewarding whether the initial presentation is in this guise or with a more overt complaint of anxiety, depression, or inability to deal with some new personal problem. Although the immediate intervention may help with the specific presenting problem the more widely-based and longer-standing demands for help are not met, while the habit for seeking it becomes stronger as it is rewarded. Thus, the seeking of help in this way becomes more vigorous in proportion to the failure of the service to provide it. A pattern of regular attendance at the doctor is established, which results in dissatisfaction for the patient and, often, frustration for the doctor. Similar patterns of relationship may develop in respect of other welfare services. Every doctor and social worker is familiar with the fully developed version of this syndrome, in which the life of the individual has become an endless round of unfulfilled requests for help and more help. The condition is truly one of addiction to help. The related theme of abnormal illness behaviour is taken up elsewhere in this volume (chaps. 6.2, 6.3, 8.2, 8.8, 8.9).

The clinician will most likely recognize inadequacy if he looks carefully into the present predicament of the individual and his past history in the broad areas of domesticity, social relationships, and working life.

Inadequacy at a domestic level is often revealed by a series of broken relationships or marriages or by a chronically unhappy marriage with frequent arguments and separations. The choice of partner may reflect the individual's problems, since inadequate individuals often seek out each other and then mutually fail to give what each is seeking from the other. Sometimes the individual may have made little or no progress towards the formation of adult sexual relationships. His need for intimacy and a supportive domestic life may be partially satisfied by continuing to live in the parental home, by seeking residence in institutions, or by finding residential employment, for example as a hotel porter or Oxford don. Sexual fulfilment may then be found at some immature level through half-hearted homosexuality, transvestism, or fetishism, or by seeking the company of sexually immature humans. Although it is only a minority of such individuals who may seek sexual relations with children or adolescents, many find a greater social ease in their company than in the company of adults and may play roles as teachers or scout leaders. Similarly, young inadequate women may become prolific producers of children with whom they seek unsuccessfully the kind of intimacy they cannot achieve elsewhere. It is not uncommon for such women to produce children who are eventually taken into care. Life then becomes a crusade to recover their children from the allegedly 'evil' authorities who have taken them away. It is from among such children that some of the next generation of inadequate personalities are likely to spring.

Other manifestations of inadequacy in parents include the physical and emotional neglect of young children who are then at risk of the consequences of such deprivation. Some of these parents may batter their children (see p. 396, 403 and chap. 11.3).

On exploring the social history of the inadequate person the clinician will often find an absence of close friendships, particularly longstanding ones, a lack of involvement with neighbourhood or community and a failure to set down roots in the form of a permanent home. Spare time, of which he may have an abundance, may be spent in walking aimlessly, solitary drinking, or mindless consumption of radio, television, or cinematic material. Such special interests or hobbies as he has developed are unlikely to require group involvement and may consist exclusively of such solitary activities as stamp-collecting or bird-watching.

In his working life the inadequate individual may have difficulty in finding employment. He has often failed to develop special skills, though he may have attempted courses of training which he has not completed. His work record may reveal frequent changes of employment, interspersed with periods out of work, a failure to progress towards better-paid jobs and often a pattern of sackings for lateness, failure to attend, or arguments with colleagues, especially superiors.

Clinical types and case histories

Typically the family and personal history of the individual will reveal some evidence of inadequacy in one or both parents or possibly early parental loss or marital breakdown. In addition to emotional deprivation there may be a background of impoverishment or other physical deprivation. There may be evidence of poor early socialization and low school achievement. This low achievement is often at variance with the level of intelligence and is evidence of a relative failure to function at an optimal level. Such discrepancy between potential ability and actual attainment may be seen to persist throughout life.

The following case histories illustrate this development while also demonstrating wider aspects of inadequacy.

Mr. A, age 33, an only child. His mother, who was an alcoholic, died when he was eight. He progressed poorly at school and barely learned to read or write. He lived a sheltered existence with his father, doing regular unskilled work, until the latter died when he was twenty-five. Subsequently he was manipulated by his landlord out of the parental home. He became unsettled, moving from job to job, with no stable home life. He married a girl whom he met through an agency. They moved from council accommodation to living with friends and relations until his wife found residential domestic work and they lived in her room. There were sexual difficulties, frequent arguments, and talk of separation. He developed duodenal ulcer symptoms, and was treated surgically. He presented with polymorphous complaints about all aspects of his existence, having previously sought help from both his family doctor and the Marriage Guidance Council. His expectations for a transformation of his lot were naíve and unrealistic. Clinic attendance came quickly to an end, presumably because he could not obtain what he sought.

The precarious situation in which the individual so often finds himself may be attended by neurotic and depressive symptomatology. This may take the form of specific phobias (commonly of travelling or crowded places), obsessional rituals which may consume much of the individual's waking life, the development of conversion symptoms which may claim much concern and attention from others, or chronic feelings of inertia, emptiness, and despair. Attempts to remove these uncomfortable feelings may result in the regular consumption of psychotropic drugs, especially sedatives of the benzodiazepine group and alcohol, with the risks attendant on such practices. Secondary problems of drug dependence and alcoholism may develop and be seen by the individual as a state preferable to the uncomfortable predicament in which he finds himself without such medication, as illustrated by the following case history.

Mr B, age 38. This patient was the only child of middle-class parents. He obtained a University place to study pharmacology but failed to complete the course on account of his 'neurosis'. He took up photography and, after marriage, obtained a residential job with the RSPCA, which he greatly enjoyed. However, his wife committed suicide and he subsequently lost both the job and his home at the age of 33. Following an unsuccessful business venture he remained continuously out of work, living in the home which he inherited from his parents. He made little contact with others, spending much time in bed, drinking heavily. Throughout adult life he had sought out and received a great deal of psychiatric help both in the form of psychotherapy and medication, especially with sedative drugs, which he was determined not to abandon. Although ostensibly seeking to obtain help, his manner was aggressive, nihilistic, and calculated to destroy any attempt to alter his mode of life. His main interest in therapeutic contact was to establish his right to continue on medication, insisting that since doctors had no other help to offer, his sedative drugs should not be withdrawn. His pharmacological expertise was used

to support his arguments, often it seemed in an attempt to achieve enhanced status in his relationship with the therapist.

The capacity to develop dependence on drugs is only one aspect of a wide-ranging propensity to form dependent relationships on a variety of people and things. Commonly neighbours, social workers, doctors, and institutions are the objects of this tendency, contact with one or several of which produces a temporary feeling of security and confidence and an alleviation of anxiety and depression. Some individuals find solace in eating and such a process may underlie or contribute to some cases of obesity.

Many inadequate individuals may recognize their inability to lead normal self-sufficient lives and resent their reliance on people and things. They may gain satisfaction in acts of self-assertion which are only understandable in terms of their long-standing feelings of deprivation and inability to assert themselves as independent adults free of parental bonds capable of looking after themselves. Their neurotic acts of self-assertion may be directed against authority in general and take the form of minor criminal acts, such as damage to public property and shoplifting; or they may take the more specific form of rejecting the help which they need and have sought out, presumably to pre-empt rejection by the therapist, which their sense of personal inferiority leads them to anticipate. The extent of the disability and the demands for help will depend on the degree of success that the individual has contrived in finding a niche for himself which meets his needs. Thus, an undemanding residential job close to the parental home may give adequate protection from the consequences of exposure of the individual's weaknesses, while the conditions last. However, those who do not or cannot achieve such situations are likely to make demands on the medical services. The following case history illustrates these features of criminality and institutional dependence.

Mr C, age 50. This patient was the unwanted son of a prostitute and was brought up by foster-parents and in an orphanage. He sought out his natural mother when he was 14 but was rejected by her and subsequently sought shelter and protection by entering into homosexual relationships with older men. Throughout adult life he was repeatedly convicted for importuning and stealing, and served several prison sentences. His thefts were often of trivial objects, commonly food in small quantities, and sometimes poorly concealed. He described great excitement associated with sexual arousal from the whole sequence of stealing, discovery, and arrest. Between offences he struggled to maintain himself and had many periods of successful employment in jobs as a steward or waiter in formal institutional settings. In time of trouble he quickly turned to the medical profession for support and sympathy. Management consisted in regular supportive interviews in a psychiatric out-patient clinic aimed at providing a forum for presenting and analysing intercurrent stresses in the hope that a resumption of impulsive criminal activity could be avoided. Intermittent criminal activity continued none the less.

Management and treatment

The disabilities of the inadequate individual illustrate, as much as any other psychiatric disorder, the conceptual problems of knowing how much allowance to make for the individual's own capacity to help himself. Inadequate individuals tend to be poorly tolerated outside the helping agencies. They often receive short shrift from employers, are treated with irritation or indulgence in the courts, and are secretly or overtly despised and resented by friends, relations, and neighbours. Given that there are few if any specific therapeutic measures which are likely to yield significant changes in the individual, at the very least the helper must ensure that his intervention does no harm and is a justifiable use of his professional time and skills. Such is the capacity of some individuals to demand help and such is the willingness of some helpers to provide it that a vicious circle may develop in which the patient's defects are progressively rewarded and strengthened and the professional life and energy of the helper is increasingly absorbed and consumed.

As always in medicine, the greatest likelihood of successful management is created by early diagnosis. In allowing the needs of the inadequate individual to develop into a secondary addiction to helpers or drugs, the doctor is not only making the condition worse but destroying his own powers of successful intervention. The latter depends on identifying the problem and in helping the individual to identify it. The argument as to whether or not he will require major psychotherapeutic treatment or the same kind of simple explanation as is being attempted in this exposition will not be conducted here.* Suffice it to say that in either endeavour the helper is in a paradoxical situation. His task is to educate the individual in the nature of his difficulties, to point out how his emotional needs interfere with normal fulfilment in life and to give guidance on how he might set about things differently. In giving this help

*For a general discussion of the indications for and value of psychotherapeutic treatment of different kinds see chapter 3

he will readily be perceived as the fulfiller of all his unfulfilled and unfulfillable wishes. Thus in helping the individual to overcome his addiction, the therapist may become the object of it. It will therefore be necessary to ensure that help is rationed and not always available on demand. The patient must be weaned towards trying to tolerate some stresses and some anxiety against a background of support. Firmness is required as well as kindness and that firmness must be seen to be resolute and not open to infection by the patient's own vacillations and anxieties. Help may be required over many years, and perhaps indefinitely, though the contact need not necessarily be frequent or prolonged. In times of extreme distress there may be a place for sedative or antidepressant medication but such occasions should be kept to a minimum and the temporary nature of the prescription and any attendant risks of habit-formation explained to the patient.

Similar principles apply to more general tactics of management. Consistency among all those (and there may be many) involved in other aspects of management is essential. It is of no advantage to the patient if, for example, the doctor is adopting the strategy described above and some other agency is entering into a ceaseless round of offering help and more help. However, there may be so many sources of help that limiting its provision is not always tactically feasible. It is essential that all concerned are aware of the pathology and overall plan so that the patient cannot play one off against another. The overall aim at a practical level is to obtain such physical framework of support as is thought likely to reduce or eliminate the risks of decompensation with recurrence of neurotic and depressive symptomatology. Translated into action this means provision of adequate accommodation and regular day-time activity of a kind which will be within the patient's tolerance and provide security. For some this may be residential employment, for others it may be hostel accommodation and sheltered employment or other undemanding work situation. For housewives and mothers regular support and supervision, in the form of home visits by social workers, health visitors, or community-based nurses may be required.

In favourable circumstances some inadequate individuals may benefit from a course of social skills training directed at increasing their capacity for assertion, initiative and self-confidence in specific social situations which they find hard to negotiate and where failure stands in the way of a richer attainment in life. Examples would be excessive timidity in asking girls out, overwhelming anxiety and inhibition in interviews for jobs, or difficulty in accepting the authority of superiors at work.

So great is the amount of interested concern which is provided by admission to hospital that great care should be exercised in taking this step with an inadequate individual. However, flexibility of approach is essential and admission should never be refused solely on the grounds of inadequacy. In times of crisis or exacerbation of neurotic and depressive symptomatology, admission may prove a useful adjunct to the more structured long-term management regime and indeed may be essential in preventing the collapse of carefully nurtured plans.

It is a sad fact that diagnosis of the problem is often long-delayed and by the time a referral is made for specialist psychiatric help, there is a well-established and unbreakable addiction to medical help. In such a situation the aims of management may be limited to containment. Sometimes this can be achieved by the referring doctor and the role of the psychiatrist may simply be to advise his colleague of the nature of the problem and how best to handle it. Colleagues in other specialities frequently share the layman's distaste for prolonged contact with such individuals and are only too ready to refer them out of their own clinics into those of the psychiatrist. However, there seems no good reason why in appropriate circumstances the care of the meek should not be shared by all who set themselves up as professional helpers.

12.2
Child sexual molestation
D. J. WEST

Among the dominant groups in our culture – Freud and Kinsey notwithstanding – parents characteristically try to discourage overtly erotic behaviour in their small children. Nowadays it is done as much by silent avoidance and unspoken disapproval as by physical restraint or punishment. This promotes secrecy, deters discussion or explanation and hampers rational learning. It might be better, as some authorities suggest (Yates, 1979), if erotic interests could be recognized and discussed in much the same way as all the other experiences that the child has to learn to deal with. An unexpected confrontation with adult sexuality must come as a greater shock to children who have been artificially shielded and kept in ignorance.

Young children can learn to enjoy sexual stimulation by an adult without being troubled by the sense of guilt that develops by the time puberty is reached. Something like a quarter of young adults of either sex, when questioned confidentially, will recall experiences of sexual approaches from adults during their early years, experiences which never get reported to parents or anyone else (Kinsey *et al.*, 1953; Landis, 1956). Casual experiences of this kind usually make no lasting impression. Nevertheless, the discovery that their child has been involved sexually with an adult male (reported female culprits are very rare) provokes in many parents a frenzied over-reaction which can be more damaging to the child than the incidents themselves. If this is followed by police interrogations, much coaching by parents in what to say, and ultimately a cross-examination in court, with family tension mounting all the while, the stress is considerable and the likelihood of adverse reactions much increased (Gibbens & Prince, 1963).

Parental over-reaction is encouraged by the exaggerated stereotype of the physically dangerous sex fiend promoted by the popular press. In reality, most of the paedophiles who seek out other people's children are pathetically lonely and socially and sexually inhibited. Their conduct rarely amounts to more than erotic fondling and perhaps genital exposure with invitations to touch. Their approaches are gently persuasive rather than deliberately frightening or aggressive. Indeed, the children are sometimes passionate initiators of the seduction. This is reflected in the prevalence of cases in which a child is known to have been involved with more than one adult, and also in the fact that (especially with girls) the offender is often a person with whom the child is normally in close contact – a family member, family friend, relative, neighbour, and so forth (Virkkunen, 1975; Ingram, 1979).

Some offenders are exclusive paedophiles, sexually aroused only by physically immature, pre-pubertal children, and may be positively repulsed by the hair, odour, and other bodily characteristics of sexual maturity. Others do not really prefer children, but are incapable of finding or coping with an adult sexual partner. Many are separated, widowed, or miserably married. Their victims are mostly girls, but homosexual paedophiles are also quite common and some will approach boys or girls indiscriminately.

Young boys are surprisingly knowing about the homosexual interests of some of their teachers or youth leaders. When homosexual scandals have broken out at boys' boarding-schools many pupils have reported experiences with the offenders and most others 'knew all about it'. Homosexual offenders entice boys with treats, with pornography, with boasts about their (imaginary) prowess with women, and with games ending up in horseplay. A boy's partiality to these adventures is more likely to reflect something missing in his home life than to portend a permanent homosexual orientation. The friendship can be more important than the sex, and many homosexuals describe how they have preserved friendly relations with happily married men who were originally boy protégés and sex-mates.

Follow up studies of children known to have been sexually involved with adults other than their parents, reveal an unexpectedly low incidence of adverse effects (Burton, 1968). The latter seem related to the age and stage of development, the relationship to the abusing person, and the reactions of the family and community. Some of the disturbances which are noted probably antedate any sexual incident. Neglected children from disorganized homes with low social standards are vulnerable because they seek attention from outsiders and are attracted by small rewards. Emotional deprivation, the result of parental preoccupation with their own problems, or sexual anxiety communicated from the parents, may also increase vulnerability. Excessive warnings against contact with strangers can be counter-productive. Accidental encounters not reported are less likely to produce trauma than repeated experiences in which the child colludes with the offender and is shamed by detection. Worst of all are the cases, fortunately rare, in which children are coerced by threats, subjected to violence, or actually raped by psychopathic assailants.

Incest offenders, (see chapter 9.4) usually fathers or stepfathers, are not true paedophiles and not liable to interfere with children outside the home. Typically, they become involved with a daughter as she is approaching puberty, although sometimes they molest much younger children. Not uncommonly, all the daughters in a household are enlisted one after the other as each one reaches the required age. Some of the offenders are tyrannical, brutal, or drunken men who terrorize the children into submission so that physical and sexual abuse may be associated. More often, they are mild men of unexceptional, even exemplary, social demeanour, caught up in a family drama of love and hate, in which the wife, by subtle or not so subtle rejection or inadequacy, and perhaps by passive collusion in the daughter's exploitation, makes a heavy contribution. Such situations may persist for many years till the daughter leaves (Maisch, 1973; Gibbens et al., 1978).

Incest victims are sometimes too bewildered to complain, or if they do tell their mothers they may meet with censure and disbelief. On the other hand many are, at least for the time being, content to find themselves the centre of their father's interest. If the situation does get reported it is often initially through some extraneous factor such as a pregnancy, a jealous sister, a quarrel between the parents or parental possessiveness when the girl begins to acquire boyfriends, contraction of venereal disease, or presentation with a psychiatric disorder. Girls are often much attached to their incestuous fathers, deeply distressed if he is prosecuted and imprisoned and further traumatized if, on his release and return home, the social services decide she is in danger and must be sent away. Although some girls are weighed down by anxiety and guilt about incest, many others appear to take it in their stride and to exhibit no sexual or marital problems subsequently. Some retrospective clinical data suggest that the effects can be long-lasting (see chapter 9.4).

Sexual involvements at or after puberty, although still legally classified as assault, incest, or unlawful sexual intercourse with a girl under sixteen, are in practice largely consensual and raise controversial moral and social issues in addition to psychiatric complications. If parents, teachers, or other adults disapprove strongly enough, adolescent infatuations, heterosexual or homosexual, can become the subject of criminal prosecution. Under-age girls absconding from home with a boy-friend or prostituting themselves, and boys wandering alone to cinemas, amusement arcades, or public conveniences for the purposes of homosexual masturbation, perhaps for monetary reward, are matters in which the police are liable to initiate action leading to prosecutions, especially if the sexual misconduct is part of a generally antisocial, delinquent life style, which is often the case. Because the age of consent for homosexuality is twenty-one, and because of anxiety that homosexual experience in boys may lead to a permanent deviant sexual orientation, male homosexual involvements are liable to be brought to psychiatric attention, either by families or via the courts, even when the youthful participant is sexually fully mature. This may account for the fact that the average age of youthful male 'victims' of sexual assault appears higher than that of female victims.

Treatment for some casual sexual incident will usually take the form of simple reassurance, perhaps directed more to the parents than to the child. Continued sexual involvement calls for more active intervention. Sympathetic, but firm, insistence on the termination of contacts with an outsider who has abused the child's friendship may be all that is necessary, provided this is accompanied by adequate explanation and no recrimination. If the offender is a family member or parent it is often preferable for psychiatrist and social worker to co-operate in dealing with the situation informally, thus avoiding the break-up of the home where this is unnecessary. Incest problems include the relationship between the parents as well as the relationship of each with the child, so all three must be taken into therapy (Walters, 1975). If full co-operation appears lacking, it may be best to leave the matter to be reported to the police and some feel that police involvement should be the rule in any intra-familial sexual activity. Unfortunately, initial co-operation by all concerned sometimes dissolves away when it becomes clear that the danger of prosecution has been averted. In other cases, official allegations will already have been made and the psychiatrist is called upon by the court for the purpose of obtaining a psychiatric assessment on a convicted offender. In this eventuality, the psychiatrist needs to investigate the family as a whole, to know the prospects of the marriage continuing, to assess the risks and benefits of trying to preserve the home intact as well as to determine the offender's amenability to advice or psychotherapy, either voluntary, or as a condition of probation. Imprisonment in these cases is not a treatment and is not decided on medical grounds.

The need for treatment of the victim is indicated by the presence of symptoms, whether these are a continuation of previous malaise and family disturbance as is usually the case in incest, or whether they date from a sexual incident occurring outside the family. Anxiety reactions, sleep disturbance, moodiness, scholastic problems, sexual phobias, and sexual misconduct are all possible danger signals (De Francis, 1969). Some children who have 'gone along with' a sexual routine, apparently without demur, have been inwardly guilty and frightened but have felt unable to resist requests from an authoritative or trusted adult. Victims too young to know what sex is all about may become anxious later as they start to appreciate the social significance of the incidents. Older children become disturbed for different reasons, because they fear criticism or ostracism, because their self-esteem is damaged by discovery, because they have been in fear of pregnancy or disease or because they are aware of the danger of rejection by parents as a result of their involvement with another adult.

References

Chapter 1.1.1

Boring, E. G. (1950) *A History of Experimental Psychology*. 2nd ed. New York: Appleton-Century-Crofts

Ellenberger, H. F. (1970) *The Discovery of the Unconscious*. London: Allen Lane, Penguin Press

World Health Organization (1978) *Mental Disorders: Glossary and Guide to their Classification in Accordance with the 9th Revision of the International Classification of Diseases*. Geneva: WHO

Zilboorg, G. & Henry G. W. (1941) *A History of Medical Psychology*. New York: Norton

Chapter 1.1.2

Achenbach, T. M. (1980) DSM III in the light of empirical research on the classification of child psychopathology. *J. Amer. Acad. child Psychiat.*, **19**, 395–412

American Psychiatric Association. (1980) *Diagnostic and statistical manual of mental disorders*. DSM–III. Washington, DC: American Psychiatric Association

Berger, M., Yule, W. & Rutter, M. (1975) Attainment and adjustment in two geographic areas: II. Prevalence of specific reading retardation. *Brit. J. Psychiat.*, **126**, 510–19

Cantwell, D. P., Russell, A. T., Mattison, R. & Will, L. (1979) A comparison of DSM II and DSM III in the diagnosis of childhood psychiatric disorders. IV. Difficulties in the use of global comparisons and conclusions. *Arch. gen. Psychiat.*, **36**, 1227–8

Chiles, J. A., Miller, M. L. & Cox, G. B. (1980) Depression in an adolescent delinquent population. *Arch. gen. Psychiat.*, **37**, 1179–86

Farrington, D. P. (1978) The family backgrounds of aggressive youth. In *Aggression and Anti-Social Behavior in Children and Adolescence*, ed. Hersov, L. A., Berger, M. & Shaffer, D. London: Pergamon Press

Field, E. (1967) *A Validation Study of Hewitt & Jenkins' Hypothesis*. London: HMSO

Gould, M. (1980) The prognostic significance of an empirically-based typology of adolescent behavior profiles. Presented at the 27th Annual Meeting of the American Academy of Child Psychiatry, October, 1980. Chicago, Illinois

Henn, F. A., Bardwell, R. & Jenkins, R. L. (1980) Juvenile delinquents revisited. *Arch. gen. Psychiat.*, **37**, 1160–5

Hersov, L. (1977) Emotional disorders. In *Child Psychiatry: Modern Approaches*, ed. Rutter, M. & Hersov, L. Oxford: Blackwell

Hewitt, L. E. & Jenkins, R. L. (1946) *Fundamental Patterns of Maladjustment, the Dynamics of their Origin*. Springfield, Ill.: State of Illinois

Jones, M. B., Offord, D. R. & Abrams, N. (1980) Brothers, sisters and anti-social behaviour. *Brit. J. Psychiat.*, **136**, 139–46

McCord, W., McCord, J. & Howard, A. (1961) Familial correlates of aggression in non-delinquent male children. *J. abnorm. soc. Psychol.*, **63**, 493–503

Martin, B. (1975) Parent–child relations. In *Review of Child Development Research*, ed. Horowitz, F. D., vol. 4. Chicago: University of Chicago Press

Robins, L. N. (1966) *Deviant Children Grown Up*. Baltimore: Williams & Wilkins

— (1978) Sturdy childhood predictors of adult anti-social behavior: Replications from longitudinal studies. *Psychol. Med.*, **8**, 611–22

Rutter, M. (1971) Parent–child separation: psychological effects on the children. *J. child Psychiat.*, **12**, 233–60

— (1972) Relation between child and adult psychiatric disorders. *Acta psychiat. scand.*, **48**, 3–21

Rutter, M. & Shaffer, D. (1980) DSM III: A step foward or back in terms of the classification of child psychiatric disorders? *J. child Psychiat.*, **19**, 371–94

Rutter, M., Tizard, J. & Whitmore, J. (1970) *Education, Health and Behaviour*. London: Longman

Shaffer, D. (1974) Suicide in childhood and early adolescence. *J. child psychol. Psychiat.*, **15**, 275–91

Shapiro, A. K., Shapiro, E., Wayne, H. *et al.* (1973) Organic factors in Giles de la Tourette's syndrome. *Brit. J. Psychiat.*, **122**, 659–64

Sturge, C., Shaffer, D. & Rutter, M. (1977) The reliability of child codes used in I.C.D.–9. Paper presented at the annual meeting of the Child Psychiatry section of Royal College of Psychiatrists. St Andrews, Scotland

World Health Organization (1978) *Mental Disorders: Glossary and Guide to their Classification in Accordance with the 9th Revision of the International Classification of Diseases*. Geneva: WHO

Chapter 1.2.1

Berke, J. (1972) 'Anti-psychiatry': an interview with Dr Joseph Berke. In *Laing and Antipsychiatry*, ed. Boyers, R. & Orrill, R., p. 210. Harmondsworth: Penguin

Brown, G. W. & Harris, T. (1978) *Social Origins of Depression: A Study of Psychiatric Disorder in Women*. London: Tavistock Publications

Cobb, S. (1963) Mind–body relationships. In *The Psychological Basis of Medical Practice*, ed. Lief, H. I., Lief, V. F. & Lief, N. R., p. 40. New York: Hoeber Medical Division, Harper & Row

Cooper, B. & Shepherd, M. (1970) Life change, stress and mental disorder: the ecological approach. In *Modern Trends in Psychological Medicine 2*, ed. Harding Price, J., pp. 104–6. London: Butterworths

Fish, F. (1974) *Fish's Clinical Psychopathology: Signs and Symptoms in Psychiatry*, ed. Hamilton M., p. 6. Bristol: Wright

Jaspers, K. (1963) *General Psychopathology*. Translated from 7th edn by Hoenig, J. & Hamilton, M. W. Manchester: Manchester University Press

Lewis, A. (1972) 'Psychogenic': a word and its mutations. *Psychol. Med.*, **2**, 209–15

Mayer-Gross, W., Slater, E. & Roth, M. (1969) *Clinical Psychiatry*, 3rd edn, ed. Slater, E. & Roth, M., p. 262. London: Baillière, Tindall & Cassell

Rycroft, C. (1972) *A Critical Dictionary of Psychoanalysis*, p. 130. Harmondsworth: Penguin

Siegler, M. & Osmond, H. (1966) Models of madness. *Brit. J. Psychiat.*, **112**, 1193–203

Sim, M. (1968) *Guide to Psychiatry*, 2nd edn, pp. 266–7. London: Livingstone

Slater, E. (1965) The diagnosis of 'hysteria'. *Brit. med. J.*, **1**, 1395–9.

Chapter 1.2.2

Brown, G. W. & Harris, T. O. (1978) *Social Origins of Depression. A Study of Psychiatric Disorder in Women*. London: Tavistock

Brown, G. W., Ní Bhrolcháin, M. & Harris, T. O. (1979) Psychotic and neurotic depression. Part 3. Aetiological and background factors. *J. affect. Dis.*, **1**, 195–211

Cooper, B. (1972) Clinical and social aspects of chronic neurosis. *Proc. Roy. Soc. Med.*, **65**, 509–12

Finlay-Jones, R. & Brown, G. W. (1981) Types of stressful life event and the onset of anxiety and depressive disorders. *Psychol. Med.*, **11**, 803–15.

Henderson, S., Byrne, D. G., Duncan-Jones, P., Scott, R. & Adcock, S. (1980) Social relationships, adversity and neurosis. A study of associations in a general population sample. *Brit. J. Psychiat.*, **136**, 574–83

Kendell, R. E. (1968) *The Classification of Depressive Illnesses*. Institute of Psychiatry, Maudsley Monograph No. 18. London: Oxford University Press

Lader, M. & Marks, I. M. (1972) *Clinical Anxiety*, pp. 155–6. London: Heinemann

Leff, M. J., Roatch, J. F. & Bunney, W. E. (1970) Environmental factors preceding the onset of severe depressions. *Psychiatry*, **33**, 293–311

Paykel, E. S. (1971) Classification of depressed patients: a cluster analysis derived grouping. *Brit. J. Psychiat.*, **118**, 278–88

Paykel, E. S., Prusoff, B. A. & Klerman, G. L. (1971) The endogenous-neurotic continuum in depression, rater independence and factor distributions. *J. psychiat. Res.*, **8**, 73–90

Thomson, K. C. & Hendrie, H. C. (1972) Environmental stress in primary depressive illness. *Arch. gen. Psychiat.*, **26**, 130–2

Weissman, M. M. & Paykel, E. S. (1974) *The Depressed Woman. A Study of Social Relationships*. Chicago: University of Chicago Press

World Health Organization (1978) *Mental Disorders: Glossary and Guide to their Classification in Accordance with the 9th Revision of the International Classification of Diseases*. Geneva: WHO

Chapter 1.2.3

Barr, M. L., Sergovitch, F. R., Carr, D. H. & Shaver, E. L. (1969) The triplo-X female: an appraisal based on a study of twelve cases and a review of the literature. *Can. Med. Ass. J.*, **101**, 247–58

Beumont, P. J. V., Bancroft, J. H. J., Beardwood, C. J. & Russell, G. F. M. (1972) Behavioural changes after treatment with testosterone: case report. *Psychol. Med.*, **2**, 70–72

Christiansen, K. O. (1974) The genesis of aggressive criminality: Implications of a study of crime in a Danish twin study. In *Determinants and Origins of Aggressive Behaviour*, ed. de Wit, J. & Hartup, W. W. pp. 233–53. The Hague: Mouton

Goodwin, D. W., Schulsinger, F., Hermansen, L., Guze, S. B. & Winokur, G. (1973) Alcohol problems in adoptees raised apart from alcoholic biological parents. *Arch. gen. Psychiat.*, **28**, 238–43

Goodwin, D. W., Schulsinger, F., Møller, N., Hermansen, L., Winokur, G. & Guze, S. B. (1974) Drinking problems in adopted and non-adopted sons of alcoholics. *Arch. gen. Psychiat.*, **31**, 164–9.

Heston, L. L. & Shields, J. (1968) Homosexuality in twins: a family study and a registry study. *Arch. gen. Psychiat.*, **18**, 149–60

Kaij, L. (1960) *Alcoholism in Twins*. (Stockholm: Almqvist & Wiksell

Lange, J. (1931) *Crime as Destiny*. (Originally published in 1929, trans. Haldane, Charlotte, 1931) London: Allen & Unwin

Ljunberg, L. (1957) Hysteria: a clinical, prognostic and genetic study. *Acta psychiat. scand.*, **32**, Supp 112

Money, J. (1975) Human behaviour cytogenetics: review of psychopathology in three syndromes – 47XXY; 47XYY; and 45X. *J. sex Res.*, **11**(3), 181–200

Money, J. & Mittenthal, S. (1970) Lack of personality pathology in Turner's syndrome: relation to cytogenetics, hormones and physique. *Behav. Genet.*, **1**, 43–56

Myhre, S. A., Ruvalcaba, R. H. A., Johnson, H. R., Thuline, H. C. & Kelley, V. C. (1970) The effects of testosterone treatment in Klinefelter's syndrome. *J. Pediat.*, **76**, 267–76

Nielsen, J. (1969) Klinefelter's syndrome and the XYY syndrome. *Acta psychiat. scand.*, **45**, Supp. 209

— (1972) Gender role identity and sexual behaviour in persons with sex chromosome aberrations. *Dan. med. Bull.*, **19**, 269–75

Partanen, J., Bruun, K. & Markkanen, T. (1966) *Inheritance of Drinking Behaviour*. Helsinki: Finnish Foundation for Alcohol Studies

Pitcher, D. R. (1981) Sex chromosome disorders: a review. *CRC Crit. Rev. clin. lab. Sci.*, **13**(4), 241–82

Polani, P. E. (1977) Abnormal sex chromosomes, behaviour and mental disorder. In *Developments in Psychiatric Research*, ed. Turner, J. M., pp. 89–128. London: Hodder & Stoughton

Schulsinger, F. (1972) Psychopathy: heredity and environment. *Int. J. ment. Health*, **1**, 190–206

Shields, J. (1962) *Monozygotic Twins Brought up Apart and Brought up Together*. London: Oxford University Press

— (1973) Heredity and psychological abnormality. In *Handbook of Abnormal Psychology*, 2nd edn, ed. Eysenck, H. J., pp. 540–603. London: Pitman Medical

— (1976) Genetic factors in neurosis. In *Research in Neurosis*, ed. van Praag, H. M., pp. 155–70. Utrecht: Bohn, Scheltema & Holkema

Slater, E. (1961) The thirty-fifth Maudsley lecture: 'Hysteria 311'. *J. ment. Sci.*, **107**, 359–81

— (1962) Birth order and maternal age of homosexuals. *Lancet*, i, 69–71

Slater, E. & Cowie, V. (1971) *The Genetics of Mental Disorders*. London: Oxford University Press

Slater, E. & Shields, J. (1969) Genetical aspects of anxiety. In *Studies of Anxiety* ed. Lader, M. H., pp. 62–71. *British Journal of*

Psychiatry Special Publication No. 3. Ashford, Kent: Headley

Theilgaard, A. (1972) Cognitive style and gender role in persons with sex chromosome aberrations. *Dan. med. Bull.*, **19**, 276–86

Witkin, H. A., Mednick, S. A., Schulsinger, F., Bakkeström, E., Christiansen, K. O., Goodenough, D. R., Hirschhorn, K., Lundsteen, C., Owen, D. R., Philip, J., Rubin, D. B. & Stocking, M. (1976) Criminality in XYY and XXY men. *Science*, **193** 547–55

Chapter 1.2.4

Ballinger, C. B. (1975) Psychiatric morbidity and the menopause; screening of general population sample. *Brit. med. J.*, **3**, 344–6

Ballinger, C. B. (1976) Psychiatric morbidity and the menopause: clinical features. *Brit. med. J.*, **1**, 1183–5

Christie Brown, J. R. W. & Christie Brown, M. E. (1976) Psychiatric disorders associated with the menopause. In *The Menopause: A Guide to Current Research and Practice*, ed. Beard, R. J., pp. 57–79. England: MTP Press

Erikson, E. (1965) *Childhood and Society*. Harmondsworth: Penguin

Graham, P. J. & Rutter M. L. (1977) Adolescent disorders. In *Child Psychiatry: Modern Approaches*, ed. Rutter, M. & Hersov, L., pp. 407–27. Oxford: Blackwell

Greene, J. G. & Cooke, P. J. (1980) Life stress and symptoms at the climacterium. *Brit. J. Psychiat.*, **136**, 486–91

Jaszman, L., Van Lith, N. D. & Zatt, J. C. A. (1969) The perimenopausal symptoms. *Med. Gynaecol. Sociol.*, **4**, 268–75

McKinlay, S. M. & Jeffreys, M. (1974) The menopausal syndrome. *Brit. J. prev. soc. Med.*, **28**, 108–15

Meyer, J. E. (1974) Psychoneurosis and neurotic reactions in old age. *J. Amer. Geriat. Soc.*, **22**, 254–7

Neugarten, B. L. & Kraines, R. J. (1965) Menopausal symptoms in women of various ages. *Psychosom. Med.*, **27**, 266–73

Offer, P. (1969) *The Psychological World of the Teenager: A Study of Normal Adolescent Boys*. New York: Basic Books

Post, F. (1965) *The Clinical Psychiatry of Late Life*. Oxford: Pergamon Press

Rutter, M. L., Graham, P. J., Chadwick, O. & Yule, W. (1976) Adolescent turmoil: fact or fiction? *J. child Psychol. Psychiat.*, **17**, 35–50

Schofield, M. (1965) *The Sexual Behaviour of Young People*. London: Longman

Studd, J., Chakavarti, S. & Okram, D. (1977) The climacterium. *Clin. Obstet. Gynaecol.*, **4**, 3–29

Thompson, B., Hart, S. A. & Durno, D. (1973) Menopausal age and symptomatology in a general practice. *J. biol. Sci.*, **5**, 71–82

Winokur, G. (1973) Depression in the menopause *Amer. J. Psychiat.*, **130**, 92–3

Chapter 1.2.5

Brozek, J. & Caster, W. O. (1957) Psychologic effects of thiamine restriction and deprivation in normal young men. *Amer. J. clin. Nutrition*, **5**, 109–20

Crow, T. J. (1978) Viral causes of psychiatric disease. *Postgrad. med. J.*, **54**, 763–7

Eitinger, L. (1959) The importance of atrophy of the brain in psychiatric disease pictures. *Nord. Med.*, **61**, 301–3

Goldstein, K. (1942) *After Effects of Brain Injuries in War*. New York: Grune & Stratton

Greenbaum, J. V. & Lurie, L. A. (1948) Encephalitis as a causative factor in behaviour disorders of children. *J. Amer. Med. Ass.*, **136**, 923–30

Haug, J. O. (1962) Pneumoencephalographic studies in mental disease. *Acta psychiat. scand.*, Supp. 165, 1–104

Hill, D. & Watterson, D. (1942) Electroencephalographic studies of psychopathic personalities. *J. Neurol. Neurosurg. Psychiat.*, **5**, 47–65

Kolansky, H. & Moore, W. T. (1971) Effects of marihuana on adolescents and young adults. *J. Amer. Med. Ass.*, **216**, 486–92

— (1972) Toxic effects of chronic marihuana use. *J. Amer. Med. Ass.*, **222**, 35–41

Lishman, W. A. (1973) The psychiatric sequelae of head injury: a review. *Psychol. Med.*, **3**, 304–18

— (1978) *Organic Psychiatry: The Psychological Consequences of Cerebral Disorder*. Oxford: Blackwell

Lycke, E., Norrby, R. & Roos, B. (1974) A serological study on mentally ill patients: with particular reference to the prevalence of herpes virus infections. *Brit. J. Psychiat.*, **124**, 273–9

Lyon, R. L. (1962) Huntington's chorea in the Moray Firth area. *Brit. med J.*, **1**, 1301–6

Mark, V. H. & Ervin, F. R. (1970) *Violence and the Brain*. New York: Harper & Rowe

Minski, L. (1933) The mental symptoms associated with 58 cases of cerebral tumour. *J. Neurol. Psychopathol.*, **13**, 330–43

Mitchell, W., Falconer, M. A. & Hill, D. (1954) Epilepsy with fetishism relieved by temporal lobectomy. *Lancet*, **ii**, 626–30

Petersen, P. (1968) Psychiatric disorders in primary hyperparathyroidism. *J. clin. Endocrinol. Metab.*, **28**, 1491–5

Reynolds, E. H. (1967) Effects of folic acid on the mental state and fit frequency of drug-treated epileptic patients. *Lancet*, **i**, 1086–8

Reynolds, E. H., Preece, J. M., Bailey, J. & Coppen, A. (1970) Folate deficiency in depressive illness. *Brit. J. Psychiat.*, **117**, 287–92

Ron, M. A. (1977) Brain damage in chronic alcoholism: a neuropathological, neuroradiological and psychological review. *Psychol. Med.*, **7**, 103–12

Shukla, G. D., Srivastava, O. N. & Katiyar, B. C. (1979) Sexual disturbances in temporal lobe epilepsy: a controlled study. *Brit. J. Psychiat.*, **134**, 288–92

Snaith, R. P., Mehta, S. & Raby, A. H. (1970) Serum folate and vitamin B12 in epileptics with and without mental illness. *Brit. J. Psychiat.*, **116**, 179–83

Spies, T. D., Aring, C. D., Gelperin, J. & Bean, W. B. (1938) The mental symptoms of pellagra: their relief with nicotinic acid. *Amer. J. med. Sci.*, **196**, 461–75

Stafford-Clark, D. & Taylor, F. H. (1949) Clinical and electroencephalographic studies of prisoners charged with murder. *J. Neurol. Neurosurg. Psychiat.*, **12**, 325–30

Taylor, D. C. (1969) Sexual behaviour and temporal lobe epilepsy. *Arch. Neurol.*, **21**, 510–16

Whitlock, F. A. (1967) The aetiology of hysteria. *Acta psychiat. Scand.*, **43**, 144–62

Williams, D. (1969) Neural factors related to habitual aggression: consideration of the differences between those habitual aggressives and others who have committed crimes of violence. *Brain*, **92**, 503–20

Chapter 1.3.1

Boden, M. (1979) *Piaget.* Glasgow: Fontana

Bower, T. G. R. (1979) *Human Development.* San Francisco: Freeman

Bowlby, J. (1975) *Attachment and Loss,* vol. 2: *Separation: Anxiety and Anger.* Harmondsworth: Penguin

Donaldson, M. (1978) *Children's Minds.* London: Fontana

Freedman, D. G. (1975) Culture, inbreeding and behavior, with some thoughts on inter-ethnic communication. In *Society, Stress and Disease,* ed Levi, L., vol. II, *Childhood and Adolescence.* London: Oxford University Press

Freud, A. (1946) *The Ego and the Mechanisms of Defence.* London: Hogarth Press

Hersov, L. (1976) School refusal. In *Child Psychiatry: Modern Approaches,* ed. Rutter, M. & Hersov, L., pp. 455–86. Oxford: Blackwell

Hill, D. & Watterson, D. (1942) Electroencephalographic studies of psychopathic personalities. *J. Neurol. Psychiat.,* **5,** 47–65

Hutt, C., (1972) Sexual differentiation in human development. In *Gender Differences, their Ontogeny and Significance,* ed. Ounsted, C. & Taylor, D. C. London: Churchill-Livingstone

Lambert, L. & Streather, J. (1980) *Children in Changing Families.* London: Macmillan

McFarlane, J. W., Allen, L. & Honzig, P. (1954) *A Developmental Study of Behaviour Problems of Normal Children between 21 months and 14 years.* Berkeley & Los Angeles: University of California Press

Newson, J. & Newson, E., (1976) *Seven Years Old in the Home Environment.* London: Allen & Unwin

Piaget, J. (1926) *The Language and Thought of the Child.* London: Routledge & Kegan Paul

— (1929) *The Child's Conception of the World.* London: Routledge & Kegan Paul

— (1932) *The Moral Judgement of the Child.* London: Routledge & Kegan Paul

Porter, R. & Collins, G. M. (Eds.) (1982) *Temperamental Differences in Infants and Young Children.* London: Pitman.

Quitkin, F. & Klein, D. F. (1969) Two behavioural syndromes in young adults related to possible minimal brain dysfunction. *J. psychiat. Res.,* **1,** 131–42

Rich, J. (1956) Types of stealing. *Lancet,* **i,** 496–8

Rutter, M. (1966) *Children of Sick Parents: An Environmental and Psychiatric Study.* Maudsley Monograph No. 16. Oxford: Oxford University Press

— (1976a) Sociocultural influences. In *Child Psychiatry, Modern Approaches,* ed. Rutter, M. & Hersov, L., pp. 109–35. Oxford. Blackwell

— (1976b) Separation, loss and family relationships. In *Child Psychiatry: Modern Approaches,* ed. Rutter, M. & Hersov, L., pp. 47–73. Oxford. Blackwell

— (1977) Brain damage syndromes in childhood: concepts and findings. *J. child Psychol. Psychiat.,* **18,** 1–21

— (1981) Stress, coping and development: some issues and some questions. *J. child Psychol. Psychiat.,* **22,** 323–53

Rutter, M., Cox, A., Tupling, C., Berger, M. & Yule, W. (1975) Attainment and adjustment in two geographical areas. I The prevalence of psychiatric disorder. *Brit. J. Psychiat.,* **126,** 493–509

Rutter, M., Graham, P., Chadwick, O. & Yule, W., (1976) Adolescent turmoil: fact or fiction. *J. child Psychol. Psychiat.,* **17,** 35–56

Rutter, M., Maughan, B., Mortimer, P. & Ousten, J. (1979) *Fifteen Thousand Hours, Secondary Schools and their effects on Children.* London: Open Books

Rutter, M., Quinton, D. & Yule, W. (1977) *Family Pathology and Disorder in Children.* London: Wiley

Rutter, M., Tizard, J. & Whitmore, L. (1970) *Education, Health and Behaviour.* London: Longman

Sandberg, S. T., Rutter, M. & Taylor, E. (1978) Hyperkinetic disorder in psychiatric clinic attenders. *Dev. Med. child Neurol.,* **20,** 279–99

Schachar, R., Rutter, M. & Smith, A. (1981) The characteristics of situationally and pervasively hyperactive children: implications for syndrome definition. *J. child Psychol Psychiat.,* **22,** 375–92

Seglow, J., Pringle, M. L. Kellmer & Wedge, P. (1972) *Growing Up Adopted.* Windsor: NFER

Shepherd, M., Oppenheim, A. N. & Mitchell, S. (1966) Childhood behaviour disorders and the child guidance clinic: and epidemiological study. *J. child Psychol. Psychiat.,* **7,** 39–52

Thomas, A., Chess, S. & Birch, H. G. (1968) *Temperament and Behaviour Disorders in Children.* London: London University Press

Tizard, B. (1977) *Adoption: A Second Chance.* London: Open Books

Toulmin, S. (1970) Reasons and causes. In *Explanation in the Behavioural Sciences,* ed. Borger, R. & Cioffi, F. Cambridge: Cambridge University Press

Wolff, S. (1967) Behavioural characteristics of primary school children referred to a psychiatric department. *Brit. J. Psychiat.,* **113,** 885–983

Wolff, S. (1981) *Children Under Stress,* 2nd edn. London: Penguin

Wolff, S. & Acton, W. P. (1968) Characteristics of parents of disturbed children. *Brit. J. Psychiat.,* **114,** 593–601

Wolkind, S. & Rutter, M. (1973) Children who have been 'in care' – an epidemiological study. *J. child Psychol. Psychiat.,* **14,** 97–105

Chapter 1.3.2

Apley, J. & Hale, B. (1973) Children with recurrent abdominal pain: how do they grow up? *Brit. med. J.,* **3,** 7–9

Bellman, M. (1966) Studies on encopresis. *Acta. paed. scand.* Supp. 170

Berg, I., Marks I., McGuire, R. & Lipsedge, M. (1974) School phobia and agoraphobia. *Psychol. Med.,* **4,** 428–34

Bindelglas, P. M. & Dee, G. (1978) Enuresis treatment with imipramine hydrochloride: a ten-year follow-up study. *Amer. J. Psychiat.,* **135,** 1549–52

Butensky, A., Faralli, V., Heebner, D. & Waldron, I. (1976) Elements of the coronary-prone behaviour pattern in children and teenagers. *J. psychosom. Res.,* **20,** 439–44

Christensen, M. F. & Mortensen, O. (1975) Long-term prognosis in children with recurrent abdominal pain. *Arch. Dis. Childh.,* **50,** 110–14

Gersten, J. C., Langner, T. S., Eisenberg, J. G., Simcha-Fagan, O. & McCarthy, E. D. (1976) Stability and change in types of behavioral disturbance of children and adolescents. *J. abn. child Psychol.,* **4,** 111–27

Graham, P. (1970) Pathology in the brain and antisocial disorder. In *The Exceptional Child,* ed. Hellmuth, J. New York: Brunner/Mazel

— (1977) Intergenerational influences on psychosocial development. *Int. J. ment. Health*, **6**, 73–89

Graham, P. & Rutter, M. (1973) Psychiatric disorder in the young adolescent: a follow-up study. *Proc. R. Soc. Med.* **66**, 1228–9

Graham, P., Rutter, M. & George S. (1973) Temperamental characteristics as predictors of behavior disorders in children. *Amer. J. Orthopsychiat.* **43**, 328–39

Kagan, J. & Moss, H. A. (1962) *Birth to Maturity: A Study in Psychological Development*. New York: Wiley

Kohlberg, L., Lacrosse, J. & Ricks, D. (1972) The predictability of adult mental health from child behavior. In *Manual of Child Psychopathology*, ed. Wolman, B. B. New York: McGraw-Hill

Lishman, A. (1974) The speed of recall of pleasant and unpleasant experiences. *Psychol. Med.*, **4**, 212–18

Marks, I. M. (1969) *Fears and Phobias*. London: Heinemann

Mellsop, G. W. (1972) Psychiatric patients seen as children and adults: childhood predictors of adult illness. *J. child Psychol. Psychiat.*, **13**, 91–101

— (1973) Adult psychiatric patients on whom information was recorded during childhood. *Brit. J. Psychiat.*, **123**, 703–10

Mendelson, W., Johnson, N. & Stewart, M. (1971) Hyperactive children as teenagers: a follow-up study. *J. nerv. ment. Dis.*, **153**, 273–9

Minde, K., Weiss, G. & Mendelson, W. (1972) A five-year follow-up study of 91 hyperactive schoolchildren. *J. Amer. Acad. Child Psychiat.*, **11**, 595–610

Pittman, F. S., Langsley, D. G. & DeYoung, C. G. (1968) Work and school phobia: a family approach to treatment. *Amer. J. Psychiat.*, **124**, 1535–41

Pritchard, M. & Graham, P. (1966) An investigation of a group of patients who have attended both the child and adult departments of the same psychiatric hospital. *Brit. J. Psychiat.*, **112**, 603–12

Robbins, L. (1963) The accuracy of parental recall of aspects of child development and child rearing practice. *J. abnorm. soc. Psychol.*, **66**, 261–70

Robins, L. N. (1966) *Deviant children grown up*. Baltimore: Williams & Wilkins

— (1978) Sturdy childhood predictors of adult antisocial disorders. *Psychol. Med.*, **8**, 611–22

Roff, M. (1972) A two factor approach to juvenile delinquency and the later histories of juvenile delinquents. In *Life History Research in Psychopathology*, ed. Roff, M., Robins, L. N. & Pollack, M., vol. 2. Minneapolis: University of Minnesota Press

— (1974) Childhood antecedents of adult neurosis, severe bad conduct and psychological health. In *Life History Research in Psychopathology*, ed. Ricks, D. F., Thomas, A. & Roff, M. vol. 3, pp. 131–62. University of Minnesota Press

Ryle, A. (1967) *Neurosis in the Ordinary Family*. London: Tavistock

Sandberg, S., Rutter, M. & Taylor, E. (1978) Hyperkinetic disorder in psychiatric clinic attenders. *Dev. Med child Neurol.*, **20**, 279–99

Thomas, A. and Chess, S. (1977) *Temperament and Development*, pp. 27–47. New York: Brunner/Mazel

Waldron, S. (1976) The significance of childhood neurosis for adult mental health. *Amer. J. Psychiat.*, **133**, 532–8

Watt, N. F. (1978) Patterns of childhood social development in adult schizophrenics. *Arch. gen. Psychiat.*, **35**, 160–5

Chapter 2.1

Balint, M. (1957) *The Doctor, his Patient and the Illness*. London: Pitman Medical

Campbell, P. G. & Russell, G. F. M. (1982) The psychiatric assessment. In *Clinical Skills: A System of Clinical Examination*, 2nd edn, ed. Bouchier, I. D. & Morris, J. S. London: Saunders

Finesinger, J. E. (1948) Psychiatric interviewing. *Amer. J. Psychiat.*, **105**, 187–95

Fletcher, C. (1979) Towards better practice and teaching of communication between doctors and patients. In *Mixed Communications: Problems and Progress in Medical Care. Essays on Current Research*, Twelfth Series, ed. McLachlan, G. London: Oxford University Press (for the Nuffield Provincial Hospitals Trust)

Glover, E. (1955) *The Technique of Psychoanalysis*. London: Baillière, Tindall & Cox

Institute of Psychiatry (1973) *Notes on Eliciting and Recording Clinical Information*. London: Oxford University Press

International Classification of Diseases (1978) *Mental Disorders: Glossary and Guide to their Classification*. Geneva: WHO

Kirby, G. H. (1921) *Guides for History-Taking and Clinical Examination of Psychiatric Cases*. New York: Abeney

Leff, J. P. & Isaacs, A. (1978) *Psychiatric Examination in Clinical Practice*. Oxford: Blackwell

Mayer-Gross, W. M., Slater, E. & Roth, M. (1969) *Clinical Psychiatry*, 3rd edn, ed. Slater, E. & Roth, M. London: Baillière, Tindall & Cassell

Schneider, K. (1950) *Psychopathic Personalities*, 9th edn. Trans. Hamilton, M. W., 1958. New York: Grune & Stratton

Sullivan, H. S. (1954) *The Psychiatric Interview*. London: Tavistock

Watzlawick, P., Beavin, J. H. & Jackson, D. D. (1968) *Pragmatics of Human Communication*. London: Faber & Faber

Wing, J. K., Cooper, J. E. & Sartorius, N. (1974) *The Description and Classification of Psychiatric Symptoms: An Instruction Manual for the PSE and Catego System*. London: Cambridge University Press

Chapter 2.2

Brown, G. W. & Rutter, M. (1966) The measurement of family activities and relationships: a methodological study. *Hum. Rel.*, **19**, 241–63

Conners, C. K. (1969) A teacher rating scale for use in drug studies with children. *Amer. J. Psychiat.*, **126**, 884–8

Cox, A. (1975) The assessment of parental behaviour. *J. child Psychol. Psychiat.*, **16**, 255–9

Cox, A., Holbrook, D. & Rutter, M. (1981) Psychiatric interviewing techniques: VI. Experimental study; eliciting feelings. *Brit. J. Psychiat.*, **139**, 144–52

Cox, A., Hopkinson, K. & Rutter, M. (1981) Psychiatric interviewing techniques: II. naturalistic study; eliciting factual information. *Brit. J. Psychiat.*, **138**, 283–91

Cox, A. & Rutter, M. (1976) Diagnostic appraisal and interviewing. In *Child Psychiatry – Modern Approaches*, ed. Rutter, M. & Hersov, L., pp. 271–305. Oxford: Blackwell

Cox, A., Rutter, M. & Holbrook, D. (1981) Psychiatric interviewing techniques: V. experimental study; eliciting factual information. *Brit. J. Psychiat.*, **139**, 29–37

Douglas, J. W. B., Lawson, A., Cooper, J. F. & Cooper, E. (1968) Family interaction and the activities of young children. *J. child Psychol. Psychiat.*, **9**, 157–71

Duehn, W. D. & Proctor, E. K. (1977) Initial clinical interaction and premature discontinuance in treatment. *Amer. J. Orthopsychiat.*, **47**, 284–90

Haley, J. (1976) Conducting the first interview. In *Problem Solving Therapy*, ed. Haley, J., pp. 9–47. New York: Harper

Hart, H., Bax, M. & Jenkins, S. (1978) The value of developmental history. *Dev. Med. child Neurol.*, **20**, 442–52

Heilbrun, A. (1974) Interviewer style, client satisfaction and premature termination following initial counselling contact. *J. couns. Psychol.*, **22**, 346–50

Hopkinson, K., Cox, A. & Rutter, M. (1981) Psychiatric interviewing techniques: III. naturalistic study; eliciting feelings. *Brit. J. Psychiat.*, **138**, 406–15

May, J. R. & Miller, P. R. (1977) Note taking and information recall: an empirical study. *J. med. Educ.*, **52**, 523–5

Rutter, M. (1967) A children's behaviour questionnaire for completion by teachers: preliminary findings. *J. child Psychol. Psychiat.*, **8**, 1–11

Rutter, M. & Brown, G. W. (1966) The reliability and validity of measures of family life and relationships in families containing a psychiatric patient. *Soc. Psychiat.*, **1**, 38–53

Rutter, M. & Cox, A. (1981) Psychiatric interviewing techniques: I. methods and measures. *Brit. J. Psychiat.*, **138**, 273–82

Rutter, M., Cox, A., Egert, S., Holbrook, D. & Everitt, B. (1981) Psychiatric interviewing techniques: IV. experimental study; four contrasting styles. *Brit. J. Psychiat.*, **138**, 456–65

Rutter, M., Cox, A., Tupling, C., Berger, M. & Yule, W. (1975a) Attainment and adjustment in two geographical areas: 1. the prevalence of psychiatric disorder. *Brit. J. Psychiat.*, **126**, 493–509

Rutter, M. & Graham, P. (1968) The reliability and validity of the psychiatric assessment of the child: 1. interview with the child. *Brit. J. Psychiatry*, **114**, 563–79

Rutter, M., Shaffer, R. D. & Sturge, C. (1975b) *A Guide to a Multiaxial Classification Scheme for Psychiatric Disorders in Childhood and Adolescence*. London: Institute of Psychiatry

Rutter, M., Tizard, J. & Whitmore, K. (1970) *Education, Health and Behaviour*. London: Longman

Satir, V. (1964) *Conjoint Family Therapy*. New York: Science & Behavioural Books

Shapiro, R. J. & Budman, S. H. (1973) Defection, termination and continuation in family and individual therapy. *Family in Process*, **12**, 55–67

Stott, D. H. (1963) *The Social Adjustment of Children*, 2nd edn. London: University of London Press

Chapter 2.3

Cavanagh, N. C. (1980) *A Scheme of Paediatric Neurological Investigation*. London: Geigy

Woodmansey, A. C. (1971) Parent guidance. *Dev. Med. child Neurol.*, **13**, 243–4

Chapter 2.4

Beck, A. T., Ward, C. H., Mendelsohn, M., Mock, J. & Erbaugh, J. (1961) An inventory for measuring depression. *Arch. gen. Psychiat.*, **4**, 561–71

Closs, S. J. & Hutchings, M. J. (1976) *APU Arithmetic Test*. London: Hodder & Stoughton

Cooper, J. (1970) The Leyton obsessional inventory. *Psychol. Med.*, **1**, 48–64

Eysenck, H. J. & Eysenck, S. B. G. (1975) *Manual of the Eysenck Personality Questionnaire, Junior and Adult*. London: Hodder & Stoughton

Hersen, M. & Bellack, A. S. (1976) *Behavioural Assessment: A Practical Handbook*. New York: Pergamon

Hodgson, R. J. & Rachman, S. (1977) Obsessional-compulsive complaints. *Behav. Res. Ther.*, **15**, 389–95

Jensen, A. R. (1959) The reliability of projective techniques: a review of the literature. *Acta psychol.*, **16**, 3–31

Kanfer, F. H. & Saslow, G. (1969) Behavioural diagnosis. In *Behavior Therapy: Appraisal and Status*, ed. Franks, C. M. New York: McGraw-Hill

Matarazzo, J. D. (1972) *Wechsler's Measurement and Appraisal of Adult Intelligence*. Baltimore: Williams & Wilkins

Mischel, W. (1968) *Personality and Assessment*. New York: Wiley

Neale, M. D. (1966) *The Neale Analysis of Reading Ability*, 2nd edn. London: Macmillan

Rachman, S. J. & Hodgson, R. J. (1980) *Obsessions and Compulsions*. Englewood Cliffs, N.J.: Prentice-Hall

Raven, J. C. (1956) *Standard Progressive Matrices*, Rev. edn. London: Lewis

— (1958) *Mill Hill Vocabulary Scale*, 2nd edn. London: Lewis

Raven, J. C., Court, J. H. & Raven, J. (1978) *Manual for the Raven's Progressive Matrices and Vocabulary Scales*. London: Lewis

Rutter, M., Shaffer, D. & Sturge, C. (1975) *A Guide to a Multi-Axial Classification Scheme for Psychiatric Disorders in Childhood and Adolescence*. London: Institute of Psychiatry

Schonell, F. J. & Schonell, F. E. (1960) *Diagnostic and Attainment Testing*. Edinburgh: Oliver & Boyd

Taylor, J. A. (1953) A personality scale of manifest anxiety. *J. abnorm. soc. Psychol.*, **48**, 285–95

Vernon, P. E. (1977) *Graded Word Spelling Test*. London: Hodder & Stoughton

Vernon, P. E. & Miller, K. M. (1976) *Graded Arithmetic-Mathematics Test*. London: Hodder & Stoughton

Wechsler, D. (1955) *Manual for the Wechsler Adult Intelligence Scale*. New York: Psychological Corporation

— (1958) *The Measurement and Approach of Adult Intelligence*. Baltimore: Williams & Wilkins

— (1974) *Manual for the Wechsler Intelligence Scale for Children* (Revised). New York: Psychological Corporation

— (1976) *Manual for the Wechsler Intelligence Scale for Children* (revised), British edn. Windsor: National Foundation for Educational Research

— (1981) *WAIS. R Manual: Wechsler Adult Intelligence Scale, Revised*. New York: The Psychological Corporation.

Wolpe, J. & Lang, P. (1964) A fear survey schedule for use in behaviour therapy. *Behav. Res. Ther.*, **2**, 27–30

Wolpe, J. & Lazarus, A. A. (1966) *Behavior Therapy Techniques*. New York: Pergamon

Chapter 3.1.1

Adler, A. (1956) *The Individual Psychology of Alfred Adler*, ed. Ansbacher, H. L. & R. R. New York: Basic Books

Barlow, W. (1973) *The Alexander Principle*. London: Gollancz

Bierer, J. (1940) Psychotherapy in mental hospital practice. *J. ment. Sci.*, **86**, 928–47

Bion, W. R. & Rickman, J. (1943) Inter-group tensions: their study as a task of the group. *Lancet*, **ii**, 678–81

Brown, J. A. C. (1961) *Freud and the Post-Freudians*. Harmonds-worth: Pelican

Fordham, F. (1953) *An Introduction to Jung's Psychology*. Harmonds-worth: Pelican

Foulkes, S. H. (1950) Group therapy: a short survey and orientation with particular reference to group-analysis. *Brit. J. med., Psychol.*, **23**, 199–205

Foulkes, S. H. & Anthony, E. J. (1957) *Group Psychotherapy*. Har-mondsworth: Penguin

Frank, J. D. (1963) *Persuasion and Healing*. New York: Schocken Books

Freud, A. (1966a) *The Ego and The Mechanisms of Defence*. London: Hogarth Press & Institute of Psychoanalysis

Freud, A. (1966b) *Normality and Pathology in Childhood*. London: Hogarth Press & Institute of Psychoanalysis

Freud, S. (1971) *The Complete Introductory Lectures on Psychoanaly-sis*, ed. Strachey, J. London: Allen & Unwin

Fromm, E. (1957) *The Art of Loving*. London: Allen & Unwin

Gelder, M. G. & Marks, I. M. (1966) Severe agoraphobia. A con-trolled prospective trial of behaviour therapy. *Brit. J. Psy-chiat.*, **112**, 309–19

Hadfield, J. A. (1950) *Psychology of Mental Health*. London: Allen & Unwin

Hall, G. S. (1920) *Translation of Freud's General Introduction to Psy-choanalysis*. New York: Boni & Liveright

Herbart, J. F. (1891) *A Textbook in Psychology*. Trans. from the orig-inal German by Smith, M. K. (1891). New York: Appleton

Horney, K. (1939) *New Ways in Psychoanalysis*. New York: Kegan Paul French Trubner

James, W. (1912) Does 'consciousness' exist? In *Essays in Radical Empiricism*, pp. 1–39. New York: Longmans Green

Jaspers, K. (1963) *The Nature of Psychotherapy*. Trans. Hoenig, J. & Hamilton, M. Manchester: Manchester University Press

Jones, E. (1954, 1955, 1957) *Sigmund Freud. Life and Work*. 3 Vols. London: Hogarth Press

Jones, M. (1957) The treatment of personality disorders in a thera-peutic community. *Psychiatry*, **20**, 211–20

Jung, C. G. Principal translated works listed in *An Introduction to Jung's Psychology*, Fordham, F. (1953), listed above

Klein, M. (1948) *Contributions to Psychoanalysis*. London: Hogarth Press

Klein, M. & Rivière, J. (1937) *Love, Hate and Reparation*. London: Hogarth Press

Lewis, A. (1956) *Price's Textbook of the Practice of Medicine*, Section XIX, Psychological Medicine, pp. 1619–20. London: Oxford University Press

Ling, T. M. (1946) Rehabilitation of British industry's neurosis cases. *J. Rehab.*, **12**, 33–5

Main, T. F. (1946) The hospital as a therapeutic institution. *Bull. Menninger Clin.*, **10**, 66–70

Rivers, W. H. R. (1920) *Instinct and the Unconscious*. Cambridge: Cambridge University Press

Sullivan, H. S. (1955) *Conceptions of Modern Psychiatry*. London: Tavistock

Suttie, I. (1935) *The Origins of Love and Hate*. London: Kegan Paul

Taylor, F. Kräupl (1958) A history of group and administrative therapy in Great Britain. *Brit. J. med. Psychol.*, **XXXI**, parts 3 & 4, 153–73

— (1969) Prokaletic measures derived from psychoanalytic technique. *Brit. J. Psychiat.*, **115**, 407–19

Whyte, Lancelot Law (1960) *The Unconscious before Freud*. New York: St Martin's Press

Chapter 3.1.2

Baker, R., Hall, J. N., Hutchinson, K. & Bridge, G. (1977) Symptom changes in chronic schizophrenic patients on a token econ-omy: a controlled experiment. *Brit. J. Psychiat.*, **131**, 381–93

Bancroft, J. (1974) *Deviant Sexual Behaviour*. Oxford: Clarendon Press

Beck, A. T. (1976) *Cognitive Therapy and Emotional Disorders*. New York: International Universities Press

Bird, J. (1979) The behavioural treatment of hysteria. *Brit. J. Psy-chiat.*, **134**, 129–37

Ellis, A. A. (1962) *Reason and Emotion in Psychotherapy*. New York: Stuart

Gambril, E. D. (1977) *Behaviour Modification: Handbook of Assess-ment, Intervention and Evaluation*. San Francisco: Jossey-Bass

Garfield, S. L. & Bergin, A. E. (Ed.) (1978) *Handbook of Psychother-apy and Behaviour Change*, 2nd edn. New York: Wiley

Gelder, M. G., Bancroft, J. H. J., Gath, D. H., Johnston, D. W., Mathews, A. M. & Shaw, P. M. (1973) Specific and non-specific factors in behaviour therapy. *Brit. J. Psychiat.*, **123**, 445–62

Jannoun, L., Munby, M., Caralan, J. & Gelder, M. (1980) A home-based treatment program for agoraphobia: Replication and controlled evaluation. *Behav. Ther.*, **11**, 294–305

Johnston, D. W. & Gath, D. H. (1973) Arousal levels and attribu-tion effects in diazepam assisted flooding. *Brit. J. Psychiat.*, **123**, 463–66

Masters, W. H. & Johnson, V. E. (1970) *Human Sexual Inadequacy*. London: Churchill

Rush, A. J., Beck, A. T., Kovacs, M. & Hollon, S. (1977) Compara-tive efficacy of cognitive therapy and pharmacotherapy in the treatment of depressed outpatients. *Cog. Ther. Res.*, **1**, 17–37

Trower, P. E., Bryant, B. & Argyle, M. (1978) *Social Skills and Men-tal Health*. London: Methuen

Wolpe, J. (1958) *Psychotherapy by Reciprocal Inhibition*. Berkeley, California: Stanford University Press

Yates, A. J. (1970) *Behaviour Therapy*. New York: Wiley.

Chapter 3.1.3.

Ackerman, N. (1966) *Treating the Troubled Family*. New York: Basic Books

Alexander, J. & Parsons, B. (1973) Short term behavioural interven-tion with delinquent families: impact on family process and recidivism. *J. abnorm. Psychol.*, **81**, 219–25

Azrin, N. H., Naster, B. J. & Jones, R. (1973) Reciprocity counsel-ing: a rapid learning-based procedure for marital counsel-ing. *Behav. Res. Ther.*, **11**, 365–82

Bateson, G. Jackson, D. D., Haley, J. & Weakland, J. H. (1956) Toward a theory of schizophrenia. *Behav. Sci.*, **1**, 251–64

Beels, C. C. & Ferber, A. S. (1969) Family therapy: a view. *Family Process*, **8**, 280–318

Bloch, D. A. (1973) *Techniques of Family Psychotherapy: A Primer*. New York: Grune & Stratton

Boszormenyi-Nagy, I. & Framo, J. (1965) (Eds.) *Intensive Family Therapy*. New York: Harper & Row

Bowen, M. (1966) The use of family theory in clinical practice. *Compr. Psychiat.*, **7**, 345–74

Byng-Hall, J. (1979) Re-editing family mythology during family therapy. *J. fam. Ther.*, **1**, 103–16

Cade, B. & Southgate, P. (1979) Honesty is the best policy. *J. fam. Ther.*, **1**, 23–32

Crowe, M. J. (1978a) Behavioural approaches to marital and family problems. In *Current Themes in Psychiatry'*, ed. Gaind, R. & Hudson, B. London: Macmillan

— (1978b) Conjoint marital therapy: a controlled outcome study. *Psychol. Med.*, **8**, 623–36

DeWitt, K. N. (1978) The effectiveness of family therapy. *Arch. gen. Psychiat.*, **35**, 549–61

Dicks, Henry V. (1967) *Marital Tensions*. London: Routledge

Gurman, A. S. (1973) The effects and effectiveness of marital therapy. A review of outcome research. *Family Process*, **12**, 145–70

Haley, J. (1976) *Problem Solving Therapy*. San Francisco: Jossey-Bass

Hendricks, W. J. (1971) Use of multi-family counselling groups in the treatment of male narcotic addicts. *Int. J. group Psychother.*, **21**, 84–90

Jackson, D. & Weakland, J. (1961) Conjoint family therapy: some considerations on theory, technique and results. *Psychiat.*, **24**, 30–45

Jacobson, N. S. (1977) Problem solving and contingency contracting in the treatment of marital discord. *J. consult. clin. Psychol.*, **45**, 92–100

— (1978) Specific and non-specific factors in a behaviour approach to marital discord. *J. consult. clin. Psychol.*, **46**, 442–52

Langsley, D. G., Flomenhaft, K. & Machotka, P. (1969) Follow-up evaluation of family crisis therapy. *Amer. J. Orthopsychia.*, **39**, 753–60

Lask, B. & Matthew, D. (1979) Childhood asthma: the results of a controlled trial of family psychotherapy. *Arch. Dis. Child.*, **54**, 116–19

Liberman, R. P., Levine, J., Wheeler, E., Sanders, N. & Wallace, C. (1976) Marital therapy in groups: a comparative evaluation of behavioural and interactional formats. *Acta psych. scand.* Supp. 266

Lidz, T., Fleck, S., Alanen, I. O. & Cornelison, A. (1963) Schizophrenic patients and their siblings. *Psychiat.*, **26**, 1–18

Madanes, C. & Haley, J. (1977) Dimensions of family therapy. *J. nerv. ment. Dis.*, **165**, 88–98

Minuchin, S. (1974) *Families and Family Therapy*. London: Tavistock

Parkes, C. M. (1972) *Bereavement: Studies of Grief in Adult Life*. London: Tavistock

Patterson, G. R. & Hops, H. (1972) Coercion, a game for two: intervention techniques for marital conflict. In *The Experimental Analysis of Social Behaviour*, ed. Ulrich, R. E. & Mountjoy, P. New York: Appleton

Paul, N. & Grosser, G. (1965) Operational mourning and its role in conjoint family therapy. *Comm. ment. Health J.*, **1**, 339–45

Pincus, L. & Dare, C. (1978) *Secrets in the Family*. London: Faber & Faber

Satir, V. (1967) *Conjoint Family Therapy: A Guide to Theory and Technique*. Palo Alto: Science & Behaviour Books

Selvini Palazzoli, M., Cecchin, G., Prata, G. & Boscolo, L. (1978) *Paradox and Counter-Paradox*. New York: Aronson

Simon, R. (1972) Sculpting the family. *Family Process*, **11**, 49–58

Skynner, A. C. R. (1976) *One Flesh, Separate Persons*. New York: Grune & Stratton

Stuart, R. B. (1969) Operant-interpersonal treatment for marital discord. *J. consult. clin. Psychol.*, **33**, 675–82

Von Bertalanffy, L. (1966) General systems theory and psychiatry. In *American Handbook of Psychiatry*, ed. Arierl, S. vol. 3. New York: Basic Books

Wynne, L. (1965) Some indications and contra-indications for exploratory family therapy. In *Intensive Family Therapy*, ed. Boszomenyi-Nagy, I. & Framo, J., New York: Harper & Row

Chapter 3.1.4

Anders, T. F. & Ciaranello, R. D. (1977) Psychopharmacology of childhood disorders. In *Psychopharmacology. From Theory to Practice*, ed. Barchas, J. et al., pp. 407–24. New York: Oxford University Press

Blackwell, B. (1973) Psychotropic drugs in use today. The role of diazepam in medical practice. *J. Amer. Med. Ass.*, **225**, 1637–41

Cohen, I. M. (1970) The benzodiazepines. In *Discoveries in Biological Psychiatry*, ed. Ayd, F. J. & Blackwell, B. Philadelphia: Lippincott

Covington, J. S. (1975) Alleviating agitation, apprehension, and related symptoms in geriatric patients: A double-blind comparison of phenothiazine and a benzodiazepine. *Southern med. J.*, **68**, 719–24

Dasberg, H. H. & van Praag, H. (1974) The therapeutic effect of short-term oral diazepam treatment of acute clinical anxiety in a crisis centre. *Acta psychiat. scand.*, **50**, 326–40

Gaind, R. N. & Jacoby, R. (1978) Benzodiazepines causing aggression. In *Current Themes in Psychiatry*, ed. Gaind, R. N. & Hudson, B. L., pp. 371–9. London: Macmillan

Greenblatt, D. J. & Shader, R. I. (1974) *Benzodiazepines in Clinical Practice*. New York: Raven Press

Hollister, L. E. (1978) *Clinical Pharmacology of Psychotherapeutic Drugs*. New York: Churchill Livingstone

Kelly, D. (1976) Neurosurgical treatment of psychiatric disorders. In *Recent Advances in Clinical Psychiatry*, ed. Granville-Grossman K., No. 2, pp. 227–61. Edinburgh: Churchill Livingstone

Lader, M. H., Bond, A. J. & James, D. C. (1974) Clinical comparison of anxiolytic drug therapy. *Psychol. Med.*, **4**, 381–7

Palmer, G. C. (1978) Use, overuse, misuse, and abuse of benzodiazepines. *Alabama J. med. Sci.*, **15**, 383–92

Rickels, K., Downing, R. W. & Winokur, A. (1978) Antianxiety drugs: clinical use in psychiatry. In *Handbook of Psychopharmacology*, ed. Iversen, L. L., Iversen, S. D. & Snyder, S. H., pp. 395–430. New York: Plenum

Solomon, K. & Hart, R. (1978) Pitfalls and prospects in clinical research on antianxiety drugs: benzodiazepines and placebo – a research review. *J. clin. Psychiat.*, **39**, 823–31

Stewart, P. B., Forgnone, M. & May, F. E. (1974) Epidemiology of acute drug intoxications: patient characteristics, drugs and medical complications. *Clinical Toxicology*, **7**, 513–30

Chapter 3.2.1.

Caudill, W. (1958) *The Psychiatric Hospital as a Small Community*. Cambridge, Mass.: Harvard University Press

Goffman, E. (1968) *Asylums*. Harmondsworth: Penguin

Hinshelwood, R. D. & Manning, N. (1979) *Therapeutic Communities*. London: Routledge & Kegan Paul

Jensen, E. (1980) (Ed.) *The Therapeutic Community*. London: Croom Helm

Jones, M. (1948) Physiological and psychological responses to stress in neurotic patients. *J. ment. Sci.* **94**, 392–427

Kreeger, L. (Ed.) (1975) *The Large Group*. London: Constable

Lorentzen, S. (1981) *J. Oslo City Hospital*, **31**, 4–6

Main, T. (1946) The hospital as a therapeutic institution. *Bull. Menninger Clin.*, **10**, 3, 66–70

Maxmen, J. (1973) Group therapy as viewed by hospitalized patients. *Arch. gen. Psychiat.* **28**, 404–8

May, P. R. A. & Simpson, G. M. (1980) Schizophrenia: overview of treatment methods. In *Comprehensive Textbook of Psychiatry*, II, ed. Freedman, A. M., Kaplan, H. I. & Sadock, B. I. Baltimore: Williams & Wilkins

Stanton, A. H. & Schwartz, M. S. (1954) *The Mental Hospital*. New York: Basic Books

Walton, H. J. (1974) Application of group methods in ward administration. In *Small Group Psychotherapy*, ed. Walton, H. J. Harmondsworth: Penguin

Chapter 3.2.2.

Beard, B. H. (1972) Patterns of utilization in a psychiatric day hospital, *Texas Med.*, **68**, 74–80

Bierer, J. (1951) *The Day Hospital: An Experiment in Social Psychiatry and Syntho-Analytic Psychotherapy*. London: Lewis

Carney, M. W., Ferguson, R. S. & Sheffield, B. P. (1970) Psychiatric day hospital and community, *Lancet*, **i**, 1218–20

Edwards, C. (1978) *A National View of Day Care Services*. DHSS Seminar Report. London: DHSS

Michaux, Mary., Chelst, M. P., Foster, S., Pruim, R. J. & Dansiger, E. (1973) Post release adjustment of day and full time psychiatric patients. *Arch. gen. Psychiat.*, **29**, 647–51

Wilder, J. F., Levin, G. & Zwerling, I. (1966) A two year follow-up evaluation of acute psychotic patients treated in a day hospital. *Amer. J. Psychiat.*, **122**, 1095–101

Chapter 3.3.1

Barker, P. (1981) *Basic Family Therapy*. London: Granada

Dare, C. (1977) Dynamic Treatments. In *Child Psychiatry: Modern Approaches*, ed. Rutter, M. & Hersov, L., pp. 949–66 Oxford: Blackwell

Frank, J. (1979) What is psychotherapy? In *An Introduction to the Psychotherapies*, ed. Bloch, S., pp. 1–22. Oxford: Oxford University Press

Glick, I. D. & Kessler, D. R. (1974) *Marital and Family Therapy*, New York: Grune & Stratton

Haley, J. (1976) *Problem-solving Therapy*. New York: Jossey-Bass

Hersov, L. & Bentovim, A. (1977) In-patient units and day-hospitals. In *Child Psychiatry: Modern Approaches*, ed. Rutter, M. & Hersov, L., pp. 880–900. Oxford: Blackwell

Holbrook, D. (1978) A combined approach to parental coping. *Brit. J. soc. Work*, **8**, 439–51

Lask, B. (1979) Family therapy: outcome research 1972–78. *J. fam. Ther.*, **1**, 87–91

Lask, B. & Kirk, M. (1979) Childhood asthma: family therapy as an adjunct to routine management. *J. fam. Ther.*, **1**, 33–9

McAuley, R. & McAuley, P. (1977) *Child Behaviour Problems. An Empirical Approach to Management*. London: Macmillan

Millar, S. (1968) *The Psychology of Play*. Harmondsworth: Penguin

Minuchin, S. (1974) *Families and Family Therapy*. London: Tavistock

Reid, W. J. & Shyne, A. W. (1969) *Brief and Extended Case Work*. New York: Columbia University Press

Reisman, J. M. (1973) *Principles of Psychotherapy with Children*, p. 10. New York: Wiley

Rosenthal, A. J. & Levine, S. J. (1971) Brief psychotherapy with children: process of therapy. *Amer. J. Psychiat.*, **128**, 141–6

Shepherd, M., Oppenheim, B. & Mitchell, S. (1971) *Childhood Behaviour and Mental Health*. London: University of London Press

Skynner, A. C. R. (1969) A group-analytic approach to conjoint family therapy. *J. child Psychol. Psychiat.*, **10**, 81–106

Sussenwein, F. (1977) Psychiatric social work. In *Child Psychiatry: Modern Approaches*, ed. Rutter, M. & Hersov, L., pp. 967–91. Oxford: Blackwell

Tizard, B. (1977) *Adoption: A Second Chance*. London: Open Books

Wilkinson, T. (1979) The problems and values of objective nursing observations in psychiatric care. *J. adv. Nursing*, **4**, 151–9

Yule, W. (1977) Behavioural approaches. In *Child Psychiatry: Modern Approaches*, ed. Rutter, M. & Hersov, L., pp. 923–48. Oxford: Blackwell

Chapter 3.3.2

Abraham, K. (1920) The applicability of psychoanalytic treatment to patients at an advanced age. In *Selected Papers of Karl Abraham*, trans. Bryan, D. & Strachey, A. (1927). *International Psychoanalytical Library*, No. 13, pp. 312–17. London: Hogarth Press

Bergmann, K. (1971) The neuroses of old age. In *Recent Developments in Psychogeriatrics*, ed. Kay, D. W. K. & Walk, A. *British Journal of Psychiatry*, Special Publications No. 6, pp. 39–50. Ashford, Kent: Headley Bros

— (1978) Neurosis and personality disorders in old age. In *Studies in Geriatric Psychiatry*, ed. Isaacs, A. D. & Post, F., pp. 41–76. Chichester: Wiley

Blau, D. & Berezin, M. A. (1975) Neuroses and character disorders. In *Modern Perspectives in the Psychiatry of Old Age*, ed. Howells, J. G., chap. 9, pp. 201–31. New York: Brunner/Mazel; Edinburgh: Churchill-Livingstone

Bowlby, J. (1969) Psychopathology of anxiety: the role of affectional bonds. In *Studies of Anxiety*, ed. Lader, M. H. *British Journal of Psychiatry*, Special Publications, No. 3, 80–6. Ashford, Kent: Headley Bros

Butler, R. N. (1975) Psychotherapy in Old Age. In *American Handbook of Psychiatry*, ed. Arieti S., 2nd edn, vol. 5, chap. 42, pp. 807–28. Washington: American Psychiatric Association

Cooper, B. & Schwartz, R. (1981) Psychiatric case identification in an elderly urban population. *Soc. Psychiat.*, **17**, 43–52

Erikson, E. H. (1959) Identity and the life cycle. In *Selected Papers. Psychological Issues*, vol. 1, No. 1, Monograph 1. New York: International Universities Press

Foster, E. M., Kay, D. W. K. & Bergmann, K. (1976) The characteristics of old people receiving or needing services: the relevance of psychiatric diagnoses, *Age and Ageing*, **5**, 245–55

Goldfarb, A. I. (1967) Geriatric psychiatry. In *Comprehensive Textbook of Psychiatry*, ed. Freedman, A. M. & Kaplan, H. I., pp. 1464–87. Baltimore: Williams & Wilkins

Hinton, J. (1967) *Dying*. London: Penguin

Hussian, R. A. (1981) *Geriatric Psychiatry – A Behavioural Perspective*. New York: Van Nostrand, Reinhold

Kay, D. W. K., Beamish, P. & Roth, M. (1964a) Old age and mental disorders in Newcastle upon Tyne, Part I: A study of prevalence. *Brit. J. Psychiat.*, **110**, 146–58

— (1964b) Old age and mental disorders in Newcastle upon Tyne, Part II: A study of possible social and medical causes. *Brit. J. Psychiat.*, **110**, 668–82

Kay, D. W. K. & Bergmann, K. (1980) Epidemiology of mental disorders among the aged in the community In *Handbook of Mental Health and Aging*, ed. Birren, J. E. & Sloane, B. R., pp. 34–56. New Jersey: Prentice Hall

Kessel, W. I. N. & Shepherd, M. (1962) Neurosis in hospital and general practice. *J. ment. Sci.*, **108**, 159–66

Parkes, C. M. (1972) *Bereavement: Studies of Grief in Adult Life.* London: Tavistock

Seligman, M. E. P. (1975) *Helplessness – on Depression, Development and Death.* San Francisco: Freeman

Shepherd, M. & Gruenberg, E. M. (1957) The age for neuroses. *Milbank Mem. Fund Q.*, **35**, 258–65

Shepherd, M., Cooper, B., Brown, A. C. & Kalton, G. W. (1966) *Psychiatric Illness in General Practice* London: Oxford University Press

Verwoerdt, A. (1981) Psychotherapy for the elderly. In *Health Care of the Elderly*, Ed Arie, T., pp. 104–17. London: Croom Helm

Chapter 3.3.3

Berg, J. M., Gilderdales, S. & Way, J. (1969) On telling parents of a diagnosis of mongolism. *Brit. J. Psychiat.*, **15**, 1195–6

Bryant, K. N. & Hirschberg, J. C. (1961) Helping parents of a retarded child. *Amer. J. Dis. Childh.*, **102**, 52–6

Carr, J. (1974) The effect of the severely subnormal on their families. In *Mental Deficiency. The Changing Outlook*, ed., Clarke, A. M. & Clarke, A. B. D., pp. 807–37. London: Methuen

Clements, J. C., Bidder, R. T., Gardner, S., Bryant, G. & Gray, O. P. (1980) A home advisory service for pre-school children with developmental delays. *Child Care Health Dev.*, **6**, 25–33

D'Arcy, E. (1968) Congenital defects: mother's reaction to first information. *Brit. med. J.*, **3**, 796–8

Farber, B. & Rykman, D. R. (1965) Effects of severely mentally retarded children on family relationships. *Ment. Retard. Abstr.*, **2**, 1–17

Gath, A. (1975) The effects of mental subnormality on the family. In *Contemporary Psychiatry*, ed. Silverstone, T. & Barraclough, B., pp. 284–8 Ashford: Headley Bros

— (1979) Parents as therapists of mentally handicapped children. *J. child Psychol. Psychiat.*, **20**, 161–5

Hill, R. (1949) *Families under Stress*, p. 275. New York: Harper

MacKeith, R. (1973) The feelings and behaviour of parents of handicapped children. *Dev. Med. child Neurol.*, **15**, 524–7

Malvia, S. N. (1973) Parents of the mentally retarded. *Soc Welf.*, **19**, 7–8

O'Dell, S. (1974) Training parents in behaviour modification. A review. *Psychol. Bull.*, **81**, 418–33

Revill, S. & Blunden, R. (1979) A home training service for preschool developmentally handicapped children. *Behav. Res. Ther.*, **17**, 207–14

San Martino, M. & Newman, M. B. (1974) Siblings of retarded children: a population risk. *Child Psychiat. Hum. Dev.*, **4**, 168–77

Schild, S. (1971) The family of the retarded child. In *The Mentally Retarded Child and his Family: A Multidisciplinary Handbook*, ed. Koch, R. & Dobson, J. C., pp. 266–84 New York: Brunner/Mazel

Tarjan, G. (1977) Mental retardation and clinical psychiatry. In *Research to Practice in Mental Retardation*, vol. 1, *Care and Intervention*, ed. Mittler, P. & de Jong, J. M., pp. 412–16 Baltimore: University Park Press

Willer, B. S., Intagliata, J. C. & Atkinson, A. C. (1978). Crises for families of mentally retarded persons including the crisis of deinstitutionalisation. *Brit. J. ment. Subnorm.*, **25**, 38–49

Wolfensberger, W. (1968) Counselling the parents of the retarded. In *Mental Retardation, Appraisal, Rehabilitation and Education*, ed. Baumeister, A. A., pp. 399–400 London: University of London Press

Chapter 3.4.1

Altschul, A. T. (1972) *Patient–Nurse Interaction. A Study of Interaction Patterns in Acute Psychiatric Wards.* Edinburgh; Churchill-Livingstone

Bird, J., Marks, I. M. & Lindley, P. (1979) Nurse therapists in psychiatry: developments, controversies and implications. *Brit. J. Psychiat.*, **125**, 321–9

Burr, J. (1970) *Nursing the Psychiatric Patient.* 2nd edn. London: Baillière Tindall & Cassell

Burton, G. (1965) *Nurse and Patient: The Influence of Human Relationships.* London: Tavistock

Groen, J. J. & Feldman-Toledano, Z. (1966) Educative treatment of patients and parents in anorexia nervosa. *Brit. J. Psychiat.*, **112**, 671–81

Leininger, M. M. (1961) Changes in psychiatric nursing. A reflection of the impact of sociocultural forces. *Can. Nurse*, **57**, 938–49

Marks, I. M., Hallam, R. S., Connolly, J. & Philpott, R. (1977) *Nursing in Behavioural Psychotherapy: An Advanced Clinical Role for Nurses.* London: Royal College of Nursing of the United Kingdom

Marks, I., Bird, J. & Lindley, P. (1978) Behavioural nurse therapists 1978 – developments and implications. *Behav. Psychother.*, **6**, 25–35

Russell, G. (1981) The current status and treatment of anorexia nervosa. In *Proceedings of the 3rd World Congress on Biological Psychiatry, Stockholm*, July, 1981, ed. Geelen, J. Amsterdam: Elsevier/North Holland

Simpson, M. A. (1976) Self-mutilation. *Brit. J. hosp. Med.*, **16**, 430–38

Chapter 3.4.2

Beck, A. T., Rush, A. J., Shaw, B. F. & Emery, A. (1979) *Cognitive Therapy for Depression.* New York: Guildford

Bellack, A. S. & Hersen, M. (1980) *Introduction to Clinical Psychology.* New York: Oxford University Press

Calhoun, K. S., Adams, H. E. & Mitchell, K. M. (1974) (Eds.) *Innovative Treatment Methods in Psychotherapy.* New York: Wiley

Corsini, R. J. (Ed.) (1981) *Handbook of Innovative Psychotherapies.* New York: Wiley

Eysenck, H. J. (Ed.) (1976) *Case Studies in Behaviour Therapy.* London: Routledge & Kegan Paul

Eysenck, H. J. & Rachman, S. (1965) *Causes and Cures of Neuroses.* London: Routledge & Kegan Paul

Mackay, D. (1975) *Clinical Psychology – Theory and Therapy*. London: Methuen

Marks, I. M., Hallam, R. S., Connolly, J. & Philpott, R. (1977) *Nursing in Behavioural Psychotherapy*. London: Royal College of Nursing

O'Dell, S. (1974) Training parents in behaviour modification: a review. *Psychol. Bull.*, **81**, 418–33

Wolpe, J. (1958) *Psychotherapy by Reciprocal Inhibition. Stanford:* Stanford University Press

Yates, A. J. (1970) *Behavior Therapy*. New York: Wiley

— (1980) *Biofeedback and Modification of Behaviour*. New York: Plenum

Yule, W. (1974) Teaching psychological principles to non-psychologists. *J. Ass. Educ. Psychol.*, **10**, 5–16

Yule, W. & Hemsley, D. R. (1977) Single-case methodology in medical psychology. In *Contributions to Medical Psychology, vol. I*, ed. Rachman, S. London: Pergamon Press

Chapter 3.4.3

Beck, A. T. (1976) *Cognitive Therapy and the Emotional Disorders*. New York: International University Press

Brown, G. W. & Harris, T. (1978) *Social Origins of Depression. A Study of Psychiatric Disorder in Women*. London: Tavistock

Cooper, B., Harwin, B. G., Depla, C. & Shepherd, M. (1975) Mental health care in the community: an evaluative study. *Psychol. Med.*, **5**, 372–80

Davis, B. M. (1977) *Community Health and Social Services*. London: Hodder & Stoughton

Ford, D. (1975) *Children, Courts and Caring*. London: Constable

Raustron, D. (1980) Child Care Law. *BAAF*, Nov.

Robinson, D. (1977) *Self Help and Health: Mutual Aid for Modern Problems*. London: Martin Robertson

Sainsbury, P., Costain, W. R. & Grad, J. (1965) The effects of a community service on the referral and admission rates of elderly psychiatric patients. In *World Psychiatric Association Symposium, Psychiatric Disorders in the Aged*. Manchester: Geigy

The Children's Act (1975) London: HMSO

The Child Care Act (1980) London: HMSO (This Act was implemented on 1 April 1981, after the original draft of this section was completed. This was not an innovatory Act as such, but a consolidation of existing legislation.)

The Children and Young Persons Act (1969) London: HMSO

Chapter 3.4.4

Bennett, D. H. (1977) The mentally ill. In *Rehabilitation Today*, Publications ed. Mattingly, S., chap. 19. London: Update

Bion, W. R. (1961) *Experiences in Groups, and Other Papers*. London: Tavistock

Bion, W. R. (1970) *Attention and Interpretation: A Scientific Approach to Insight in Psycho-analysis and Groups*. London: Tavistock

Clark, D. H. (1964) *Administrative Therapy*. London: Tavistock

Foulkes, S. H. & Anthony, E. J. (1957) *Group Psychotherapy*. London: Penguin

Jennings, S. (1975) *Creative Therapy*. London: Pitman

Jung, C. G. (1934) *Modern Man in Search of a Soul*. London: Kegan Paul, Trench & Trubner

Lowen, A. (1958) *Physical Dynamics of Character Structure*. New York: Grune & Stratton. (Reprinted 1971, as *The Language of the Body*, New York: Macmillan)

Lyddiatt, E. M. (1970) *Spontaneous Painting and Modelling – A Practical Approach in Therapy*. London: Constable

Mare, P. B. de & Kreeger, L. C. (1974) *Introduction to Group Treatments in Psychiatry*. London: Butterworths

Moreno, J. L. (1946) *Psychodrama I* (Revised 1964). New York: Beacon House

— (1959) *Psychodrama II*. New York: Beacon House

— (1969) *Psychodrama III*. New York: Beacon House

Perls, F. S. (1969) *Gestalt Therapy Verbatim*, ed. O'Stevens, J. California: Real People Press

Rogers, C. (1965) *Client Centred Therapy*. London: Constable

Rogers, C. (1973) *Encounter Groups*. London: Penguin

Schulz, W. B. (1973) *Joy*. London: Penguin

Westman, H. (1961) *The Springs of Creativity*. New York: Atheneum

Chapter 3.4.5

Douglas, J. W. B. (1964) *The Home and the School*. London: McGibbon & Kee

Kolvin, I., Garside, R. F., Nicol, A. R., Macmillan, A., Wolstenholme, F. & Leitch, I. M. (1981) *Help Starts Here: The Maladjusted Child in the Ordinary School*. London: Tavistock

Rutter, M., Maughan, B., Mortimore, P. & Ouston, J. (1979) *Fifteen Thousand Hours*. London: Open Books

Rutter, M., Tizard, J. & Whitmore, K. (1970) *Education, Health and Behaviour*. London: Longman

Special Educational Needs, (1978) *Report of the Committee of Enquiry into the Education of Handicapped Children and Young People* London: HMSO

Wolff, S. & Chick, J. (1980) Schizoid personality in childhood: a controlled follow-up study. *Brit. J. Psychiat.*, **10**, 85–100

Chapter 3.5.1

Dell, S. (1980) Transfer of Special Hospital patients to the NHS. *Brit. J. Psychiat.*, **136**, 222–34

Gunn, J., Robertson, G., Dell, S., & Way, C. (1978) *Psychiatric Aspects of Imprisonment*. London: Academic Press

Home Office (1979) *Report of the Work of the Prison Department 1978*. London: HMSO

Orr, J. (1978) The imprisonment of mentally abnormal offenders. *Brit. J. Psychiat.*, **133**, 194–9

Chapter 3.5.2

Clarke, C. S. (1979) The COHSE Report on the management of violent patients. Counsel's opinion. *Bullet Roy. Coll. Psychiatrists*, February, 1979, 21–5

DHSS, Home Office, Welsh Office. Lord Chancellor's Department (1978) *Review of the Mental Health Act, 1959*. Cmd. Report No. 7320. London: HMSO

Gunn, J. (1974) Management of patients who have committed offences. *Medicine*, **30**, 1783–9

Mental Health Act (1959) 7 & 8 Eliz. 2. Ch. 72. London: HMSO

Royal College of Psychiatrists (1977) The College's comments on 'A Review of the Mental Health Act, 1959'. *Brit. J. Psychiat., News and Notes*, January, 1977, 9–17

Chapter 4.1.1

Baldwin, J. A. & Oliver, J. C. (1975) Epidemiology and family characteristics of severely abused children. *Brit. J. prev. soc. Med.*, **29**, 205–21

Lynch, M. (1978) The prognosis of child abuse. *J. child Psychol. Psychiat.*, **19**, 175–80

Richman, N. (1977a) Behaviour problems in preschool children: family and social factors. *Brit. J. Psychiat.*, **131**, 523–7

— (1977b) Disorders in preschool children. In *Child Psychiatry – Modern Approaches*, ed. Rutter, M. & Hersov, L., pp. 387–406. Oxford: Blackwell

Richman, N., Stevenson, J. E. & Graham, P. J. (1975) Prevalence of behaviour problems in preschool children – an epidemiological study in a London borough. *J. child Psychol. Psychiat.*, **16**, 272–87

— (1982) *Preschool to School: A Behavioural Study*. London: Academic Press

Rogers, D., Tripp, J., Bentovim, A. & Robinson, A. (1976) Non-accidental poisoning: an extended syndrome of child abuse. *Brit. med. J.*, **1**, 793–6

Wolff, S. (1961a) Social and family background of preschool children with behaviour disorders attending a child guidance clinic. *J. child Psychol. Psychiat.*, **2**, 260–8

— (1961b) Symptomatology and outcome of preschool children with behaviour disorders attending a child guidance clinic. *J. child Psychol. Psychiat.*, **2**, 269–76

Wolkind, S. N. & Rutter, M. (1973) Children who have been 'in care': an epidemiological study. *J. child Psychol. Psychiat.*, **14**, 97–105

Chapter 4.1.2

Bernstein, B. (1962) Social class, linguistic codes and grammatical elements. *Lang. Speech*, **5**, 221–40

Brain, Lord (1965) *Speech Disorders – Aphasia and Agnosia*, 2nd edn. London: Butterworth

Brodbeck, A. J. & Irwin, O. C. (1946) The speech behaviour of infants without families. *Child Dev.*, **17**, 145–56

Brown, J. B. & Lloyd, H. (1975) A controlled study of children not speaking at school. *J. Ass. Workers Maladj. Children*, **3**, 49–63

Brown, R., Cazden, C. & Bellugi-Klima, U. (1969) The child's grammar from I to III. In *Minnesota Symposia on Child Psychology*, ed. Hill, J. P., vol. 2, pp. 28–73. Minnesota: University of Minnesota Press

Browne, E., Wilson, V. & Laybourne, P. C. (1963) Diagnosis and treatment of elective mutism in children. *J. Amer. Acad. Child Psychiat.*, **2**, 605–17

Bruner, J. S., Oliver, R. R. & Greenfield, P. M. (1966) *Studies in Cognitive Growth*. New York: Wiley

Cazden, C. (1966) Subcultural differences in child language. *Merrill-Palmer Q.*, **12**, 185–219

Chomsky, N. (1957) *Syntactic Structures*. The Hague: Mouton

— (1965) *Aspects of the Theory of Syntax*. Cambridge, Mass.: MIT Press

— (1969) *The Acquisition of Syntax in Children from 5 to 10*. Cambridge, Mass.: MIT Press

Conrad, R. (1977) The reading ability of deaf school-leavers. *Brit. J. educ. Psychol.*, **47**, 138–48

Critchley, E. (1967) Language development of hearing children in a deaf environment. *Dev. Med. child Neurol.*, **9**, 274–80

Fundudis, T., Kolvin, I. & Garside, R. F. (1979) *Psychological Development of Speech-Retarded and Deaf Children*. London: Academic Press

Ingram, T. T. S. (1959a) A description of classification of common disorders of speech in childhood. *Arch. Dis. Childh.*, **34**, 444–55

— (1959b) Specific developmental disorders of speech in childhood. *Brain*, **32**, 450–67

— (1963) Delayed development of speech with special reference to dyslexia. *Proc. R. Soc. Med.*, **56**, 199–203

— (1972) The classification of speech and language disorders in young children. In *The Child with Delayed Speech* ed. Rutter, M. & Martin, J. A. M. *Clin. dev. Med.* No. **43**, 13–32. London: SIMP/Heinemann

Irwin, O. C. (1960) Infant speech: effect of systematic reading of stories. *J. speech hearing Res.*, **3**, 187–90

Klaus, R. A. & Gray, S. W. (1968) The early training project for disadvantaged children: a report after five years. Monograph, *Soc. Res. Child Dev.*, No. 120

Kolvin, I. & Fundudis, T. (1981) Elective mute children: Psychological development and background factors. *J. child Psychol. Psychiat.*, **22**:3:219–32

Lenneberg, E. H. (1967) *Biological Foundations of Language*. New York: Wiley

Lewis, M. (1968) Language and mental development. In *Development in Human Learning, II*, ed. Lunzer, A. E. & Morris, J. F., p. 68. London: Staples Press

Lotter, V. (1966) Epidemiology of autistic conditions in young children: I – Prevalence. *Soc. Psychiat.*, **1**, 124–37

McCready, E. B. (1962) Defects in the zone of language (word deafness and word blindness) and their influence in education and behaviour. *Amer. J. Psychiat.*, **6**, 267–78

Meadow, K. P. (1975) The development of deaf children. In *Review of Child Development Research*, ed. Hetherington, E. M., Hagen, J. W., Kron, R. & Stein, A. H., vol. 5, pp. 439–506. Chicago: University of Chicago Press

Menyuk, P. & Looney, P. A. (1972) A problem of language disorder: length versus structure. *J. speech hearing Res.*, **15**, 264–79

Mittler, P. (1972) Psychological assessment of language abilities. In *The Child with Delayed Speech*, ed. Rutter, M. & Martin, J. A. M. *Clin. dev. Med.*, No. **43**, 106–19. London: SIMP/Heinemann

Moores, D. (1972) Language disabilities of hearing-impaired children. In *Principles of Childhood Language Disabilities*, ed. Irwin, J. V. & Marge, M. pp. 159–83. Englewood Cliffs, N.J.: Prentice-Hall

Morley, M. (1965) *The Development and Disorders of Speech in Childhood*, 2nd edn (3rd edn 1972). Edinburgh: Churchill-Livingstone

Myklebust, H. R. (1964) *The Psychology of Deafness*, 2nd edn. New York: Grune & Stratton

Orton, S. T. (1934) Some studies in the language function. *Res. Pub. Ass. Res. Nerv. Ment. Dis.*, **13**, 614–33

Orton, S. T. (1937) *Reading, Writing and Speech Problems in Children*. London: Chapman & Hall

Parker, E. B., Olsen, T. F. & Throckmorton, M. C. (1960). Social casework with elementary school children who do not talk in school. *Soc. Work*, **5**, 64–70

Provence, S. & Lipton, R. C. (1962) *Infants in Institutions*. New York: International Universities Press

Reed, M. (1970) Deaf and partially hearing children. In *The Psycho-*

logical *Assessment of Mental and Physical Handicaps,* ed. Mittler, P., pp. 403–37 London: Methuen

Routh, D. K. (1969) Conditioning of social response differentiation in infants. *Dev. Psychol.,* **1,** 219–26

Rutter, M. (1972) Clinical assessment of language disorder in the young child. In *The Child with Delayed Speech,* ed. Rutter, M. & Martin, J. A. M. *Clin. dev. Med.* No. **43,** 33–47 London: SIMP/Heinemann

— (1977) Speech delay. In *Child Psychiatry,* ed. Rutter, M. & Hersov, L., pp. 688–716. Oxford: Blackwell

Rutter, M. & Yule, W. (1970) Neurological aspects of intellectual retardation and specific reading retardation. In *Education, Health and Behaviour,* ed. Rutter, M., Tizard, J. & Whitmore, K., pp. 54–74. London: Longman

Rutter, M. & Mittler, P. (1972) Environmental influences on language development. In *The Child with Delayed Speech,* ed. Rutter, M. & Martin, J. A. M. *Clin. dev. Med.,* No. **43,** 52–67. London: SIMP/Heinemann

Salfield, D. J. (1950) Observations of elective mutism in children. *J. ment. Sci.,* **96,** 1024–32

Stevenson, J. & Richman, N. (1976) The prevalence of language delay in a population of three-year-old children and its association with general retardation. *Dev. Med. child Neurol.,* **18,** 431–41

— (1978) Behaviour, language and development in three-year-old children. *J. Autism child Schiz.,* **8,** 299–314

Tizard, J. (1964) *Community Services for the Mentally Handicapped.* Oxford: Oxford University Press

— (1970) The role of social institutions in the causation, prevention and alleviation of mental retardation. In *Socio-Cultural Aspects of Mental Retardation,* ed. Haywood, H. C., pp. 281–340 New York: Appleton-Century-Crofts

Tramer, M. (1934) Electiver Mutismus bei Kindern. *Z. Kinderpsychiat.,* **1,** 30–5

U.S. Office of Demographic Studies (1973) *Further Studies in Achievement Testing, Hearing-Impaired Students. Data from the annual survey of hearing-impaired children and youth* (Series D, No. 13). Washington DC: Gallaudet College

Vernon, M. (1976) Communication and the education of deaf and hard of hearing children. In *Methods of Communication Currently Used in the Education of Deaf Children,* ed. Henderson, P., pp. 99–109. London: RNID

Wiley, J. (1971) A psychology of auditory impairment. In *Psychology of Exceptional Children and Youth,* ed. Cruickshank, W. M., pp. 414–39 Englewood Cliffs, N.J.: Prentice-Hall

Wright, H. L. (1968) A clinical study of children who refuse to talk in school. *J. Amer. Acad. Child Psychiat.,* **7,** 603–17

Chapter 4.1.3

Barkley, R. (1977) A review of stimulant drug research with hyperactive children. *J. child Psychol. Psychiat.,* **18,** 137–65

Brown, G., Chadwick, O., Shaffer, D., Rutter, M. & Traub, M. (1981) A prospective study of children with head injuries. III. Psychiatric sequelae. *Psychol. Med.,* **11,** 63–78

Cantwell, D. (1977) Hyperkinetic syndrome. In *Child Psychiatry: Modern Approaches,* ed. Rutter, M. & Hersov, L., pp. 524–55. Oxford: Blackwell

Mendelson, W., Johnson, N. & Stewart, M. (1971) Hyperactive children as teenagers: a follow-up study. *J. nerv. ment. Dis.,* **153,** 273–9

Menkes, M., Rowe, J. & Menkes, J. (1967) A twenty-five year follow-up study on the hyperkinetic child with minimal brain dysfunction. *Pediat.,* **39,** 393–9

Ounsted, C. (1955) The hyperkinetic syndrome in epileptic children. *Lancet,* **2,** 303–11

Rapoport, J., Buchsbaum, M. S., Zahn, T. P., Weingartner, H., Lindlow, C. & Mikkelsen, E. J. (1978) Dextroamphetamine: cognitive and behavioral effects in normal prepubertal boys. *Science,* **199,** 560–63

Rutter, M., Graham, P. & Yule, W. (1970) *A Neuropsychiatric Study in Childhood.* Clinics in Developmental Medicine No. 35/36. London: SIMP/Heinemann

Safer, D. J. & Allen, R. P. (1976) *Hyperactive Children: Diagnosis and Management.* Baltimore: University Park Press

Sandberg, S., Rutter, M. & Taylor, E. (1978) Hyperkinetic disorder in psychiatric clinic attenders. *Dev. Med. child Neurol.,* **20,** 279–99

Shaffer, D. & Greenhill, L. (1979) A critical note on the predictive validity of 'The Hyperkinetic Syndrome'. *J. child Psychol. Psychiat.,* **20,** 61–72

Shaffer, D., McNamara, N. & Pincus, J. H. (1974) Controlled observations on patterns of activity, attention and impulsivity in brain damaged and psychiatrically disturbed boys. *Psychol. Med.,* **4,** 4–18

Sprague, R. & Sleator, E. (1975) What is the proper dose of stimulant drugs in children? *Int. J. ment. Health,* **4,** 75–118

Taylor, E. (1980) Development of attention. In *Scientific Foundations of Developmental Psychiatry,* ed. Rutter, M., pp. 185–97. London: Heinemann

Tizard, B. & Rees, J. (1975) The effect of early institutional rearing on the behaviour problems and affectional relationships of four-year-old children. *J. child Psychol. Psychiat.,* **16,** 61–74

Weiss, B. & Laties, V. (1962) Enhancement of human performance by caffeine and the amphetamines. *Pharmacol. Rev.,* **14,** 1–36

Weiss, G., Minde, K., Werry, J., Douglas, V. & Nemeth, E. (1971) Studies on the hyperactive child, viii: five-year follow-up. *Arch. gen. Psychiat.,* **24,** 409–14

Weiss, G., Hechtman, L., Perlman, T., Hopkins, J. & Wener, A. (1979) Hyperactives as young adults. A controlled prospective ten-year follow-up of 75 children. *Arch. gen. Psychiat.,* **36,** 675–81

Chapter 4.1.4

Anthony, E. J. (1957) An experimental approach to the psychopathology of childhood: encopresis. *Brit. J. med. Psychol.,* **30,** 146–75

Baker, B. L. (1969) Symptom treatment and symptom substitution in enuresis. *J. abnorm. Psychol.,* **74,** 42–9

Bakwin, H. (1973) The genetics of bed-wetting. In *Bladder Control and Enuresis,* ed. Kolvin, I., MacKeith, R. & Meadow, S. R. *Clin. dev. Med.,* Nos. 48/49. London: SIMP/Heinemann

Bellman, M. (1966) Studies on encopresis. *Acta paediat. scand.,* Supp. 170

Bemporad, J. L., Pfeifer, C. M., Gibb, L., Cortner, R. H. & Bloom, W. (1971) Characteristics of encopretic patients and their families. *J. Amer. Acad. Child Psychiat.,* **10,** 272–92

Berg, I. (1979) Day wetting in children. *J. child Psychol. Psychiat.,* **20,** 167–73

Berg, I., Fielding, D. & Meadow, R. (1977) Psychiatric disturbance, urgency and bacteriuria in children with day and night wetting. *Arch. Dis. Childh.*, **52**, 651–7

Brazelton, T. B. (1962) A child-oriented approach to toilet training. *Pediat.*, **29**, 121–8

Coekin, M. and Gairdner, D. (1960) Faecal incontinence in children. *Brit. med. J.*, **2**, 1175–80

De Jonge, G. A. (1973) Epidemiology of enuresis: A survey of the literature. In *Bladder Control and Enuresis*, ed. Kolvin, I., MacKeith, R. & Meadow, S. R. *Clin. dev. Med.*, Nos. 48/49. London: SIMP/Heinemann

deVries, M. W. & deVries, M. R. (1977) Cultural relativity of toilet training readiness: perspective from East Africa. *Pediat.*, **60**, 170–7

Dische, S. (1973) Treatment of enuresis with an enuresis alarm. In *Bladder Control and Enuresis*, ed. Kolvin, I., MacKeith, R. & Meadow, S. R. *Clin. dev. Med.*, Nos. 48/49. London: SIMP/Heinemann

Dominian, J. (1961) A Study of Adult Enuresis. D.P.M. Dissertation, University of London

Douglas, J. W. B. (1973) Early disturbing events and later enuresis. In *Bladder Control and Enuresis*, ed. Kolvin, I., MacKeith, R. & Meadow, S. R. *Clin. dev. Med.*, Nos. 48/49. London: SIMP/Heinemann

Foxx, R. M. & Azrin, N. H. (1973) Dry pants. A rapid method of toilet training children. *Behav. Res. Ther.*, **11**, 435–42

Hallgren, B. (1956) Enuresis II: a study with reference to certain physical, mental and social factors possibly associated with enuresis. *Acta psychiat. neurol. scand.*, **31**, 405–36

Hallgren, B. (1957) Enuresis: a clinical and genetic study. *Acta psychiat. neurol. scand. Suppl.* 114.

Hersov, L. (1960) Persistent non-attendance at school. *J. child Psychol. Psychiat.*, **1**, 130–6

Hersov, L. (1977) Faecal soiling. In *Child Psychiatry: Modern Approaches*, ed. Rutter, M. & Hersov, L., pp. 613–27. Oxford: Blackwell

Hetherington, E. M. & Brackbill, Y. (1963) Etiology and covariation of obstinacy, orderliness and parsimony in young children. *Child Dev.*, **34**, 919–43

Kaffman, M. & Elizur, E. (1977) Infants who become enuretics: A Longitudinal Study of 161 Kibbutz children. *Monogr. Soc. Res. Child Dev.*, **42**, Serial No. 170

Levine, A. (1943) Enuresis in the navy. *Amer. J. Psychiat.*, **100**, 320–25

Michaels, J. J. (1955) *Disorders of Character: Persistent Enuresis, Juvenile Delinquency and Psychopathic Personality*. Springfield, Ill.: Thomas

Miller, F. J. W., Court, S. D. M., Walton, W. S. & Knox, W. G. (1960) *Growing Up in Newcastle-upon-Tyne*. London: Oxford University Press

Olatawura, M. (1973) Encopresis: a review of thirty-two cases. *Acta paediat. scand.*, **62**, 358–64

Pinkerton, P. (1958) Psychogenic megacolon in children: the implications of bowel negativism. *Arch. Dis. Childh.*, **33**, 371–80

Rutter, M., Yule, W. & Graham, P. (1973) Enuresis and behavioural deviance: some epidemiological considerations. In *Bladder Control and Enuresis* ed. Kolvin, I., MacKeith, R. & Meadow, S. R. *Clin. dev. Med.* Nos. 48/49. London: SIMP/Heinemann

Shaffer, D. (1977) Enuresis. In *Child Psychiatry: Modern Approaches*, ed. Rutter, M. & Hersov, L. pp. 581–612. Oxford: Blackwell

Shaffer, D., Stephenson, J. D. & Thomas, D. V. (1979) Some effects of imipramine on micturition and their relevance to

its anti-enuretic activity. *Neuropharmacol.*, **18**, 33–7

Stalker, H. & Band D. (1946) Persistent enuresis: a psychosomatic study. *J. ment. Sci.*, **92**, 324–42

Stein, Z. & Susser, M. (1967) Social factors in the development of sphincter control. *Dev. Med. child Neurol.*, **9**, 692–706

Thorne, F. C. (1943) The incidence of nocturnal enuresis after age five. *Amer. J. Psychiat.*, **100**, 686–9

Wender, E. H., Palmer, F. B., Herbst, J. J. & Wender, P. H. (1976). Behavioural characteristics of children with chronic non-specific diarrhoea. *Amer. J. Psychiat.*, **133**, 20–5

Werry, J. S. & Cohrssen, J. (1965) Enuresis: an etiologic and therapeutic study. *J. Pediat.*, **67**, 423–31

Yeates, W. K. (1973) Bladder function: increased frequency and nocturnal incontinence. In *Bladder Control and Enuresis*, ed. Kolvin, I., MacKeith, R. & Meadow, S. R. *Clin. dev. Med.*, Nos. 48/49. London: SIMP/Heinemann

Chapter 4.2.1

Baker, H. & Wills, U. (1978) School phobia: classification and treatment. *Brit. J. Psychiat.*, **132**, 492–9

Belson, W. A. (1975) *Juvenile Theft: The Causal Factors*. London: Harper & Row

Berg, I. (1970) A follow-up study of school phobic adolescents admitted to an inpatient unit. *J. child Psychol. Psychiat.*, **11**, 37–47

— (1974) A self administered dependency questionnaire (S.A.D.Q.) for use with the mothers of school children. *Brit. J. Psychiat.*, **124**, 1–9

Berg, I. & Collins, A. (1974) Wilfulness in school phobic adolescents. *Brit. J. Psychiat.*, **125**, 468–9

Berg, I. & Fielding, D. (1978) An evaluation of hospital inpatient treatment in adolescent school phobia. *Brit. J. Psychiat.*, **132**, 500–5

Berg, I. & McGuire, R. (1971) Are school phobic adolescents over-dependent? *Brit. J. Psychiat.*, **119**, 167–8

— (1974) Are mothers of school phobic adolescents over-protective? *Brit. J. Psychiat.*, **124**, 10–13

Berg, I., Butler, A. & Hall, G. (1976) The outcome of adolescent school phobia. *Brit. J. Psychiat.*, **128**, 80–5

Berg, I., Butler, A. & Pritchard, J. (1974a) Psychiatric illness in the mothers of school phobic adolescents. *Brit. J. Psychiat.*, **125**, 466–7

Berg, I., Butler, A. & McGuire, R. (1972) Birth order and family size of school phobic adolescents. *Brit. J. Psychiat.*, **121**, 509–14

Berg, I., Butler, A., Fairbairn, I. & McGuire R. (1981) The parents of school phobic adolescents – a preliminary investigation of family life variables. *Psychol. Med.*, **11**, 79–83

Berg, I., Collins, T., McGuire R. & O'Melia, J. (1975) Educational attainment in adolescent school phobia. *Brit. J. Psychiat.*, **126**, 435–8

Berg, I., Marks, I., McGuire, R. & Lipsedge, M. (1974b) School phobia and agoraphobia. *Psychol. Med.*, **4**, 428–34

Berg, I., Nichols, K. & Pritchard, C. (1969) School phobia – its classification and relationship to dependency. *J. child Psychol. Psychiat.*, **10**, 123–41

Berg, I., Butler, A., Hullin, R., Smith, R. & Tyrer, S. (1978a) Features of children taken to juvenile court for failure to attend school. *Psychol. Med.*, **8**, 447–53

Berg, I., Consterdine, M., Hullin, R., McGuire, R. & Tyrer, S. (1978b) The effect of two randomly allocated court procedures on truancy. *Brit. J. Criminol.*, **18**, 232–44

Berg, I., Hullin, R., Allsop, M., O'Brien, P. & MacDonald, R. (1974c) Biopolar manic-depressive psychosis in early adolescence: a case report. *Brit. J. Psychiat.*, **125**, 416–17

Berney, T., Kolvin, I., Bhate, S. R., Garside, R. F., Jeans, J., Kay, B. & Scarth, L. (1981) School phobia: a therapeutic trial with clomipramine and short term outcome. *Brit. J. Psychiat.*, **138**, 110–18

Cameron, H. (1978) Unpublished work, presented at Monte Carlo Conference: Children under stress

Chazan, H. (1962) School phobia. *Brit. J. educ. Psychol.*, **32**, 209–17

Coolidge, J. C., Brodie, R. D. & Feeney, B. (1964) A ten-year follow-up of 66 school phobic children. *Amer. J. Orthopsychiat.*, **34**, 675–84

Coolidge, J. C., Hahn, P. B. & Peck, A. L. (1957) School phobia: neurotic crisis or way of life. *Amer. J. Orthopsychiat.*, **27**, 296–306

Eisenberg, L. (1958) School phobia: a study in the communication of anxiety. *Amer. J. Psychiat.*, **114**, 712–18

Farrington, D. (1980) Truancy, delinquency, the home and the school. In *Out of School: Modern Perspectives in School Refusal and Truancy*, ed. Hersov, L. & Berg, I. Chichester: Wiley

Fogelman, K., Tibbenham, A. & Lambert, L. (1980) Absence from school: findings from the National Child Development Study. In *Out of School: Modern Perspectives in School Refusal and Truancy*, ed. Hersov, L. & Berg, I. Chichester: Wiley

Galloway, D. (1980) Problems in the assessment and management of persistent absenteeism from school. In *Out of School: Modern Perspectives in School Refusal and Truancy*, ed. Hersov, L. & Berg, I. Chichester: Wiley

Gath, D., Cooper, B. & Gattoni, F. E. G. (1972) Child guidance and delinquency in a London borough. *Psychol. Med.*, **2**, 185–91

Gittelman-Klein, R. & Klein, D. F. (1980) Separation anxiety in school refusal and its treatment with drugs. In *Out of School: Modern Perspectives in School Refusal and Truancy*, ed. Hersov, L. & Berg, I. Chichester: Wiley

Herbert, M. (1978) *Conduct Disorders of Childhood and Adolescence*, pp. 257–63. Chichester: Wiley

Hersov, L. A., (1960a) Persistent non-attendance at school. *J. child Psychol. Psychiat.*, **1**, 130–6

— (1960b) Refusal to go to school. *J. child Psychol. Psychiat.*, **1**, 137–45.

— (1976) School refusal. In *Child Psychiatry – Modern Approaches*, ed. Rutter, M. & Hersov, L. Oxford: Blackwell

Johnson, A. M., Falstein, E. I., Szureck, S. A. & Svendsen, M. (1941) School phobia. *Amer. J. Orthopsychiat.*, **11**, 702–11

Kahn, J. H. (1958) School refusal – some clinical and cultural aspects. *Med. Off.*, **100**, 337–40

Kahn, J. H. & Nursten, J. P. (1962) School refusal: a comprehensive view of school phobia and other failures of school attendance. *Amer. J. Orthopsychiat.*, **32**, 707–18

Kennedy, W. A. (1965) School phobia: a rapid treatment of fifty cases. *J. abnorm. Psychol.*, **70**, 285–9

Klein, E. (1945) The reluctance to go to school. *Psycho-anal. Study Child*, **1**, 263–79

Lassers, E., Nordan, R. & Bradholm, S. (1973) Steps in the return to school of children with school phobia. *Amer. J. Psychiat.*, **130**, 265–8

Leventhal, T., Weinberger, G., Stander, R. J. & Stearns, R. P. (1967) Therapeutic strategies with school phobias. *Amer. J. Orthopsychiat.*, **37**, 64–70

Lewis, M. (1980) Psychotherapeutic treatment in school refusal. In *Out of School: Modern Perspectives in School Refusal and Truancy*, ed. Hersov, L. & Berg, I. Chichester: Wiley

Miller, L. C., Barrett, C. L., Hampe, E. & Nobel, E. (1971) Children's deviant behaviour within the general population. *J. consult. clin. Psychol.*, **37**, 16–22

Mitchell, S. & Shepherd, M. (1980) Reluctance to go to school. In *Out of School: Modern Perspectives in School Refusal and Truancy*, ed. Hersov, L. & Berg, I. Chichester: Wiley

Moore, T. (1966) Difficulties of the ordinary child in adjusting to primary school. *J. child Psychol. Psychiat.*, **7**, 17–38.

Morgan, G. A. V. (1959) Children who refuse to go to school. *Med. Off.*, **102**, 221–4

Reporter (1979) Private school boy shot himself. *The Daily Telegraph*, 3 February

Reynolds, D., Jones, D., St Leger, S. & Murgatroyd, S. (1980) School factors and truancy. In *Out of School: Modern Perspectives in School Refusal and Truancy*, ed. Hersov, L. & Berg, I. Chichester: Wiley

Robins, L. N. (1978) Sturdy childhood predictors of adult antisocial behaviour: replications from longitudinal studies. *Psychol. Med.*, **8**, 611–22

Rodriguez, A., Rodriguez, M. & Eisenberg, L. (1959) The outcome of school phobia: A follow-up study based on 41 cases. *Amer. J. Psychiat.*, **116**, 540–4

Rutter, M. (1966) *Children of Sick Parents*. Maudsley Monograph No. 16. London: Oxford University Press

Rutter, M., Tizard, J. & Whitmore, K. (1970) *Education, Health and Behaviour*. London: Longman

Rutter, M., Graham, P., Chadwick, O. F. D. & Yule, W. (1976) Adolescent turmoil: fact or fiction? *J. child Psychol. Psychiat.*, **17**, 35–56

Smith, S. L. (1970) School refusal with anxiety: a review of sixty-three cases. *Can. Psychiat. Ass. J.*, **15**, 257–64

Tennent, T. G. (1969) School non-attendance and delinquency. D.M. thesis, University of Oxford

Tyrer, P. & Tyrer, S. (1974) School refusal, truancy and adult neurotic illness. *Psychol. Med.*, **4**, 416–21

Waldfogel, S. J. C., Coolidge, J. C. & Hahn, P. B. (1957) The development, meaning and management of school phobia. *Amer. J. Orthopsychiat.*, **27**, 754–76

Waller, D. & Eisenberg, L. (1980) School refusal in childhood: a psychiatric-paediatric perspective. In *Out of School: Modern Perspectives in School Refusal and Truancy*, ed. Hersov, L. & Berg, I. Chichester: Wiley

Warren, W. (1948) Acute neurotic breakdown in children with refusal to go to school. *Arch. Dis. Childh.*, **23**, 266–72

Yule, W., Hersov, L. & Treseder, J. (1980) Behavioural treatment in school refusal. In *Out of School: Modern Perspectives in School Refusal and Truancy*, ed. Hersov, L. & Berg, I. Chichester: Wiley

Chapter 4.2.2

Adult Literacy: Progress in 1975/6. (1976) *Report to the Secretaries of State for Education and Science and for Scotland by the Adult Literacy Resource Agency's Management Committee on the First Year's Operation.* London: HMSO

Bradley, L. & Bryant, P. E. (1978) Difficulties in auditory organization as a possible cause of reading backwardness. *Nature, London*, **271**, 746–7

Bullock Report: A Language for Life (1975) Report of the Committee of Inquiry appointed by the Secretary of State for Education and Science under the Chairmanship of Sir Alan Bullock. London: HMSO

Chall, J. S. (1967) *Learning to Read: The Great Debate*. New York: McGraw-Hill

Children with specific reading Difficulties (1972) Report of the Advisory Committee on Handicapped Children under the chairmanship of Professor J Tizard. Department of Education and Science. London: HMSO

Critchley, M. (1964) *Developmental Dyslexia*. London: Heinemann

Elkonin, D. B. (1963) The psychology of mastering the elements of reading. In *Educational Psychology in the USSR*, ed. Simon, B. & Simon, J., pp. 165–79. London: Routledge & Kegan Paul

— (1973) Comparative reading – USSR. In *Comparative Reading. Cross-National Studies of Behavior and Processes in Reading and Writing*, ed. Downing, J., pp. 551–79. New York: Macmillan

Finlayson, J. (1973) First we must recognize the complaint. *The Times*, London, 28 November

Finucci, J. M., Guthrie, J. T., Childs, A. L., Abbey, H. & Childs, B. (1976) The genetics of specific reading disability. *Ann. hum. Genet., London*, 40, 1–23

Gerstmann, J. (1924) Fingeragnosie: eine umschreibene Störung der Orienterung am eigener Körper. *Wien. klin. Wochenschr.*, 37, 110–12

Guttmann, E. (1937) Congenital arithmetic disability and acalculia (Henschen). *Brit. j. med. Psychol.*, 16, 16–35

Hallgren, B. (1950) Specific dyslexia: a clinical and genetic study. *Acta psychiat. neurol. scand.*, Supp. 65

Henschen, S. E. (1919) Über Sprach- Musik- und Rechenmechanismen und ihre Lokalisation im Gehirn. *Zeitschr. ges. Neurol. Psychiat.*, 52, 273–98

Hinshelwood, J. (1895) Word-blindness and visual memory. *Lancet*, i, 1564–70

— (1917) *Congenital Word-Blindness*. London: Lewis

Klasen, E. (1972) *The Syndrome of Specific Dyslexia*. Baltimore: University Park Press

Landsdown, R. (1978) Annotation: retardation in mathematics: a consideration of multifactorial determination. *J. child Psychol. Psychiat.*, 19, 181–5

Liberman, I. Y., Shankweiler, D., Fischer, F. W. & Carter, B. (1974) Explicit syllable and phoneme segmentation in the young child. *J. exper. child Psychol.*, 18, 201–12

Mattingly, I. G. (1972) Reading, the linguistic process and linguistic awareness. In *Language by Ear and by Eye: The Relationship between Speech and Reading*, ed. Kavanagh J. F. & Mattingly, I. G., pp. 133–47 Cambridge, Mass: MIT Press

Orton, S. T. (1937) *Reading, Writing and Speech Problems in Children*. London: Chapman & Hall

Pringle Morgan, W. (1896) A case of congenital word blindness. *Brit. med. J.*, 2, 1378

Russell, G. (1982a) Writing and dyslexia – an historical analysis. *J. child Psychol. Psychiat.*, 23, 383–400

— (1982b) Impairment of phonetic reading in dyslexia and its persistence beyond childhood. *J. child Psychol. Psychiat.*, 23, 459–75

Rutter, M., Tizard, J. & Whitmore, K. (1970) *Education, Health and Behaviour*. London: Longman

Rutter, M. & Yule, W. (1975) The concept of specific reading retardation. *J. child Psychol. Psychiat.*, 16, 181–97

Rutter, M., Yule, W., Tizard, J. & Graham, P. (1967) Severe reading retardation: its relationship to maladjustment, epilepsy and neurological disorders (Isle of Wight survey). In *Proceedings of the First International Conference of the Association for Special Education*, 1, 280–93

Shankweiler, D. & Liberman, I. Y. (1976) Exploring the relations between reading and speech. In *The Neuropsychology of Learning Disorders – Theoretical Approaches*, ed. Knights, R. M. & Bakker, D. J., pp. 297–313. Baltimore: University Park Press

Slade, P. D. & Russell, G. F. M. (1971) Developmental dyscalculia: a brief report on four cases. *Psychol. Med.*, 1, 292–8

Snowling, M. J. (1980) The development of grapheme–phoneme correspondence in normal and dyslexic readers. *J. exper. child Psychol.*, 29, 294–305

Vellutino, F. R. (1979) *Dyslexia, Theory and Research*. Cambridge, Mass.: MIT Press

Williams, J. P. (1980) Teaching decoding with an emphasis on phoneme analysis and phoneme blending. *J. educ. Psychol.*, 72, 1–15

World Health Organization (1978) *Manual of the International Statistical Classification of Diseases, Injuries and Causes of Death (ICD–9)*. Geneva: WHO

Yule, W. (1967) Predicting reading ages on Neale's analysis of reading ability. *Brit. J. educ. Psychol.*, 37, 252–5

Zerbin-Rudin, E. (1967) Congenital world blindness. *Bull. Orton Soc.*, 17, 47–54

Chapter 4.2.3

Brown, G. W. & Harris, T. (1978) Social origins of depression. *A Study of Psychiatric Disorder in Women*. London: Tavistock

Carr, J. (1970) Mongolism: telling the parents. *Dev. Med. child Neurol.*, 12, 213–21

Chess, S. (1977) Evolution of behaviour disorder in a group of mentally retarded children. *J. Amer. Acad. Child Psychiat.*, 16, 5–13

Chess, S., Fernandez, P., & Korn, S. (1978) Behavioural consequences of congenital rubella. *J. Pediat.*, 93, 699–703

Chess, S. & Hassibi, M. (1970) Behaviour deviations in mentally retarded children. *J. Amer. Acad. child Psychiat.*, 9, 282–97

Corbett, J. (1976) Mental retardation – psychiatric aspects. In *Child Psychiatry – Modern Approaches*, ed. Rutter, M. & Hersov, L., pp. 829–55. Oxford: Blackwell

Drotar, D., Baskiewicz, A., Irvin, N., Kennell, J. & Klaus, M. (1975) The adaptation of parents to the birth of an infant with a congenital malformation: a hypothetical model. *Pediat.*, 56, 710–17

Edgerton, R. (1979) Mental Retardation. In *The Developing Child Series*, ed. Bruner, J., Cole, M. & Lloyd, B. London: Open Books

Gath, A. (1977) The impact of an abnormal child upon the parents. *Brit. J. psychiat.*, 130, 405–10

Gibson, D. (1978) *Down's Syndrome: The Psychology of Mongolism*. Cambridge: Cambridge University Press

Goodman, N. & Tizard, J. (1962) Prevalence of imbecility and idiocy among children. *Brit. med. J.*, 1, 216–19

Heber, R. (1961) A manual on terminology and classification in mental retardation. *Amer. J. ment. Def.*, Supp. No. 64

Kushlick, A. (1961) Subnormality in Salford. In *A Report on the Mental Health Services of the City of Salford for the Year 1960*, by Susser, M. W. & Kushlick, A. Salford: Salford Health Department

— (1964) The prevalence of recognized mental subnormality of IQ under 50 among children in the South of England, with reference to the demand for places for residential care. Paper to the International Copenhagen Conference on the Scientific Study of Mental Retardation, Copenhagen

Lambert, N., Windmiller, M. & Cole, L. (1974) *The AAMN Adaptive Behaviour Scale*. Washington: American Association on Mental Deficiency

Oswin, M. (1978) *Children Living in Long-stay Hospitals*. Spastics International Medical Publications Research Monograph No 5. London: Heinemann

Paget-Gorman Sign System. The Association for Experiment in Deaf Education Limited.

Philips, I. & Williams, N. (1975) Psychopathology and mental retardation – a study of 100 mentally retarded children. I Psychopathology. *Amer. J. Psychiat.*, **132**, 1265–71

— (1977) Psychopathology and mental retardation – a study of 100 mentally retarded children. II Hyperactivity *Amer. J. Psychiat.*, **134**, 418–19

Rutter, M. (1971) Psychiatry. In *Mental Retardation. An Annual Review*, vol. III, ed. Wortis, J. pp. 186–221. New York: Grune & Stratton

Rutter, M., Graham, P. and Yule, M. (1970) *A Neuropsychiatric Study in Childhood*. London: Spastics International Medical Press, Heinemann

Rutter, M., Tizard, J. & Whitmore, K. (1970) *Education, Health and Behaviour*. London: Longman

Seidel, U. P., Chadwick, O. F. D. & Rutter, M. (1975) Psychological disorders in crippled children. A comparative study of children with and without brain damage. *Dev. Med. child Neurol.*, **17**, 563–73

Susser, M. W. & Kushlick, A. (1961) *Subnormality in Salford. A Report on the Mental Health Services in the City of Salford in the Year 1960*. Salford: Salford Health Department

Tizard, J. & Grad, J. C. (1961) *The Mentally Handicapped and their Families*. Maudsley Monograph No. 7. London: Oxford University Press

Walker, M. (1980) *Revised Makaton Vocabulary*. Farnborough: Makaton Vocabulary Development Project

Warnock, H. M. (1978) *Special Educational Needs – Report of the Committee of Enquiry into the Education of Handicapped Children and Young People*. London: HMSO

Webster, T. G. (1970) Emotional development in mentally retarded children. In *Psychiatric Approaches to Mental Retardation*, ed. Menolascino, F. pp. 3–54. New York: Basic Books

Chapter 4.2.4

Agle, D. P. (1964) Psychiatric studies of patients with haemophilia and related states. *Arch. int. Med.*, **114**, 76–82

Bakwin, H. & Bakwin, R. M. (1972) *Behaviour Disorders in Children*, 4th edn. Philadelphia: Saunders

Broadbent, V. (1980) Acute leukaemia in childhood – the problems of modern treatment. *Ass. Child Psychol. Psychiat., News*, No. 5

Burton, L. (1975) *The Family Life of Sick Children – A Study of Families coping with Chronic Childhood Disease*. London: Routledge & Kegan Paul

Churven, P. (1977) A group approach to the emotional needs of parents with leukaemic children. *Aus. paediat. J.*, **13**, 290–4

Davis, F. (1963) *Passage Through Crisis*. New York: Bobbs-Merrill

Dorner, S. (1975) The relationship of physical handicap to stress in families with an adolescent with spina bifida. *Dev. Med. child Neurol.*, **17**, 765–776

Douglas, J. W. B. (1975) Early hospital admissions and later disturbances of behaviour and learning. *Dev. Med. child Neurol.*, **17**, 456–81

Freeman, R. D. (1977) Psychosocial problems associated with childhood hearing impairment. In *Hearing and Hearing Impairment*, ed. Bradford, L. J. & Hardy, W. G., pp 405–15. New York: Grune & Stratton

Gath, A. (1972) The mental health of siblings of a congenitally abnormal child. *J. child Psychol. Psychiat.*, **13**, 211–18

Gath, A., Smith, M. A. & Baum, J. D. (1980) Emotional, behavioural and educational disorders in diabetic children. *Arch. Dis. Childh.*, **55**, 371–5

Halverson, C. F. & Victor, J. B. (1976) Minor physical anomalies and problem behaviour in elementary school children. *Child Dev.*, **47**, 281–5

Heffron, W. A., Bommelacre, K. & Masters, R. (1973) Group discussions with the parents of leukaemic children. *Paediat.*, **52**, 831–45

Landtman, B., Valanne, E. H. & Aukee, M. (1968) Emotional implications of heart disease. *Ann. Paediat. Fenn.*, **14**, 71–92

Lavigne, J. V. & Ryan, M. (1979) Psychologic adjustment of siblings of children with chronic illness. *Pediat.*, **63**, 616–27

Mattsson, A. & Gross, S. (1966) Social and behavioural studies on haemophiliac children and their families. *J. Paediat.*, **68**, 952–64

Minuchin, S., Baker, L., Rosman, B. L., Liebman, R., Milman, L. & Todd, T. C. (1975) A conceptual model of psychosomatic illness in children. *Arch. gen. Psychiat.*, **32**, 1031–8

Offord, D. R. & Aponte, J. T. (1967) Distortion of disability and effect on family life. *J. Amer. Acad. Child Psychiat.*, **6**, 499–511

Paquay-Weinstock, M., Appelboom-Fondu, J. & Dopchie, N. (1979) Influence of a chronic disease on the evolution of the family dynamics. A study of 25 families of haemophiliac children. *Acta paedopsychiatr.*, **44**, 219–28

Pinkerton, P. (1967) Correlating physiologic with psychodynamic data in the study and management of childhood asthma. *J. Psychosom. Res.*, **11**, 11–25

Quinton, D. & Rutter, M. (1976) Early hospital admission and later disturbances of behaviour: an attempted replication of Douglas' findings. *Dev. Med. child Neurol.*, **18**, 447–59

Rapin, I. (1978) Consequences of congenital hearing loss – a long term view. *J. Otolaryngol.*, **7**, 473–83

Reddihough, D. S., Landau, L., Jones, H. J. & Rickards, W. S. H. (1977) Family anxieties in childhood asthma *Aus. paediat. J.*, **13**, 295–8

Richards, M. P. M. (1978) Possible effects of early separation on later development of children – a review. In *Separation and Special Care Baby Units*, ed. Brimblecome, F. S. W., Richards, M. P. M. & Roberton, N. R. C., pp. 12–32. London: SIMP/Heinemann

Richman, L. & Harper, D. (1978) School adjustment of children with observable disabilities. *J. abnorm. child Psychol.*, **6**, 11–18

Roskies, E. (1972) *Abnormality and Normality. The Mothering of Thalidomide Children*. Ithaca, New York: Cornell University Press

Rutter, M., Tizard, J. & Whitmore, K. (1970) *Education, Health and Behaviour*. London: Longman

Rutter, M., Graham, P. & Yule, M. (1970) *A Neuropsychiatric Study in Childhood*. London: SIMP/Heinemann

Sandberg, S. (1976) Psychiatric disorder in children with birth anomalies. *Acta psychiat. scand.*, **54**, 1–16

Satterwhite, B. B. (1978) Impact of chronic illness on child and family: an overview based on five surveys with implications for management. *Int. J. rehab. Res.*, **1**, 7–17

Seidel, U. P., Chadwick, O. F. D. & Rutter, M. (1975) Psychological disorders in crippled children. A comparative study of children with and without brain damage. *Dev. Med. child Neurol.*, **17**, 563–73

Steg, J. P. & Rapoport, L. (1975) Minor physical anomalies in normal, neurotic, learning disabled and severely disturbed children. *J. Autism childh. Schiz.*, **5**, 299–307

Swift, C., Seidman, F. & Stein, J. (1967) Adjustment problems in juvenile diabetes. *Psychosom. Med.*, **29**, 555–71

Tavormina, J. B., Kastren, L. S., Slater, P. M. & Watt, S. L. (1976) Chronically ill children. A psychologically and emotionally deviant population? *J. of abnorm. child Psychol.*, **4**, 99–110

Tew, B. J., Payne, H. & Laurence, K. M. (1974) Must a family with a handicapped child be a handicapped family? *Dev. Med. child Neurol.*, **16**, Supp., **32**, 95–8

Warnock, H. M. (1978) *Special Educational Needs – Report of the Committee of Enquiry into the Education of Handicapped Children and Young People.* London: HMSO

Welbourn, M. (1975) Spina bifida children attending ordinary schools. *Brit. med. J.*, **1**, 142–5

Werry, J. S. (1972) Psychosomatic disorders. In *Psychopathological Disorders of Childhood*, ed. Quay, H. C. & Werry, J. S., pp. 134–84. New York: Wiley

Chapter 5.1.1

Albert, N. & Beck, A. T. (1975) Incidence of depression in early adolescence: a preliminary study. *J. Youth Adol.*, **4**, 301–7

Anthony, E. J. & Scott, P. D. (1960) Manic-depressive psychosis in childhood. *J. child Psychol. Psychiat.*, **1**, 53–72

Beck, A. T. (1967) *Depression: Clinical, Experimental and Theoretical Aspects.* New York: Harper and Row

Brown, G. & Harris, T. (1978) *Social Origins of Depression.* London: Tavistock

Caplan, M. G. & Douglas, V. I. (1969) Incidence of parental loss in children with depressed mood. *J. child Psychol. Psychiat.*, **10**, 225–32

Frommer, E. (1968) Depressive illness in childhood. In *Recent Developments in Affective Disorders*, ed. Coppen, A. & Walk, A., pp. 117–36. Ashford, Kent: Headley Bros

Gittelman-Klein, R. (1977) Definitional and methodological issues concerning depressive illness in childhood. In *Depression in childhood: diagnosis, treatment and conceptual models*, ed. Schulterbrandt, J. G. & Raskin, A., pp. 69–80. New York: Raven Press

Graham, P. & Rutter, M. (1973) Psychiatric disorder in the young adolescent: a follow-up study. *Proc. Roy. Soc. Med.*, **66**, 1226–9

Heinicke, C. M. & Wertheimer, I. J. (1965) *Brief Separations.* London: Longman

Heisel, J. S., Ream, S., Raitz, R., Rappaport, S. & Coddington, R. D. (1973) The significance of life events as contributory factors in the diseases of children. III: A study of paediatric patients. *J. Paediatrics*, **89**, 119–23

Kovacs, M. & Beck, A. T. (1977) An empirical-clinical approach towards a definition of childhood depression. In *Depression in childhood: diagnosis, treatment and conceptual models*, ed.

Schulterbrandt, J. G. & Raskin, A., pp. 1–25. New York: Raven Press

Kreitman, N. (1977) *Parasuicide.* London: Wiley

McKnew, D. H., Cytryn, L., Efron, A. M., Gershon, E. S. & Bunney, W. E. (1979) Offspring of patients with affective disorders. *Brit. J. Psychiat.*, **134**, 148–52

O'Callaghan, M. J. & Hull, D. (1978) Failure to thrive or failure to rear? *Arch. Dis. Childh.*, **53**, 788–93

Petti, T. A. (1978) Depression in hospitalised child psychiatric patients: approaches to measuring depression. *J. Amer. Acad. Child Psychiat.*, **17**, 49–59

Rapoport, J. L. (1977) Report of sub-committee on the treatment of depression in children. In *Depression in childhood: diagnosis, treatment and conceptual models*, ed. Schulterbrandt, J. G. & Raskin, A., pp. 163–4. New York: Raven Press

Robins, L. N. (1966) *Deviant children grown up.* Baltimore: Williams & Wilkins

Rutter, M. (1966) *Children of sick parents.* London: Oxford University Press

Rutter, M., Tizard, J. & Whitmore, K. (1970) *Education, Health and Behaviour.* London: Longman

Shaffer, D. (1974) Suicide in childhood and early adolescence. *J. child Psychol. Psychiat.*, **15**, 275–92

Thomas, A. & Chess, S. (1977) *Temperament and Development.* New York: Brunner/Mazel

Weinberg, W., Rutman, J., Sullivan, L., Penick, E. & Dietz, S. G. (1973) Depression in children referred to an educational diagnostic center: diagnosis and treatment. *J. Pediat.*, **83**, 1065–72

Whitten, C. F., Pettit, M. G. & Fischhoff, J. (1969) Evidence that growth failure from maternal deprivation is secondary to undereating. *J. Amer. Med. Ass.*, **209**, 1675–82

Youngerman, J. & Canino, I. A. (1978) Lithium carbonate use in children and adolescents. *Arch. gen. Psychiat.*, **35**, 216–27

Chapter 5.1.2

Abraham, K. (1924) A short study of the development of the libido viewed in the light of mental disorders. Reprinted in *Selected Papers on Psychoanalysis.* (1953) New York: Basic Books

Andrews, G., Kiloh, L. & Kehoe, L. (1978) Asthenic personality, myth or reality. *Aus. N. Z. J. Psychiat.*, **12**, 95–8

Beard, G. (1880) *American Nervousness.* Richmond, Virginia

Beck, A. (1974) Depressive Neurosis. In *American Handbook of Psychiatry* ed. Arieti, S. vol. III, 2nd ed. New York: Basic Books

Blum, G. & Miller, D. (1952) Exploring the psychoanalytic theory of the 'oral character'. *J. Personal.*, **20**, 287–304

Bonime, W. (1966) The psychodynamics of neurotic depressions. In *American Handbook of Psychiatry* ed. Arieti, S., vol. III, 1st ed. New York: Basic Books

Brown, G. & Harris, T. (1978) *Social Origins of Depression.* London: Tavistock

Chodoff, P. (1972) The depressive personality. *Arch. gen. Psychiat.*, **27**, 666–73

Essen-Moller, E. (1956) Individual traits and morbidity in a Swedish rural population *Acta psychiat.*, Second Supp. **100**

Eysenck, H. (1959) *Manual of the Maudsley Personality Inventory.* London: University of London Press

Foulds, G. A. (1965) *Personality and Personal-Illness.* London: Tavistock

— (1976) *The Hierarchical Nature of Personal Illness.* London: Academic Press

Gottheil, E. & Stone, G. (1968) Factor analytic study of orality and anality. *J. nerv. ment. Dis.*, **146**, 1–17

Grinker, R. (1961) *The Phenomenon of Depressions*. New York: Hoeber

Gruhle, H. (1935) *Psychopathy. Textbook of Nervous and Mental Illness*. Halle, Germany

Hagnell, O. (1966) *A Prospective Study of the Incidence of Mental Disorder*. Norstedts: Svenska Boleforlagets

Hirschfeld, R. & Klerman, G. (1979) Personality attributes and affective disorders. *Amer. J. Psychiat.*, **136**, 67–70

Hurry, J., Tennant, C. & Bebbington, P. (1980). The selective factors leading to psychiatric referral. *Acta psychiat. scand.*, **62**, Supp. 285, 315–23

Imboden, J, Canter, A. & Cluff, L. (1961) Convalescence from influenza. *Arch. int. Med.*, **108**, 393–9

Janet, P. (1908) *Les obsessions et la psychasthénie*. 2nd ed. Paris: Masson

Koch, J. (1891) *Psychopathic Inferiorities*. Ravensburg

Lazare, A. & Klerman, G. (1978) Hysteria and depression. *Amer. J. Psychiat.*, **124**, 48–56

Lazare, A., Klerman, G. & Armor, D. (1966) Oral, obsessive and hysterical patterns. *Arch. gen. Psychiat.*, **14**, 624–30

Lundquist, G. A. (1973) Alcohol dependence. *Acta psychiat. scand.*, **49**, 332–40

Mendelson, M. (1967) Neurotic depressive reaction. In *Comprehensive Textbook of Psychiatry*, ed. Freedman, A. & Kaplan, H. Baltimore: Williams & Wilkins

Nyman, G. (1956) Variations in personality. *Acta psychiat. neurol. scand.*, Supp. **107**

Paykel, E. & Prusoff, B. (1973) Relationships between personality dimensions: neuroticism and extraversion against obsessive hysterical and oral personality. *Brit. J. soc. clin. Psychol.*, **12**, 309–18

Perris, C. (1966) Personality traits. *Acta psychiat. scand.*, Supp. **194**, 68–82

Schneider, K. (1950) *Die Psychopathischen Persönlichkeiten*. Trans. into English by Hamilton, M. W., 1958. Springfield, Ill.: Thomas

Sjöbring, H. (1973) Personality structure and development, a model and its application. *Acta psychiat. scand.*, Supp. 244

Standage, K. (1979) The use of Schneider's typology for the diagnosis of personality disorders – an examination of reliability. *Brit. J. Psychiat.*, **135**, 238–42

Tolle, R. (1968) The mastery of life by psychopathic personalities. *Psychiat. Clin.*, **1**, 1–8

Weissman, M. & Myers, J. (1978) Rates and risks of depressive symptoms in a United States urban community. *Acta psychiat. scand.*, **57**, 219–31

Weissman, M. M., Prusoff, B. A. & Klerman, G. L. (1978) Personality and the prediction of long-term outcome of depression. *Amer. J. Psychiat.*, **135**: 7, 797–9

Chapter 5.1.3

Akiskal, H., Bitar, A., Puzantian, V., Rosenthal, T. & Walker, P. (1978) The nosological status of neurotic depression. *Arch. gen. Psychiat.*, **35**, 756–66

Beck, A. (1967) *Depression: Clinical, Experimental and Theoretical Aspects*. New York: Hoeber

— (1976) *Cognitive Therapy and the Emotional Disorders*. New York: International University Press

Bornstein, P., Clayton, P., Halikas, J., Maurice, W. & Robins, E.

(1973) The depression of widowhood after 13 months. *Brit. J. Psychiat.*, **122**, 561–6

Brown, G. & Harris, T. (1978) *Social Origins of Depressions*. London: Tavistock

Brown, G., Sklair, F., Harris, T. & Birley, J. (1973) Life events and psychiatric disorders. *Psychol. Med.*, **3**, 74–87

Carrol, B., Fielding, J. & Blashri, T. (1973) Depression rating scales: a critical review. *Arch. gen. Psychiat.*, **28**, 361–6

Clayton, P. J., Halikas, J. A. & Maurice, W. L. (1971) The bereavement of the widowed. *Dis. nerv. Syst.*, **32** (9), 597–604

— (1972) The depression of widowhood. *Brit. J. Psychiat.*, **120**, 71–7

Downing, R. & Rickels, K. (1974) Mixed anxiety-depression: fact or myth? *Arch. gen. Psychiat.*, **30**, 312–20

Ey, H. (1963) *Manuel de psychiatrie*. 2nd ed. Paris: Masson

Foulds, G. (1973) The relationship between the depressive illnesses. *Brit. J. Psychiat.*, **123**, 531–4

Freud, S. (1917) Mourning and melancholia. In *Complete works of Sigmund Freud*, vol. 4, pp. 143–258. London: Hogarth Press

Goldberg, D. (1979) Detection and assessment of emotional disorders in a primary care setting. *Int. J. ment. Health*, **8**, No. 2, 30–48

Goldberg, D. & Huxley, P. (1980) *Mental Illness in the Community*. London: Tavistock

Goldberg, D., Rickels, K., Downing, R. & Hesbacher, P. (1976) A comparison of two psychiatric screening tests. *Brit. J. Psychiat.*, **129**, 61–7

Hagnell, O. (1966) *A Prospective Study of the Incidence of Mental Disorder*. Norstedts: Svenska Bokfortajet

Henderson, S., Duncan-Jones, P. Byrne, D., Scott, R. & Adcock, S. (1979) A standardised study of prevalence. *Acta psychiat. scand.*, **60**, 355–74

Jacobs, S., Prusoff, B. & Paykel, E. (1974) Recent life events in schizophrenia and depression. *Psychol. Med.*, **4**, 444–53

Kendell, R. E. (1976) The classification of depression: a review of contemporary confusion. *Brit. J. Psychiat.*, **129**, 15–28

Kerr, T., Schapira, K., Roth, M. & Garside, R. (1970) The relationship between the MPI and the course of affective disorders. *Brit. J. Psychiat.*, **116**, 11–19

Kessel, N. (1971) Psychiatric aspects of barbiturate poisoning. In *Acute Barbiturate Poisoning*, ed. Mathew, H., pp. 269–90. Amsterdam: Excerpta Medica

Kiloh, L. Andrews, G., Neilson, M. & Bianchi, G. (1972) The relationship between the syndromes called endogenous and neurotic depression. *Brit. J. Psychiat.*, **121**, 183–96

Klerman, G. (1977) Anxiety and depression. In *Handbook of Studies on Depression*, ed. Burrows, G. Amsterdam: Excerpta Medica

Klerman, G., Rounsaville, B., Chevron, E., Neu, C. & Weissman, M. (1979) *Manual for Short-term Interpersonal Psychotherapy*, 4th ed. New Haven–Boston Collaborative Project. Unpublished manuscript obtained from Dr Weissman

Lewis, A. (1956) Affective disorders. In *Prices Textbook of Medicine*, ed. Hunter, D., 9th ed., p. 649. London: Oxford University Press

Lieberman, S. (1978) Nineteen cases of morbid grief. *Brit. J. Psychiat.*, **132**, 159–63

Maddison, D. (1968) The relevance of conjugal bereavement for preventative psychiatry. *Brit. J. med. Psychol.*, **41**, 223–32

Overall, J., Hollister, L., Johnson, M. & Pennington, V. (1966) Nosology of depression and differential response to drugs. *J. Amer. Med. Assoc.*, **195**, 946–50

Parkes, C. (1970) The first year of bereavement. *Psychiatry*, **33**, 444–67

Parkes, C. & Brown, R. (1972) Health after bereavement. *Psychosom. Med.*, **34**, 449–61

Paykel, E. (1971) Classification of depressed patients: a cluster analysis derived group. *Brit. J. Psychiat.*, **118**, 275–88

Paykel, E., Myers, J., Dienelt, M., Klerman, G., Rosenthal, J. & Pepper, M. (1969). Life events and depression: a controlled study. *Arch. gen. Psychiat.*, **21**, 753–60

Price, J. (1968) The genetics of depressive behaviour. In *Recent Developments in Affective Disorders*, ed. Cooper, A. J. & Wade, A. Brit. J. Psychiat. Special Publication No. 2. Ashford, Kent: Headley Bros

Robins, E., Gassner, J., Kayes, J., Wilkinson, R. & Murphy G. (1959) Communication of suicidal intent. *Amer. J. Psychiat.*, **115**, 724–32

Roth, M., Gurney, C., Garside, R. & Kerr, T. (1972) Studies in the classification of affective disorders. The relationship between anxiety states and depressive illnesses – 1. *Brit. J. Psychiat.*, **121**, 147–61

Rush, A., Beck, A., Kovacs, M. & Hollon, S. (1977) Comparative efficiency of cognitive therapy and pharmacotherapy in the treatment of depressed outpatients. *Cognit. Ther. Res.*, **1**, 17–37

Schmidt, E., O'Neal, P. & Robins, E. (1954) Evaluation of suicide attempts as a guide to therapy. *J. Amer. Med. Assoc.*, **155**, 549–54

Shields, J. (1971) Heredity and psychological abnormality. In *Handbook of Abnormal Psychology*, 2nd edn., ed. Eysenck, H. J. London: Pitman

Schneidman, E., & Farberon, N. (1957) *Clues to Suicide*. New York: McGraw-Hill

Slater, E. & Cowie, V. (1971) *The Genetics of Mental Disorders*. London: Oxford University Press

Slater, E. & Roth, M. (1977) *Clinical Psychiatry*. London: Baillière, Tindall & Cassell

Spitzer, R., Endicott, J. & Robins, E. (1978) *Research Diagnostic Criteria for a Selected Group of Functional Disorders* 3rd edn. New York: New York State Psychiatric Institute

Stenstedt, A. (1966) Genetics of neurotic depression. *Acta psychiat. scand.*, Supp. **127**

Surtees, P. & Kendell, R. (1979) The hierarchy model of psychiatric symptomatology: an investigation based on PSE ratings. *Brit. J. Psychiat.*, **135**, 438–43

Weissman, M. & Myers, J. (1978) The rates and risks of mental disorders in the US urban community. *Acta psychiat. scand.*, **57**, 219–31

Weissman, M., Prusoff, B., Dimascio, A., Neu, C., Goklaney, M. & Klerman, G. (1979) The efficacy of drugs and psychotherapy in the treatment of acute depressive episodes. *Amer. J. Psychiat.*, **136**, 555–8

WHO (1978) *Mental Disorders: Glossary and Guide to their Classification in Accordance with the 9th Revision of the International Classification of Diseases*. Geneva: WHO

Wing, J. K. (1980) The use of the PSE in general population surveys *Acta psychiat. scand.*, **62**, Supp. **285**, 230–40

Wing, J., Mann, S., Leff, J. & Nixon, J. (1978) The concept of a 'case' in psychiatric population surveys. *Psychol. Med.*, **8**, 203–17

Chapter 5.1.4

Brown, G. W., Bhrolchain, M. N. & Harris, T. (1975) Social class and psychiatric disturbance among women in an urban population. *Sociology*, **9**, 225–54

Pitt, B. (1975) Psychiatric illness following childbirth. In *Contemporary Psychiatry*, ed. Silverstone, T. & Barraclough, B. British Journal of Psychiatry Special Publication No 9. London: Headley Bros

Richman, N. (1977) Behaviour problems in pre-school children: family and social factors. *Brit. J. Psychiat.*, **131**, 523–7

Rutter, M. (1966) *Children of Sick Parents: an Environmental & Psychiatric Study*. Institute of Psychiatry, Maudsley Monograph, No 16. London: Oxford University Press

Rutter, M., Graham, P. & Yule, W. (1970) A neuropsychiatric study in childhood. *Clin. Dev. Med.*, No. 35–6. London: SIMP/Heinemann

Weissman, M. M., Paykel, E. S. & Klerman, G. L. (1972) The depressed woman as mother. *Soc. Psychiat.*, **7**, 98–108

Wolff, S. & Acton, W. P. (1968) Characteristics of parents of disturbed children. *Brit. J. Psychiat.*, **114**, 593–601

Wolkind, S. N. (1982) Infant temperament, maternal depression and child behaviour problems. In *Temperamental Differences in Infants and Young Children*, ed. Porter, R. & Collins, G. M., pp. 221–30. Ciba Symposium 89. London: Pitman

Wrate, R. M., Rooney, A., Thomas, P. F. & Cox, J. L. (1983) Postnatal depression, and subsequent child behaviour. (To be published)

Chapter 5.2.1

Ackner, B. (1954) Depersonalisation: II Clinical syndromes. *J. ment. Sci.*, **100**, 854–72

Anthony, E. J. (1967) Psychiatric disorders of childhood: psychoneurotic, psychophysiological and personality disorders. In *Comprehensive Textbook of Psychiatry*, ed. Freedman, A. M., Kaplan, H. I. & Kaplan, H. S., chap. 41. Baltimore: Williams & Wilkins

Beard, G. M. (1880) *American Nervousness*. London: Putnam

Beck, A. T., Laude, R. & Bohnert, M. (1974) Ideational components of anxiety neurosis. *Arch. gen. Psychiat.*, **31**, 319–25

Bentovim, A. (1979) Family therapy. In *An Introduction to the Psychotherapies*, ed. Bloch, S., chap. 8. Oxford: Oxford University Press

Berg, I., Marks, I., McGuire, R. & Lipsedge, M. (1974) School phobia and agoraphobia. *Psychol. Med.*, **4**, 428–34

British National Formulary (1981)

Brown, F. W. (1942) Heredity in the psychoneuroses. *Proc. R. Soc. Med.*, **30**, 895–904

Brown, G. W. & Harris, T. (1978) *Social Origins of Depression*. London: Tavistock

Buglass, D., Clarke, J., Henderson, A. S., Kreitman, N. & Presley, A. S. (1977) A study of agoraphobic housewives. *Psychol. Med.*, **7**, 73–86

Cummings, J. D. (1944) The incidence of emotional symptoms in school children. *Brit. J. educ. Psychol.*, **14**, 151–61

Cummings, J. D. (1946) A follow-up study of emotional symptoms in school children. *Brit. J. educ. Psychol.*, **16**, 163–77

Deutsch, H. (1929) The genesis of agoraphobia. *Int. J. Psychoanal.*, **10**, 51–69

Eisenberg, L. (1958) School phobia: a study of the communication of anxiety. *Amer. J. Psychiat.*, **114**, 712–18

Ey, H., Bernard, P. & Brisset, C. (1974) *Manuel de psychiatrie*. Paris: Masson

Freud, S. (1895a) The justification for detaching from neurasthenia eurasthenia a particular syndrome: the anxiety neurosis. In *Collected Works*, 2nd edn, vol. I, pp. 76–106. London: Hogarth Press & Institute of Psychoanalysis (1940)

— (1895b) A reply to criticisms on the anxiety neurosis. In *Collected Works*, 2nd edn, vol. I, pp. 107–27. London: Hogarth Press & Institute of Psychoanalysis (1940)

Friedman, J. H. (1950) Short-term psychotherapy of 'phobia of travel'. *Amer. J. Psychother.*, **4**, 259–78

Friedman, P. & Goldstein, J. (1974) Phobic reactions. In *American Handbook of Psychiatry*, ed. Arieti, S., 2nd edn, vol. III, chap. 6. New York: Basic Books

Greer, S. (1969) The prognosis of anxiety states. In *Studies in Anxiety*, ed. Lader, M. H., chap. 25. *British Journal of Psychiatry* Special Publication No. 3. Ashford, Kent: Headley Bros

Hersov, L. (1976) Emotional disorders. In *Child Psychiatry: Modern Approaches*, ed. Rutter, M. & Hersov, L., chap. 18. Oxford: Blackwell

Holmes, T. H. & Rahe, R. H. (1967) The social adjustment rating scale. *J. psychosom. Res.*, **11**, 213–18

Kedward, H. (1969) The outcome of neurotic illness in the community. *Soc. Psychiat.*, **4**, 1–4

Klein, D. F. (1964) Delineation of two drug responsive anxiety syndromes. *Psychopharmacol.*, **5**, 397–408

Lader, M. & Wing, L. (1964) Habituation of the psychogalvanic reflex in patients with anxiety states and in normal subjects. *J. Neurol., Neurosurg. Psychiat.*, **27**, 210–18

Lader, M. H. (1969) Psychophysiological aspects of anxiety. In *Studies of Anxiety*, chap. 8. *British Journal of Psychiatry*, Special Publication No. 3. Ashford, Kent: Headley Bros

Lazarus, R. S. (1966) *Psychological Stress and the Coping Process*. New York: McGraw-Hill

Lewis, A. J. (1966) Psychological medicine: In *Prices Textbook of the Practice of Medicine*, 10th ed., ed. Bodley Scott, R. London: Oxford University Press

Lief, H. I. (1967) Anxiety reaction. In *Comprehensive Textbook of Psychiatry*, ed. Friedman, A. M. & Kaplan, H. I., chap. 23. Baltimore: Williams & Wilkins

Marks, I. M. (1969) *Fears and Phobias*. London: Heinemann

Mayer-Gross, W., Slater, E. & Roth, M. (1960) *Clinical Psychiatry*, 3rd edn, ed. Slater, E. & Roth, M. London: Baillière Tindall & Cassell

Meyer, J. E. (1961) Depersonalisation in adolescence. *Psychiat.*, **24**, 357–60

Miller, E. R. (1953) On street fear. *Int. J. Psychoanal.*, **34**, 232–52

Miner, G. D. (1973) The evidence for genetic components in the neuroses. *Arch. gen. Psychiat.*, **29**, 111–18

Mountjoy, C. Q., Roth, M., Garside, R. F. & Leitch, I. M. (1977) A clinical trial of phenelzine in anxiety, depressive and phobic neuroses. *Brit. J. Psychiat.*, **131**, 486–92

Roberts, A. H. (1964) Housebound housewives – a follow-up study of a phobic anxiety state. *Brit. J. Psychiat.*, **110**, 191–7

Roth, M. (1959) The phobic anxiety–depersonalisation syndrome. *Proc. R. Soc. Med.*, **52**, 587–9

Roth, M., Carney, C., Garside, R. F. & Kerr, T. A. (1972) Studies in the classification of affective disorders: the relation between anxiety states and depressive illnesses. *Brit. J. Psychiat.*, **121**, 147–61

Rutter, M. (1966) *Children of Sick Parents: An Environmental and Psychiatric Study*. Maudsley Monograph, No. 16. Oxford: Oxford University Press

Rutter, M., Tizard, J. & Whitmore, K. (eds.) (1970) *Education, Health and Behaviour*. London: Longman

Schapira, K., Roth, M., Kerr, T. A. & Gurney, C. (1972) The prognosis of affective disorders: the differentiation of anxiety states from depressive illnesses. *Brit. J. Psychiat.*, **121**, 175–81

Schilder, P. (1935) *The Image and Appearance of the Human Body*. Psyche Monograph, No. 4. London

Sedman, G. (1966) Depersonalisation in a group of normal subjects. *Brit. J. Psychiat.*, **112**, 907–12

Shaw, P. M. (1979) A comparison of three behaviour therapies in the treatment of social phobia. *Brit. J. Psychiat.*, **134**, 620–3

Shorvon, H. J., Hill, J. D. N., Burkitt, E. & Halstead, H. (1946) The depersonalisation syndrome. *Proc. R. Soc. Med.*, **39**, 779–92

Slater, E. & Shields, J. (1969) Genetical aspects of anxiety. In *Studies in Anxiety*, ed. Lader, M. H., chap. 9. *British Journal of Psychiatry* Special Publication No. 3. Ashford, Kent: Headley Bros

Terhune, W. (1949) The phobic syndrome: a study of 86 patients with phobic reactions. *Arch. Neurol. Psychiat.*, **62**, 162–72

Tyrer, P. & Tyrer, S. (1974) School refusal truancy and neurotic illness. *Psychol. Med.*, **4**, 416–21

Westphal, C. (1871) Die Agoraphobie: Eine neuropathische Erscheinung. *Arch. Psychiat. Nervenkr.*, **3**, 138–61

Chapter 5.2.2

Berg, I. (1982) When truants and school refusers grow up. *Brit. J. Psychiat.*, **141**, 208–10

Berg, I., Butler, A. & Pritchard, J. (1974) Psychiatric illness in the mothers of school phobic adolescents. *Brit. J. Psychiat.*, **125**, 466–7

Pritchard, M. & Graham, P. (1966) An investigation of a group of patients who have attended both the child and adult departments of the same psychiatric hospital. *Brit. J. Psychiat.*, **112**, 603–12

Rutter, M. (1966) *Children of Sick Parents*. Maudsley Monograph No 16. London: Oxford University Press

Tyrer, P. & Tyrer, S. (1974) School refusal, truancy and adult neurotic illness *Psychol. Med.*, **4**, 416–21

Chapter 6.1

Caplan, H. (1970) Hysterical 'Conversion' Symptoms in Childhood. M. Phil. thesis, University of London

Chodoff, P. (1974) The diagnosis of hysteria: an overview. *Amer. J. Psychiat.*, **131**, 1073–8

Creak, M. (1969) Hysteria in childhood. *Acta paedopsychiat.*, **36**, 269–74

Dubowitz, V. & Hersov, L. (1976) Management of children with non-organic (hysterical) disorders of motor function. *Dev. Med. child Neurol.*, **18**, 358–68

Robins, E. & O'Neal, P. (1953) Clinical features of hysteria in children, with a note on prognosis. A two to seventeen year follow-up study of 41 patients. *Nerv. Child*, **10**, 246–71

Sirois, F. (1974) Epidemic hysteria. *Acta psychiat. scand.*, Supp. **252**

Chapter 6.2

Asher, R. (1951) Munchausen's syndrome. *Lancet*, **i**, 339–41

Barham Carter, A. (1949) The prognosis of certain hysterical symptoms. *Brit. med. J.*, **1**, 1076–9

Breuer, J. & Freud, S. (1896) Studies on hysteria. In *Standard Edition of the Complete Psychological Works of Sigmund Freud*, vol. 2, pp. 3–17. London: Hogarth Press (1955)

Chodoff, P. (1974) The diagnosis of hysteria: an overview. *Amer. J. Psychiat.*, **131**, 1073–8

Janet, P. (1907) *The Major Symptoms of Hysteria*. New York: Macmillan

Lewis, A. (1975) The survival of hysteria. *Psychol. Med.*, **5**, 9–12

Ljungberg, L. (1957) Hysteria: a clinical, prognostic and genetic study. *Acta psychiat. neurol. scand.*, Supp. **112**

Miller, H. (1961) Accident neurosis. *Brit. med. J.*, **1**, 919–25 & 992–8

Moss, P. D. & McEvedy, C. P. (1966). An epidemic of overbreathing among schoolgirls. *Brit. med. J.*, **2**, 1295–302

Purtell, J. J. (1951) Observations on clinical aspects of hysteria. *J. Amer. Med. Ass.*, **146**, 902–9

Slater, E. (1965) Diagnosis of hysteria. *Brit. med. J.*, 1395–9

Sylvester, J. & Liversedge, L. A. (1960) Conditioning and the occupational cramps. In *Behaviour Therapy and the Neuroses*, ed. Eysenck, H. J. Oxford: Pergamon Press

Chapter 6.3

American Psychiatric Association (1980) *Diagnostic and Statistical Manual*, 3rd edn. Washington, DC: APA

Chodoff, P. (1974) The diagnosis of hysteria: an overview. *Am. J. Psychiat.*, **131**, 1073–8

Kräupl Taylor, F. (1969) Prokaletic measures derived from psychoanalytic technique. *Brit. J. Psychiat.*, **115**, 407–19

Murphy, G. E. & Guze, S. B. (1960) Setting limits: the management of the manipulative patient. *Amer. J. Psychother.*, **14**, 30–47

Chapter 6.4

Tyrer, P. & Alexander, J. (1979) Classification of personality disorder. *Brit. J. Psychiat.*, **135**, 163–7

Wolff, S. & Acton, W. P. (1968) Characteristics of parents of disturbed children. *Brit. J. Psychiat.*, **114**, 593–601

Chapter 7.1

Adams, P. L. (1973) *Obsessive Children: A Sociopsychiatric Study*. London: Butterworth

Andrews, G. & Harris, M. (1964) *The Syndrome of Stuttering*. London: Heinemann

Asperger, H. (1944) Die autistichen Psychopathen im Kindesalter. *Arch. Psychiat. Nervenkr.*, **117**, 76–142

Azrin, N. H. & Nunn, R. G. (1974) A rapid method for eliminating stuttering by a regulated breathing approach. *Behav. Res. Ther.*, **12**, 279–86

Baumeister, A. A. & Forehand, R. (1973) Stereotyped acts. In *International Review of Research in Mental Retardation*, ed. Ellis, N. R., vol. 6, pp. 55–92. New York: Academic Press

Boniface, D. & Graham, P. (1979) The three year old and his attachment to a special soft object. *J. child Psychol. Psychiat.*, **20**, 217–24

Cherry, C. & Sayers, B. McA. (1956) Experiments upon the total inhibition of stammering by external control and some clinical results. *J. psychosom. Res.*, **1**, 233–6

Cohen, D. J., Young, J. G., Nathanson, J. A. & Shaywitz, B. A. (1979) Clonidine in Tourette's syndrome. *Lancet*, **ii**, 551–3

Corbett, J. A., Matthews, A. M., Connell, P. H. & Shapiro, D. A. (1969) Tics and Gilles de la Tourette's syndrome: a followup study and critical review. *Brit. J. Psychiat.*, **115**, 1229–41

Corbett, J. A. (1975) Aversion for the treatment of self-injurious behaviour. *J. ment. def. Res.*, **19**, 79–95

— (1977) Tics & Tourette's syndrome. In *Child Psychiatry: Modern Approaches*, ed. Rutter, M. & Hersov, L., pp. 829–55. Oxford: Blackwell

Craven, E. M. (1969) Gilles de la Tourette's syndrome treated with haloperidol. *J. Amer. Med. Ass.*, **210**, 134–5

Fransella, F. (1975) *Need to Change?* London: Methuen

Hollingsworth, F. E., Tanguay, P. E., Grossman, L. & Pabst, P. (1980) Long term outcome of obsessive compulsive disorder in childhood. *J. Amer. Acad. Child Psychiat.*, **19**, 134–44

Jones, H. G. (1960) Continuation of Yates' treatment of ticquer. In *Behaviour Therapy and the Neuroses*, ed. Eysenck, H. J., pp. 250–9. London: Pergamon

Judd, L. (1965) Obsessive compulsive neurosis in children. *Arch. gen. Psychiat.*, **12**, 136–43

Kanner, L. (1943) Autistic disturbances of affective contact. *Nerv. Child*, **2**, 217–24

Kellmer Pringle, M. L., Butler, N. R. & Davie, R. (1967) *11 000 Seven-Year-Olds*. National Bureau for Co-operation in Child Care. London: Longman

Marchant, R., Howlin, P., Yule, W. & Rutter, M. (1974) Graded change in the treatment of the behaviour of autistic children. *J. child Psychol. Psychiat.*, **15**, 221–7

Morley, M. E. (1957) *The Development and Disorders of Speech in Childhood*. Edinburgh: Livingstone

Opie, I. & Opie, P. (1969) *Children's Games in Street and Playground*. Oxford: Clarendon Press

Rustin, L. (1978) An intensive group programme for adolescent stammerers. *Brit. J. Disord. Commun.*, **13**, 85–92

Ryan, B. (1971) Operant procedures applied to stuttering therapy for children. *J. speech hearing Disord.*, **36**, 264–80

Shapiro, A. K., Shapiro, E., Bruun, R. D., & Sweet, R. D. (1978) *Gilles de la Tourette's Syndrome*. New York: Raven Press

Warren, W. (1965) A study of adolescent psychiatric inpatients and the outcome six or more years later. ii. The follow up study. *J. child Psychol. Psychiat.*, **6**, 141–60

Weiner, I. B. (1967) Behaviour therapy in obsessive compulsive neurosis. Treatment of an adolescent boy. *Psychother. Theory Res. Pract.*, **4**, 27–9

Wells, P. G. & Malcolm, M. T. (1971) Controlled trial of treatment in 36 stutterers. *Brit. J. Psychiat.*, **119**, 603–5

West, R. (1958) An agnostic's speculations about stuttering. In *Stuttering: A Symposium*, ed. Eisenson, J., pp. 167–222. New York: Harper Bros

Wing, L. (1976) Early childhood autism. Oxford: Pergamon

Wohl, M. (1968) The electronic metronome – an evaluative study. *Brit. J. Disord. Commun.*, **3**, 89–98

Chapter 7.2

Abraham, K. (1921) Contribution to the theory of the anal character. In *Selected Papers on Psycho-analysis* (1948). London: Hogarth

Black, A. (1974) The natural history of obsessional neurosis. In *Obsessional States*, ed. Beech, H. R. London: Methuen

Blacker, C. P. & Gore, A. T. (1955) *Triennial Statistical Report, Bethlem Royal and Maudsley Hospitals*

Brown, F. W. (1942) Heredity in the psychoneuroses. *Proc. R. Soc. Med.*, **35**, 785–90

Cawley, R. (1971) Evaluation of psychotherapy. *Psychol. Med.*, **1**, 101–3
— (1974) Psychotherapy and obsessional disorders. In *Obsessional State*, ed. Beech, H.R. London: Methuen
Cooper, J. E., Gelder, M. G. & Marks, I. M. (1965) Results of behaviour therapy in 77 psychiatric patients. *Brit. med. J.*, **1**, 1222–5
Cooper, J. E. & Kelleher, M. J. (1973) The Leyton Obsessional Inventory: a principal components analysis on normal subjects. *Psychol. Med.*, **3**, 204–8
Emmelkamp, P. M. G. & Kwee, K. G. (1977) Obsessional ruminations: comparison between thought stopping and prolonged exposure in imagination. *Behav. Res. Ther.*, **15**, 441–4
Fenichel, O. (1945) *The Psychoanalytic Theory of Neurosis.*, New York: Norton
Freud, A. (1966) Obsessional neurosis. *Int. J. Psychoanal.*, **47**, 116–22
Freud, S. (1895) Obsessions and phobias – their psychical mechanisms and their aetiology. In *Collected Papers*, vol. 2. (1948) London: Hogarth
— (1908) Character and anal eroticism. In *Collected Papers*, vol. 2, (1948). London: Hogarth
— (1913) The predisposition to obsessional neurosis. In *Collected Papers*, vol. 2. (1948) London: Hogarth
Gittleson, N. L. (1966) The effects of obsessions in depressive psychoses. *Brit. J. Psychiat.*, **112**, 253–9
Greer, H. S. & Cawley, R. H. (1966) *Some Observations on the Natural History of Neurotic Illness.* Mervyn Archdall Medical Monograph. No. 3. Sydney: Australian Medical Association
Grimshaw, L. (1964) Obsessional disorders and neurological illness. *J. neurol. Neurosurg. Psychiat.*, **27**, 229–31
Hodgson, R., Rachman, S. & Marks, I. M. (1972) The treatment of chronic obsessional compulsive neurosis: follow-up and further findings. *Behav. Res. Ther.*, **10**, 181–9
Ihda, S. (1965) Psychiatrische Zwillingforschung in Japan. *Arch. Psychiat. Nervenkr.*, **207**, 209–20
Ingram, I. M. (1961) Obsessional illness in mental hospital patients. *J. ment. Sci.*, **107**, 382–402
Inouye, E. (1965) Similar and dissimilar manifestations of obsessive compulsive neurosis in monozygotic twins. *Amer. J. Psychiat.*, **121**, 1171–5
Janet, P. (1903) *Les obsessions et la psychasthénie.* Paris: Alcan
Jones, E. (1918) Anal erotic character traits. In *Papers on Psychoanalysis*, (1938). London: Baillière, Tindall & Cox
Kelleher, M. J. (1972) Cross-national (Anglo-Irish) differences in obsessional symptoms and traits of personality. *Psychol. Med.* **2**, 33–41
Kretschmer, E. (1927) *Der sensitive Beziehungswahn.* Berlin: Springer
— (1974) The sensitive delusion of reference. In *Themes and Variations in European Psychiatry*, ed. Hirsch, S. & Shepherd, M. Bristol: Wright
Kringler, E. (1965) Obsessional neurotics: a long term follow-up. *Brit. J. Psychiat.*, **111**, 709–22
Lewis, A. J. (1936) Problems of obsessional illness. *Proc. R. Soc. Med.*, **29**, 325–36
— (1946) Psychological medicine. In *A Textbook of Medicine*, 7th ed., ed. Price, F. W. London: Oxford University Press
— (1957) Obsessional illness. *Acta neuropsiquiat. arg.*, **3**, 323–35
Lo, W. H. (1967) A follow-up study of obsessional neurotics, in Hong-Kong Chinese. *Brit. J. Psychiat.*, **113**, 823–32

Marks, I. M., Crowe, M., Drew, E., Young, J. & Dewhurst, W. G. (1969) Obsessive-compulsive neurosis in identical twins. *Brit. J. Psychiat.*, **115**, 991–8
Marks, I. M., Hodgson, R. & Rachman, S. (1975) Treatment of chronic obsessional neurosis by in vivo exposure. A two-year follow-up and issues in treatment. *Brit. J. Psychiat.*, **127**, 349–64
Marks, I. M., Hallam, R. S., Philpott, R. & Connolly, J. (1977) *Behavioural Psychotherapy for Neurosis: An Advanced Clinical Role for Nurses.* Book for Research Series of Royal College of Nursing. London: Whitefriars Press
Meyer, V. (1966) Modification of expectancies in cases with obsessional rituals. *Behav. Res. Ther.*, **4**, 273–80
Mitchell-Heggs, N., Kelly, D. & Richardson, A. (1976) Stereotactic limbic leucotomy – follow-up at sixteen months. *Brit. J. Psychiat.*, **128**, 226–40
Murray, R. M., Cooper, J. E. & Smith, A. (1979) The Leyton Obsessional Inventory: an analysis of the responses of 73 obsessional patients. *Psychol. Med.*, **9**, 305–11
Pollitt, J. (1957) Natural history of obsessional states. *Brit. med. J.*, **1**, 194–8
Rachman, S. (1974) Primary obsessional slowness. *Behav. Res. Ther.*, **12**, 9–18
Rin, H. & Lin, T. Y. (1962) Mental illness among Formosan aborigines as compared with the Chinese in Taiwan. *J. ment. Sci.*, **108**, 134–46
Rosen, K. (1947) The clinical significance of obsessions in schizophrenia. *J. ment. Sci.*, **103**, 773–86
Rosenberg, C. M. (1957) Familial aspects of obsessional neurosis. *Brit. J. Psychiat.*, **113**, 405–13
— (1968) Obsessional neurosis. *Aus. N. Z. J. Psychiat.*, **2**, 33–8
Rüdin, E. (1953) Ein Beitrag zur Frage der Zwangskrankheit, insbesondere ihrere hereditären Beziehungen. *Arch. Psychiat. Nervenkr.*, **191**, 14–54
Sandler, J. & Joffe, W. G. (1965) Notes on obsessional manifestations in children. *Psychoanal. Stud. Child*, **20**, 428–38
Schilder, P. (1938) Organic background to obsessions and compulsions. *Amer. J. Psychiat.*, **94**, 1397–9
Schneider, K. (1925) Schwangzustande und Schizophrenie. *Arch. Psychiat. Nervenkr.*, **74**, 93–107
Skoog, G. (1959) The anancastic syndrome and its relation to personality attitudes, *Acta psychiat. scand.*, Supp. **134**
— (1965) Onset of anancastic conditions: a clinical study. *Acta psychiat. scand.*, Supp. **184**
Stekel, W. (1949) *Compulsion and Doubt.* University lib. ed., 1962. New York: Grosset & Dunlop
Stengel, E. (1945) A study on some clinical aspects of the relationship between obsessional neurosis and psychotic reaction types. *J. ment. Sci.*, **91**, 166–87
— (1948) Some clinical observations on the psycho-dynamic relationship between depression and obsessive compulsive symptoms. *J. ment. Sci.*, **94**, 650–52
Stern, R. S. & Cobb, J. P. (1978) The phenomenology of obsessive-compulsive neurosis. *Brit. J. Psychiat.*, **132**, 233–9
Stern, R., Lipsedge, M., & Marks, I., (1973) Thought-stopping of obsessional thoughts: a controlled trial. *Behav. Res. Ther.*, **11**, 659–62
Straus, E. W. (1966) *Phenomenological Psychology: Selected Papers.* London: Tavistock
Sykes, K., & Tredgold, R. F. (1964) Restricted orbital undercutting. A study of its effect on 350 patients over 10 years 1951–60. *Brit. J. Psychiat.*, **110**, 609–40

Taylor, F. K. (1979) *Psychopathology: Its Causes and Symptoms.* London: Quartermaine House

Tiernari, P. (1963) Psychiatric illness in identical twins. *Acta psychiat. scand.,* **39,** Supp. **171**

WHO (1978) *Mental Disorders: Glossary and Guide to their Classification in accordance with the Ninth Revision of the International Classification of Diseases.* Geneva: WHO

Westphal, C. (1878) Zwangsvorstellung. *Arch. Psychiat. Nervenkr.,* **8,** 734–50

Wolpe, J. (1958) *Psychotherapy by Reciprocal Inhibition.* Stanford: Stanford University Press

Woodruff, R. & Pitts, F. N. (1964) Monozygotic twins with obessional neurosis. *Amer. J. Psychiat.,* **120,** 1075–80

Chapter 7.3

Anthony, E. J. (1957) An experimental approach to the psychopathology of childhood: encopresis. *Brit. J. med. Psychol.,* **30,** 146–75

Olatawura, M. (1973) Encopresis: a review of thirty-two cases. *Acta paediat. scand.,* **62,** 358–64

Chapter 8.1

Alexander, F. (1950) *Psychosomatic Medicine.* New York: Norton

American Psychiatric Association (1980) *Diagnostic and Statistical Manual of Mental Disorders.* Washington DC.: APA

Brady, J. V., Porter, R. W., Conrad, D. G. & Mason, J. W. (1958) Avoidance behaviour and the development of gastroduodenal ulcers. *J. exp. Anal. Behav.,* **1,** 69–73

Cannon, W. B. (1920) *Bodily changes in Pain, Hunger, Fear and Rage,* 2nd edn. New York: Appleton-Century-Crofts

Crisp, A. H. (1968) The role of the psychiatrist in the general hospital. *Postgrad. Med. J.,* **44,** 268–76

Deutsch, F. (1939) The choice of organ in organ neurosis. *Int. J. Psychoanal.,* **20,** 252–62

Dunbar, H. F. (1935) *Emotions and Bodily Changes.* 3rd edn. New York: Columbia University Press

Engel, G. L. (1958) Studies of ulcerative colitis. V. Psychological aspects and their implications for treatment. *Amer. J. digest. Dis.,* **3,** 315–37

Feinstein, A. R. (1970) What kind of basic science for clinical medicine? *New Eng. J Med.,* **283,** 847–52

Friedman, M. & Rosenman, R. H. (1960) Overt behaviour in coronary disease. *J. Amer. Med. Ass.,* **173,** 1320–25

Friedman, M., Byers, A. & Rosenman, R. H. (1970) Coronary-prone individuals (type A behaviour pattern): some biochemical characteristics. *J. Amer. Med. Ass.,* **212,** 1030–7

Gantt, W. H. (1944) *Experimental Basis for Neurotic Behaviour: Origin and Development of Artificially Produced Disturbances of Behaviour in Dogs.* New York: Hoeber

Grinker, R. R. (1973) *Psychosomatic Concepts.* New York: Aronson

Havens, L. L. (1973) *Approaches to the Mind.* Boston: Harvard University Press

Hinkle, L. E. & Wolff, H. G. (1957) The stature of man's adaption to his total environment and the relation of this to illness. *Arch. int. Med.,* **99,** 442–60

Holmes, T. H. & Rahe, R. H. (1967) The social readjustment rating scale. *J. psychosom. Res.,* **11,** 213–18

Kasl, S. V. & Cobb, S. (1970) Blood pressure changes in men undergoing job loss. *Psychosom. Med.,* **32,** 19–38

Lipowski, Z. J. (1967) Review of consultation psychiatry and psychosomatic medicine. *Psychosom. Med.,* **29,** 153–71; 201–24

MacLeod, J. G. & Walton, H. J. (1969) Liaison between physicians and psychiatrists in a teaching hospital. *Lancet,* **ii,** 789–92

Maguire, G. P., Julier, D. L., Hawton, K. E. & Bancroft, J. H. J. (1974) Psychiatric referral and morbidity in two general wards. *Brit. med. J.,* **1,** 268–70

O'Shaughnessy, B. (1980) *The Will,* 2 vols. Cambridge: Cambridge University Press

Shepherd, M., Davies, B. & Culpen, R. (1960) Psychiatric illness in the general hospital. *Acta psychiat. neurol. scand.,* **35,** 518–25

Wolf S. & Wolff, H. G. (1943) *Human Gastric Function.* New York: Oxford University Press

World Health Organization (1978) *Ninth Edition of the International Classification of Diseases.* Geneva: WHO

Chapter 8.2

Bonica, J. J. (1974) Organization and function of a pain clinic. In *Advances in Neurology,* ed. Bonica, J. J., vol. 4, pp. 433–43. New York: Raven Press

Bradley, J. J. (1963) Severe localised pain associated with the depressive syndrome. *Brit. J. Psychiat.,* **109,** 741–5

Cowden, R. C. & Brown, J. E. (1956) The use of a physical symptom as a defence against psychosis. *J. abnorm. soc. Psychol.,* **53,** 133–5

Engel, G. (1959) Psychogenic pain and the pain prone patient. *Amer. J. Med.,* **26,** 899–918

Fordyce, W. E. (1976) *Behavioural Methods for Chronic Pain and Illness.* St Louis: Mosby

Hallett, E. C. & Pilowsky, I. (1982) The response to treatment in a multidisciplinary pain clinic. *Pain,* **12,** 365–74

Merskey, H. & Spear, F. G. (1967) *Pain: Psychological and Psychiatric Aspects.* London: Baillière, Tindall & Cassell

Pilowsky, I. (1970) Primary and secondary hypochondriasis. *Acta psychiat. scand.,* **46,** 273–85

— (1976) The psychiatrist and the pain clinic, *Amer. J. Psychiat.,* **133,** 752–6

— (1978a) Psychodynamic aspects of the pain experience. In *The Psychology of Pain,* ed. Sternbach, R. A., pp. 203–17. New York: Raven Press

— (1978b) A general classification of abnormal illness behaviours. *Brit. J. med. Psychol.,* **51,** 131–7

Pilowsky, I. & Bassett, D. L. (1982) Individual dynamic psychotherapy for chronic pain. In *Chronic Pain,* ed. Roy, R. & Tunks, E., pp. 107–25. London: Williams & Wilkins

Sternbach, R. A. (1968) *Pain: A Psychophysiological Analysis.* New York: Academic Press

Wall, P. D. (1979) On the relation of injury to pain. The John H. Bonica Lecture. *Pain,* **6,** 253–64

Chapter 8.3

Agras, S. & Werne, J. (1977) Behaviour modification in anorexia nervosa: research foundations. In *Anorexia Nervosa,* ed. Vigersky, R. A., pp. 291–303. New York: Raven Press

Anand, B. K. & Brobeck, J. R. (1951) Localization of a 'feeding center' in the hypothalamus of the rat. *Proc. Soc. exp. Biol. Med.,* **77,** 323–4

Bell, E. T., Harkness, R. A., Loraine, J. A. & Russell, G. F. M. (1966) Hormone assay studies in patients with anorexia nervosa. *Acta endocrin.,* **51,** 140–8

Beumont, P. J. V., Beardwood, C. J. & Russell, G. F. M. (1972) The occurrence of the syndrome of anorexia nervosa in male subjects. *Psychol. Med.*, **2**, 216–31

Bruch, H. (1974) *Eating Disorders: Obesity, Anorexia Nervosa and the Person Within*. London: Routledge & Kegan Paul

— (1978) *The Golden Cage: The Enigma of Anorexia Nervosa*. London: Open Books

Crisp, A. H. (1980) *Anorexia Nervosa: Let Me Be*. London: Academic Press

Crisp, A. H., Chen, C., Mackinnon, P. C. B. & Corker, C. (1973) Observations of gonadotrophic and ovarian hormone activity during recovery from anorexia nervosa. *Postgrad. med. J.*, **49**, 584–90

Crisp, A. H., Harding, B. & McGuinness, B. (1974) Anorexia nervosa. Psychoneurotic characteristics of parents: relationship to progress. A quantitative study. *J. psychosom. Res.*, **18**, 167–73

Crisp, A. H. & Kalucy, R. S. (1974) Aspects of the perceptual disorder in anorexia nervosa. *Brit. J. med. Psychol.*, **74**, 349–61

Crisp, A. H., Palmer, R. L. & Kalucy, R. S. (1976) How common is anorexia nervosa? A prevalence study. *Brit. J. Psychiat.*, **128**, 549–54

Dally, P., Gomez, J. with Isaacs, A. J. (1979) *Anorexia Nervosa*. London: Heinemann Medical Books

Fairburn, C. G. (1981) A cognitive behavioural approach to the management of bulimia. *Psychol. Med.*, **11**, 707–11

Garner, D. M. & Garfinkel, P. E. (1980) Socio-cultural factors in the development of anorexia nervosa. *Psychol. Med.*, **10**, 647–56

Goldberg, S. C., Halmi, K. A., Casper, R., Eckert, E. & Davis, J. M. (1977) Pretreatment predictors of weight change in anorexia nervosa. In *Anorexia Nervosa*, ed. Vigersky, R.A., pp. 31–41. New York: Raven Press

Groen, J. J. & Feldman-Toledano, Z. (1966) Educative treatment of patients and parents in anorexia nervosa. *Brit. J. Psychiat.*, **112**, 671–81

Gull, W. W. (1874) Anorexia nervosa (apepsia hysterica, anorexia hysterica). *Trans. Clin. Soc. London*, **7**, 22–8

Hsu, L. K. G., Crisp. A. H. & Harding, B. (1979) Outcome of anorexia nervosa. *Lancet*, **i**, 61–5

Kay, D. W. K. & Leigh, D. (1954) The natural history, treatment and prognosis of anorexia nervosa based on a study of 38 patients. *J. ment. Sci.*, **100**, 411–31

Kendell, R. E., Hailey, A. & Babigian, H. M. (1973) The epidemiology of anorexia nervosa. *Psychol. Med.*, **3**, 200–3

Lasègue, E. C. (1873) On hysterical anorexia. *Med. Times Gaz.*, **2**, 265–6, 367–9. Translated in *Evolution of Psychosomatic Concepts, Anorexia Nervosa: A Paradigm*, ed. Kaufman, M. R. & Heiman, M., pp. 141–55, (1965) London: Hogarth Press

Lewin, K., Mattingly, D. & Millis, R. R. (1972) Anorexia nervosa associated with hypothalamic tumour. *Brit. med. J.*, **2**, 629–30

Liebman, R., Minuchin, S. & Baker, L. (1974). An integrated treatment program for anorexia nervosa. *Amer. J. Psychiat.*, **131**, 432–6

Loudon, I. S. L. (1980) Chlorosis, anaemia, and anorexia nervosa. *Brit. med. J.*, **2**, 1669–75

Marshall, J. F. (1976) Neurochemistry of central monoamine systems as related to food intake. In *Appetite and Food Intake*, ed. Silverstone, T. Report of the Dahlem Workshop on Appetite and Food Intake, Berlin, 8–12 December 1975, pp. 43–63. Life Sciences Research Report, 2. Berlin: Abakon Verlagsgesellschaft, for Dahlem Konferenzen

Minuchin, S., Baker, L., Rosman, B. L., Liebman, R., Milman, L. & Todd, T. C. (1975) A conceptual model of psychosomatic illness in children. *Arch. gen. Psychiat.*, **32**, 1031–8

Morgan, H. G. & Russell, G. F. M. (1975) Value of family background and clinical features as predictors of long-term outcome in anorexia nervosa: four-year follow-up study of 41 patients. *Psychol. Med.*, **5**, 355–71

Mortimer, C. H., Besser, G. M., McNeilly, A. S., Marshall, J. S., Harsoulis, P., Tunbridge, W. M. S., Gomez-Pan, A. & Hall, R. (1973) Luteinizing hormone and follicle stimulating hormone releasing test in patients with hypothalamic-pituitary-gonadal dysfunction. *Brit. med. J.*, **iv**, 73–7

Morton, R. (1694). *Phthisiologia: Or A Treatise of Consumptions*. London: Princes Arms Press

Nillius, S. J. & Wide, L. (1977) The pituitary responsiveness to acute and chronic administration of gonadotrophin-releasing-hormone in acute and recovery stages of anorexia nervosa. In *Anorexia Nervosa*, ed. Vigersky, R. A., pp. 225–41. New York: Raven Press

Pertschuk, M. J. (1977) Behaviour therapy: extended follow-up. In *Anorexia Nervosa*, ed. Vigersky, R. A., pp. 305–13. New York: Raven Press

Russell, G. F. M. (1965) Metabolic aspects of anorexia nervosa. *Proc. roy. Soc. Med.*, **58**, 811–14

— (1972) Premenstrual tension and 'psychogenic' amenorrhoea: psycho-physical interactions. *J. psychosom. Res.*, **16**, 279–87

— (1977) Editorial: The present status of anorexia nervosa. *Psychol. Med.*, **7**, 363–7

— (1979) Bulimia nervosa: an ominous variant of anorexia nervosa. *Psychol. Med.*, **9**, 429–48

Russell, G. F. M., Campbell, P. G. & Slade, P. D. (1975) Experimental studies on the nature of the psychological disorder in anorexia nervosa. *Psychoneuroendocrinol.*, **1**, 45–56

Russell, G. F. M. & Mezey, A. G. (1962) An analysis of weight gain in patients with anorexia nervosa treated with high calorie diets. *Clin. Sci.*, **23**, 449–61

Slade, P. D. & Russell, G. F. M. (1973) Awareness of body dimensions in anorexia nervosa: cross-sectional and longitudinal studies. *Psychol. Med.*, **3**, 188–99

Theander, S. (1970) Anorexia nervosa: a psychiatric investigation of 94 female patients. *Acta psychiat. scand.*, Supp. **214**

Wakeling, A., DeSouza, V. A. & Beardwood, C. J. (1977) Assessment of the negative and positive feedback effects of administered oestrogen on gonadotrophin release in patients with anorexia nervosa. *Psychol. Med.*, **7**, 397–405

Waller, J. V., Kaufman, M. R. & Deutsch, F. (1940) Anorexia nervosa. A psychosomatic entity. *Psychosom. Med.*, **2**, 3–16

Chapter 8.4

Allon, N. I. (1975) Fat is a dirty word: fat as a sociological and social problem. In *Recent Advances in Obesity Research I*. Proceedings of the 1st International Congress on Obesity, 8–14 October 1974, London, ed. Howard, A., pp. 244–7. London: Newman

Bierman, E. L. (1979) Obesity. In *Cecil Textbook of Medicine*, ed. Beeson, P. B., McDermott, W. & Wyngaarden, J. B., pp. 1692–9. Philadelphia, London, Toronto: Saunders

Brook, C. G. D., Lloyd, J. K. & Wolf, O. H. (1972) Relation between age of onset of obesity and size and number of adipose cells. *Brit. med. J.*, **2**, 25–7

Bruch, H. (1974) *Eating Disorders: Obesity, Anorexia Nervosa and the Person Within*. London: Routledge & Kegan Paul

Bruch, H. & Touraine, G. (1940). The family frame of obese children. *Psychosom Med.*, **11**, 141–206

Crisp, A. H., Kalucy, R. S., Pilkington, T. R. E. & Gazet, J.-C. (1977) Some psychosocial consequences of ileojejunal bypass surgery. *Amer. J. clin. Nutrition*, **30**, 109–20

Crisp, A. H. & McGuiness, B. (1976) Jolly fat: relation between obesity and psychoneuroses in general population. *Brit. med. J.*, **1**, 7–9

Crisp, A. H. & Stonehill, E. (1970) Treatment of obesity with special reference to seven severely obese patients. *J. psychosom. Res.*, **14**, 327–45

Donald, D. W. A. (1973) Mortality rates among the overweight. In *Anorexia Nervosa and Obesity*, symposium, ed. Robertson, R. F., pp. 63–70. Edinburgh: Royal College of Physicians

Foch, T. T. & McClearn, G. E. (1980) Genetics, body wieght and obesity. In *Obesity*, ed. Stunkard, A. J., pp. 48–71. Philadelphia, London & Toronto: Saunders

Garb, J. L., Garb, J. R. & Stunkard, A. J. (1975) Social factors and obesity in Navajo Indian children. In *Recent Advances in Obesity Research 1*. Proceedings of the 1st International Congress on Obesity, 8–14 October 1974, London, ed. Howard, A., pp. 37–9. London: Newman

Garrow, J. S. (1974) *Energy Balance and Obesity in Man*. Amsterdam: North-Holland

Glucksman, M. L. & Hirsch, J. (1973) The perception of body size. In *The Psychology of Obesity: Dynamics and Treatment*, ed. Kiell, N., pp. 48–54. Springfield, Ill.: Thomas

Goldman, R., Jaffa, M. & Schachter, S. (1968) Yom Kippur, Air France, dormitory food, and the dating behaviour of obese and normal persons. *J. Pers. soc. Psychol.*, **10**, 117–23

Hetherington, A. W. & Ranson, S. W. (1940) Adiposity in the rat. *Anat. Records*, **78**, 149

Hirsch, J. & Knittle, J. L. (1970) Cellularity of obese and nonobese human adipose tissue. *Federal Proc.*, **29**, 1516–21

Kannel, W. B. & Gordon, T. (1975) Some determinants of obesity and its impact as a cardiovascular risk factor. In *Recent Advances in Obesity Research 1*. Proceedings of the 1st International Congress on Obesity, 8–14 October 1974, London, ed. Howard, A., pp. 14–27. London: Newman

Kaplan, H. I. & Kaplan, H. S. (1957) The psychosomatic concept of obesity. *J. nerv. ment. Dis.*, **125**, 181–201

Kekwick, A. & Pawan, G. L. S. (1956) Calorie intake in relation to body weight changes in the obese. *Lancet*, **ii**, 155–61

Levitz, L. E. & Stunkard, A. J. (1974) A therapeutic coalition for obesity: behaviour modification and patient self-help. *Amer. J. Psychiat.*, **131**, 423–7

Lipinski, B. G. (1975) Life change events as correlates of weight gain. In *Recent Advances on Obesity Research I*. Proceedings of the 1st International Congress on Obesity, 8–14 October 1974, London, ed. Howard, A., pp. 210–12. London: Newman

McCance, C. (1961) *Psychiatric factors in obesity*. Dissertation for the Academic Diploma of Psychological Medicine of the University of London

Mayer, J. (1965) Genetic factors in human obesity. *Ann. N. Y. Acad. Sci.*, **131**, 412–21

Mendelson, M. (1966) Psychological aspects of obesity. *Int. J. Psychiat.*, **2**, 599–612

Metropolitan Life Insurance Company (1959) New weight standards for men and woman. *Stat. Bull.*, **40**, 1–4

Miller, F.J.W., Billewicz, W. Z. & Thomson, A. M. (1972) Growth from birth to adult life of 442 Newcastle-upon-Tyne children. *Brit. J. prev. soc. Med.*, **26**, 224–30

Miller, N. E. (1955) Shortcomings of food consumption as a measure of hunger: results from other behavioural techniques. *Ann. N.Y. Acad. Sci.*, **63**, 141–43

Mills, M. J. & Stunkard, A. J. (1976) Behavioural changes following surgery for obesity. *Amer. J. Psychiat.*, **133**, 527–31

Munro, J. F. (1979) Drug treatment of obesity. *Prescribers J.*, **19**, 106–12

Newman, H. H., Freeman, F. N. & Holzinger, K. J. (1937) *Twins: A Study of Heredity and Environment*. Chicago: University of Chicago Press

Nisbett, R. E. (1968) Determinants of food intake in obesity. *Science*, **159**, 1254–5

Pilkington, T. R. E., Gazet, J.-C., Ang, L., Kalucy, R. S., Crisp, A. H. & Day, S. (1976) Explanations for weight loss after ileojejunal bypass in gross obesity. *Brit. med. J.*, **1**, 1504–5

Robinson, R. G., Folstein, M. F., & McHugh, P. R. (1979) Reduced caloric intake following small bowel bypass surgery: a systematic study of possible causes. *Psychol. Med.*, **9**, 37–53

Russell, G.F.M. (1962) The effect of diets of different composition on weight loss, water and sodium balance in obese patients. *Clin. Sci.*, **22**, 269–77

Schachter, S., Goldman, R. & Gordon, A. (1968) Effects of fear, food deprivation, and obesity on eating. *J. Pers. soc. Psychol.*, **10**, 91–7

Shapiro, B. (1973) Regulation of adipose tissue size. In *Energy in Man*, ed. Apfelbaum, M., pp. 247–59. Paris: Masson

Shields, J. (1962) *Monozygotic Twins, Brought Up Apart and Brought up Together. An Investigation into the Genetic and Environmental Causes of Variation in Personality*, chap. 7. London: Oxford University Press

Shipman, W. G. & Plesset, M. R. (1963) Anxiety and depression in obese dieters. *Arch. gen. Psychiat.*, **8**, 530–5

Silverstone, J. T. (1973) Psychosocial aspects of obesity. In *The Psychology of Obesity: Dynamics and Treatment*, ed. Kiell, N., chap. 6, pp. 67–74. Springfield, Ill.: Thomas

Silverstone, J. T., Gordon, R. P. & Stunkard, A. J. (1969) Social factors in obesity in London. *Practitioner*, **202**, 682–8

Srole, L., Langner, T. S., Michael, S. T., Opler, M. R. & Rennie, T.A.C. (1962) *Mental Health in the Metropolis: Midtown Manhattan Study 1*. New York: McGraw-Hill

Stunkard, A. J. (1957) The 'dieting depression'. *Amer. J. Med.*, **23**, 77–86

— (1975) Obesity and the social environment. In *Recent Advances in Obesity Research 1*. Proceedings of the 1st International Congress on Obesity, 8–14 October 1974, London, ed. Howard, A., chap. 4, pp. 178–90. London: Newman

— (1977) Behavioral treatments of obesity: failure to maintain weight loss. In *Behavioral Self-Management: Strategies, Techniques and Outcomes*, ed. Stuart, R. B., pp. 317–50. New York: Brunner/Mazel

Stunkard, A. J. & Koch, L. (1964) The interpretation of gastric motility. *Arch. gen. Psychiat.*, **11**, 74–82

Stunkard, A. J. & McLaren-Hume, M. (1959) The results of treatment for obesity. *Arch. int. Med.*, **103**, 79–85

Van Itallie, T. B. & Campbell, R. G. (1972) Multidisciplinary approach to the problem of obesity. *J. Amer. Dietet. Ass.*, **61**, 385–90

Withers, R.F.J. (1964) Problems in the genetics of human obesity. *Eugen. Rev.*, **56**, 81–90

Chapter 8.5

Altschule, M. D. & Brem, J. (1963) Periodic psychosis of puberty. *Amer. J. Psychiat.*, **119**, 1176–8

Appleby, B. P. (1960) A study of premenstrual tension in general practice. *Brit. med. J.*, **1**, 391–3

Backstrom, T. & Carstensen, H. (1974) Estrogen and progesterone in plasma in relation to premenstrual tension. *J. ster. Biochem.*, **5**, 257–60

Benedek-Jaszmann, L. F. & Hearn-Sturtevant, M. D. (1976) Premenstrual tension and functional infertility: aetiology and treatment. *Lancet*, **i**, 1095–8

Bickers, W. & Woods, M. (1951) Premenstrual tension: rational treatment. *Texas Rep. biol. Med.*, **9**, 406–19

Birtchnell, J. & Floyd, S. (1974). Attempted suicide and the menstrual cycle – a negative conclusion. *J. psychosom. Res.*, **18**, 361–9

Bruce, J. & Russell, G.F.M. (1962) A study of weight changes and balance of water, sodium and potassium. *Lancet*, **ii**, 267–71

Carroll, M. & Steiner, M. (1978) The psychobiology of premenstrual dysphoria: the role of prolactin. *Psychoneuroendocrinol.*, **3**, 171–80

Clare, A. W. (1977) Psychological problems of women complaining of premenstrual symptoms. *Curr. med. Res. Opinion*, **4**, (4), 23–8

— (1979) The treatment of premenstrual symptoms. *Brit. J. Psychiat.*, **135**, 567–79

— (1981) *Psychiatric and Social Aspects of Premenstrual Complaint.* M.D. Thesis, National University of Ireland, University College, Dublin

Coppen, A. (1965) The prevalence of menstrual disorders in psychiatric patients. *Brit. J. Psychiat.*, **111**, 155–67

Dalton, K. (1959) Menstruation and acute psychiatric illness. *Brit. med. J.*, **1**, 148–9

— (1960) Menstruation and accidents. *Brit. med. J.*, **2**, 1425–6

— (1961) Menstruation and crime. *Brit. med. J.*, **2**, 1752–3

— (1966) The influence of mother's menstruation on her child. *Proc. R. Soc. Med.*, **59**, 1014–16

— (1968) Menstruation and examination. *Lancet*, **ii**, 1386–8

— (1969) *The Menstrual Cycle.* Harmondsworth: Penguin

— (1970) Children's hospital admissions and mother's menstruation. *Brit. med. J.*, **2**, 27–8

— (1977) *The Premenstrual Syndrome and Progesterone Therapy.* London: Heinemann

— (1980) Cyclical criminal acts in premenstrual syndrome. *Lancet*, **ii**, 1070–1

— (1981) Discussion on treatment. In *The Premenstrual Syndrome*, ed. van Keep, P. & Utian, W. H. Lancaster: MTP

Day, J. B. (1979) Clinical trials in the premenstrual syndrome. *Curr. med. Res. Opinion*, **6**, (5), 40–5

Diamond, S. B., Rubinstein, A. A., Dunner, D. L. & Fieve, R. R. (1976) Menstrual problems in women with primary affective illness. *Compr. Psychiat.*, **17**, 4, 541–8

d'Orbán, P. T. & Dalton, J. (1980) Violent crime and the menstrual cycle. *Psychol. Med.*, **10**, 353–9

Ellis, D. P. & Austin, P. (1971) Menstruation and aggressive behaviour in a correction center for women. *J. crim Law, Criminol. Police Sci.*, **62**, 3, 388–95

Fortin, J. N., Wittkower, E. D. & Kalz, F. (1958) Psychosomatic approach to premenstrual tension syndrome: A preliminary report. *Can. Med. Ass. J.*, **79**, 978–81

Frank, R. T. (1931) The hormone causes of premenstrual tension. *Arch. Neurol. Psychiat.*, **26**, 1053–7

Goldzieher, J. W., Moses, L. E., Averkin, E. *et al.* (1971) Nervousness and depression attributed to oral contraceptives: a double-blind placebo-controlled study. *Amer. J. Obstet. Gynaecol.*, **111**, 1013–20

Golub, L. J., Menduke, H. & Conley, S. S. (1965) Weight changes in college women during the menstrual cycle. *Amer. J. Obstet. gynaecol.*, **91**, 89–94

Grant, E.C.G. & Mears, E. (1967) Mental effect of oral contraceptives. *Lancet*, **ii**. 945–6

Grant, E.C.G. & Pryse-Davies, J. (1968) Effects of oral contraceptives on depressive mood changes and on endometrial monoamine oxidase and phosphatases. *British med. J.*, **3**, 777–80

Gregory, B.A.J.C. (1957) The menstrual cycle and its disorders in psychiatric patients. 1. Review of the literature. *J. Psychosom. Res.*, **2**, 199–224

Herzberg, B. & Coppen, A. (1970) Changes in psychological symptoms in women taking oral contraceptives. *Brit. J. Psychiat.*, **116**, 161–4

Horrobin, D. (1973) *Prolactin: Physiology and Clinical Significance.* Lancaster: MTP.

Janowsky, D. S., Gorney, R. & Mandell, A. J. (1967) Psychiatric and ovarian-adrenocortical hormone correlates: case study and literature review. *Arch. gen. Psychiat.*, **17**, 459–69

Kerr, G. D. (1977) The management of the premenstrual syndrome. *Curr. med. Res. Opin.*, **4**, Supp. 4, 29–34

Kessel, N. & Coppen, A. (1963) The prevalence of common menstrual symptoms. *Lancet*, **ii**, 61–4

Klaiber, E. L., Kobayashi, Y., Broverman, D. M. & Hall, F. (1971) Plasma monoamine oxidase activity in regularly menstruating women and in amenorrheic women receiving cyclic treatment with oestrogens and a progestin. *J. clin. endocrin. Metab.*, **33**, 630–7

Koeske, R. K. & Koeske, G. F. (1975) An attributional approach to moods and the menstrual cycle. *J. Pers. soc. Psychol.*, **31**, 3, 473–8

Kopell, B. S., Lunde, D. T., Clayton, R. B. & Moos, R. H. (1969) Variations in some measures of arousal during the menstrual cycle. *J. nerv. ment. Dis.*, **148**, 180–7

Kramp, J. L. (1968) Studies on the premenstrual syndrome in relation to psychiatry. *Acta psychiat. scand.*, Supp. **203**, 261–7

Kutner, S. J. & Brown, W. L. (1972) Types of oral contraceptives, depression, and premenstrual symptoms. *J. nerv. ment. Dis.*, **155**, 3, 153–62

Lamb, W. M., Ulett, G. A., Masters, W. H. & Robinson, D. W. (1953) Premenstrual tension, EEG, hormonal and psychiatric evaluation. *Amer. J. Psychiat.*, **109**, 840–8

Lever, J., Brush, M. & Haynes, B. (1979) *PMT. The Unrecognised Illness.* London: Melbourne House

Linghaerde, P. & Bredland, R. (1954) Hyperestrogenic cyclic psychosis. *Acta psychiat. scand.*, **29**, 355–64

MacKinnon, P.C.B. & MacKinnon, I. L. (1956) Hazards of the menstrual cycle. *Brit. med J.*, **1**, 555

MacKinnon, I. L., MacKinnon P.C.B. & Thomson, A. D. (1959) Lethal hazards of the luteal phase of the menstrual cycle. *Brit. med. J.*, **1**, 1015–17

Mattsson, B. & von Schoultz, B. (1974) A comparison between lithium placebo and a diuretic in premenstrual tension. *Acta psychiat. scand.*, Supp. **255**, 75–84

McClure, J. N. Jr., Reich, T. & Wetzel, R. D. (1971) Premenstrual symptoms as an indicator of bipolar affective disorder. *Brit. J. Psychiat.*, **119**, 527–8

Moos, R. H. (1969) Typology of menstrual cycle symptoms. *Amer. J. Obstet. Gynaecol.*, **103**, 390–402

Moos, R. H., Kopell, B. S., Melges, R. R., Yalom, I. D., Lunde, D.T., Clayton, R. B. & Hamburg, D. A. (1969) Fluctuations in symptoms and moods during the menstrual cycle. *J. psychosom. Res.*, **13**, 37–44

Munday, M. (1977) Hormone levels in severe premenstrual tension. *Curr. med. Res. Opin.*, **4**, (4), 16–22

O'Brien, P.M.S., Craven, D., Selby, C. & Symonds, E. M. (1979) Treatment of premenstrual syndrome by spironolactone. *Brit. J. Obstet. Gynaecol.*, **86**, 142–7

Parlee, M. B. (1973) The premenstrual syndrome. *Psychol. Bull.*, **80**, 6, 454–65

— (1974) Stereotypic beliefs about menstruation: A methodological note on the Moos Menstrual Distress Questionnaire and some new data. *Psychosom. Med.*, **36**, 3, 229–40

Pennington, V. M. (1957) Meprobamate (Miltown) in premenstrual tension. *J. Amer. Med. Ass.*, **164**, 638–40

Rees, L. (1953) The premenstrual tension syndrome and its treatment. *Brit. med. J.*, **1**, 1014–16

Reeves, B. D., Garvin, J. E. & McElin, T. W. (1971) Premenstrual tension. Symptoms and weight changes related to potassium therapy. *Amer. J. Obstet. Gynaecol.*, **109**, 1036–41

Rodin, J. (1976) Menstruation, reattribution and competence. *J. Pers. soc. Psychol.*, **3**, 345–53

RCGP (Royal College of General Practitioners) (1974) *Oral Contraceptives and Health*, p. 29. London: Pitman Medical

ROSPA (Royal Society for the Prevention of Accidents) (1977), *PMT – Premenstrual Tension*. Pamphlet

Singer, K., Cheng, R. & Schou, M. (1974) A controlled evaluation of Lithium in the premenstrual tension syndrome. *Brit. J. Psychiat.*, **124**, 50–1

Sletton, I. W. & Gershon, S. (1966) The premenstrual syndrome: A discussion of its physiology and treatment with lithium ion. *Compr. Psychiat.*, **7**, 197–206

Smith, S. L. (1975) Mood and the menstrual cycle. In *Topics in Psychoendocrinology*, ed. Sacher, E. J. New York: Grune & Stratton

Sommer, B. (1973) The effect of menstruation on cognitive and perceptual-motor behaviour: A review. *Psychosom. Med.*, **35**, 515–34

Steiner, M., Haskett, R. F., Osmun, J. N. & Carroll, B. J. (1980) Treatment of premenstrual tension with lithium carbonate. *Acta psychiat. scand.*, **61**, 96–102

Steiner, M., Haskett, R. F. & Carroll, B. J. (1980) Premenstrual tension syndrome. *Acta psychiat. scand.*, **62**, 177–90

Stieglitz, E. J. & Kimble, S. T. (1949) Premenstrual intoxication. *Amer. J. med. Sci.*, **218**, 616–23

Taylor, J. W. (1979) The timing of menstruation – related symptoms assessed by a daily symptom rating scale. *Acta psychiat. scand.*, **60**, 87–105

Tonks, C. M., Rack, P. H. & Rose, M. J. (1968) Attempted suicide and the menstrual cycle. *J. psychosom Res.*, **11**, 319–23

Tuch, R. H. (1975) The relationship between a mother's menstrual status and her response to illness in her child. *Psychosom. Med.*, **37**, 5, 388–94

Udry, J. R. & Morris, N. M. (1968) Distribution of coitus in the menstrual cycle. *Nature* (Lond.), **200**, 593–6

Valins, S. & Nisbett, R. E. (1971) *Attribution Processes in the Development and Treatment of Emotional Disorders.* Morristown, New Jersey: General Learning Corporation

van Keep, P. A. & Haspels, A. A. (1979) Het premenstruele syndroom, een epidemiologisch onderzoek. *J. drug Res.*, **4**, 568

van Keep, P. A. & Lehert, P. (1981) The premenstrual syndrome – an epidemiological and statistical exercise. In *The Premenstrual Syndrome*, ed. van Keep, P. A. & Utian, W. H., chap. 2, pp. 31–42. Lancaster: MTP

Wearing, M. P., Yuhosz, M. D., Campbell, R. & Love, E. J. (1972) The effect of the menstrual cycle on tests of physical fitness. *J. sports Med. phys. Fitness*, **12**, 38–41

Williams, J.G.P. & Sperryn, P. N. (1976) Women in Sport. In *Sports Medicine*, chap 10, 210–25. London: Arnold

Winston, F. (1973) Oral contraceptives, pyridoxine and depression. *Amer. J. Psychiat.*, **130**, 1217–21

Zaharieva, E. (1965) Survey of Sportswomen at the Tokyo Olympics. *J. sports Med. phys. Fitness*, **5**, 215–19

Chapter 8.6

Bleuler, M. (1967) Endocrinological psychiatry and psychology. *Henry Ford Hosp. med. J.*, **15**, 309–17

Christie Brown, J.R.W. (1968) Mood changes following parathyroidectomy. *Proc. R. Soc. Med.*, **61**, 1121–3

— (1972) Psychological and dietary aspects of secondary amenorrhoea. *Psychosom. Med. Obstet. Gynaecol.*, ed. Morris, N., pp. 579–81 Basle: Karger

Cohen, S. I. (1980) Cushing's syndrome: a psychiatric study of 29 patients. *Brit. J. Psychiat.*, **130** 120–4

Drew, F. L. & Stifel, E. N. (1968) Secondary amenorrhoea among young women entering religious life. *Obstet. Gynaecol.*, **32**, 47–50

Drillien, C. M. (1946) A study of normal and abnormal menstrual function in the auxiliary territorial services. *J. Obstet. Gynaecol. Brit. Commonwealth*, **53**, 228–34

Jeffcoate, W. J., Silverstone, J. T., Edwards, C. R. W. & Besser, G. M. (1979) Psychiatric manifestations of Cushing's syndrome. *Q. J. Med.*, **191**, 465–72

Kelly, W. F., Checkley, S. A. & Bender, D. A. (1980) Cushing's Syndrome, tryptophan and depression. *Brit. J. Psychiat.*, **136**, 125–32

Lishman, W. A. (1978) *Organic Psychiatry*, chap. 11, p. 596. Oxford: Blackwell

White, G. H. & Walmsley, R. N. (1978) Can the clinical assessment of thyroid function be improved? *Lancet*, **ii** (8096), 933–5

Whybrow, P. C., Prange, A. J. & Treadway, C. R. (1969) Mental changes accompanying thyroid gland dysfunction. *Arch. gen. Psychiat.*, **20**, 48–63

van Keep, P. A. & Utian, W. H. (Eds.) (1981) *The Premenstrual Syndrome*. Lancaster: MTP Press

Chapter 8.7

Brown, F. W. (1938) The psychological investigation of a case of dermatitis artefacta. *Guy's Hosp. Reports*, **88**, 356–66

Calnan, J. (1980) Dermatitis artefacta. *World Med.*, **15**, 97–9

Cotterill, J. A. (1981) Dermatological non-disease: a common and potentially fatal disturbance of cutaneous body image. *Brit. J. Dermatol.*, **104**, 611–19

Ebling, F. J. & Rook, A. (1968) Hair. In *Textbook of Dermatology,* ed. Rook, A., Wilkinson, D. S. & Ebling, F. J. G., chap. 46, pp. 1384–9. Oxford: Blackwell

Edwards, K. C. S. (1954) Pruritis in melancholia. *Brit. med. J.*, **2**, 1527–9

Gillespie, R. D. (1938) Dermatitis artefacta. *Guy's Hosp. Reports*, **88**, 172–84

Hollender, M. H. & Abram, H. S. (1973) Dermatitis factitia. *South. med. J.*, **66**, 1279–85

Kenyon, F. E. (1962) A psychiatric survey of a random sample of out-patients attending a dermatological hospital. *J. psychosom. Res.*, **6**, 129–35

Lyell, A. (1972) Dermatitis artefacta and self-inflicted disease. *Scot. med. J.*, **17**, 187–96

Macalpine, I. (1953) Pruritis ani: a psychiatric study. *Psychosom. Med.*, **15**, 499–508

Menninger, K. (1947) Observations of a psychiatrist in a dermatology clinic. *Bull. Menninger Clin.*, **11**, 141–7

Prosser Thomas, E. (1937) Dermatitis artefacta: a note on an unusual case. *British med. J.*, **1**, 804–6

Rook, A. & Wilkinson, D. S. (1968) Psychocutaneous disorders. In *Textbook of Dermatology*, ed. Rook, A., Wilkinson, D. S. & Ebling, F. J. G., chap. 54, pp. 1587–9. Oxford: Blackwell

Shuster, S. (1981) Reason and the rash. *Proc. R. Inst. Great Britain*, **53**, 136–63

Sneddon, I. & Sneddon, J. (1975) Self-inflicted injury: a follow-up study of 43 patients. *Brit. med. J.*, **3**, 527–30

Stokes, J. H. & Garner, V. C. (1929) The diagnosis of self-inflicted lesions of the skin. *J. Amer. Med. Ass.*, **93**, 438–43

Whitlock, F. A. (1976) *Psychophysiological Aspects of Skin Disease*, pp. 21–3, 118–27, 148, 211–17. London: Saunders

Zaidens, S. H. (1951) Self-inflicted dermatoses and their psychodynamics. *J. nerv. ment Dis.*, **113**, 395–404

Chapter 8.8.

Alexander, F. (1949) *Fundamentals of Psychoanalysis*. London: Allen & Unwin

Alvarez, W. C. (1944) A gastro-intestinal hypochondriac and some lessons he taught. *Gastroenterology*, **2**, 265–9

Bianchi, G. N. (1973) Patterns of hypochondriasis: A principal components analysis. *Brit. J. Psychiat.*, **122**, 541–8

Gehring, E. W. (1932) Painful women. *Maine med. J.*, **23**, 139–43

Kenyon, F. E. (1964) Hypochondriasis: A clinical study. *Brit. J. Psychiat.*, **110**, 478–88

Langner, T. S. & Michael, S. T. (1963) *Life Stress and Mental Health*. London: Collier-Macmillan

Perley, M. J. & Guze, S. B. (1962) Hysteria – the stability and usefulness of clinical criteria. *New Eng. J. Med.*, **266**, 421–6

Pilowsky, I. (1967). Dimensions of hypochondriasis. *Brit. J. Psychiat.*, **113**, 89–94

— (1968) The response to treatment in hypochondriacal disorders. *Aus. N. Z. J. Psychiat.*, **2**, 88–94

— (1970) Primary and secondary hypochondriasis. *Acta psychiat. scand.*, **46**, 273–85

— (1978) A general classification of abnormal illness behaviours. *Brit. J. med. Psychol.*, **51**, 131–7

Pilowsky, I. & Spence, N. D. (1977) Ethnicity and illness behaviour. *Psychol. Med.*, **7**, 447–52

Chapter 8.9

Bergmann, T. (1965) *Children in the Hospital*. New York: International Universities Press

Campbell, J. (1978) The child in the sick role: Contributions of age, sex, parental status and parental values. *J. Health soc. Behav.*, **19**, 35–51

Creak, M. (1969) Hysteria in childhood. *Acta paedopsychiat.*, **36**, 269–74

Dubowitz, V. & Hersov, L. (1976) Management of children with non-organic (hysterical) disorders of motor function. *Dev. Med. child Neurol.*, **3**, 358–68

Freud, A. (1952) The role of bodily illness in the mental life of children. In *The Psychoanalytic Study of the Child*, **7**, pp. 69–81.

Kellner, R. (1963) *Family Ill Health*. London: Tavistock

Kendell, R. E. (1974) A new look at hysteria. *Medicine:* (London), **30**, 1780–3

Kessel, N. & Shepherd, M. (1965) The health and attitude of people who seldom consult the doctor. *Med. Care*, Jan–March

Kleinman, A., Eisenberg, L. & Good, B. (1978) Culture illness and care. *Ann. int. Med.* **88**, 251–8

Mechanic, D. (1962) The concept of illness behaviour. *J. Chron. Dis.*, **15**, 189–94

— (1964) The influence of mothers on their children's health attitudes and behaviour. *Paediatrics*, **33**, 444–53

Mechanic, D. & Volkart, E. A. (1961) Stress, illness behaviour and the sick role. *Amer. sociol. Rev.*, **26**, 51–8

Mrazek, D. (1976) Integration or segregation of theoretical frameworks: a challenge in psychiatric education. *Compr. Psychiat.*, **17**, 249–57

Parsons, T. (1952) *The Social System*, pp. 437, 446 London: Tavistock

Pickering, G. W. (1974) *Creative Malady*, p. 33. London: Allen & Unwin

Pilowsky, I. (1969) Abnormal illness behaviour. *Brit. J. med. Psychol.*, **42**, 347–51

Robinson, D. (1972) Illness behaviour and children's hospitalization. A schema of parents' attitudes toward authority. *Soc. Sci. Med.*, **6**, 447–68

Twaddle, A. (1972) The concepts of sick role and illness behaviour. In *Advances in Psychosomatic Medicine*, ed. Lipowski, Z., vol. 8, pp. 162–79. Basel: Karger

Zola, I. K. (1972) Studying decision to see the doctor. In *Advances in Psychosomatic Medicine*, ed. Lipowski, Z., vol. 8, pp. 216–36. Basel: Karger

Chapter 9.1

Bancroft, J. (1977) The behavioural approach to treatment. In *Handbook of Sexology*, ed. Money, J. & Musaph, H. Amsterdam: Excerpta Medical

— (1980a) Psychophysiology of sexual dysfunction. In *Handbook of Biological Psychiatry. Part II. Brain mechanisms and Abnormal Behavior – Psychophysiology*, ed. van Praag, H. New York: Marcel Dekker

— (1980b) Endocrinology of sexual function. In *Clin. Obstet. Gynaecol.*, vol. 7, No. 2, 253–81, ed. M. Ebstein. Philadelphia: Saunders

— (1980c) Treatment of sexual problems. In *Psychiatric Ethics*, ed. Bloch, S. & Chodoff, P. Oxford: Oxford University Press

Bancroft, J. & Coles, L. (1976) Three years experience in a sexual problems clinic. *Brit. med. J.*, **1**, 1575–77

Barbach, L. C. (1974) Group treatment of pre-orgasmic women. *J. sex. marit. Ther.*, **1**, 139–45

Beaumont, G. (1979). Sexual side-effects of psychotropic drugs. *Brit. J. Clin. Pract.*, symposium supp., **4**, 45–47

Carney, A., Bancroft, J. & Mathews, A. (1978) Combination of hormonal and psychological treatment for female sexual unresponsiveness: a comparative study. *Brit. J. Psychiat.*, **133**, 339–46

Chesser, E. (1956) *The Sexual, Marital and Family Relationship of the English Woman*. London: Hutchinson

Fisher, S. (1973) *The Female Orgasm*. New York: Basic Books

Franks, E., Anderson, C. & Rubinstein, D. (1978) Frequency of sexual dysfunction in 'normal' couples. *New Eng. J. Med.*, **299**, 111–15

Frenken, J. (1976) *Afkeer van Seksualiteit*. Van Loghum, Slaterius-Darenter

Gebhard, P. H. & Johnson, A. B. (1979) *The Kinsey Data: Marginal Tabulation of the 1938–1963 Interviews conducted by the Institute for Sex Research*. Philadelphia: Saunders

Ginestie, J. F. & Romieu, A. (1978) *Radiologic Exploration of Impotence*. The Hague: Martinus Nijhoff Medical Division

Golden, J. S., Price, S., Heinrich, A. G. & Lobitz, W. C. (1978) Group vs couple treatment of sexual dysfunction. *Arch. sex. Behav.*, **7**, 593–602

Hunt, M. (1974) *Sexual Behavior in the 1970s*. Chicago: Playboy Press

Kaplan, H. S., Kohl, R. N., Pomeroy, W. B., Offit, A. N. & Hogan, B. (1974) Group treatment of premature ejaculation. *Arch. sex. Behav.*, **3**, 443–52

Kinsey, A. C., Pomeroy, W. B. & Martin, C. F. (1948) *Sexual Behavior in the Human Male*. Philadelphia: Saunders

Kinsey, A. C., Pomeroy, W. B., Martin, C. F. & Gebhard, P. H. (1953) *Sexual Behavior in the Human Female*. Philadelphia: Saunders

Leiblum, S. R., Rosen, R. & Pierce, D. (1976) Group treatment format: mixed sexual dysfunctions. *Arch. sex. Behav.*, **5**, 313–22

Masters, W. H. & Johnson, V. E. (1970) *Human Sexual Inadequacy*. Boston: Little Brown

Mears, E. (1978) Sexual problems clinics. An assessment of the work of 26 doctors trained by the Institute of Psychosexual Medicine. *Pub. Health (Lond.)*, **92**, 218–23

Michal, V. (1978) Vascular surgery in the treatment of impotence. *Brit. J. sex. Med.*, **5**, (40), 13–18

Rainwater, L. (1966) Some aspects of lower class sexual behaviour. *J. soc. Issues*, **22**, 96–108

Renshaw, D. (1980) Diabetic importance – inevitable or imposed? *Brit. J. sex. Med.*, **6**, (55) 35–7

Riley, A. J. & Riley, E. J. (1978) A controlled study to evaluate directed masturbation in the management of primary orgasmic failure in women. *Brit. J. Psychiat.*, **133**, 404–9

Schiavi, R. C. (1979) Some problems in the differential diagnosis of erectile disorders. *Sexuality & Disability*, **2**, 66–70

Schmidt, G. (1977) Working class and middle class adolescents. In *Handbook of Sexology*, Ed. Money, J. & Musaph, H. Amsterdam: Elsevier/North Holland

Skakkebaek, N. E., Bancroft, J., Davidson, D. W. & Warner, P. (1980) Androgen relacement with oral testosterone undecanoate in hypogonald men: a double blind controlled study. *Clin. Endocrinol.*, **14**, 49–61

Zilbergeld, B. (1975) Group treatment of sexual dysfunction in men without partners. *J. sex. marit. Ther.*, **1**, 204–14

Chapter 9.2

Bancroft, J. (1974) *Deviant Sexual Behaviour: Modification and Assessment*. Oxford: Clarendon Press

— (1977) The behavioural approach to treatment. In *Handbook of Sexology*, ed. Money, J. & Musaph, H. Amsterdam: Elsevier

— (1978) The relationship between hormones and sexual behaviour in humans. In *Biological Determinants of Sexual Behaviour*, ed. Hutchinson, J. B. Chichester: Wiley

— (1980) Modification of homosexual preferences: some ethical considerations. In *Medical Sexology*, ed. Forleo, R. & Pasini, W. Amsterdam: Elsevier

Bell, A. P. & Weinberg, M. S. (1978) *Homosexualities. A Study of Diversity among Men and Women*. London: Mitchell Beazley

Blumstein, P. W. & Schwartz, P. (1976) Bisexuality in women. *Arch. sex. Behav.*, **5**, 171–82

Bullough, V. L. (1976) *Sexual Variance in Society and History*. New York: Wiley

Dörner, G., Rohde, W., Stahl, F., Krell, L. & Masins, W. G. (1975) A neuroendocrine predisposition for homosexuality in men. *Arch. sex. Behav.*, **4**, 1–8

Ford, C. S. & Beach, F. A. (1952) *Patterns in Sexual Behaviour*. London: Eyre & Spottiswoode

Freeman, M. D. A. (1979) The law and sexual deviation. In *Sexual Deviation*, ed. Rosen, I. Oxford: Oxford University Press

Gagnon, J. & Simon, W. (1973) *Sexual Conduct: The Social Sources of Human Sexuality*. Chicago: Aldine

Green, R. (1980) Sex-typed boyhood behaviour and adolescent sexuality. *Medical Sexology*, ed. Forleo, R. & Pasini, W., pp. 318–20. Amsterdam: Elsevier

Heston, L. L. & Shields, J. (1968) Homosexuality in twins: a family study and a register study. *Arch. gen. Psychiat.*, **18**, 149–60

Hoffman, M. (1968) *The Gay World*. New York: Basic Books

Hooker, E. (1967) The homosexual community. In *Sexual Deviance*, ed. Gagnon, J. H. & Simon, W. New York: Harper & Row

Humphreys, R. A. L. (1970) *Tearoom Trade*. Chicago: Aldine

Hunt, M. (1974) *Sexual behavior in the 1970s*. Chicago: Playboy Press

Masters, W. H. & Johnson, V. E. (1979) *Homosexuality in Perspective*. Boston: Little, Brown

Pietropinto, A. & Simenauer, J. (1977) *Beyond the Male Myth. A Nationwide Survey*. New York: Times

Schofield, M. (1965) *Sociological Aspects of Homosexuality. A Comparative Study of Three Types of Homosexuals*. London: Longman

Siegelman, M. (1972) Adjustment of male homosexuals and heterosexuals. *Arch. sex. Behav.*, **2**, 9–25

— (1978) Psychological adjustment of homosexual and heterosexual men: a cross national replication. *Arch. sex. Behav.*, **7**, 1–12

Weinberg, M. S. & Williams, C. J. (1974) *Male Homosexuals: Their Problems and Adaptations*. New York: Oxford Univ. Press

Whitam, F. (1977) Childhood indications of male homosexuality. *Arch. sex. Behav.*, **6**, 89–96

Zuger, B. (1978) Effeminate behavior present in boys from childhood: ten additional years of follow-up. *Compr. Psychiat.*, **19**, 363–9

Chapter 9.3

Bancroft, J. H. J. (1977) The behavioural approach to treatment. In *Handbook of Sexology*, section xvi, ed. Money, J. & Mustaph H., pp. 1197–225. Amsterdam: Excerpta Medica

Blumer, D. (1969) Transsexualism, sexual disfunction and temporal lobe disorder. In *Transsexualism and Sex Reassignment*, pp. 213–19. Baltimore: Johns Hopkins Press

Edgerton, M. T., Jr. & Meyer, J. K. (1973) Surgical and psychiatric aspects of transsexualism. In *Surgery of the External Genitalia*, ed. Horton, C., pp. 117–61. New York: Little, Brown

Erikson, E. H. (1968) *Identity: Youth and Crisis*. London: Faber & Faber

Gebhard, P. H. (1965) *Sex Offenders*. New York: Harper & Row

Gelder, M. G. & Marks, I. M. (1969) Aversion treatment in transvestism and transsexualism. In *Transsexualism and Sex Reassignment*, ed. Green R. & Money, J. Baltimore: Johns Hopkins Press

Gibbens, T. C. N., Way, C. & Soothill, K. L. (1977) Behavioural types of rape. *Brit. J. Psychiat.*, **130**, 32–42

Green, R. (1977) Atypical psychosexual development. In *Child Psychiatry*, ed. Rutter, M. & Hersov, L., pp. 788–806. Oxford: Blackwell

Greenacre, P. (1979) Fetishism. In *Sexual Deviation*, 2nd ed. ed. Rosen, I., pp. 79–108. Oxford: Oxford University Press

Hoenig, J. & Kenna, J. C. (1974) The prevalence of transsexualism in England and Wales. *Brit. J. Psychiat.*, **124**, 181–90

Maguire, R. J., Carlisle, J. M. & Young, B. G. (1965) Sexual deviation as conditioned behaviour: a hypothesis. *Behav. Res. Ther.*, **2**, 185–90

Meyer, J. K. & Reter, D. J. (1979) Sex reassignment. *Arch. Gen. Psychiat.*, **36**, 1010–15

Mohr, J. W., Turner, R. E. & Jerry, M. B. (1964) *Paedophilia and Exhibitionism*. Toronto: Toronto University Press

Money, J. & Walker, P. A. (1977) Counselling the transsexual. In *Handbook of Sexology*, section xvi, ed. Money, J. & Mustaph, H., pp. 1289–301. Amsterdam: Excerpta Medica

Prince, V. & Bentler, P. (1972) Survey of 504 cases of transvestism. *Psychol. Rep.*, **31**, 903–17

Radzinowicz, L. (1957). *Sexual Offences*, ed. Radzinowicz, L. London: Macmillan

Rooth, F. G. (1971) Indecent exposure and exhibitionism. *Brit. J. Hosp. Med.*, **5**, 521–33

Rooth, F. G. & Marks, I. M. (1974) Persistent exhibitionism: short term responses to self regulation and relaxation treatment. *Arch. sex. Behav.*, **3**, 227–48

Rosen, I. (1979a) The general psychoanalytical theory of perversion: a critical and clinical review. In *Sexual Deviation*, 2nd ed., ed. Rosen, I., pp. 29–64. Oxford: Oxford University Press

— (1979b) Exhibitionism, scopophilia and voyeurism. In *Sexual Deviation*, 2nd ed., ed. Rosen, I., pp. 139–94. Oxford: Oxford University Press

Stoller, R. J. (1971) The term 'transvestism'. *Arch. gen. Psychiatry*, **24**, 230–7

Stoller, R. J. (1979) The gender disorders. In *Sexual Deviation*, 2nd edn, ed. Rosen, I., pp. 109–38. Oxford: Oxford University Press

Wakeling, A. (1977) Antilibido agents. In *Psychotherapeutic Drugs*, Part ii: *Applications*, ed. Usdin, E. & Forrest, I. S., pp. 1413–53. New York: Marcel Dekker

— (1979) A general psychiatric approach to sexual deviation.

In *Sexual Deviation*, 2nd edn, ed. Rosen, I., pp. 1–28. Oxford: Oxford University Press

Wålinder, J. (1968) Transsexualism: definition, prevalence and sex distribution. *Acta. psychiat. scand.*, Supp. **203**, 255–8

Chapter 9.4

Bluglass, R. (1979) Incest. *Brit. J. hosp. Med.*, **24/2**, 152–7

Cowie, J., Cowie, V. & Slater, E. (1968) *Delinquency in Girls*, London: Heinemann

Gebhard, P. H., Gagnon, J. H., Pomeroy, W. B. & Christenson, C. V. (1965) *Sex Offenders*. London: Heinemann

Herman, J. & Hirschmann, L. (1981) families at risk for father–daughter incest. *Amer. J. Psychiat.*, **138**, 967–70

Meiselman, K. C. (1978) *Incest*. London: Jossey-Bass

Mrazek, P. B. & Kempe, C. H. (Eds.) (1981) *Sexually Abused Children and their Families*. Oxford: Pergamon

Peters, J. J. (1976) Children who are victims of sexual assault. *Amer. J. Psychother.*, **30**, 398–421

Scottish Law Commission (1980) *The Law of Incest in Scotland*. Edinburgh: Scottish Law Commission

Weinberg, S. K. (1955) *Incest Behaviour*. New York: Citadel

Chapter 10.1

Cadoret, R. J. & Gath, A. (1978) Inheritance of alcoholism in adoptees. *Brit. J. Psychiat.*, **132**, 252–8

d'Orbán, P. T. (1970) Heroin dependence and delinquency in women – a study of heroin addicts in Holloway Prison. *Brit. J. Addiction*, **65**, 67–78

— (1973) Female narcotic addicts: a follow-up study of criminal and addiction careers. *Brit. med. J.*, 4, 435–7

Foulds, G. A. & Hassall, C. (1969) The significance of age of onset of excessive drinking in male alcoholics. *Brit. J. Psychiat.*, **115**, 1027–32

Glatt, M. M. (1974) *A Guide to Addiction and its Treatment*. Lancaster: MTP

Goodwin, D., Schulsinger, F., Hermansen, L., Guze, S. & Winokur, G. (1975) Alcoholism and the hyperactive child syndrome. *J. nerv. ment. Dis.*, **160**, 349–53

Jones, M. C. (1968) Personality correlates and antecedents of drinking patterns in adult males. *J. consult. clin. Psychol.*, **32**, 2–12

Kandel, D. (1974) Interpersonal influences on adolescent illegal drug use. In *Drug Use: Epidemiological and Sociological Approaches*, ed. Josephson E., & Carroll, E. E., pp. 207–46. Washington DC: Hemisphere

Kessel, N. & Walton, H. (1974) *Alcoholism*. Harmondsworth: Penguin

McCord, W. & McCord, J. (1960) *Origins of Alcoholism*. London: Tavistock

Mehryar, A. H. & Moharreri, M. R. (1978) A study of authorized opium addiction in Shiraz City and Fars Province, Iran. *Brit. J. Addiction*, **73**, 93–102

Noble, P. J. (1970) Drug-taking in delinquent boys. *Brit. med. J.*, **1**, 102–5

Noble, P. & Barnes, G. G. (1971) Drug taking in adolescent girls: factors associated with the progression to narcotic use. *Brit. med. J.*, **2**, 620–3

O'Connor, J. (1978) *The Young Drinkers*. London: Tavistock

Plant, M. A. (1975) *Drug Takers in an English Town*. London: Tavistock

Robins, L. N. (1966) *Deviant Children Grown Up*. Baltimore: Williams & Wilkins

Schuckit, M., Rimmer, J. Reich, T. & Winokur, G. (1970) Alcoholism: antisocial traits in male alcoholics. *Brit. J. Psychiat.*, **117**, 575–6

Scott, P. D. & Willcox, D. R. (1965) Delinquency and the amphetamines. *Brit. J. Psychiat.*, **111**, 865–75

Wiepert, G. D., D'Orbán, P. T. & Bewley, T. H. (1979) Delinquency of opiate addicts treated at two London Clinics. *Brit. J. Psychiat.*, **134**, 14–23

Chapter 10.2

Bass, M. (1970) Sudden sniffing death. *J. Amer. Med. Ass.*, **212**, 2075–9

Blumberg, H. H., Cohen, S. D., Dronfield, B. E., Mordecai, E. A., Roberts, J. C. & Hawks, D. (1974) British opiate users: II Differences between those given an opiate script and those not given one. *Int. J. Addictions*, **9**, 205–20

Brook, R. Kaplun, J. & Whitehead, P. C. (1974) Personality characteristics of adolescent amphetamine users as measured by the MMPI. *Brit. J. Addiction*, **69**, 61–6

De Leon, G., Holland, S. & Rosenthal, M. S. (1972) Phoenix House. Criminal activity of dropouts. *J. Amer. Med. Ass.*, **222**, 686–9

De Leon, G., Skodol, A. & Rosenthal, M. S. (1973) Phoenix House. Changes in psychopathological signs of resident drug addicts. *Arch. gen. Psychiat.*, **28**, 131–5

DHSS (Department of Health and Social Security) (1977) *Guide to the Misuse of Drugs Act 1971 and to Certain Regulations Made Under The Act*. London: DHSS

Gardner, R. & Connell, P. H. (1970) One year's experience in a drug-dependence clinic. *Lancet*, **ii**, 455–9

Ghodse, A. H. (1977) Drug dependent individuals dealt with by London casualty departments. *Brit. J. Psychiat.*, **131**, 273–80

Goto, I., Matsumura, M., Inoue, N., Murai, Y., Shida, K., Santo, T. & Kuroiwa, Y. (1974) Toxic polyneuropathy due to glue sniffing. *J. Neurol. Neurosurg. Psychiat.*, **38**, 838–53

Harding, G. T. (1975) Psychotherapy in the treatment of drug dependence. A survey of the scientific literature. In *Drug Dependence – Treatment and Treatment Evaluation*, pp. 59–80. Skandia International Symposia. Stockholm: Almqvist & Wiksell

Jaffe, J. H. (1975) Drug addiction and drug abuse. In *The Pharmacological Basis of Therapeutics*, ed. Goodman, L. S. & Gilman, A., 5th edn, pp. 245–83. New York: Macmillan

James, I. P. (1973) Drug abuse in Britain. *Med. Sci. Law*, **13**, 246–51

King, M. D., Day, R. E., Oliver, J. S., Lush, M. & Watson, J. M. (1981) Solvent encephalopathy. *Brit. med. J.*, **283**, 663–5

Kosviner, A., Hawks, D. & Webb, M. G. (1974) Cannabis use amongst British university students. *Brit. J. Addiction*, **69**, 35–60

Ogborne, A. C. & Melotte, C. (1977) An evaluation of a therapeutic community for former drug users. *Brit. J. Addiction*, **72**, 75–82

Oliver, J. S. & Watson, J. M. (1977) Abuse of solvents 'for kicks'. A review of 50 cases. *Lancet*, **i**, 84–6

Oppenheimer, E., Stimson, G. V. & Thorley, A. (1979) Seven-year follow-up of heroin addicts: abstinence and continued use compared. *Brit. med. J.*, **2**, 627–30

Robins, L. N. (1966) *Deviant Children Grown Up*. Baltimore: Williams & Wilkins

Smart, R. G. (1976) Outcome studies of therapeutic community and halfway house treatment for addicts. *Int. J. Addictions*, **11**, 143–59

Stimson, G. V. (1972) Patterns of behaviour of heroin addicts. *Int. J. Addictions*, **7**, 671–91

Tyrer, P. (1980). Dependence on benzodiazepines. *Brit. J. Psychiat.*, **137**, 576–7

Wikler, A. (1975) Opioid antagonists and deconditioning in addiction treatment. In *Drug Dependence – Treatment and Treatment Evaluation*, pp. 157–84. Skandia International Symposia. Stockholm: Almqvist & Wiksell

Winick, C. A. (1962) Maturing out of narcotic addiction. *Bull. Narcot.*, **14**, 1–7

World Health Organization (1974) *Expert Committee on Drug Dependence: Twentieth Report*. W.H.O. Technical Report Series, No. 551. Geneva: WHO

Chapter 10.3

Bruun, K., Edwards, G., Lumio, M., Makela, K., Pan, L., Popham, R. E., Room, R., Schmidt, W., Skog, O-J., Sulkunnen, P. & Osterberg, E. (1975) *Alcohol Control Policies in Public Health Perspective*. Helsinki: Finnish Foundation for Alcohol Studies

Caetano, R., Edwards, G., Oppenheim, A. N. & Taylor, C. (1978) Building a standardized alcoholism interview schedule. *Drug Alc. Depend.*, **3**, 185–97

Camberwell Council on Alcoholism (1980) (Ed.) *Women and Alcohol*. London: Tavistock

Coid, J. (1979) Mania a potu: a critical review of pathological intoxication. *Psychol. Med.*, **9**, 709–19

Cook, T. (1975) *Vagrant Alcoholics*. London: Routledge & Kegan Paul

Cutting, J. (1979) Alcohol dependence and alcohol-related disabilities. In *Recent Advances in Clinical Psychiatry, No. 3*, ed. Granville-Grossman, K., chap. 7, pp. 225–50. Edinburgh: Churchill-Livingstone

Davies, D. L. (1962) Normal drinking in recovered alcoholics. *J. Stud. Alcohol*, **23**, 94–104

DHSS (Department of Health and Social Security) (1978) The pattern and range of services for problem drinkers. *Report of the Advisory Committee on Alcoholism*. London: HMSO

Edwards, G. (1980) Drinking problems: putting the Third World on the map. *Lancet*, **ii**, 402–4

Edwards, G. & Grant, M. (eds.) (1980) *Alcoholism Treatment in Transition*. London: Croom Helm

Edwards, G. & Gross, M. M. (1976) Alcohol dependence: provisional description of a clinical syndrome. *Brit. med. J.*, **1**, 1058–61

Edwards, G., Gross, M. M., Keller, M., Moser, J. & Room, R. (eds.) (1977) *Alcohol-related disabilities*. WHO Offset publication No. 32. Geneva: WHO

Edwards, G. & Guthrie, S. (1967) A controlled trial of in-patient and out-patient treatment of alcohol dependence. *Lancet*, **i**, 555–9

Edwards, G., Hawker, A., Hensman, C., Peto, J. & Williamson, V. (1973) Alcoholics known or unknown to agencies: epidemiological studies in a London suburb. *Brit. J. Psychiat.*, **123**, 169–83

Edwards, G., Hensman, C. & Peto, J. (1971) Drinking problems among recidivist prisoners. *Psychol. Med.*, **5**, 388–99

Gillies, H. (1965) Murder in the west of Scotland. *Brit. J. Psychiat.*, **111**, 1087–94

Glatt, M. M. (1970) *The Alcoholic – and The Help He Needs* (2 vols). London: Priory Press

Goodwin, D. W. Schulsinger, F., Møller, N., Hermansen, L., Winokur, G. & Guze, S. B. (1974) Drinking problems in adopted and non-adopted sons of alcoholics. *Arch. gen. Psychiat.*, **31**, 164–9

Hodgson, R., Stockwell, T., Rankin, H. & Edwards, G. (1978) Alcohol dependence: the concept, its utility and measurement. *Brit. J. Addiction*, **73**, 339–42

Hore, B. D. (1976) *Alcohol Dependence*. London: Butterworths

Jellinek, E. M. (1946) Phases in the drinking history of alcoholics. *J. Stud. Alcohol*, **7**, 1–88

— (1960) *The Disease Concept of Alcoholism*. New Haven: Hillhouse Press

Ledermann, S. (1956) Alcool, alcoolisme, alcoolisation (Alcohol, alcoholism, alcoholisation). Données scientifiques de caractère physiologique, économique et social. Institut National d'Études Démographiques, Travaux et Documents, No. 29. Paris: Presses Universitaires de France

Litman, G. K., Eiser, J. R., Rawson, N. S. B. & Oppenheim, A. N. (1979) Differences in relapse precipitants and coping behaviour between alcohol relapsers and survivors. *Behav. Res. Ther.*, **17**, 89–94

Madden, J. S. (1979) *A Guide to Alcohol and Drug Dependence*. Bristol: J Wright

Mendelson, J. H. & Mello, N. K. (Eds.) (1979) *The Diagnosis and Treatment of Alcoholism*. New York: McGraw Hill

Nathan, P. E., Marlatt, G. A. & Løberg, T. (Eds.) (1978) *Alcoholism: New Directions in Behavioral Research and Treatment*. New York: Plenum

Nicholls, P., Edwards, G. & Kyle, E. (1974). A study of alcoholics admitted to four hospitals: II General and cause-specific mortality during follow-up. *Q. J. Stud. Alcohol*, **35**, 841–55

Orford, J. (1975) Alcoholism and marriage. *J. Stud. Alcohol*, **36**, 1537–63

— (1976). Aspects of the relationship between alcohol and drug abuse. In *Drugs and Drug Dependence*, ed. Edwards, G., Russell, M. A. H., Hawks, D. & MacCafferty, M., chap. 19, pp. 188–98. Farnborough: Saxon House

Orford, J. & Edwards, G. (1977) *Alcoholism*. Maudsley Monograph, No. 26. Oxford: Oxford University Press

Orford, J. & Guthrie, S. (1976) Coping behaviour used by wives of alcoholics: a preliminary investigation. In *Alcohol Dependence and Smoking Behaviour*, ed. Edwards, G., Russell, M. A. H., Hawks, D. & MacCafferty, M., chap. 21, pp. 136–43. Farnborough: Saxon House

Orford, J. & Hawker, A. (1974) Note on the ordering of onset of symptoms in alcohol dependence. *Psychol. Med.*, **4**, 281–8

Otto, S. & Orford, J. (1978) *Not Quite Like Home: Small Hostels for Alcoholics and Others*. Chichester: Wiley

Pittman, D. J. & Snyder, C. R. (Eds.) (1962) *Society, Culture and Drinking Patterns*. New York: Wiley

Plant, M. A. & Hore, B. (Eds.) (1980) *Alcohol Problems in Employment*. London: Croom Helm

Polich, J. M., Armor, D. J. & Braiker, H. B. (1980) Patterns of alcoholism over four years. *J. Stud. Alcohol*, **41**, 397–416

Robinson, D. (1979) *Talking Out of Alcoholism: The Self-Help Process of Alcoholics Anonymous*. London: Croom Helm

Ron, M. A. (1979) Organic psychosyndromes in chronic alcoholics. *Brit J Addiction*, **74**, 353–8

Schmidt, W. (1977) Cirrhosis and alcohol consumption: an epidemiological perspective. In *Alcoholism: New Knowledge and New Responses*, ed. Edwards, G. & Grant, M., chap. 1, pp. 15–47. London: Croom Helm

Schuckit, M. A. (1979) *Drug and Alcohol Abuse: A Clinical Guide to Diagnosis and Treatment*. New York: Plenum

Shaw, S., Cartwright, A., Spratley, T. & Harwin, J. (1978) *Responding to Drinking Problems*. London: Croom Helm

Shields, J. (1977) Genetics and alcoholism. In *Alcoholism: New Knowledge and New Responses*, ed. Edwards, G., & Grant, M., chap. 8, pp. 117–35. London: Croom Helm

Stockwell, T., Hodgson, N. R., Edwards, G., Taylor, C. & Rankin, H. (1979) The development of a questionnaire to measure severity of alcohol dependence. *Brit. J. Addiction*, **74**, 79–87

Vaillant, G. E. (1979) Natural history of alcoholism 1; a preliminary report. In *Human functioning in longitudinal perspective*, ed. Sells, S. B. & Strauss, J., chap. 11, pp. 147–54. Baltimore: Williams & Wilkins

Wilson, C. & Orford, J. (1978) Children of alcoholics. *J. Stud. Alcohol*, **39**, 121–42

WHO (World Health Organization) (1952) Expert committee on mental health: alcohol subcommittee second report. *Technical Report Series No. 48*. Geneva: WHO

WHO (World Health Organization) (1981) Memorandum on the nomenclature and classification of drug- and alcohol-related problems. *Bull. WHO*, **59**, 225–42

Chapter 10.4

Bohman, M. (1978) Some genetic aspects of alcoholism and criminality. *Arch. gen. Psychiat.*, **35**, 269–76

Davies, J. & Stacey, B. (1972) *Teenagers and Alcohol: A Developmental Study in Glasgow*, vol. II. London: HMSO

Goodwin, D., Schulsinger, F., Hermansen, L., Guze, S. & Winokur, G. (1973) Alcohol problems in adoptees raised apart from alcoholic biological parents. *Arch. gen. Psychiat.*, **28**, 238–43

Goodwin, D., Schulsinger, F., Moller, N., Hermansen, L., Winokur, G. & Guze, S. (1974) Drinking problems in adopted and non-adopted sons of alcoholics. *Arch. gen. Psychiat.*, **31**, 164–9

Hawker, A. (1978) *Adolescents and Alcohol*. London: Edsall

Jahoda, G. & Cramond, J. (1972) *Children and Alcohol: A Developmental Study in Glasgow*, vol. I. London: HMSO

Lancet (1980) Annotation, **ii**, 188

Nylander, I. (1960) The children of alcoholic fathers. *Acta paediat. scand.*, **49**, Supp. **121**

O'Connor, J. (1978) *The Young Drinkers*. London: Tavistock

Plant, M. A. (1979) *Drinking Careers*. London: Tavistock

Smithells, R. W. (1979) Fetal alcohol syndrome. *Dev. Med. child Neurol.*, **21**, 244–8

Chapter 10.5

Bergler, E. (1970) *The Psychology of Gambling*. New York: International Universities Press

Dickerson, M. G. (1974) *The Effect of Betting Shop Experience on Gambling Behaviour*. Unpublished thesis for degree of Doctor of Philosophy in Psychology, University of Birmingham.

Dickerson, M. G. & Weeks, D. (1979) Controlled gambling as a therapeutic technique for compulsive gamblers. *J. behav. Ther. exp. Psychiat.*, **10**, 139–41

Freud, S. (1928) Dostoevsky and Parricide. In *Complete Psychological Works of Sigmund Freud*, ed. Strachey, J., Vol. 21, p. 177 (1961) London: Hogarth Press

HMSO (1978) *Final Report of the Royal Commission on Gambling, 1976–78.* Cmnd 7200. London: HMSO

— (1980) *Gambling Statistics: Great Britain: 1968–78.* Cmnd 7897. London: HMSO

Moran, E. (1970 a) Gambling as a form of dependence. *Brit. J. Addict.*, **64**, 419–27

— (1970 b) Clinical and social aspects of risk-taking. *Proc. Roy. Soc. Med.*, **63**, 1273–7

— (1975) Pathological gambling. In *Contemporary Psychiatry*, ed. Silverstone, T. & Barraclough, B. *Brit. J. Psychiat.*, Special publication No. 9, 416–28

— (1979) An assessment of the Report of the Royal Commission on Gambling 1976–78. *Brit. J. Addict.*, **74**, 3–9

Moran, J. (1979) *Mind Out: Six Topics for Social Education.* London: Arnold

Royal College of Psychiatrists (1977) *Submission of Evidence to the Royal Commission on Gambling.* London: Royal College of Psychiatrists

Seager, C. P. (1970) Treatment of compulsive gamblers by electrical aversion. *Brit. J. Psychiat.*, **117**, 545–53

US Commission on the Review of the National Policy Toward Gambling. (1976) *Gambling in America: Final Report.* US Government Printing Office Washington.

Wray, I. & Dickerson, M. G. (1981) Cessation of high frequency gambling and 'withdrawal' symptoms. *Brit. J. Addict.*, **76** (4), 528–31

Chapter 11.1

Alexander, J. F., Barton, C., Schiavo, R. S. & Parsons, B. V. (1976) Systems-behavioural intervention with families of delinquents. *J. consult. clin. Psychol.*, **44**, 656–64

Berkowitz, L. (1969) (ed.) *Roots of Aggression.* New York: Atherton Press

Bohman, M. (1978) Some genetic aspects of alcoholism and criminality: a population of adoptees. *Arch. gen. Psychiat.*, **35**, 269–76

Brody, S. R. (1976) *The Effectiveness of Sentencing.* (Home Office Research Studies, 35.) London: HMSO

Bowlby, J. (1951) *Maternal Care and Mental Health.* Geneva: WHO

Cantwell, D. (1977) Hyperkinetic syndrome. In *Child Psychiatry – Modern Approaches*, ed. Rutter M. & Hersov, L., pp. 524–55. Oxford: Blackwell

Christiansen, K. O. (1977) A preliminary study of criminality among twins. In *Biosocial Bases of Criminal Behavior*, (ed. Mednick, S. A. & Christiansen, K. O. pp. 89–108. New York: Garden Press

David, O. J., Hoffman, S. P., Sverd, J., Clark, J. & Voeller, K. (1976) Lead and hyperactivity. Behavioral response to chelation. *Amer. J. Psychiat.*, **133**, 1155–8

Davie, R., Butler, N. & Goldstein, H. (1972) *From Birth to Seven.* London: Longman

Emery, R. E. & Marholin, D. (1977) An applied behavior analysis of delinquency. *Amer. Psychol.*, **32**, 860–73

Eysenck, H. J. (1977) *Crime and Personality.* London: Paladin

Farrington, D. P. (1973) Self-reports of deviant behaviour: predic-tive and stable? *J. Criminal Law & Criminology*, **64**, 99–110

— (1979) Delinquent behaviour modification in the natural environment. *Brit. J. Criminol.*, **19**, 353–72

Freeman, J. M., Aron, A. M., Collard, J. E. & Mackay, M. C. (1965) The emotional correlates of Sydenham's chorea. *Pediat.*, **35**, 42–9

Glueck, S. & Glueck, E. T. (1959) *Predicting Delinquency and Crime.* Cambridge, Mass.: Harvard University Press

Gregory, R. J. & Mohan, P. J. (1977) Effect of asymptomatic lead exposure on childhood intelligence: A critical review *Intelligence*, **1**, 381–400

Hood, R. & Sparks, R. (1970) *Key Issues in Criminology*, pp. 46–79 London: Weidenfeld & Nicolson

Hutchings, B. & Mednick, S. A. (1977) Criminality in adoptees and in their adoptive and biological parents. In *Biosocial Bases of Criminal Behavior*, ed. Mednick, S. A. & Christiansen, K. O., pp. 127–42. New York: Gardner Press

Knoblock, H. & Pasamanick, B. (1966) Prospective studies in the epidemiology of reproductive casualty. *Merrill-Palmer Q.*, **12**, 27–43

McClintock, F. H. & Bottoms, A. E. (1973) *Criminals Coming of Age.* London: Heinemann

McCord, J. (1978a) A thirty year follow up of treatment effects. *Amer. Psychol.*, **33**, 284–9

— (1978b) A longitudinal view of the relationship between paternal absence and crime. Paper given at *American Society of Criminology* Nov. 1978

Martinson, R., Palmer, T. & Adams, S. (1976) *Rehabilitation, Recidivism and Research.* Hackensack, N.J.: Nat. Counc. Crime & Delinquency

Osborn, S. G. & West, D. J. (1978) The effectiveness of various predictors of criminal careers. *J. Adolescence*, **1**, 101–17

Quay, H. C. (1977) The three faces of evaluation. *Crim. Just. Behav.*, **4**, 341–54

Rachman, S. J. (1973) The effects of psychological treatment. In *Handbook of Abnormal Psychology*, ed. Eysenck, H. J., pp. 805–61. London: Pitman

Ratcliffe, J. M. (1977) Developmental and behavioural functions in young children with elevated blood lead levels. *Brit. J. prev. soc. Med.*, **31**, 258–64

Robins, L. N. (1966) *Deviant Children Grown Up.* Baltimore: Williams & Wilkins

Roth, M. (1972) Human violence as viewed from the psychiatric clinic. *Amer. J. Psychiat.*, **128**, 1043–56

Rutter, M. (1972) *Maternal Deprivation Reassessed.* Harmondsworth: Penguin

— (1980) Raised lead levels and impaired cognitive/behavioural functioning: a review of the evidence. *Dev. Med. child Neurol.*, **22**(1), Supp. 42

Rutter, M. L., Graham, P. & Yule, W. (1970) *A Neuropsychiatric Study in Childhood.* London: Heinemann

Sandberg, S. T., Rutter, M. & Taylor, E. (1978) Hyperkinetic disorder in psychiatric clinic attenders. *Dev. Med. child Neurol.* **20**, 279–99

Shaffer, D., Chadwick, O. & Rutter, M. (1975) Psychiatric outcome of localised head injury in children. In *Outcome of Severe Damage to the Central Nervous System*, Symposium 34. London: Ciba Foundation

Slater, E. & Roth, M. (1969) *Clinical Psychiatry.* London: Ballière, Tindall & Cassell

Stott, D. H. (1966) *Studies of Troublesome Children.* London: Tavistock

Trasler, G. (1973) Criminal behaviour. In *Handbook of Abnormal Psychology*, H. J. Eysenck, ed., pp. 67–96. London: Pitman

Wadsworth, M. (1979) *Roots of Delinquency: Infancy, Adolescence and Crime*. Oxford: Martin Robertson

Wender, P. H. & Eisenberg, L. (1974) Minimal brain dysfunction in children. In *American Handbook of Psychiatry*, ed. Arieti, S., pp. 130–46. New York: Basic Books

West, D. J. (1969) *Present Conduct and Future Delinquency*, pp. 108–15. London: Heinemann

West, D. J. & Farrington, D. P. (1973) *Who Becomes Delinquent?* London: Heinemann

— (1977) *The Delinquent Way of Life*. London: Heinemann

Chapter 11.2

Cleckley, H. (1955) *The Mask of Sanity*, 3rd ed. St. Louis: Mosby

Durbin, J. R., Pasewark, R. A. & Albers, D. (1977) Criminality and mental illness: A study of arrest rates in a rural state *Amer. J. Psychiat.*, **134**, 80–3

Durkheim, E. (1901) The normal and the pathological. Reprinted in *The Sociology of Crime and Delinquency*, 2nd ed. (1970) ed. Wolfgang, M. E., Savitz, L. & Johnston, N., pp. 11–14, New York: Wiley, as an extract from *Les Règles de la méthode sociologique* 2nd edn., Paris: Alcan. Trans. Solovary, S. A. & Mueller, J. H. as *The Rules of Sociological Method* (1960). Glencoe, Ill.: Free Press

Eysenck, H. J. & Eysenck, S.B.G. (1978) Psychopathy, personality and genetics. In *Psychopathic Behaviour: Approaches to Research*, ed. Hare, R. D. & Schalling, D., pp. 197–224. Chichester: Wiley

Farrington, D. P., Gundry, G. & West, D. J. (1975) The Familial Transmission of Criminality. *Med., Sci. Law*, **15**, 177–86

Gibbens, T. C. N. (1963) *Psychiatric Studies of Borstal Lads*. Maudsley Monograph, No. 11. London: Oxford University Press

Glueck, S. & Glueck, E. (1956) *Physique and Delinquency* New York: Harper

Gunn, J. (1974) Disasters, asylums and plans: forensic psychiatry today. *British med. J.*, **3**, 611–13

— (1978) *Epileptic Prisoners*. London: Academic Press

Gunn, J. & Robertson, G. (1976) Psychopathic personality: a conceptual problem. *Psychol. Med.*, **6**, 631–4

Gunn, J., Robertson, G., Dell, S. & Way, C. (1978) *Psychiatric Aspects of Imprisonment*. London: Academic Press

Hare, R. D. & Cox, D. N. (1978) Clinical and empirical conceptions of psychopathy and the selection of subjects for research. In *Psychopathic Behaviour: Approaches to Research*, ed. Hare, R. D. & Schalling, D., pp. 1–22. Chichester: Wiley

Hare, R. D. & Schalling, D. (1978) *Psychopathic Behaviour: Approaches to Research*. Chichester: Wiley

King, L. N. & Young, Q. D. (1978) Increased prevalence of seizure disorders among prisoners. *J. Amer. Med. Ass.*, **239**, 2674–5

Lewis, A. (1974) Psychopathic personality: a most elusive category. *Psychol. Med.*, **4**, 133–40

Lewis, D. O. & Balla, D. (1975) Sociopathy and its synonyms: inappropriate diagnoses in child psychiatry. *Amer., J. Psychiat.*, **132**, 720–2

Masuda, M., Cutler, D. L., Hein, L. & Holmes, J. H. (1978) Life events and prisoners. *Arch. gen. Psychiat.*, **35**, 197–203

McClintock, F. M. & Avison, N. H. (1968) *Crime in England & Wales*. London: Heinemann

National Advisory Commission on Civil Disorders (1968) *Report*. Washington: U.S. Government Printing Office

Pichot, P. (1978) Psychopathic behaviour: a historical overview. In *Psychopathic Behaviour: Approaches to Research*, ed. Hare, R. D., & Schalling, D., pp. 55–70 Chichester: Wiley

Prichard, J. C. (1835) *A Treatise on Insanity and other Disorders Affecting the Mind*. London: Sherwood, Gilbert & Piper

Rappeport, J. R. & Lassen, G. (1965) Dangerousness – arrest rate comparisons of discharged patients and the general population. *Amer. J. Psychiat.*, **123**, 413–19

Robins, L. N. (1966) *Deviant Children Grown Up*. Baltimore: Williams & Wilkins

Rutter, M. & Madge, N. (1976) *Cycles of Disadvantage*. London: Heinemann

Sosowsky, L. (1978) Crime and violence amongst mental patients reconsidered *Amer. J Psychiat.*, **135**, 33–42

Steele, B. F. & Pollock, C. B. (1968) A psychiatric history of parents who abuse infants and small children. In *The Battered Child*, ed. Helfer, R. E. & Kempe, C. H., pp. 103–48. Chicago: University of Chicago Press

Sutherland, E. H. (1947) Differential association. In *The Sociology of Crime and Delinquency*, 2nd ed. (1970), ed. Wolfgang, M. E., Savitz, L. & Johnston, N., pp. 208–10. New York: Wiley

Taylor, P. J. (1982) Schizophrenia and violence. In *Contemporary Aspects of Forensic Psychiatry and Psychology*, ed. Gunn, J. & Farrington, D., pp. 269–84. Chichester: Wiley

Walker, N. (1968a) *Crime and Punishment in Britain* (rev. edn) Edinburgh: Edinburgh University Press

— (1968b) *Crime and Insanity in England*, vol. 1. Edinburgh: Edinburgh University Press

Walker, N. & McCabe, S. (1973) *Crime and Insanity in England*, vol. 2. Edinburgh: Edinburgh University Press

Walton, H. J. & Presly, A. S. (1973) Use of a category system in the diagnosis of abnormal personality. *Brit. J. Psychiat.*, **122**, 259–68

Watts, F. N. & Bennett, D. H. (1978) Social deviance in a day hospital. *Brit. J. Psychiat.*, **132**, 455–62

West, D. J. (1963) *The Habitual Prisoner* London: Macmillan

West, D. J. & Farrington, D. P. (1973) *Who Becomes Delinquent?* London: Heinemann

Chapter 11.3

Biller, H. B. (1970) Father absence and the personality development of the male child. *Dev. Psychol.*, **2**, 181–201

Hall, F., Pawlby, S. J. & Wolkind, S. (1980) Early life experiences and later mothering behaviour: a study of mothers and their 20-week old babies. In *The Importance of the First Year of Life*, ed. Shaffer, D. & Dunn, J. pp. 153–74. London: Wiley

Quinton, D. & Rutter, M. (1976) Early hospital admissions and later disturbances of behaviour: an attempted replication of Douglas' findings. *Dev. Med. child Neurol.*, **18**, 447–59

Robins, L. N. (1966) *Deviant Children Grown Up*. Baltimore: Williams & Wilkins

Rutter, M. (1966) *Children of Sick Parents: An Environmental & Psychiatric Study*. Institute of Psychiatry Maudsley Monograph No. 16. London: Oxford University Press.

— (1970) Sex differences in children's responses to family stress. In *The Child in His Family*, ed. Anthony, E. J. & Koupernik, C., pp. 165–96. New York: Wiley

Rutter, M. (1976) Separation, loss and family relationships. In *Child Psychiatry: Modern Approaches*, ed. Rutter, M. & Hersov, L., pp. 47–73. Oxford: Blackwell

Rutter, M. & Madge, N. (1977) *Cycles of Disadvantage*. London: Heinemann

Rutter, M., Maughan, B., Mortimore, P. & Ouston, J. (1979) *15 000 Hours: Secondary Schools and their Effects on Children*. London: Open Books

Rutter, M. & Mrazek, D. (1982) personal communication

Shields, J. (1976) Polygenic Influences. In *Child Psychiatry: Modern Approaches*, ed. Rutter, M. & Hersov, L., pp. 22–47. London: Blackwell

Tonge, W. L., James, D. S., & Hillam, S. M. (1975) *Families without Hope: A Controlled Study of 33 Problem Families*. British Journal of Psychiatry, Special Publication No 11. London: Headley Bros

Tuckman, J. & Regan, R. A. (1966) Intactness of the home and behaviour problems in children. *J. child Psychol. Psychiat.*, **7**, 225–33

West, D. H. & Farrington, D. P. (1977) *The Delinquent Way of Life*. London: Heinemann

Whalley, L., Robinson, T. J., McIsaac, M. & Wolff, S. (1978) Psychiatric referrals from Scottish Children's Hearings: a comparative study. *J. child Psychol. Psychiat.*, **19**, 269–78

Wolff, S. & Acton, W. P. (1968) Characteristics of parents of disturbed children. *Brit. J. Psychiat.*, **114**, 593–601

Wolkind, S., Hall, F. & Pawlby, S. (1977) Individual differences in mothering behaviour: a combined epidemiological and observational approach. In *Epidemiological Approaches in Child Psychiatry*, ed. Graham, P. J., pp. 107–25 London: Academic Press

Chapter 12.1

Monro, A. B. (1954) A rating scale developed for use in clinical psychiatric investigations. *J. ment. Sci.*, **100**, 657–69

— (1959) The inadequate personality in psychiatric practice. *J. ment. Sci.*, **105**, 44–50

Walton, H. J. & Presley, A. S. (1973) dimensions of abnormal personality. *Brit. J. Psychiat.*, **122**, 269–76

Chapter 12.2

Burton, L. (1968) *Vulnerable Children*. London: Routledge & Kegan Paul

De Francis, V. (1969) *Protecting the Child Victim of Sex Crimes*. Denver, Colorado: American Humane Association Children's Division

Gibbens, T. C. N. & Prince, J. (1963) *Child Victims of Sex Offences*. London: Institute for the Study and Treatment of Delinquency

Gibbens, T. C. N., Soothill, K. L. & Way, C. K. (1978) Sibling and parent child incest offenders. *Brit. J. Criminol.*, **18**, 40–52

Ingram, M. (1979) Paedophilia. *Brit. J. sex. Med.* **6**, (No. 44) 22–6; (No. 45) 25–26, 60

Kinsey, A. C., Pomeroy, W. B., Martin, C. E. & Gebhard, P. H. (1953) *Sexual Behavior in the Human Female*. Philadelphia: Saunders

Landis, J. T. (1956) Experiences of 500 children with adult sexual deviation. *Psychiatric Quarterly*, Supp., **30**, 91–109

Maisch, H. (1973) *Incest*. London: Deutsch

Virkkunen, M. (1975) Victim-precipitated pedophilia offences. *Brit. J. Criminol.* **15**, 175–80

Walters, D. R. (1975) *Physical and Sexual Abuse of Children*. Bloomington: Indiana University Press

Yates, A. (1979) *Sex without Shame*. London: Temple Smith

Cross-references to other volumes in the series

CROSS-REFERENCES

In addition to specific references given below, the reader is referred to volume 1 for a discussion of the concepts, descriptive and developmental phenomena, principles of classification, iagnosis, assessment and treatment, and neuropsychological, socio-cultural, and forensic aspects of general psychopathology, to volume 2 for the relationship between mental disorder and somatic illness, to volume 3 for a study of psychoses of uncertain aetiology, with particular reference to schizophrenias, affective psychoses, paranoid states, and psychoses with origin specific to childhood, and to volume 5 for a discussion of the scientific foundations of psychiatry.

(See also the key to volumes and chapters.)

Author index

Subject index